D0164254

Interventions, Effects, and Outcomes in Occupational Therapy

ADULTS AND OLDER ADULTS

Interventions, Effects, and Outcomes in Occupational Therapy
ADULTS AND OLDER ADULTS

Mary Law, PhD, FCAOT
Professor and Associate Dean
Rehabilitation Science
McMaster University
Hamilton, Ontario, Canada

Mary Ann McColl, PhD, MTS
Associate Director, Centre for Health Services and Policy Research
Professor, Community Health and Epidemiology/Rehabilitation Therapy
Queen's University
Kingston, Ontario, Canada

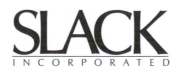

SLACK
INCORPORATED

RM735
.L39
.2010
0430443034

www.slackbooks.com

ISBN: 978-1-55642-880-7

Copyright © 2010 by SLACK Incorporated

Interventions, Effects, and Outcomes in Occupational Therapy: Adults and Older Adults, Instructor's Manual, is also available from SLACK Incorporated. Don't miss this important companion to *Interventions, Effects, and Outcomes in Occupational Therapy: Adults and Older Adults*. To obtain the *Instructor's Manual*, please visit www.efacultylounge.com.

All rights reserved. No part of this book may be reproduced, stored in a retrieval system or transmitted in any form or by any means, electronic, mechanical, photocopying, recording or otherwise, without written permission from the publisher, except for brief quotations embodied in critical articles and reviews.

The procedures and practices described in this book should be implemented in a manner consistent with the professional standards set for the circumstances that apply in each specific situation. Every effort has been made to confirm the accuracy of the information presented and to correctly relate generally accepted practices. The authors, editor, and publisher cannot accept responsibility for errors or exclusions or for the outcome of the material presented herein. There is no expressed or implied warranty of this book or information imparted by it. Care has been taken to ensure that drug selection and dosages are in accordance with currently accepted/recommended practice. Due to continuing research, changes in government policy and regulations, and various effects of drug reactions and interactions, it is recommended that the reader carefully review all materials and literature provided for each drug, especially those that are new or not frequently used. Any review or mention of specific companies or products is not intended as an endorsement by the author or publisher.

SLACK Incorporated uses a review process to evaluate submitted material. Prior to publication, educators or clinicians provide important feedback on the content that we publish. We welcome feedback on this work.

Published by: SLACK Incorporated
                  6900 Grove Road
                  Thorofare, NJ 08086 USA
                  Telephone: 856-848-1000
                  Fax: 856-853-5991
                  www.slackbooks.com

Contact SLACK Incorporated for more information about other books in this field or about the availability of our books from distributors outside the United States.

Library of Congress Cataloging-in-Publication Data

Interventions, effects, and outcomes in occupational therapy : adults and older adults / [edited by] Mary Law, Mary Ann McColl.
    p. ; cm.
  Includes bibliographical references and index.
  ISBN 978-1-55642-880-7 (alk. paper)
  1. Occupational therapy. 2. Meta-analysis. I. Law, Mary C. II. McColl, Mary Ann, 1956-
  [DNLM: 1. Occupational Therapy--methods--Meta-Analysis. 2. Adult. 3. Treatment Outcome--Meta-Analysis. WB 555 L416i 2010]
  RM735I58 2010
  615.8′515--dc22
                            2009033228

For permission to reprint material in another publication, contact SLACK Incorporated. Authorization to photocopy items for internal, personal, or academic use is granted by SLACK Incorporated provided that the appropriate fee is paid directly to Copyright Clearance Center. Prior to photocopying items, please contact the Copyright Clearance Center at 222 Rosewood Drive, Danvers, MA 01923 USA; phone: 978-750-8400; website: www.copyright.com; email: info@copyright.com

Printed in the United States of America.

Last digit is print number: 10 9 8 7 6 5 4 3 2 1

CONTENTS

About the Authors vii
Contributors ix
Preface xi

Chapter 1   Occupational Therapy: Interventions, Effects, and Outcomes 1
             Mary Law, PhD, FCAOT and Mary Ann McColl, PhD, MTS

Chapter 2   Occupational Therapy-Sensitive Outcomes: Literature Search and Study Selection 15
             Briano Di Rezze, MSc (OT), OT Reg. (Ont.); Laura Bradley, MSc (OT), OT Reg. (Ont.);
             Mary Law, PhD, FCAOT; and Mary Ann McColl, PhD, MTS

Chapter 3   Participation in Daily Occupations 23
             Mary Law, PhD, FCAOT and Mary Ann McColl, PhD, MTS

Chapter 4   Self-Care Outcomes 47
             Laura Bradley, MSc (OT), OT Reg. (Ont.) and Brenda H. Vrkljan, PhD, OT Reg. (Ont.)

Chapter 5   Productivity—Work and Volunteer Work Outcomes 119
             Mary Law, PhD, FCAOT and Rebecca Gewurtz, MSc (OT), OT Reg. (Ont.)

Chapter 6   Leisure Outcomes 145
             Mary Ann McColl, PhD, MTS

Chapter 7   Environmental Change to Improve Outcomes 155
             Mary Law, PhD, FCAOT; Briano Di Rezze, MSc (OT), OT Reg. (Ont.); and
             Laura Bradley, MSc (OT), OT Reg. (Ont.)

Chapter 8   Physical Determinants of Occupation 183
             Mary Ann McColl, PhD, MTS and Wendy Pentland, PhD, OT Reg. (Ont.)

Chapter 9   Socio-Cultural Determinants of Occupation 247
             Mary Ann McColl, PhD, MTS

Chapter 10   Psycho-Emotional Outcomes 261
             Mary Law, PhD, FCAOT and Rebecca Gewurtz, MSc (OT), OT Reg. (Ont.)

Chapter 11   Interventions to Improve Cognitive-Neurological Outcomes 285
             Briano Di Rezze, MSc (OT), OT Reg. (Ont.)

Chapter 12   Conclusion and Recommendations 325
             Mary Law, PhD, FCAOT and Mary Ann McColl, PhD, MTS

Annotated Bibliography 331
Index 363

Interventions, Effects, and Outcomes in Occupational Therapy: Adults and Older Adults, Instructor's Manual, is also available from SLACK Incorporated. Don't miss this important companion to *Interventions, Effects, and Outcomes in Occupational Therapy: Adults and Older Adults.* To obtain the *Instructor's Manual,* please visit www.efacultylounge.com.

ABOUT THE AUTHORS

Mary Law, PhD, FCAOT, is Professor and Associate Dean (Health Sciences) of Rehabilitation Science and Associate Member of the Department of Clinical Epidemiology and Biostatistics at McMaster University, Hamilton, Ontario, Canada. She holds the John and Margaret Lillie Chair in Childhood Disability Research. Mary, an occupational therapist by training, is co-founder of CanChild Centre for Childhood Disability Research, a multidisciplinary research center at McMaster University. Mary's research centers on the development and validation of client-centered outcome measures, evaluation of occupational therapy interventions with children, the effect of environmental factors on the participation of children with disabilities in day-to-day activities, and transfer of research knowledge into practice. She has had a long interest in outcome measurement and is the lead author of the Canadian Occupational Performance Measure, an outcome measure for occupational therapy now translated into 30 languages and used in more than 40 countries around the world. Mary has received many honors nationally and internationally including the Muriel Driver Lectureship, the top award in Canadian occupational therapy, election to the American Occupational Therapy Foundation Academy of Research, and Fellow, Canadian Association of Occupational Therapists. Mary has also been elected to the membership of the Canadian Academy of Health Sciences and serves on their board representing rehabilitation science.

Mary Ann McColl, PhD, MTS, is Professor in Rehabilitation Therapy and Community Health and Epidemiology and Associate Director of the Centre for Health Services and Policy Research at Queen's University. Before coming to Queen's, she was Director of Research at Lyndhurst Spinal Cord Centre and taught at the University of Toronto. She is an author of several books on disability and disability policy, as well as several occupational therapy textbooks and resources. She is a co-author on the Canadian Occupational Performance Measure, along with Mary Law and several other prominent Canadian occupational therapists. Mary Ann is a Fellow of the Canadian Association of Occupational Therapists. In addition to graduate work in epidemiology and biostatistics, she has recently completed a Master's of Theological Studies and does part-time community chaplaincy. Her research interests include occupational therapy theory and measurement, disability studies and disability policy, access to health services for people with disabilities, aging and disability, community integration, social support, and spirituality and health.

CONTRIBUTORS

Laura Bradley, MSc (OT), OT Reg. (Ont.)
(Chapters 2, 4, 7)
Occupational Therapist
Ottawa Children's Treatment Center
Ottawa, Ontario, Canada

Briano Di Rezze, MSc (OT), OT Reg. (Ont.)
(Chapters 2, 7, 11)
PhD Student
School of Rehabilitation Science
McMaster University
Hamilton, Ontario, Canada

Rebecca Gewurtz, MSc (OT), OT Reg. (Ont.)
(Chapters 5, 10)
McMaster University
Hamilton, Ontario, Canada

Wendy Pentland, PhD, OT Reg. (Ont.)
(Chapter 8)
Associate Professor
Occupational Therapy
School of Rehabilitation Therapy
Queen's University
Kingston, Ontario, Canada

Brenda H. Vrkljan, PhD, OT Reg. (Ont.)
(Chapter 4)
Assistant Professor
Occupational Therapy
School of Rehabilitation Science
Faculty of Health Sciences
McMaster University
Hamilton, Ontario, Canada

PREFACE

The growth of evaluative research in occupational therapy over the past few decades is remarkable. Over the past 15 years, occupational therapy has embraced the development and use of evidence in practice. It has also recognized that the use of research results alone does not constitute evidence-based practice. Our profession has been enriched by many studies exploring the experiential nature of occupational therapy intervention and examining specific outcomes after intervention. Research findings together with client goals and values and therapists' clinical wisdom lead to best practices. In this way, evidence-based practice becomes a powerful tool that helps practitioners provide higher quality services for clients and their families.

While evidence-based practice may appear straightforward, implementation in everyday occupational therapy practice remains challenging for several reasons. To incorporate research about current therapy approaches into practice, therapists need to access relevant research studies, appraise their quality, synthesize the findings, and apply the results to their specific client population. Likewise, student occupational therapists need to have ready access to critically appraised research across the domains of therapy intervention. While the availability of systematic reviews has helped this process, few evidence-based resources have synthesized research information specific to occupational therapy practice.

The purpose of the book is to assemble for students, practitioners, administrators, educators, researchers, and policymakers the evidence for the effectiveness of occupational therapy for adults and older adults. This book contributes the unique function of linking eight types of occupational therapy **intervention** with the **effects** that can be expected from those interventions, with the measures most commonly used to demonstrate **outcomes**. The book provides the results of a comprehensive scoping review of research on occupational therapy intervention with adults and older adults. The focus of the book is not just on evaluative research but the outcomes that measure the effects of occupational therapy intervention. We were impressed by the amount of research that has been completed over the past 28 years. Our hope is that this book provides guidance for future research on occupational therapy outcomes. For faculty, please go to www.efacultylounge.com to examine the Instructor's Manual and PowerPoint slides that we have developed to accompany this book.

We are grateful to the Health Outcomes for Better Information and Health committee of the Ontario Ministry of Health and Long Term Care for providing research funding to undertake this scoping review. A very special thank you to Briano Di Rezze, the research coordinator on this project. Briano ensured that all the literature searches were thorough and carefully documented. Thanks to all of the student occupational therapists who were hired to critically appraise specific studies. Finally, we thank the authors who contributed their expertise to specific chapters.

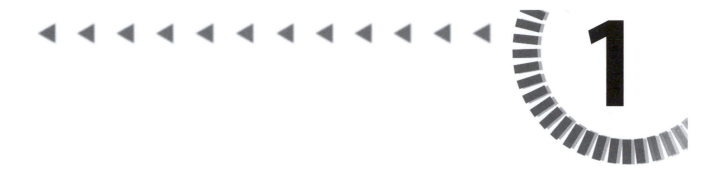

OCCUPATIONAL THERAPY: INTERVENTIONS, EFFECTS, AND OUTCOMES

Mary Law, PhD, FCAOT and Mary Ann McColl, PhD, MTS

Occupational therapy is a health profession that focuses on "promoting health and well-being through occupation. Occupation refers to everything that people do during the course of everyday life" (Canadian Association of Occupational Therapists [CAOT], 2003). Occupational therapists focus on enabling a client's participation in occupations of daily life that are meaningful to him or her and bring purpose to his or her life (American Occupational Therapy Association [AOTA], 2008). Occupational therapists work with people who are at risk or have problems participating in daily occupations because of illness or disability or environmental barriers.

Occupational therapy, over the past decade, has embraced the development and use of evidence in practice. Evidence-based occupational therapy has been supported by national professional organizations and has been taught in occupational therapy educational programs. The goal of such endorsement is to ensure that evidence-based practice becomes a powerful tool that helps practitioners provide higher quality services for their clients and families.

Evidence-based practice has been defined by Rosenberg and Donald (1995) as "the process of systematically finding, appraising, and using contemporaneous research findings as the basis for clinical decisions. Evidence-based medicine asks questions, finds and appraises the relevant data, and harnesses that information for everyday clinical practice" (p. 1122). As evidence-based practice evolved and was applied to occupational therapy, there was a recognition that research knowledge is combined with clinical reasoning and clients' values and desires to inform clinical decision making (Haynes, 2002; Law, Pollock & Stewart, 2004).

While evidence-based practice may appear straightforward, implementation in everyday occupational therapy practice remains challenging for several reasons. To incorporate research about current therapy approaches into practice, therapists need to access relevant research studies, appraise their quality, synthesize the findings with other research, and apply the results to their specific client population. Students in occupational therapy apply the same approach to clinical cases studied within their programs. For both practitioners and students, the time and skills required to accurately synthesize evidence for application to practice is prohibitive. While the

M. Law & M. A. McColl (Eds.)
Interventions, Effects, and Outcomes in Occupational Therapy:
Adults and Older Adults (pp. 1-13)
© 2010 SLACK Incorporated

availability of systematic reviews has helped this process, few evidence-based resources have synthesized research information specific to occupational therapy practice.

Purpose of This Book

This book has been developed to assist with the development of evidence-based occupational therapy. The purpose of the book is to assemble for students, practitioners, administrators, educators, researchers, and policymakers the evidence for the effectiveness of occupational therapy for adults and older adults. The book provides the results of a comprehensive systematic review of research on occupational therapy intervention with adults and older adults (Law & McColl, 2006). The information in this book does not focus on therapy for children or youth.

The book brings together, for the first time, the most recently published peer-reviewed literature, conceptual approaches, outcome measures, and intervention approaches to address three main areas of occupational therapy for adults and older adults:

▲ **Interventions**: The ways occupational therapists purposefully interact with and provide treatment to their clients in attempts to improve occupation; these interventions can be provided by occupational therapists alone or by occupational therapists working within an interprofessional team

▲ **Effects:** The outcomes that occupational therapy can be successful in achieving as a result of intervention

▲ **Outcomes:** The indicators and assessments that occupational therapists use to show where occupational therapy has made a difference

The specific objectives for this book are:

▲ To identify a finite set of **interventions** with which occupational therapists are most often associated and to provide details of those intervention approaches.

▲ To identify where the research evidence shows that occupational therapists can achieve specific **effects** as a result of those interventions.

▲ To identify the **outcome** measures most commonly and reliably used by researchers in occupational therapy to demonstrate the effects of interventions.

In Chapter 1, we discuss key background information on each of these three topics. Occupational therapy intervention is discussed within the context of the International Classification of Functioning, Disability, and Health (ICF). We then outline characteristics of occupational therapy intervention and the theoretical frameworks that underpin this scoping review.

Interventions

Occupational therapy interventions focus on engagement in everyday occupations (AOTA, 2008; CAOT, 1997; Canadian Institute for Health Information, 2007). When occupations are disrupted, occupational therapists provide assessment and intervention to determine the cause of these difficulties and to design an intervention to enable the development and performance of occupations meaningful to that person, group, or organization. Occupational therapists intervene in five main sectors of the health care system, particularly acute care, home care, long-term care, rehabilitation, and primary care. Occupational therapy interventions are underpinned by several key conceptual approaches, which provide a context for practice. This section explores the ideas of enabling client-centered practice, and goal setting. An understanding of these concepts is important to understanding occupational therapy interventions. Finally, occupational therapy interventions fall into nine main categories, which will be described at the end of this section.

Enabling Process

Occupational therapists perform assessments of a person's participation in daily occupations, identify underlying reasons for difficulties with occupational performance, and plan intervention to improve occupational participation. Frameworks and processes have been developed to guide therapy practice. Two widely used frameworks will be discussed.

The AOTA (2008) has published the Occupational Therapy Practice Framework to delineate the domain and process of occupational therapy assessment and intervention. As described in the Framework, the domain of occupational therapy is to enhance citizens' health and participation in daily life through occupation (AOTA, 2008). Areas of occupation include activities of daily living (ADL), instrumental activities of daily living (IADL), rest and sleep, education, work, play, leisure, and social participation. Worldwide, these areas of occupation have been categorized into the areas of self-care (ADL, IADL, rest, sleep), productivity (education, work, volunteer work), and leisure (leisure, play, social participation). In the Framework, the process of occupational therapy service provision includes evaluation, intervention, and outcome monitoring (AOTA, 2008). Specific steps in the occupational therapy process include development of an occupational profile and analysis of occupational performance (under evaluation); development, implementation, and review of an intervention plan (under intervention); and use of outcomes to support participation through engagement in occupation (AOTA, 2008). Because the Framework is not a theory, it is

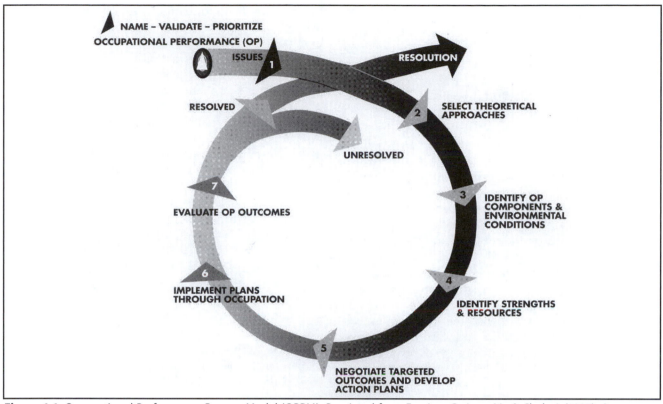

Figure 1-1. Occupational Performance Process Model (OPPM). Reprinted from Fearing, G., Law, M., & Clark, J. (1997). An occupational performance process model: Fostering client and therapist alliances. *Canadian Journal of Occupational Therapy, 64*(1), 7-15 with permission of CAOT Publications ACE.

designed to be used together with conceptual and practice models for occupational therapy.

Developed in Canada and used internationally, the Occupational Performance Process Model (OPPM) (Figure 1-1) provides a detailed description of the occupational therapy assessment and intervention process (Fearing, Law, & Clark, 1997). This model provides a guideline for the steps in occupational therapy practice.

Client-Centered Practice

Occupational therapy intervention puts client-centeredness at the forefront of practice. Occupational therapists work with clients to establish meaningful goals for therapy. People receiving occupational therapy services want to be partners in the therapy process and have their individual needs met. Occupational therapists support the active engagement of people in their chosen occupations of daily life. Since 1980, Canadian occupational therapists have been leading the development of client-centered occupational therapy, and these concepts are now embraced worldwide. Basic to this approach is the recognition that clients of occupational therapy use their unique background and life experiences to determine their needs for participation in daily occupations. Therapists using a client-centered approach show respect for the choices that clients have made and will make.

Goal Setting

At the heart of client-centered occupational therapy practice is the process of goal setting. The impact of occupational therapy on client outcomes is believed to be a function of the responsiveness and accuracy of the goal-setting process. Effective goal setting facilitates the ability of clients to engage in therapy and to be successful in attaining their therapy goals. Studies in occupational therapy by Gagne and Hoppes (2003) and Howell (1986) indicate that goal setting can have a positive impact on client motivation and outcomes. Other research also supports a positive effect of goal setting on outcomes (Baker, Marshak, Rice, & Zimmerman, 2001; Ponte-Allan & Giles, 1999). Based on these results, the inclusion of a validated approach to goal setting within occupational therapy practice is suggested. Validated methods to set goals include the Canadian Occupational Performance Measure (COPM) (Law, Baptiste, Carswell, McColl, Polatajko, & Pollock, 1991, 2005) and Goal Attainment Scaling (GAS) (Hurn, Kneebone, & Cropley, 2007). As well, more research into the process and outcomes of collaborative goal setting is warranted.

Areas of Practice

Occupational therapy practices within all areas of health care, including acute care, long-term care, community care, rehabilitation, and primary care. For the research reviews completed for this book, we have used the following definitions to delineate these areas of occupational therapy practice:

▲ Long-term care provides continuing, medically complex and specialized services to adults, sometimes over extended periods of time within a hospital or rehabilitation setting. Examples include long-term care facilities (nursing homes), musculoskeletal programs, chronic care hospitals, seating, prosthetics and orthotics, return to work, adult day care, attendant care, and homes for the aged.

▲ Acute care services are specialized short-term services delivered within a hospital setting. Examples include brief inpatient stay, cardiac, orthopedic surgery (day, elective, or emergency room discharge), urgent/emergent care, and trauma unit.

▲ Home care includes a wide range of health services delivered at home or in community programs other than a hospital for recovering, disabled, or chronically or terminally ill people in need of therapeutic treatment and/or assistance with participation in daily occupations. Examples include community mental health day programs, clubhouse, sheltered workshops, community occupational therapy, and home assessments.

▲ Rehabilitation refers to adult inpatient and outpatient services provided by hospitals or rehabilitation settings. Examples include splinting and institution-based group teaching (programs with defined timelines).

▲ An emerging field for occupational therapy is primary health care, defined as health services provided at the first point of contact with the health care system. Primary care focuses on health promotion, illness and injury prevention, and the diagnosis and treatment of illness and injury (Health Canada, 2006).

Types of Occupational Therapy Interventions

Previous work attempting to classify occupational therapy theory led us to conclude that occupation can change in three ways (development, adaptation, and accommodation) and that occupational therapists seek to change occupation in three ways (remediation, compensation, and advocacy).

The goal of occupational therapy intervention is to change occupational performance either by enhancing development, promoting adaptation, or changing the environment to better accommodate disability (McColl, Law, Stewart, Doubt, Pollock, & Krupa, 2002). Occupation changes by:

▲ Development—the intrinsic processes of maturation, growth, recovery, and healing that occur within the human organism over time

▲ Adaptation—the responses that the individual makes to internal and external stimuli to optimize function

▲ Accommodation—the changes in the environment that permit increased functioning by individuals

Occupational therapists act to change occupation through three processes:

▲ Remediation—directly addressing dysfunction to alleviate it

▲ Compensation—addressing the task or the way the individual approaches the task to optimize function

▲ Advocacy—seeking changes in the environment to permit optimal function

These approaches correspond in a one-to-one fashion, as follows:

▲ When occupational therapists believe there is development (i.e., for function to actually change, for the individual to recover, develop, or improve either a specific occupation or the component skills necessary for that occupation), they tend to act in a remedial capacity to improve function to its optimal level. This type of occupational therapy focuses on the **person**.

▲ When occupational therapists discern that actual changes in the organism are unlikely, they adapt the task, the approach, the tools, or the supports to compensate for lost function. This type of occupational therapy focuses on the **occupation**.

▲ When occupational therapists see that accommodations are necessary for optimal functioning, they advocate on behalf of their client to seek the necessary changes. This type of occupational therapy focuses on the **environment**.

Our review of the literature for this book has indicated that these three broad categories of intervention can be further differentiated into eight categories of occupational therapy interventions, as shown in Table 1-1. This list has arisen out of the literature, and it serves to classify the types of interventions found in the body of evidence for the purpose of this book.

Effects

Occupational therapy is a health profession that focuses on promoting health and well-being through occupation. Occupational therapists help individuals to participate in the daily occupations that they need

Table 1-1
OCCUPATIONAL THERAPY INTERVENTIONS

Focus of Intervention	Occupational Therapy Interventions	Description
Person	1. Training	Enhancing performance of physical, psychological, cognitive, social components—e.g., strengthening, exercises, rehearsing, practicing.
	2. Skill development	Improving performance of complete tasks, such as ADL skills, social interactions, and organizational abilities. Skill development builds on training of performance components.
	3. Education	Learning more about one's condition, options for improvement, and ways of preventing difficulties or improving function.
Occupation	4. Task adaptation	Modifying or changing a task to permit it to be accomplished despite diminished component performance.
	5. Occupational development	Optimizing participation in occupations, such as vocational training or leisure programs.
Environment	6. Environmental modification	Modifying the task environment to enhance function, such as adding adaptive tools, devices.
	7. Support provision	Enhancing personal and environmental support (e.g., environmental cueing, adaptive equipment).
	8. Information and support enhancement	Providing education and information to caregivers or other important people in the environment to improve functioning.

to do, want to do, or are expected to do (Law et al., 1991, 2005). Occupational therapists focus on enabling occupations of daily life that are meaningful to their clients and bring purpose to their lives (CAOT, 2002). Occupational therapists work with people who are at risk or have problems participating in daily occupations because of illness or disability or environmental barriers.

The effects of occupational therapy are understood as an interaction of the person with the environment through the medium of occupation. Several conceptual theories and models of occupational therapy emphasize these concepts (CAOT, 1997; Christiansen, Baum, & Bass-Haugen, 2005; Dunn, Brown, & McGuigan, 1994; Kielhofner, 2006; Law, Cooper, Strong, Stewart, Rigby, & Letts, 1996a; Townsend & Polatajko, 2007). As an application example, we will discuss the Person-Environment-Occupation (PEO) Model (Figure 1-2) (Law et al., 1996a). Within the PEO Model, occupation is a function of the fit (or lack of fit) between the person's abilities and skills, the demands of a particular occupation, and the environmental conditions in which occupation takes place. Occupational performance refers to the ability to choose, organize,

and satisfactorily perform meaningful occupations that are culturally defined and age appropriate for looking after oneself, enjoying life, and contributing to the social and economic fabric of a community (CAOT, 1997).

The Canadian Model of Occupational Performance (CMOP) (Figure 1-3) (CAOT, 1997; Townsend & Polatajko, 2007) also describes the dynamic relationship between people, environment, and occupation. This model further contributes an elaboration of the contribution of the person. It allows for the idea that the effects of occupational therapy may be seen at the level of personal components such as the physical, affective, cognitive, and spiritual components.

Occupation

The primary *effect* of occupational therapy is on occupation. Occupation refers to everything that people do during the course of everyday life (AOTA, 2002; CAOT, 2003). Occupation has been shown to have a significant influence on health and well-being (Christiansen et al., 2005; Law, Steinweinder, & Leclair, 1998; McColl et al., 2002).

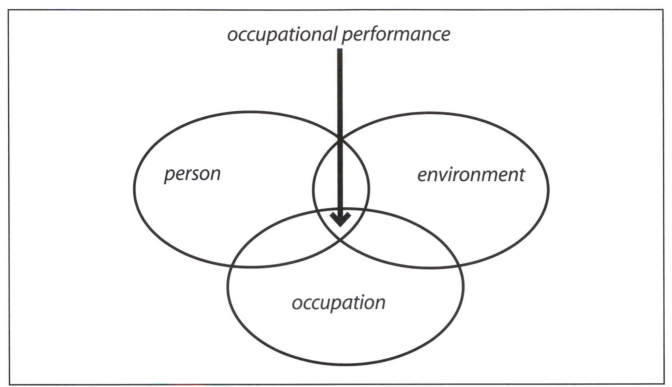

Figure 1-2. Person-Environment-Occupation (PEO) Model. Reprinted from Law, M., Cooper, B., Strong, S., Stewart, D., Rigby, P., & Letts, L. (1996b). The person-environment-occupation model: A transactive approach to occupational performance. *Canadian Journal of Occupational Therapy, 63*(1), 9-23 with permission of CAOT Publications ACE.

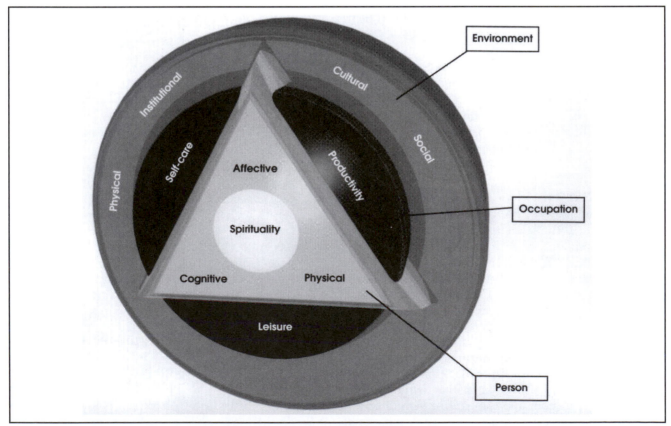

Figure 1-3. Canadian Model of Occupational Performance (CMOP). Reprinted from Canadian Association of Occupational Therapists. (2002). *Enabling occupation: An occupational therapy perspective* (Rev. ed.). Ottawa, Ontario, Canada: CAOT Publications with permission of CAOT Publications ACE.

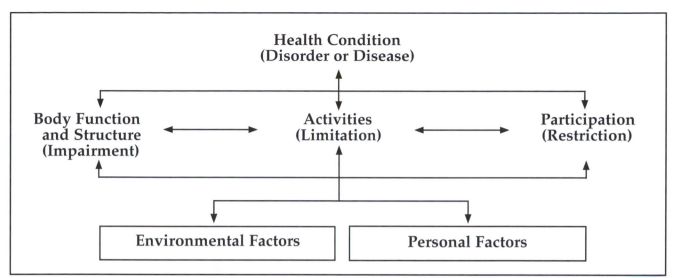

Figure 1-4. International Classification of Functioning, Disability, and Health (ICF). Reprinted with permission from World Health Organization. (2001). *International classification of functioning, disability, and health.* Geneva, Switzerland: Author.

Self-Care, Productivity, and Leisure

More specifically, occupational therapy is expected to produce effects on the three main components of occupation: self-care, work/productivity, and leisure.

▲ **Self-Care**—"Includes activities that the individual performs for the purpose of maintaining the self in a condition that allows for function" (McColl et al., 2002). Examples of areas of self-care outcomes include personal care (ADL), functional mobility, and community management.

▲ **Work/Productivity**—"Refers to the activities that customarily fill the bulk of one's day and which contribute to economic preservation, home and family maintenance, and service or personal development" (McColl et al., 2002). Examples of productivity outcomes include paid or unpaid work, household management, and school.

▲ **Leisure**—"Includes activities that one engages in when one is freed from the obligation to be productive. Leisure activities are defined by personal preferences and interests of the individual" (McColl et al., 2002). Examples of leisure outcomes include quiet recreation, active recreation, and socialization.

Participation

There are many meaningful life situations in which occupational therapists are interested that do not fit neatly into the three occupational performance categories of self-care, productivity, and leisure. For this reason, occupational therapists also focus on participation (Hammal, Jarvis, & Colver, 2004; WHO, 2002). Examples of participation outcomes in which occupational therapists might be interested include

organizing and carrying out daily tasks, functional indoor and/or outdoor mobility, driving, caring for oneself, household tasks, community living, parenting, social relationships, work, volunteer work, and leisure activities.

International Classification of Functioning, Disability, and Health

Occupational therapists provide intervention for people with and without disabilities who have difficulties performing daily occupations. Occupational therapists worldwide are increasingly using the ICF developed by the World Health Organization ([WHO], 2001) as a communication tool for intervention focus and outcome assessment. The ICF (Figure 1-4) focuses on the relationship between health conditions, health, and well-being. This classification system is being used as a common communication tool to understand health domains. The ICF provides a standard language and framework for the description of health and health-related issues as it relates to functioning (WHO, 2002).

The discipline of occupational therapy has taken this classification system into consideration when establishing practice frameworks and models of practice (AOTA, 2008; Townsend & Polatajko, 2007). In the United States, the AOTA has developed the Occupational Therapy Practice Framework to articulate the way in which occupational therapy impacts on the outcomes of occupational performance, health, and participation (AOTA, 2002, 2008). Within the Framework, its purpose is described using the language of participation from the ICF. The Framework "was developed to articulate occupational therapy's contribution to promoting the health and participation of people, organizations, and populations through engagement in occupation" (AOTA, 2008, p. 625). As well, client factors such as body function and body structure are described using definitions from the ICF (AOTA, 2008).

Determinants of Occupation

In an extensive review of theory in occupational therapy, McColl and colleagues (2002) developed taxonomy for the effects of occupational therapy, based on five determinants of occupation:

▲ The **physical** determinants of occupation refer to the musculoskeletal abilities required to achieve certain occupations. Thus, occupational therapists may seek to affect strength, range of motion, and endurance in their attempts to promote occupation.

▲ The **cognitive-neurological** determinants of occupation refer to the processing of information by the central nervous system. Occupational therapists may also seek to affect how cognitive, sensory, perceptual, and neurological information are processed to permit patients to carry out daily activities with success and satisfaction.

▲ The **psycho-emotional** determinants of occupation refer to thoughts and feelings that may assist or impede occupation. Occupational therapists may seek to produce effects on affect, coping, and behavior.

▲ The **socio-cultural** determinants of occupation include the socially constructed beliefs, attitudes, roles, and expectations that form a part of who we are. Occupational therapists may confront time use, roles, values, and spirituality as means to occupation.

▲ Occupational therapists understand that disability may be caused by inadequacies in the **environment** that cannot always be remedied by changing the individual's capabilities (Law, 1991). Occupational therapists may, therefore, seek to affect the environment by removing barriers and increasing supports in order to maximize an individual's occupational performance. Of interest to occupational therapists are three categories of environment:

△ The **physical** environment—composed of the natural and built surroundings, including safety, accessibility, and social supports (Law et al., 1996a).

△ The **social** environment—including social priorities, relationships, social values, attitudes and beliefs, role expectations, and educational attainment.

△ The **cultural-institutional** environment—including ethnic, racial, ceremonial routines, societal institutions and practices, policies, processes, and accessibility.

Outcomes

The incorporation of a valid outcome measurement process is an essential part of evidence-based occupational therapy. In a health system with increasing costs, the provision of evidence regarding the effects of services is vitally important. An approach to measurement in occupational therapy must fit with a client-centered practice in which people, their families, and therapists collaborate to define issues of occupational dysfunction and desired outcomes. Outcome measurement in any health profession can improve the decision-making process regarding specific clients or programs. We have an obligation to use interventions based on knowledge gained from measurement of outcomes. Decision makers and policymakers can use outcome measurement data to implement the most cost-effective programs.

In occupational therapy, the outcomes of interest come directly from our conceptual models of practice (Law, Baum, & Dunn, 2005). Outcomes sensitive to occupational therapy intervention center primarily on the outcomes of occupational performance and participation. As stated earlier, these outcomes include a focus on the daily occupations of self-care, productivity, and leisure.

In reviewing the outcome measures sensitive to occupational therapy interventions, we have used the studies reviewed for this book as well as current measurement literature as the basis for our recommendations. There has been considerable work completed to date on describing and critically reviewing outcome measures used in occupational therapy practice (Asher, 2007; Law, Baum, & Dunn, 2005). These works provide an excellent foundation to delineate the most appropriate outcome measures for each section of this report.

The inclusion of these measures is based on a review of their content, reliability, validity, and clinical utility. Established criteria for the evaluation of outcome measures have been used to ensure that the measures delineated in each chapter are the best that are currently available (CanChild, 2004) (Table 1-2).

Client Satisfaction With Occupational Therapy Services

One general area of outcome after therapy intervention is client satisfaction. With the emphasis on client-centered (and family-centered) practice, occupational

Table 1-2
Effects and Outcomes

Effects		Outcomes
Occupation	Participation	Overall daily occupations including:
		Community integration
		Domestic life
		Health-related quality of life
		Occupational performance
		Personal care
		Social and civic life
	Self-Care	Personal care
		Functional mobility
		Community management
	Productivity—	Knowledge of ergonomics and body mechanics
	Work and Volunteer Work	Strength, physical demand capacity
		Work endurance
		Work/return to work
		Volunteer work
		Work satisfaction
	Leisure	Leisure participation
		Satisfaction with leisure
		Perceptions of leisure participation
Environment	Cultural-Institutional, Physical, and Social Environment	Safety hazards and safety knowledge
		Use of adaptive devices and equipment
		Physical adaptations
		Client satisfaction with environmental modification and equipment/devices
		Social attitudes
		Caregiver skills in adapting home environment
		Caregiver self-efficacy
		Caregiver burden and stress
		Need for extra assistance in the home
Person	Physical	General physical health and well-being (including falls prevention)
		Pain (musculoskeletal)
		Joint protection
		Energy conservation
		Upper extremity function
		Lower extremity function (includes hip impairment)
		Positioning/seating
	Socio-Cultural	Social abilities and engagement
		Role performance
		Time use
	Psycho-Emotional	Pain
		Depressive symptoms
		Anxiety
		Interpersonal interactions
		Motivation
	Cognitive-Neurological	Cognitive abilities
		Perceptual abilities
		Neuro-motor abilities
		Sensory abilities
		Pain (neuro-motor)

therapy has focused on considering the client's needs and goals to enhance his or her quality of life. Implicit in the practice of occupational therapy is the satisfaction of the client with occupational therapy services. Within a literature review of health and social science research, the results indicated that the "evidence supports that a client-centred occupational therapy practice will lead to improved client satisfaction and outcomes" (Law, 1998, p. 25). However, few empirical studies have exclusively measured satisfaction of occupational therapy services for outcome evaluation due to the subjective nature of client perceptions of "satisfaction" and challenges in generalizing these outcomes across client populations. Nevertheless, there is indeed value in evaluating client satisfaction in conjunction with other outcome measures in anticipation that higher client satisfaction is often associated with increased compliance to influence outcomes in rehabilitation (Keith, 1998). Furthermore, satisfaction outcomes of occupational therapy services can differentiate the effects from the impact of other disciplines within multidisciplinary treatment (Keith, 1998; Whiteneck, 1994). Satisfaction outcomes were not exclusively searched within this review. However, several studies were captured in the search that we believe provide valuable insight about how occupational therapy services are perceived by clients, are evaluated (based on client satisfaction), and impact client satisfaction.

Client Perception of Occupational Therapy Services

Several qualitative studies have documented the perception of occupational therapy as a valuable health care service across different client groups and practice settings (Boutin Lester & Gibson, 2002; Case-Smith & Nastro, 1993; Darragh, Sample, & Krieger, 2001). In the phenomenological study by Boutin Lester and Gibson (2002), the perceptions of home health occupational therapy in five patients were generally positive. The main theme describing patient perception of the characteristics of occupational therapy service provision was the "therapeutic use of self by the therapist." This theme includes the perception that the relationship with the occupational therapist was like a friendship by way of the therapist's "...expressing empathy, flexibility, understanding, tolerance, kindness and optimism, and other such personal qualities, in addition to objective therapeutic skills, to help clients move toward independence in their individual way" (Boutin Lester & Gibson, 2002, p. 152).

In the study by Case-Smith and Nastro (1993), occupational therapy was an overall positive experience received by middle class mothers of children with cerebral palsy. The study was an ethnographic design, interviewing five mothers within their homes. One prominent theme on overall satisfaction with occupational therapy detailed the mothers' experience with occupational therapy in a variety of settings (e.g., hospital, early intervention and preschool programs, and private home-based occupational therapy). The mothers commonly saw occupational therapists *as agents of change* to effectively facilitate improvement in their child's function; *a source of information* regarding development, therapy, and community resources; and *a source of support* within the provision of service.

In a phenomenological study examining the client perception of occupational therapy for people receiving service post-acquired brain injury (ABI), 51 participants reported a positive role that occupational therapists played as an advocate, friend, mentor, and team member (Darragh et al., 2001). One specific theme highlighted the helpfulness of occupational therapy services. Within this theme, many of the participants indicated that occupational therapy offered services that were relevant to the subjects, with practical suggestions/strategies, and found it helpful that occupational therapy provided periodic feedback on their treatment progress.

Outcome Measures Evaluating Client Satisfaction of Occupational Therapy Services

In the literature, the measures documented to evaluate satisfaction of occupational therapy services range from program-specific questionnaires to more formal client satisfaction tools. Program-specific measures of satisfaction can involve a simple questionnaire of service components using a Likert scale for quantitative outcomes (Kealey & McIntyre, 2005). A more in-depth evaluation of services can involve the use of general models of program evaluation, such as the Programme Logic Model (Rush & Ogborne, 1991) or models specific to a client service such as the Cycle of Services for Wheelchair Seating Clinic Clients (Suzuki & Lockette, 2000). Adapting specific client satisfaction tools developed for general health care or discipline-specific services is another way the satisfaction of occupational therapy services has been measured. Tools such as the Client Satisfaction Questionnaire (Larsen, Attkisson, Hargreaves, & Nguyen, 1979) and the Physician Satisfaction Questionnaire (renamed as the Therapist Evaluation Form) (Cope, Linn, Leake, & Barrett, 1986) have been used to evaluate client satisfaction with occupational therapy services.

Characteristics of Occupational Therapy Services Impacting on Client Satisfaction

The literature reports evidence of the impact of occupational therapy services on the satisfaction of clients who have received short-term services, as well as longer term services relevant to people with disabilities.

In a cross-sectional research design, a sample of 107 adults who have accessed occupational therapy services (outpatient or community) from a regional health care facility in Canada were interviewed by a telephone survey (McKinnon, 2000). The results indicated client satisfaction with health care outcomes attributed to occupational therapy services, specifically in the importance placed by clients on interpersonal manners, communication skills, and competency of therapists, as well as the availability and accessibility of services, and outcomes related to the interventions provided.

For longer term occupational therapy services provided to clients with disabilities, two studies provide insight on similar characteristics applicable to client satisfaction. In a study by Huebner and colleagues (2003), follow-up data of 25 clients who were 21 months post-ABI assessed a variety of outcomes including an adapted version of the Client Satisfaction Questionnaire (Larsen et al., 1979) specific to occupational therapy. The overall results indicated that satisfaction with occupational therapy was generally high, in that 87% of clients were "satisfied" to "very satisfied" with occupational therapy, and 91.7% would recommend occupational therapy to a friend or family member in need of similar help. Furthermore, most respondents spontaneously had a desire to have more rehabilitation including occupational therapy. The results in high satisfaction of occupational therapy services were unrelated to most functional outcomes. Similar results indicating a high degree of satisfaction of occupational therapy services among a sample of clients with multiple sclerosis was evident in total score and item analysis using the Therapist Evaluation Form (Roush, 1995). In addition, the content of two open-ended questions within the evaluation form indicated that the clients valued therapist characteristics of being friendly and caring. Clients also reported less satisfaction with therapist technical skills as opposed to rapport issues.

In sum, it is evident that, regardless of the disability population, client satisfaction can be largely influenced by the interpersonal skills demonstrated by the occupational therapist, which can be unrelated to intervention outcomes. This is consistent with other evidence in the general health care literature, which cites the importance of interpersonal aspects of patient-professional relationships for people with disabilities (Keith, 1998). For occupational therapy services, although likely independent of measurable functional gain, the therapeutic environment that includes empathy, compassion, affirmation, and education can produce a strong sense of satisfaction (Halstead, 2001).

Outline of This Book

In Chapter 1, we provide information about the focus and conceptual underpinnings of occupational therapy practice. Chapter 2 outlines the systematic review process that was undertaken for this research.

Chapters 3 through 11 provide the results of the reviews in specific areas of outcomes that are sensitive to occupational therapy intervention:

▲ Chapter 3. Occupation/Participation
▲ Chapter 4: Self-Care
▲ Chapter 5: Productivity
▲ Chapter 6: Leisure
▲ Chapter 7: Environment
▲ Chapter 8: Physical
▲ Chapter 9: Socio-Cultural
▲ Chapter 10. Psycho-Emotional
▲ Chapter 11. Cognitive-Neurological

Chapter 12 details the authors' conclusions and recommendations, based on the findings of the scoping review.

Uses of the Book

For Students

This book provides students with a comprehensive synthesis of evaluation research in occupational therapy over the past 30 years. Student occupational therapists will learn about the most effective occupational therapy interventions for adults and older adults and how to measure outcomes after these interventions.

For Clinicians

This book is intended to assist clinicians in identifying the practices for which most evidence exists of effectiveness. The book provides a comprehensive synthesis of evaluation research in occupational therapy over almost three decades. Using strict criteria for inclusion, this book assembles and evaluates the research evidence in the published literature for occupational therapy programs that can be shown to be effective.

For Researchers

This book provides researchers with a synthesis of methods, approaches, measures, and results of intervention studies in occupational therapy in the modern period. Any researcher planning to conduct studies of the effectiveness of occupational therapy interventions would benefit from consulting the appropriate section of this book to find a summary of the strengths and weakness of previous research on the topic, as well as a guide to the most common and appropriate outcome measures in the area. The book also makes specific suggestions for further research and notes areas where research evidence is lacking for common practices and programs.

For Decision Makers

Decision makers at various levels will find this book a valuable tool in assessing the effectiveness of occupational therapy programs and making strategic investments in occupational therapy to achieve the greatest benefit for their clients. Occupational therapy managers, institutional administrators, and government funders will find information in this book to support investments in the most effective occupational therapy practices to ensure the maximum occupational performance, health, and well-being for their constituents.

For Educators

Education and training programs for occupational therapists will find this book useful for themselves and their students in that it brings together the research evidence that is currently spread over many years and sources. It assembles the best evidence available for the effectiveness of occupational therapy programs and shows how programs have been developed and evaluated over the past 30 years. It does so within the context of contemporary occupational therapy theory and provides solid rationales for the classification of evidence.

References

American Occupational Therapy Association. (2002). Occupational therapy practice framework: Domain and process. *American Journal of Occupational Therapy, 56,* 609-639.

American Occupational Therapy Association. (2008). Occupational therapy practice framework: Domain and process (2nd ed.). *American Journal of Occupational Therapy, 62,* 625-683.

Asher, I. E. (2007). *Occupational therapy assessment tools: An annotated index.* Bethesda, MA: American Occupational Therapy Association.

Baker, S. M., Marshak, H. H., Rice, G. T., & Zimmerman, G. J. (2001). Patient participation in physical therapy goal setting. *Physical Therapy, 81*(5), 1118-1126.

Boutin Lester, P., & Gibson, R. W. (2002). Patients' perceptions of home health occupational therapy. *Australian Occupational Therapy Journal, 49*(3), 146-154.

Canadian Association of Occupational Therapists. (1997). *Enabling occupation: An occupational therapy perspective.* Ottawa, Ontario, Canada: CAOT Publications.

Canadian Association of Occupational Therapists. (2002). *Enabling occupation: An occupational therapy perspective* (Rev. ed.). Ottawa, Ontario, Canada: CAOT Publications.

Canadian Association of Occupational Therapists. (2003). Position statement on everyday occupations and health, 2003. Retrieved from: www.caot.ca/default.asp?pageid=699 on May 20, 2008.

Canadian Institute for Health Information. (2007). *Workforce trends of occupational therapists in Canada, 2006.* Ottawa, Ontario, Canada: Author.

CanChild Centre for Childhood Disability Research. (2004). Outcomes measures rating form and guidelines. Retrieved from: www.canchild.ca/Default.aspx?tabid=192 on July 28, 2008.

Case-Smith, J., & Nastro, M. A. (1993). The effect of occupational therapy intervention on mothers of children with cerebral palsy. *American Journal of Occupational Therapy, 47*(9), 811-817.

Christiansen, C., Baum, C., & Bass-Haugen, J. (2005). *Occupational therapy: Performance, participation, and well-being* (3rd ed.). Thorofare, NJ: SLACK Incorporated.

Cope, D. W., Linn, L. S., Leake, B. D., & Barrett, P. A. (1986). Modification of resident's behavior by preceptor feedback of patient satisfaction. *Journal of General Internal Medicine, 1,* 394-398.

Darragh, A. R., Sample, P. L., & Krieger, S. R. (2001). Tears in my eyes 'cause somebody finally understood: Client perceptions of practitioners following brain injury. *American Journal of Occupational Therapy, 55*(2), 191-199.

Dunn, W., Brown, C., & McGuigan, A. (1994). The ecology of human performance: A framework for considering the effect of context. *American Journal of Occupational Therapy, 48,* 595-607.

Fearing, G., Law, M., & Clark, J. (1997). An occupational performance process model: Fostering client and therapist alliances. *Canadian Journal of Occupational Therapy, 64*(1), 7-15.

Gagne, D., & Hoppes, S. (2003). The effects of collaborative goal-focused occupational therapy on self-care skills: A pilot study. *American Journal of Occupational Therapy, 57*(2), 215-219.

Halstead, L. S. (2001). The power of compassion and caring in rehabilitation healing. *Archives of Physical Medicine and Rehabilitation, 82,* 149-154.

Hammal, D., Jarvis, S. N., & Colver, A. F. (2004). Participation of children with cerebral palsy is influenced by where they live. *Developmental Medicine and Child Neurology, 46,* 292-298.

Haynes, B. (2002). What kind of evidence is it that evidence-based medicine advocates want health care providers and consumers to pay attention to? *BMC Health Services Research, 2,* 1-7. www.biomedicalcentral.com/1472-6963/2/3.

Health Canada. (2006). Primary health care. Retrieved from www.hc-sc.gc.ca/hcs-sss/prim/phctf-fassp/index_e.html on July 2, 2008.

Howell, C. (1986). A controlled trial of goal setting for long-term community psychiatric patients. *British Journal of Occupational Therapy, 49*(8), 264-268.

Huebner, R. A., Johnson, K., Bennett, C. M., & Schneck, C. (2003). Community participation and quality of life outcomes after adult traumatic brain injury. *American Journal of Occupational Therapy, 57*(2), 177-185.

Hurn, J., Kneebone, I., & Cropley, M. (2007). Goal setting as an outcome measure: A systematic review. *Clinical Rehabilitation, 21*(3), 284-285.

Kealey, P., & McIntyre, I. (2005). An evaluation of the domiciliary occupational therapy service in palliative cancer care in a community trust: A patient and carers perspective. *European Journal of Cancer Care, 14*(3), 232-243.

Keith, R. A. (1998). Patient satisfaction and rehabilitation service. *Archives of Physical Medicine and Rehabilitation, 79,* 1122-1128.

Kielhofner, G. (2006). *Model of human occupation.* Philadelphia, PA: Lippincott Williams & Wilkins; 2006.

Larsen, D. L., Attkisson, C. C., Hargreaves, W. A., & Nguyen, T. D. (1979). Assessment of client/patient satisfaction: Development of a general scale. *Evaluation and Program Planning, 2,* 197-207.

Law, M. (1991). The Muriel Driver Lecture: The environment: A focus for occupational therapy. *Canadian Journal of Occupational Therapy, 58*, 171-179.

Law, M. (1998). Does client-centred practice make a difference? In M. Law (Ed.), *Client-centred occupational therapy* (pp. 19-27). Thorofare, NJ: SLACK Incorporated.

Law, M., Baptiste, S., Carswell, A., McColl, M., Polatajko, H., & Pollock, N. (1991). *Canadian Occupational Performance Measure Manual.* Toronto, Canada: CAOT Publications.

Law, M., Baptiste, S., Carswell, A., McColl, M., Polatajko, H., & Pollock, N. (2005). *Canadian Occupational Performance Measure Manual* (4th ed.). Toronto, Canada: CAOT Publications.

Law, M., Baum, C., & Dunn, W. (2005). *Measuring occupational performance: Supporting best practice in occupational therapy* (2nd ed.). Thorofare, NJ: SLACK Incorporated.

Law, M. L., Cooper, B. A., Strong, S., Stewart, D., Rigby, P., & Letts, L. (1996a). Theoretical contexts for practice of occupational therapy. In C. H. Christiansen, & C. M. Baum (Eds.), *Occupational therapy: Enabling function and well-being* (2nd ed.). Thorofare, NJ: SLACK Incorporated.

Law, M., Cooper, B., Strong, S., Stewart, D., Rigby, P., & Letts, L. (1996b). The person-environment-occupation model: A transactive approach to occupational performance. *Canadian Journal of Occupational Therapy, 63*(1), 9-23.

Law, M., & McColl, M. A. (2006). Grant funded by the Ontario Ministry of Health and Long-Term Care. January 2007-December 2008. *Health outcomes for better information and care: A scoping review of occupational therapy intervention for adults and older adults.*

Law, M., Pollock, N. & Stewart, D. (2004). Evidence-based occupational therapy: Concepts and strategies. *New Zealand Journal of Occupational Therapy, 51*(1), 14-22.

Law, M., Steinweinder, S., & Leclair, L. (1998). Occupation, health and well-being. *Canadian Journal of Occupational Therapy, 65*(2), 81-91.

McColl, M., Law, M., Stewart, D., Doubt, L., Pollock, N., & Krupa, T. (2002). *Theoretical basis of occupational therapy* (2nd ed.). Thorofare, NJ: SLACK Incorporated.

McKinnon, A. (2000). Client values and satisfaction with occupational therapy. *Scandinavian Journal of Occupational Therapy, 7*(3), 99-106.

Ponte-Allan, M., & Giles, G. M. (1999). Goal setting and functional outcomes in rehabilitation. *American Journal of Occupational Therapy, 53*, 646-649.

Rosenberg, W., & Donald, A. (1995). Evidence-based medicine: An approach to clinical problem solving. *British Medical Journal, 310*(6987), 1122-1126.

Roush, S. E. (1995). The satisfaction of patients with multiple sclerosis regarding services received from physical and occupational therapists. *International Journal of Rehabilitation and Health, 1*(3), 155-166.

Rush, B., & Ogborne, A. (1991). Program logic models: Expanding their role and structure in program planning and evaluation. *Canadian Journal of Program Evaluation, 6*, 95-106.

Suzuki, K. M., & Lockette, G. (2000). Client satisfaction survey of a wheelchair seating clinic. *Physical and Occupational Therapy in Geriatrics, 17*(2), 55-65.

Townsend, E., & Polatajko, H. (2007). *Enabling occupation II: Advancing an occupational therapy vision for health, well-being and justice through occupation.* Ottawa, Ontario, Canada: CAOT Publications.

Whiteneck, G. G. (1994). Measuring what matters: Key rehabilitation outcomes. *Archives of Physical Medicine and Rehabilitation, 75*, 1073-1076.

World Health Organization. (2001). *International classification of functioning, disability, and health.* Geneva, Switzerland: Author.

World Health Organization. (2002). *Towards a common language for functioning, disability, and health* (ICF). Geneva, Switzerland: Author.

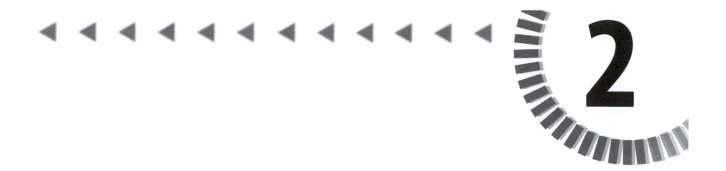

OCCUPATIONAL THERAPY-SENSITIVE OUTCOMES: LITERATURE SEARCH AND STUDY SELECTION

Briano Di Rezze, MSc (OT), OT Reg. (Ont.); Laura Bradley, MSc (OT), OT Reg. (Ont.); Mary Law, PhD, FCAOT; and Mary Ann McColl, PhD, MTS

Conducting a scoping review on the outcomes of occupational therapy intervention for the adult population is a challenging task, given the breadth of clinical practice and research areas. The goal of the search was to capture the most rigorous research related to occupational therapy outcomes published internationally across areas of adult-oriented practice. This search does not claim to have captured all occupational therapy research, but it has collected the most significant studies relevant to the field of occupational therapy. The methodology for this scoping review will be discussed in this chapter within a typical five-stage framework: Identifying the research question, identifying all relevant studies, selecting the studies for detailed analysis, charting the data according to key concepts, and collating and summarizing the findings of the selected studies (Arksey & O'Malley, 2005).

Identifying the Research Question

The research question guiding this scoping review was "What occupational therapy interventions for an adult population are most successful in achieving important occupational therapy outcomes?"

Identifying All Relevant Studies

The relevant studies were identified by searching the following electronic health databases:
▲ AMED (Allied and Complementary Medicine) 1985-2008
▲ CINAHL (Cumulative Index to Nursing and Allied Health Literature) 1982-2008
▲ EMBASE 1980-2008
▲ HAPI (Health and Psychosocial Instruments) where appropriate 1980-2008
▲ MEDLINE 1980-2008
▲ PsychInfo 1980-2008
▲ The Cochrane Library 1980-2008

To ensure that study selection was complete, the reviewers hand searched through a broad range of separate occupational therapy and health care databases containing systematic reviews and meta-analyses that focused on occupational therapy outcomes. These databases were:
▲ Occupational Therapy Critically Appraised Topics (CATs), Queens University, Kingston, Canada

M. Law & M. A. McColl (Eds.)
Interventions, Effects, and Outcomes in Occupational Therapy: Adults and Older Adults (pp. 15-21)
© 2010 SLACK Incorporated

▲ Occupational Therapy Critically Appraised Topics (CATs), University of Western Sydney, Australia
▲ OT Seeker
▲ OTD Base
▲ Campbell Collaboration
▲ Agency for Health Care Policy and Research
▲ American Occupational Therapy Association (AOTA) Evidence Briefs
▲ Canadian Occupational Therapy Foundation (COTF) Critical Research Literature Reviews

The researchers also hand searched the content and references of several unpublished or commissioned critical and systematic reviews implementing occupational therapy intervention and evaluating outcomes. The selected reviews, which were completed at McMaster University, included unpublished critical literature reviews (1985-2000) on home-based occupational therapy intervention for children and adults (Law, Pollock, Stewart, Harms, & Lammi, 2004) and goal setting (Pollock, 2004). Research titled *The Canadian Occupational Performance Measure: An Annotated Bibliography and Research Resource* (McColl, Carswell, Law, Pollock, Baptiste, & Polatajko, 2006) was also used to identify studies. Another annotated bibliography was reviewed for relevant studies by Klassen (2008) on occupational therapy in primary health care (studies spanning 2003-2008).

An initial set of keywords was established by the research team, which consisted of occupational therapy faculty, experienced occupational therapists, and occupational therapy researchers. Search terms for the initial search were drawn from prominent areas of adult occupational therapy practice, intervention, assessment, and populations (diagnoses or disabilities). The reviewers used relevant descriptors, which included "OCCUPATION(S)" (which includes all suffixes, including occupational therapy and therapist), and nine search terms identified a priori from the theory base for occupational therapy. They are:
▲ **Participation** from the World Health Organization's (WHO) International Classification of Functioning, Disability, and Health (ICF) (2001)
▲ **Self-Care, Productivity, and Leisure** from the Canadian Model of Occupational Performance (CMOP) (Canadian Association of Occupational Therapists, 1997)
▲ **Physical, Psycho-Emotional, Cognitive-Neurological, Socio-Cultural, and Environmental** from McColl and colleagues' *Theoretical Basis of Occupational Therapy, Second Edition* (2002)

These nine search terms ultimately were used as the themes of each chapter. Specific search terms within each chapter were identified, and searches were conducted consistently for each database by two independent occupational therapy reviewers. These search terms are outlined within each chapter. Also included within the searches across all chapters was a range of terms used to capture studies that exclusively evaluated therapy, measured outcomes of treatment, and/or involved multidisciplinary approaches to intervention. Keyword subject headings were entered and the "explode" feature was used to capture a wide range of studies. This search yielded more than 1,500 studies relevant to occupational therapy outcomes.

RefWorks (2008) was used to manage the large database of selected studies. RefWorks is a Web-based bibliography and database manager that enabled us to create our own personal database by importing references from text files or online databases. Study references were allocated into the nine themes (or chapters) relevant to occupational therapy-sensitive outcomes.

Selecting the Studies for Detailed Analysis

Initial Study Selection Criteria

The next step was to review the titles and abstracts of the search output for the following initial inclusion criteria:
▲ The study had to contain an intervention and an evaluation of that intervention
▲ The study had to include an adult population that was at least 18 years old
▲ The study had to be published between 1980 and 2008
▲ The study was available in English and accessible by the authors
▲ The study had to be related to occupational therapy—that is, it had to be at least one of the following:
△ Written by an occupational therapist
△ Published in an occupational therapy journal
△ Referring to an intervention delivered by an occupational therapist (independently or on a multidisciplinary team)

If the study selection was unclear after reading the title and abstract (or title only without an abstract), then the full article was retrieved online. If the article described a study where the health care professional of the intervention was not reported and the practice area was within the scope of occupational therapy practice (e.g., splinting or environmental modifications), then the article was included. Furthermore, studies were included in which multidisciplinary team members carrying out the intervention were not described, but where occupational therapy involvement has been evident in general practice (e.g., assertive community treatment [ACT]). If the article was difficult to retrieve online, the article was not published in an occupational therapy journal, and none of the authors were faculty in a department of occupational therapy (or an occupational therapist), the article was excluded. The researchers were cautious about eliminating studies. In cases where not enough information was provided, the study remained in the database and was judged once the full article could be reviewed. If full text online articles were difficult to retrieve and if the abstract or title seemed descriptive and the keywords did not indicate outcomes or research methods, the articles were excluded.

In summary, studies that were considered appropriate for this review included relevant occupational therapy research that examined practice or program evaluation, outcomes measurement, impact of practice, effectiveness of a specific occupational therapy treatment, rehabilitation of a particular deficit/disability, preventative intervention/education, effect of occupational therapy on quality of life, and/or general effects/efficacy of occupational therapy treatment.

The occupational therapy reviewers inspected all of these studies together and were required to reach consensus to determine whether studies were admissible based on the inclusion criteria. Upon completion of the initial review, approximately 1,000 studies were retained based on the consensus of occupational therapy reviewers and elimination of duplicates.

Secondary Study Selection Criteria

For those articles that remained in the dataset after the initial inclusion criteria were applied, the full article was obtained, and a further review was conducted based on the following secondary inclusion criteria:

▲ The article conformed to one of the following levels of evidence (Greenhalgh, 2006):
  △ Level 1—Systematic reviews and meta-analyses
  △ Level 2—Randomized controlled trials with definitive results
  △ Level 3—Randomized controlled trials with nondefinitive results
  △ Level 4—Cohort studies
▲ The article was a before-and-after study design
▲ The article was a single-case study design
The exclusion criteria of studies included:
▲ Descriptive or opinion articles, PhD theses
▲ Articles published by non-peer-reviewed journals
▲ Quantitative studies with levels of evidence 5 to 7 (Greenhalgh, 2006):

  △ Level 5—Case-control studies
  △ Level 6—Cross-sectional surveys
  △ Level 7—Case reports

Given the vast number of quantitative studies, it was necessary to label the study designs in an attempt to collect the most rigorous quantitative evidence. The most appropriate scale to categorize the most relevant studies was a level of evidence rating scale by Greenhalgh (2006). She characterized the levels of evidence in order from most to least rigorous, as listed previously.

A brief description of each level of evidence, adapted from Greenhalgh's *How to Read a Paper: The Basics of Evidence-Based Medicine* (2006), is included in Table 2-1. We determined that studies within Levels 1 to 4 provided the most rigorous outcomes. A priori, it was determined that single-case design studies, cross-over randomized trials, and before-and-after studies would be included in the review, because they were deemed distinct from the definition of studies within Levels 5 to 7. These studies were considered valuable to this scoping review and were decided to be included in study selection, labeled as Level 4 studies.

Through RefWorks, descriptors for each specific level of evidence were established in order to search the database for articles possessing descriptors of levels of evidence 5 to 7 so that they could be excluded from the final study list. All the studies (titles and abstracts) earmarked for removal from our database were reviewed to ensure they were appropriate for elimination. The remaining studies were reviewed to ensure the articles possessed the qualities of the levels of evidence (1 to 4).

One last review of the selected studies to ensure appropriate labeling was conducted by the research assistants (student occupational therapists) who summarized each study. For studies that did not specifically describe the health care professional(s) who carried out the intervention (i.e., whether occupational therapy was involved), research assistants excluded the articles unless they provided reasonable grounds for occupational therapy involvement, such as the author(s) being an occupational therapist, working through the department or school of occupational therapy, or if the article was published in a peer-reviewed occupational therapy journal.

Qualitative studies were also captured in the literature searches and were included in the database.

The research assistants' reviews did reveal some studies that did not meet inclusion criteria. For this book, the final number of eligible studies up to June 30, 2008 amounted to 467 studies.

Table 2-1
DESCRIPTION OF LEVELS OF EVIDENCE

Level of Evidence	Description of Studies Included
Level 1—Systematic reviews and meta-analyses	Studies reviewing the literature that use methodology that is rigorous, transparent, and auditable.
Level 2—Randomized controlled trials with definitive results	Studies randomly allocating subjects to different intervention groups with results that demonstrate no overlap between confidence intervals relating to a clinically significant effect.
Level 3—Randomized controlled trials with nondefinitive results	Studies randomly allocating subjects to different intervention groups with results that demonstrate a clinically significant effect but show an overlap between relevant confidence intervals.
Level 4—Cohort studies	Two (or more) groups of subjects selected on the basis of their involvement within a particular group or intervention often comparing outcomes.
Level 5—Case-control studies	Subjects within a specific group (cohort) are identified and matched with controls (e.g., general population group), and data collection is retrospective in nature.
Level 6—Cross-sectional surveys	Data collected at a single point in time, often retrospectively about an experience.
Level 7—Case reports	A study giving a description of the medical history of a single subject in the form of a story, often understandable by a layperson.

Adapted from Greenhalgh, T. (2006). *How to read a paper: The basics of evidence-based medicine* (3rd ed.). London, England: Blackwell Publishing Ltd.

Charting the Data According to Key Concepts

The remaining 467 articles were classified by chapter for further review and reporting, which included review studies (130), Levels 2 to 4 quantitative studies (325), and qualitative studies (12) (Table 2-2). Classification was conducted on the basis of the outcomes measured or the effects sought in the studies. The emphasis for the studies was on the outcomes achieved through occupational therapy intervention.

All studies with Level 1 study design and other literature reviews were grouped within each chapter of the column titled "Review Studies." For each chapter, the reviews were used by our research team to describe the scope of outcomes impacted by occupational therapy practice. Qualitative studies, where available within each chapter, as seen in the "Descriptive Studies" column (see Table 2-2), were also used to provide insight on the scope of occupational therapy practice as it related to outcomes measured.

Quantitative studies determined to be at levels of evidence 2 to 4 were summarized by research assistants and tabled within each category to display the available empirical evidence.

Collating and Summarizing the Findings of the Selected Studies

The results of the scoping review are summarized in chapters, corresponding to the nine areas in which occupational therapy is effective. The remaining chapters of the book will provide the results of the reviews of interventions associated with the following occupational therapy-sensitive outcomes:

▲ Occupation factors
   △ Participation
   △ Self-care (personal care, functional mobility, and community management)
   △ Productivity
   △ Leisure
▲ Environmental factors
   △ Environment (physical modification, social support, devices, and equipment)
▲ Person factors
   △ Physical components
   △ Socio-cultural components
   △ Psycho-emotional components
   △ Cognitive-neurological components

The details of the defined topic areas included within each chapter can be seen in Table 2-3.

Table 2-2
CHAPTER STUDY INCLUSIONS

OT-Sensitive Outcomes Chapters—Category	Review Studies	Levels 2-4 Studies (Quantitative)	Descriptive Studies (Qualitative)	Totals
3—Participation	13	27	1	41
4—Self-Care	29	57	4	90
5—Productivity	16	22	0	38
6—Leisure	3	9	1	13
7—Environment	14	34	2	50
8—Physical	33	97	2	132
9—Socio-Cultural	0	15	0	15
10—Psycho-Emotional	9	22	1	32
11—Cognitive-Neurological	13	42	1	56
Total	130	325	12	467

Table 2-3
DESCRIPTION OF CHAPTER CONTENT WITHIN THIS BOOK

Chapter	Chapter Focus
3—Participation	This chapter includes outcomes that are related to occupational goals, occupational performance issues, and involvement in occupations (at a community level). If an article dealt with overall functional involvement or did not specifically fit into one of self-care, productivity, or leisure, it was also included in this chapter.
4—Self-Care	This chapter includes research related to all aspects of self-care such as personal care (ADL and functional ability), functional mobility (mobility aids, wheelchair use), and community management (IADL independence, driving).
5—Productivity	This chapter describes outcomes that are related to evaluating aspects of (or abilities in) paid work, volunteer work, and home management.
6—Leisure	This chapter relates to leisure outcomes, such as leisure participation, satisfaction, number of leisure activities, time spent in leisure, and leisure attitudes and skills.
7—Environment	This chapter contains articles dealing with outcomes related to the physical environment, social environment (caregiver support for safety in home), home modifications, equipment (assistive devices, EADL), and architectural adaptations (e.g., universal design).
8—Physical	This chapter contains articles evaluating specific physical outcomes related to interventions such as overall physical health and well-being, prosthetics/orthotics, joint protection, energy conservation, seating, falls prevention, and musculoskeletal pain.
9—Socio-Cultural	This chapter focuses on socio-cultural outcomes, including social skills, time use, values, spirituality, habits, and roles.
10—Psycho-Emotional	This chapter contains articles involving mental health-related outcomes dealing with maladaptive thoughts through behavioral approaches, pain management, and psycho-educational theory.
11—Cognitive-Neurological	This chapter contains articles dealing with outcomes related to cognitive, sensory, and neurological components, including pain.

The important data from each study were abstracted and placed into the evidence tables. The empirical studies were abstracted and summarized into tables within each chapter to demonstrate the majority of research that exists on each topic area.

The description of the column headings from the summary table are explained here. In the Interventions tables, the authors of the study and the study publication date is indicated in the first column, shown as "Author (Date)." The second column indicates the population age group within the study ("Pop"). The numbers provided in this column indicate the following age groups: 1=geriatric (65+ years); 2=adult (25 to 64 years); 3=young adult (18 to 24 years); 4=adult and geriatric; and 5=young adult, adult, and geriatric. The diagnosis of client population within each study is provided in the column labeled "DX." A list of common diagnoses from the reviewers' guideline is provided in Table 2-4.

The "Setting" column in the Interventions tables details the location of where the occupational therapy intervention took place. Examples include long-term care, acute care, community care/home care, rehabilitation, and primary care. The definitions of each type of setting, with examples, are provided below.

1 = Long-term care refers to care that provides continuing, medically complex and specialized services to adults, and sometimes over extended periods of time within a hospital or rehabilitation setting. Examples include long-term care facilities (nursing homes), musculoskeletal programs, chronic care hospitals, seating, prosthetics and orthotics, return to work, adult day care, attendant care, homes for the aged.

2 = Acute care generally refers to health care services that are specialized and short-term in nature within a hospital setting. Examples include brief inpatient stay, cardiac, orthopedic surgery (day, elective, or emergency room discharge), urgent/emergent care, and trauma unit.

3 = Community care/home care refers to a wide range of nonhospital health services delivered at home or in community programs other than a hospital for recovering, disabled, or chronically or terminally ill people in need of therapeutic treatment and/or assistance with the participation in daily occupations. Examples include community mental health day programs (clubhouse, sheltered workshops, or mental health programs), community occupational therapy (home assessments, etc.).

4 = Rehabilitation refers to adult inpatient and outpatient services in rehabilitation care provided by hospitals or rehabilitation settings. Examples include splinting, institution-based group teaching (programs with defined timelines).

Table 2-4

DIAGNOSIS OR HEALTH CHARACTERISTICS OF STUDY POPULATION

1=Developmental delay
2=Autism
3=Stroke
4=Parkinson's disease
5=Multiple sclerosis
6=Spinal cord injury
7=Acquired brain injury
8=Dementia or Alzheimer's disease
9=Burns
10=Amputations
11=Anxiety
12=Depression
13=Bipolar
14=Schizophrenia
15=Addiction/substance abuse
16=Upper extremity injury
17=Lower extremity injury
18=Other diagnosis
19=Arthritis
20=Chronic pain
21=No diagnosis
22=Joint injury (includes fracture and arthroplasty of hip/knee)
23=Back pain
24=Frail elderly, at-risk older adults, older adult acute hospital intake, acute inpatient geriatric admission
25=Sensory impairment (i.e., visual, hearing, tactile, gustatory, vestibular impairment)
26=Cardiac conditions
27=Chronic obstructive pulmonary disease

5 = Primary care refers to health care that is provided as a team, which includes a medical doctor, nurse, and allied health professionals to maximize strengths of the different professionals for better health outcomes.

The final column, "Intervention," indicates the intervention(s) used within the summarized study that aimed to impact on the outcome(s) investigated.

Columns in the Effects and Outcomes tables are self-explanatory in terms of the information that was collected for the empirical studies reviewed.

In summary, the search strategy for this scoping review was described that aimed to select a breadth of rigorous research to illustrate the impact of adult occupational therapy services on a range of health and participation outcomes. Using a systematic search strategy, we were able to identify and analyze more than 460 studies evaluating the impact of adult occupational therapy services. The results of this scoping review are discussed in the remaining chapters of this book.

References

Arksey, H., & O'Malley, L. (2005). Scoping studies: Towards a methodological framework. *International Journal of Social Research Methodology, 8*, 19-32.

Canadian Association of Occupational Therapists. (1997). *Enabling occupation: An occupational therapy perspective.* Ottawa, Ontario, Canada: CAOT Publications.

Greenhalgh, T. (2006). *How to read a paper: The basics of evidence-based medicine* (3rd ed.). London, England: Blackwell Publishing Ltd.

Klassen, B. *Annotated bibliography on occupational therapy in primary health care* (from 2003-2008). Occupational therapy in primary health care poster presentation. Accelerating Primary Care 2008: Gaining Momentum conference. Alberta, Canada, February 12-14, 2008.

Law, M., Pollock, N., Stewart, D., Harms, S., & Lammi, B. (2004). McMaster University unpublished critical literature review on home-based occupational therapy intervention for children and adults. Unpublished manuscript. McMaster University, Hamilton, Canada.

McColl, M. A., Carswell, A., Law, M., Pollock, N., Baptiste, S., & Polatajko, H. (2006). *Canadian Occupational Performance Measure: An annotated bibliography and research resource.* Ottawa, Ontario, Canada: CAOT Publications.

McColl, M. A., Law, M., Stewart, D., Doubt, L., Pollock, N., & Krupa, T. (2002). *Theoretical basis of occupational therapy* (2nd ed.). Thorofare, NJ: SLACK Incorporated.

Pollock, N. (2004). Critical review on goal setting. Unpublished manuscript. McMaster University, Hamilton, Canada.

RefWorks, McMaster University. (2008). RefWorks Login Centre. Retrieved from http://refworks.scholarsportal.info.libaccess.lib.mcmaster.ca/Refworks/login.asp?WNCLang=false on July 4th, 2008.

World Health Organization. (2001). *International classification of functioning, disability, and health.* Geneva, Switzerland: Author.

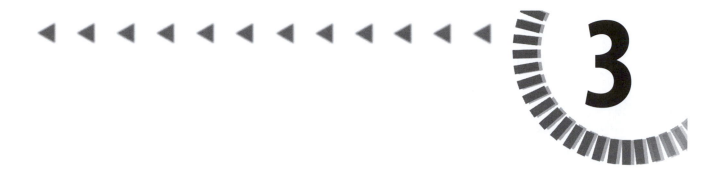

PARTICIPATION IN DAILY OCCUPATIONS

Mary Law, PhD, FCAOT and Mary Ann McColl, PhD, MTS

Occupational therapy, as noted in Chapter 1, focuses on enabling individuals and groups to participate fully in meaningful daily occupations. "Occupations are what we do. They provide the basis for feelings about ourselves. They engage us in the world around us to survive and maintain ourselves" (Christiansen, Baum, & Bass-Haugen, 2005, p. 4). Daily occupations include "everything people do to occupy themselves, including looking after themselves (self-care), enjoying life (leisure), and contributing to the social and economic fabric of their communities (productivity)" (Canadian Association of Occupational Therapists [CAOT], 2002).

Disease or illness can impact on a client's participation in daily occupations, starting from the acute stages of disease and moving to chronic disease management. For instance, Parkinson's disease can begin with mild impairments and result in high levels of disability and greatly reduced participation and quality of life (Yarrow, 1999).

This chapter includes outcomes that are related to an individual's overall engagement in daily occupations within the environment in which he or she lives. Such occupations include self-management, personal care, community mobility, household and community-based tasks, and participation in social and community life. Outcomes that focus on overall participation or several categories of participation are captured in this chapter. The studies summarized in this chapter deal with interventions that build skills and lead to improved participation in meaningful occupation(s).

Conceptual Background

As described in Chapter 1, occupational therapy focuses on enabling a client's participation in occupations of daily life that are meaningful to him or her and bring purpose to his or her life. The most important outcome of occupational therapy intervention is to maintain or improve a person's occupational performance (defined as a person's ability to perform specific occupations, as well as satisfaction with his or her performance).

The World Health Organization's ([WHO], 2001) International Classification of Functioning, Disability, and Health (ICF), also described in Chapter 1, focuses on the relationship between health conditions,

M. Law & M. A. McColl (Eds.)
Interventions, Effects, and Outcomes in Occupational Therapy:
Adults and Older Adults (pp. 23-45)
© 2010 SLACK Incorporated

Table 3-1

INTERNATIONAL CLASSIFICATION OF FUNCTIONING, DISABILITY, AND HEALTH PARTICIPATION CATEGORIES

Learning and Applying Knowledge: Learning, applying knowledge, thinking, solving problems, and making decisions.

General Tasks and Demands: Carrying out single or multiple tasks, organizing routines, and handling stress.

Communication: Communicating by language, signs, and symbols, including receiving and producing messages, carrying on conversations, and using communication devices and techniques.

Mobility: Moving from one place to another; carrying, moving, or manipulating objects; walking, running, or climbing; and using various forms of transportation.

Self-Care: Caring for oneself, washing and drying oneself, caring for one's body and body parts, dressing, eating and drinking, and looking after one's health.

Domestic Life: Carrying out domestic and everyday actions and tasks, including acquiring a place to live, food, clothing, and other necessities; household cleaning and repairing; caring for personal and other household objects; and assisting others.

Interpersonal Interactions: Carrying out basic and complex interactions with people in a contextually and socially appropriate manner.

Major Life Areas: Carrying out the tasks and actions required to engage in education, work, and employment and to conduct economic transactions.

Community, Social, and Civic Life: Doing the actions and tasks required to engage in organized social life outside the family, in community, social, and civic areas of life.

Adapted from World Health Organization. (2001). *International classification of functioning, disability, and health.* Geneva, Switzerland: Author.

health, and well-being. Within the ICF, functioning encompasses all of a person's activities within his or her community. Domains of interest in this classification system center on the person (body function and structure), his or her functioning (activities and participation), and the influence of contextual factors (personal and environmental). Participation in the ICF is defined as "involvement in a life situation" (WHO, 2001, p. 10).

The ICF categories for participation are outlined in Table 3-1. The focus of participation in the ICF is very similar to the outcome of occupational performance for the profession of occupational therapy. Thus, this chapter focuses on participation in occupations, the ultimate outcome goal for occupational therapy intervention.

Search Strategy

The methodology to search the literature, identify studies, and select them based on the inclusion criteria was discussed in Chapter 2. A systematic search of health care and occupational therapy databases, as well as hand-searched relevant references, yielded critical reviews (e.g., systematic reviews or meta-analyses) and qualitative and quantitative studies that addressed occupational therapy outcomes when providing intervention related to improving clients' participation in daily occupation. Selected studies met specific inclusion criteria, which consisted of study publication between 1980 and 2008, adult population, study intervention involving occupational therapists independently or on a multidisciplinary team, and study categorized as level of evidence 1 to 4 based on criteria by Greenhalgh (2006). For this chapter, the search terms used to capture occupational therapy-sensitive outcomes are listed in Table 3-2. A total of 27 empirical articles met the inclusion criteria and are reviewed in this chapter.

Five systematic reviews of occupational therapy interventions for specific client groups were identified as relevant to this chapter (Dixon et al., 2007; Hasselkus, 1992; Murphy & Tickle Degnen, 2001; Trombly & Ma, 2002; Wilkins, Jung, Wishart, Edwards, & Gamble Norton, 2003). Nineteen empirical articles report occupational therapy outcomes research

Table 3-2

SEARCH TERMS FOR OCCUPATIONAL THERAPY INTERVENTIONS TO IMPROVE PARTICIPATION OUTCOMES

Occupation, occupational therapy (therapist), OR multidisciplinary team AND...

Primary terms: activities, advocacy, community living, functional status, group(s), independence, independent living, life skills, motivation, participation, social adjustment, social environment, social skills.

Secondary terms: adaptation, client participation, community participation, community programs, community reintegration, consumer participation, encounter group therapy, group counseling, group discussion, group dynamics, group instruction, group processes, group structure, health promotion, independence (personality), independent living programs, interpersonal interaction, interpersonal relations, leisure activities, motivation, occupational, patient advocacy, patient participation, role, role change, self-determination, self-help groups, skills training, social behavior, social groups, social integration, socialization, social skills training, support groups.

Additional terms used to focus the search included clinical effectiveness, community health services, health care delivery, health care services, health service, health services for the aged, home care, home care services, home health care, home occupational therapy, home rehabilitation, interdisciplinary education, interdisciplinary research, interdisciplinary treatment approach, intervention treatment approach, multidisciplinary care team, outcomes, outcomes assessment patient care, outcomes (health care), outcomes research, patient care team, psychotherapeutic outcomes, rehabilitation, rehabilitation care, rehabilitation centre, rehabilitation outcomes, teamwork, treatment effectiveness evaluation, treatment outcomes.

focused on participation in occupations. Another eight multidisciplinary studies focus on the same outcomes. A summary of key findings is reported in this chapter with tables. Bibliographic summaries for each study are in the Annotated Bibliography at the end of the book.

Interventions Used to Improve Participation Outcomes

Occupational therapists are educated to support individuals with long-term diseases or acute impairments to optimize their levels of participation in daily occupations. Because clients are referred because of difficulty in maintaining or changing their usual meaningful occupations, occupational therapists support individuals in changing and adapting their role over time (Gauthier, Dalziel, & Gauthier, 1987). Interventions may include support in re-organizing daily routines, learning new skills for alternative or adaptive ways to conduct occupations, or providing and advising on resources to participate in daily occupations (Deane, Ellis Hill, Playford, Ben Shlomo, & Clarke, 2001). Research indicates that participation in occupation has a significant influence on health and well-being (Christiansen et al., 2005; Law, Steinweinder, & Leclair, 1998; McColl, Law, Stewart, Doubt, Pollock, & Krupa, 2002).

The occupational therapy interventions used in studies reviewed for this chapter focused on changing participation through changing body function/structure, improving clients' skills and performance, or optimizing participation in specific occupations. Because the goal of occupational therapy is to enable individuals to perform the tasks that are essential to their unique areas of role performance, their role within a health care team is to focus on minimizing disability related to role-related task performance (Shapero Sabari, 2001).

Intervention approaches to change body function/structure consisted of physical programs (aerobic/non-aerobic exercise, general mobilization, physical rehabilitation) or psycho-emotional programs (e.g., socialization programs) designed to lead to improvements in participation.

Occupational therapy intervention to improve skills and performance typically employed functional skill development strategies (e.g., general self-care, general disability education, domestic life) to change participation. Programs typically used education strategies, structured practice of specific occupations, and/or adaptation of activities to aid in enhancing performance of daily occupations.

Optimizing participation in specific occupations was addressed through clients' participation in occupation-based activities. Within this intervention, therapy focused on enhancing participation through adaptation to the occupation or changes to the environment in which the occupation was performed.

Effects of Occupational Therapy in Promoting Participation Outcomes

Systematic Reviews

The majority of empirical studies and systematic reviews focused on participation in daily occupations center on the participation outcomes of self-care, mobility, and domestic life. Self-care outcomes include all tasks and activities in the areas of dressing, toileting and hygiene, eating and drinking, and maintaining one's health. Mobility outcomes from these studies include indoor and community mobility, transfers or change of body position from one location to another, moving or manipulating objects, and using transportation. Domestic life includes all tasks and activities related to maintaining a place to live. This category includes finding a place to live, household cleaning, repairs, food shopping and preparation, and caring for others.

A meta-analysis was completed to synthesize evidence from 16 studies addressing the effectiveness of occupational therapy interventions for people with Parkinson's disease. Outcomes evaluated included functional abilities as well as impact of physical and psycho-emotional treatment on the client's occupations (Murphy & Tickle Degnen, 2001). Overall, the results from the study revealed small to moderate positive effects of intervention on outcomes related to the client's participation. Nine of 13 studies showed a positive effect of occupational therapy intervention on outcomes at the level of participation of the ICF (transfers, activities of daily living [ADL], and functional mobility) (Murphy & Tickle Degnen, 2001).

One critical review synthesized 15 studies regarding the effects of occupational therapy on task and activity performance for people who have had a stroke (Trombly & Ma, 2002). Eleven studies found that role participation and mobility, self-care, and domestic life participation improved significantly after occupational therapy intervention.

Within a Cochrane Review that demonstrated the efficacy of occupational therapists working with people with Parkinson's disease, two cohort studies were analyzed related to the effects of treatment on the self-care and domestic life areas of the ICF as well as quality of life (Deane et al., 2001). One of the studies demonstrated occupational therapy intervention through general mobilization activities, socialization, dexterity, and functional and educational activities (Gauthier et al., 1987). The other study described occupational therapy intervention that consisted of occupation-based activities such as handicrafts, picture drawing, basketry, folk singing, dancing, and games (Fiorani, Mari, Bartolini Ceravolo, & Provinciali, 1997). Both trials indicated positive effects of occupational therapy in people with Parkinson's disease, but improvements were small. These results are difficult to generalize because both studies demonstrated methodological flaws and had small sample sizes (Deane et al., 2001).

A critical review by Wilkins and colleagues (2003) reviewed educational and functional training interventions provided by occupational therapists. Results of the review indicate that these programs are effective in preventing decline in participation in role functioning, domestic life, and community/civic life for older adults. Such occupational therapy intervention strategies not only prevent debilitating circumstances, which can impact physical, social, or role functioning, but can also enable clients to succeed in participation of occupations through programming for people with chronic illness. As well, occupational therapy intervention is effective in improving participation outcomes for people with stroke or rheumatoid arthritis.

Empirical Studies

Empirical studies reviewed for this book provide substantial evidence that occupational therapy intervention improves participation in the daily occupations of self-care, mobility, and domestic life. Positive outcomes from intervention have been demonstrated for people with cardiac conditions (Austin, Williams, Ross, Moseley, & Hutchison, 2005), chronic obstructive pulmonary disease (Bendstrup, Ingemann Jensen, Holm, & Bengtsson, 1997), dementia (Dooley & Hinojosa, 2004; Graff, Vernooij-Dassen, Thijssen, Dekker, Hoefnagels, & Rikkert, 2006), hip fracture (Tippet, 2001), macular degeneration (Dahlin Ivanoff, Sonn, & Svensson, 2002), multiple sclerosis (Logan, Ahern, Gladman, & Lincoln, 1997), traumatic brain injury (Huebner, Johnson, Bennett, & Schneck, 2003; Wheeler, Lane, & McMahon, 2007), general medical conditions (Wressle, Filipsson, Andersson, Jacobsson, Martinsson, & Engel, 2006), rheumatoid arthritis (Helewa et al., 1991), schizophrenia (Liberman, Wallace, Blackwell, Kopelowicz, Vaccaro, & Mintz, 1998), and stroke (Egan, Kessler, Laporte, Metcalfe, & Carter, 2007; Gilbertson & Langhorne, 2000; Ng, Chu, Wu, & Cheung, 2005). These interventions were carried out in a range of settings including acute hospitals (Tippet, 2001; Wressle et al., 2006), community/home care (Dahlin Ivanoff et al., 2002; Dooley & Hinojosa, 2004; Egan et al., 2007; Gilbertson & Langhorne, 2000; Gillen, Berger, Lotia, Morreale, Siber, & Trudo, 2007; Graff et al., 2006; Helewa et al., 1991), long-term care (Yuen, Huang, Burik, & Smith, 2008), and rehabilitation centers (Austin et al., 2005; Bendstrup et al., 1997; Logan et al., 1997; Ng et al., 2005).

Of the studies reviewed by Trombly and Ma (2002), 11 demonstrated that role participation and instrumental activities of daily living (IADL) performance improved significantly more with training than within controlled conditions. These findings indicate that occupational therapy intervention can effectively improve participation and activity post-stroke by using client-chosen activities in a familiar context and provision of necessary adaptations and training in the use of adaptations (Trombly & Ma, 2002).

A large randomized controlled trial conducted by Clark and colleagues (1997) and a follow-up study of this trial (Clark et al., 2001) demonstrated that older adults living in the community benefited significantly from an occupational therapy program using lifestyle redesign to improve participation through promotion of health-relevant behaviors, transportation, personal safety, social relationships, cultural awareness, and management of finances. Older adults receiving this program improved significantly in physical and mental health function, role functioning, and vitality as compared to attention placebo and control groups. A before-and-after study of older adults also found significant differences in vitality, social functioning, mental health, and frequency of community participation after a 6-month occupational therapy wellness program (Matuska, Giles-Heinz, Flinn, Neighbor, & Bass-Haugen, 2003). Another study randomly allocated older adults from a long-term care facility to participate in a volunteer program to mentor students who use English as a second language (Yuen et al., 2008). The results from this study reported that participants in the volunteer program demonstrated higher levels of well-being than those not involved in mentoring students.

Gilbertson and Langhorne (2000) studied the effects of providing people with stroke with 10 occupational therapy in-home sessions (30 to 40 minutes) for the first 6 weeks following discharge from the hospital. The group who received these services improved significantly more than the control group on participation in daily occupations identified as important by each participant. Johansson and Bjorklund (2005) studied occupational therapy home care services based on an occupational adaptation theoretical model (treatment focused on three meaningful activities that clients wanted to master) or regular occupational therapy using a mix of approaches. Findings indicated that the regular care group had significantly greater improvement on ADL items of the Functional Independence Measure (FIM) while the occupational

adaptation group improved significantly on outcomes of general health, physical role-emotional, and physical well-being. Outcomes of general well-being, participation, and satisfaction with valued activities were evaluated in another home setting study for people with stroke by Egan and colleagues (2007). The results of this study showed clinically and statistically significant differences on client satisfaction of their occupational performance.

Two studies have also demonstrated improvement in participation in self-care and domestic life outcomes after occupational therapy intervention for people with dementia in a community setting (Dooley & Hinojosa, 2004; Graff et al., 2006). A third study involving community occupational therapy intervention showed significant improvements in post-test scores for task-specific performance in various environments (e.g., department store) for a cohort of clients who had a joint-related injury (Gillen et al., 2007).

Liberman and colleagues (1998) in a study comparing a psychosocial occupational therapy group with occupational therapy skills training found statistically significant changes for both groups over time for the outcomes of community and social life participation. People in the occupational therapy skills groups improved significantly more than the psychosocial group on ability to adapt to life circumstances.

A multidisciplinary program for people with multiple sclerosis led to significant changes in health-related quality of life and physical and mental function (DiFabio, Choi, Soderberg, & Hansen, 1997). In a before-and-after design, Helfrich and colleagues (2006) found that an occupational therapy intervention of four weekly group sessions to examine housing options and life skills led to statistically significant changes in life skills for participants who had experienced domestic violence. Another life skills intervention program involving a multidisciplinary team demonstrated an increase in community integration compared to a nonrandomized control group (Wheeler et al., 2007).

Studies of two multidisciplinary education-focused pain management programs that included occupational therapy found significant differences in achievement of participation goals (Fisher & Hardie, 2002; Persson, Rivano Fischer, & Eklund, 2004) and in activity level, general health, and vitality (Persson et al., 2004).

The specific results of the 19 empirical studies of occupational therapy intervention and eight studies of multidisciplinary intervention including occupational therapy to improve participation in daily occupations are outlined in Tables 3-3 through 3-5.

text continues on page 43

Table 3-3

OCCUPATIONAL THERAPY INTERVENTIONS PROMOTING PARTICIPATION OUTCOMES

Author (Date)	Pop	DX	Setting	Intervention
Yuen, H. K., Huang, P., Burik, J. K., & Smith, T. G. (2008)	1	18	1	**Intervention:** Along with participating in usual care and social and recreational activities, participants mentored an English-as-a-second-language student twice a week for 12 consecutive weeks. **Control:** Received usual care and participated in the usual social and recreational activities available at their residence facility.
Egan, M., Kessler, D., Laporte, L., Metcalfe, V., & Carter, M. (2007)	5	3	3	**Intervention:** Participants received up to 8 home visits from an OT to work on problems with participation in valued activities identified by the patient. The therapist and patient worked together to develop a plan to address the issues identified by the patient. Methods to carry out the plan included coaching, education, changes to the physical environment, and use of resources to enable the client to achieve a goal. **Control:** Participants received usual home rehabilitation (does not typically include OT).
Gillen, G., Berger, S. M., Lotia, S., Morreale, J., Siber, M. I., & Trudo, W. J. (2007)	1, 2	22	3, 4	**Intervention:** Along with usual rehabilitative care (individual and group OT and PT), participants completed a Community Skills Evaluation (CSE). They were accompanied by their OT and transported to a community location (pharmacy, supermarket, or department store) where they received task-specific training in safely transferring in and out of the vehicle, managing outdoor obstacles, and ambulating throughout the destination. The CSE was completed once during the rehabilitation process and took approximately 45 minutes.
Wheeler, S. D., Lane, S. J., & McMahon, B. T. (2007)	2, 3	7	3, 4	**Intervention:** Participants received usual care (1 to 3 hours of OT per week, PT and speech therapy when needed) plus an intensive life skills training program (6 hours a day for 6 weeks—delivered by a life skills trainer). **Control:** Usual rehabilitative care only (no life skills program).
Graff, M. J., Vernooij-Dassen, M. J., Thijssen, M., Dekker, J., Hoefnagels, W. H., & Rickkert, M. G. (2006)	1	8	3	**Intervention:** 10 1-hour in-home OT sessions aimed at identifying and implementing compensatory strategies and environmental approaches to address issues in participation in daily occupations in which patients and caregivers identified and prioritized the daily occupation issues. **Control:** Usual care.
Helfrich, C., Aviles, A., Badiani, C., Walens, D., & Sabol, P. (2006)	5	18	3	**Intervention:** 4 weekly and group intervention sessions (based on Model of Human Occupation) with an OT to examine housing options and life skills.
Wressle, E., Filipsson, V., Andersson, L., Jacobsson, B., Martinsson, K., & Engel, K. (2006)	1	24	2	**Intervention:** OT intervention took place during acute care stay (2 to 3 days) and included prescription of assistive devices, reports to primary care or community care, ADL training, providing education and information, discharge planning, physical function training. **Control:** Usual care.
Austin, J., Williams, R., Ross, L., Moseley, L., & Hutchison, S. (2005)	4	26	4	**Intervention:** Standard clinic-based care plus cardiac rehabilitation (8 weeks), which consisted of educational material about medication, diet, and exercise from a multidisciplinary team. Post 8-weeks, patients in the experimental group attended a 16-week exercise class that was based on the standards set for cardiac rehabilitation. **Control:** Outpatient clinic-based standard care for 8 weekly visits with cardiologist and specialist nurse. Subjects were monitored and given education on heart failure and its treatment for early detection and dietary advice.

continued

Table 3-3 (continued)
OCCUPATIONAL THERAPY INTERVENTIONS PROMOTING PARTICIPATION OUTCOMES

Author (Date)	Pop	DX	Setting	Intervention
Johansson, A., & Bjorklund, A. (2005)	4	24	3	*Intervention:* Home-based OT based on occupational adaptation theoretical model (treatment focused on 3 meaningful activities that clients wanted to master). *Control:* Home-based OT providing regular care using a mix of approaches from different conceptual models in relation to identified occupational performance issues.
Ng, S., Chu, M., Wu, A., & Cheung, P. (2005)	5	3	4	*Intervention:* Pre-post study of OT intervention provided in home post-discharge after stroke that included caregiver skills training, on-site safety advice and training, assistive device prescription, home modifications, referral to other services, and community-living skills training.
Dooley, N. R., & Hinojosa, J. (2004)	4	8	3	*Intervention:* 30-minute OT home visit to provide recommendations to caregivers and clients (included environmental modifications, caregiver approaches, and community support groups). *Control:* Usual care.
Horowitz, B. P., & Chang, P. F. (2004)	1	18, 24	4	*Intervention:* A 16-week group program to maximize performance in self-identified occupations through lifestyle redesign OT program that consisted of a 1.5-hour group every week and optional home visits once per month. *Control:* Usual care.
Persson, E., Rivano Fischer, M., & Eklund, M. (2004)	5	20	4	5-week multidisciplinary pain rehabilitation program designed to increase knowledge about pain and training in alternative ways to self-help. Individual and group treatment by OT, psychologist, physician, PT, and social worker.
Huebner, R. A., Johnson, K., Bennett, C. M., & Schneck, C. (2003)	1, 5	7	4	*Intervention:* Patients received standard comprehensive inpatient rehabilitation that included OT for a minimum of 7 days as part of their stay in a rehabilitation hospital's brain injury unit.
Matuska, K., Giles-Heinz, A., Flinn, N., Neighbor, M., & Bass-Haugen, J. (2003)	1	21	3	Participants took part in a life wellness program that included 6 months of weekly educational classes taught by at least 2 OT faculty. The program focused on teaching the importance of meaningful occupations for better quality of life and strategies to remove barriers preventing participation.
Dahlin Ivanoff, S., Sonn, U., & Svensson, E. (2002)	1	25	4	*Intervention:* Health education program: 8 2-hour group sessions led by an OT that addressed occupational performance in a variety of areas (self-care, meals, communication, orientation, mobility, shopping, food preparation, financial management, and cleaning). Modeling techniques, skills training, providing information, and teaching problem-solving strategies. *Control:* Usual care.
Fisher, K., & Hardie, R. J. (2002)	2	20	4	Multidisciplinary structured educational program of PT, OT, and clinical psychology.
Clark, F., Azen, S. P., Carlson, M., Mandel, D., LaBree, L., Hay, J., et al. (2001)	1	21	3	*Intervention:* 9 months of OT focused on health relevant behaviors, transportation, personal safety, social relationships, cultural awareness, and finances. *Control:* Usual care.

continued

Table 3-3 (continued)
OCCUPATIONAL THERAPY INTERVENTIONS PROMOTING PARTICIPATION OUTCOMES

Author (Date)	Pop	DX	Setting	Intervention
Tippet, C. (2001)	1	17	2	**Intervention:** Patients in an acute-care unit participated in a multidisciplinary rehabilitation treatment that varied in length depending on individual needs. OT was received 5 days per week and consisted of advice and demonstration on ADL. Education groups were run by OT and PT regarding how to protect from falls within the home and the psychosocial and mobility issues that occur with falls. PT was received 6 days per week and focused on exercises to promote muscle power, range of motion, and pain control. Nursing was available 24 hours per day.
Gilbertson, L., & Langhorne, P. (2000)	2	3	3	**Intervention:** Treatment group received 10 OT in-home sessions (30 to 40 minutes) for the first 6 weeks following discharge from hospital. **Control:** Usual care.
Liberman, R. P., Wallace, C. J., Blackwell, G., Kopelowicz, A., Vaccaro, J. V., & Mintz, J. (1998)	5	14	4	**Intervention:** 3 2-hour OT sessions per week for 6 months. **Group 1:** Psychosocial OT (comprised of expressive, artistic, and recreational activities). **Group 2:** Skills training provided by 1 OT and 3 paraprofessionals.
Bendstrup, K. E., Ingemann Jensen, J., Holm, S., & Bengtsson, B. (1997)	4	27	4	**Intervention:** Participants were followed for 24 weeks. The intervention group had a 12-week program in a hospital that included exercise training with a PT (1 hour, 3 times a week), 2 group lessons from an OT to learn techniques to overcome identified ADL impairments, 12 education sessions about a variety of physical and psychosocial issues related to COPD, and free nicotine patches and smoking education sessions for participants who wanted to stop smoking. **Control:** Usual care.
Clark, F., Azen, S. P., Zemke, R., Jackson, J., Carlson, M., Mandel, D., et al. (1997)	4	18	3	**Intervention:** The treatment group received usual OT while the attention control received social programming. **Control:** The control received no treatment.
DiFabio, R. P., Choi, T., Soderberg, J., & Hansen, C. R. (1997)	2	5	4	**Intervention:** 5 hours of outpatient rehabilitation care for chronic progressive MS, 1 time per week for a year. OT and PT aimed to assist patients in maintaining both physical and mental function rather than to restore to "normal" function. Counseling, help with recreational and community services, and social work services were also offered. **Control:** On waitlist for the outpatient program.
Hartman, D., Borrie, M. J., Davison, E., & Stolee, P. (1997)	1	8	1	Various IADL and therapeutic recreation activities selected by clients and their families.
Logan, P. A., Ahern, J., Gladman, J. R., & Lincoln, N. B. (1997)	5	3	4	**Intervention:** Enhanced home-based OT provided by a research OT (no waitlist, increased number of visits). **Control:** Standard OT services (prioritized waitlist) provided by a senior OT.

continued

Table 3-3 (continued)
OCCUPATIONAL THERAPY INTERVENTIONS PROMOTING PARTICIPATION OUTCOMES

Author (Date)	Pop	DX	Setting	Intervention
Helewa, A., Goldsmith, C. H., Lee, P., Bombardier, C., Hanes, B., Smythe, H. A., et al. (1991)	4	19	3	**Intervention:** Compared OT services provided in-home to no treatment control. OT provided included education (joint protection, proper positioning, energy conservation), provision of assistive devices, wheelchairs, splints, and workplace interventions (task modification, adaptations to work station, etc.). **Control:** No treatment group (received treatment after 6 weeks).

Population: 1=geriatric (65+); 2=adult (25 to 64); 3=young adult (18 to 24); 4=adult and geriatric; 5=young adult, adult, and geriatric.

Diagnosis: 3=stroke; 5=multiple sclerosis; 7=acquired brain injury; 8=dementia or Alzheimer's disease; 14=schizophrenia; 17=lower extremity; 18=other; 19=arthritis; 20=chronic pain; 21=no diagnosis; 22=joint injury; 24=at-risk older adults; 25=sensory impairment; 26=cardiac condition; 27=chronic obstructive pulmonary disease.

Setting: 1=long-term care; 2=acute care; 3=home care; 4=rehabilitation; 5=primary care.

Table 3-4
EVIDENCE OF EFFECTIVENESS OF OCCUPATIONAL THERAPY ON PARTICIPATION OUTCOMES

Author (Date)	Major Results	Study Design	Sample Size	Conclusions and Limitations
Positive Effects—Randomized Controlled Trial				
Yuen, H. K., Huang, P., Burik, J. K., & Smith, T. G. (2008)	Scores from each test were analyzed together as a composite measure of well-being. Significant differences were found between intervention and control groups from baseline to post-intervention (p=0.047) and baseline to 3-month follow-up (p=0.029). The intervention group demonstrated higher levels of well-being at both post-intervention and 3-month follow-up. No significant change was found in either group between post-intervention and 3-month follow-up.	RCT	28	**Conclusions:** Participating in a volunteer program had a positive impact on the general well-being of residents in a long-term care facility and acted as a protective factor against health deterioration. **Limitations:** A high dropout rate (28.2%) significantly reduced the sample size and power of the study.
Graff, M. J., Vernooij-Dassen, M. J., Thijssen, M., Dekker, J., Hoefnagels, W. H., & Rickkert, M. G. (2006)	At 12 weeks: Statistically significant (p<0.0001) improvement for members of treatment group on all 3 outcome measures.	RCT	105	**Conclusions:** In-home OT is effective at both improving care-recipient ADL performance and care-provider confidence. **Limitations:** Method of data collection not described.
Austin, J., Williams, R., Ross, L., Moseley, L., & Hutchison, S. (2005)	Significant improvements in health-related quality of life, functional status, and functional performance at 24 weeks between the groups (p<0.001). Functional status scores did not change in the control group, whereas significant improvements were evident at 8 and 24 weeks in the experimental group. Functional performance increased significantly by 16% in the experimental group, compared to a slight decrease in standard care group. Experimental group had fewer admissions (11 vs. 33, p<0.01) and spent fewer days in hospital (41 vs. 187, p<0.001).	RCT	179	**Conclusions:** The multidisciplinary cardiac rehabilitation program offers an effective model of care for older patients with heart failure as it can improve symptoms, functional performance, and health-related quality of life and decrease hospital admissions due to heart disease. **Limitations:** Some outcome measures lacked psychometric properties.
Dooley, N. R., & Hinojosa, J. (2004)	Statistically significant effect was obtained for: Caregiver burden (F=15.5, p<0.001) Positive affect (F [1, 34]=6.54, p=0.015) Self-care status (F [1, 34]=4.92, p=0.03).	RCT	40	**Conclusions:** OT intervention can significantly increase aspects of care recipients' quality of life and functioning, while decreasing caregiver burden. **Limitations:** Small sample size.

continued

Table 3-4 (continued)

EVIDENCE OF EFFECTIVENESS OF OCCUPATIONAL THERAPY ON PARTICIPATION OUTCOMES

Author (Date)	Major Results	Study Design	Sample Size	Conclusions and Limitations
Positive Effects—Randomized Controlled Trial				
Dahlin Ivanoff, S., Sonn, U., & Svensson, E. (2002)	At 4 months: Statistically significant improvement for members of treatment group on 13 daily occupations.	RCT	187	**Conclusions:** OT-led groups are effective at improving perceived security in ADL performance for adults with macular degeneration. **Limitations:** Outcomes measure was only tested for test-retest reliability and content validity prior to use in the trial. Intervention not described in enough detail to reproduce.
Clark, F., Azen, S. P., Carlson, M., Mandel, D., LaBree, L., Hay, J., et al. (2001)	Statistically significant improvement: Quality of Interaction Subscale (p=0.05) Subscales (p<0.05) of: Physical functioning Role functioning Vitality Social functioning Role emotional General mental health	RCT	285	**Conclusions:** The study identified long-term health benefits related to preventative OT. **Limitations:** Reasons for dropouts not reported, no record of preventing contamination or co-intervention, no reports of evaluators or participants blinded to treatment.
Gilbertson, L., & Langhorne, P. (2000)	At 7 weeks, the intervention group had significantly greater changes: COPM—Occupational performance (p=0.0006) and satisfaction (p=0.0001) D-COOP-CHARTS emotional condition (p=0.02) LHS—occupation (work/leisure) (p=0.04) At 6 months, the intervention group had significantly greater changes: Satisfaction with preparations for discharge (p=0.03), the quantity of information received about rehabilitation and recovery (p=0.04), and having a person to contact about problems related to their stroke (p=0.05).	RCT	123	**Conclusions:** The treatment group showed increases in perceived occupational performance and performance satisfaction, emotional condition, and satisfaction with service. **Limitations:** Reasons for dropouts not reported, no record of preventing contamination or co-intervention.
Liberman, R. P., Wallace, C. J., Blackwell, G., Kopelowicz, A., Vaccaro, J., & Mintz, J. (1998)	Statistically significant change was found for both groups measuring frequency of social activity, general psychological function, and symptoms of schizophrenia. OT skills training group showed statistically significant improvement over psychosocial OT group on frequency of IADL and ADL, self-esteem, symptoms of mental illness, and ability to adapt to life.	RCT	70	**Conclusions:** The skills training group scored significantly better on all scales that indicated improvement in both groups and on some scales where the psychosocial group did not improve. **Limitations:** No record of preventing contamination or co-intervention.

continued

Table 3-4 (continued)

Evidence of Effectiveness of Occupational Therapy on Participation Outcomes

Author (Date)	Major Results	Study Design	Sample Size	Conclusions and Limitations
Positive Effects—Randomized Controlled Trial				
Bendstrup, K. E., Ingemann Jensen, J., Holm, S., & Bengtsson, B. (1997)	Significant differences in the improvements in quality of life between the control and the treatment groups at 12 and 24 weeks, and at 24 weeks, respectively. At 6, 12, and 24 weeks, improvements in exercise tolerance were 21.6 vs. 79.8, 36.1 vs. 113.1, and 21.4 vs. 96.2 for control and treatment groups, respectively (p<0.004). Quality of life scores did not change in the control group but did show improvements in the intervention group.	RCT	32	**Conclusions:** A comprehensive outpatient rehabilitation program can produce long-term improvement on ADL, quality of life, and exercise tolerance in patients with moderate to severe COPD. **Limitations:** Some outcome measures lacked strong psychometric properties. Measures were translated into a different language for the study. Changes in some outcomes did not show significance. High baseline values for measures did not leave much room for improvement.
Clark, F., Azen, S. P., Zemke, R., Jackson, J., Carlson, M., Mandel, D., et al. (1997)	Significant benefit attributable to OT treatment observed with: Quality of life interaction (p=0.03) Life satisfaction (p=0.03) Health perception (p=0.05) Perceived health subscales: Bodily pain (p=0.03) Physical functioning (p=0.008) Role limitations attributable to health problems (p=0.02) Vitality (p=0.004) Social functioning (p=0.02) General mental health (p=0.02)	RCT	361	**Conclusions:** The study demonstrates that preventative OT is helpful in improving the quality of life for aging people. **Limitations:** No record of preventing contamination or co-intervention.
Logan, P. A., Ahern, J., Gladman, J. R., & Lincoln, N. B. (1997)	At 3 months: Significant improvement in ADL/IADL for treatment group (p<0.01). At 6 months: Significant improvement on care-provider perceived overall health (p<0.01). No significant difference at 6 months between ADL/IADL performance.	RCT	111	**Conclusions:** The OT program was effective in increasing function and reducing health declines for care-providers. **Limitations:** Intervention not described in enough detail to reproduce; effect sizes not provided.
Helewa, A., Goldsmith, C. H., Lee, P., Bombardier, C., Hanes, B., Smythe, H. A., et al. (1991)	At 6 weeks: Statistically significant improvement on the functional capacity score for treatment group. (F [1, 91]=6.59, p<0.012) At 12 weeks: No significant differences between groups crossover design, with crossover at 6 weeks.	RCT	105	**Conclusions:** This program is effective at increasing the functional status of adults affected with RA. **Limitations:** Reasons for dropouts not reported. Small sample size so high potential for type II error.

continued

Table 3-4 (continued)
EVIDENCE OF EFFECTIVENESS OF OCCUPATIONAL THERAPY ON PARTICIPATION OUTCOMES

Author (Date)	Major Results	Study Design	Sample Size	Conclusions and Limitations
Positive Effects—Non-Randomized Controlled Trial				
Gillen, G., Berger, S. M., Lotia, S., Morreale, J., Siber, M. I., & Trudo, W. J. (2007)	Significant improvements in post-test scores were observed in performance of community skills, satisfaction with performance, and confidence in ability to perform community skills (p<0.0001). Post-test scores were also significantly higher in all 5 community skills evaluated.	Non-RCT	107	**Conclusions:** Practicing community skills in an environment outside the clinical setting allowed subjects to generalize their skills and was effective in increasing functional ability, satisfaction with performance, and confidence in performance. **Limitations:** The study took place at one hospital, and all subjects in the study were elective surgery patients; self-reported data only—no therapist ratings were included.
Wheeler, S. D., Lane, S. J., & McMahon, B. T. (2007)	The treatment group showed significant improvements in total CIQ scores (p=0.01) and in the home integration (p=0.01) and productivity (p=0.02) subscales. The control showed no significant improvement in these scores, and neither group showed any change in the social integration subscale. Mean SWLS scores showed an overall decrease in the treatment and improvement in the control but neither of these changes reached statistical significance (p<0.05).	Non-RCT	36	**Conclusions:** The life skills training program was effective in increasing community integration and participation, but improved community participation did not have an impact on life satisfaction. **Limitations:** Small sample size and baseline differences between groups limited direct between-group comparisons. Collecting data on the treatment group retrospectively limited the ability of researchers to limit bias.
Johansson, A., & Bjorklund, A. (2005)	Control group (p<0.05) showed significantly greater improvement in 6 items on FIM. Experimental group (p<0.05) showed significantly greater improvement in 3 items on SF-36: General health, physical role-emotional, and physical well-being.	Non-RCT	19	**Conclusions:** The study indicates that the investigated model of practice generates superior outcomes on the measures employed. **Limitations:** Reasons for dropouts not reported. Small sample size, so high potential for type II error.
Ng, S., Chu, M., Wu, A., & Cheung, P. (2005)	After completion of home visits (2.76 days on average): No statistical significance from baseline. At 28 days, significant improvement on ADL/IADL; caregiver's perception of personal strain and ability to provide care; perceived ability to cope with disability; and environmental hazards. At 3-month follow-up (compared to 28 days): No significant change on the Telephone Survey (p>0.05)	Non-RCT	144	**Conclusions:** The OT program was effective at increasing function and reducing environmental risk for patients discharged after acute stroke. **Limitations:** No reports of evaluators masked to treatment, some outcome measures lacked testing of psychometric properties.

continued

Table 3-4 (continued)

EVIDENCE OF EFFECTIVENESS OF OCCUPATIONAL THERAPY ON PARTICIPATION OUTCOMES

Author (Date)	Major Results	Study Design	Sample Size	Conclusions and Limitations
Positive Effects—Non-Randomized Controlled Trial				
Persson, E., Rivano Fischer, M., & Eklund, M. (2004)	Statistically significant (p<0.001) positive changes in occupational performance; patients with sickness compensation had statistically significant (p=0.032) higher changes in occupational performance than those without sickness compensation.	Non-RCT	188	**Discussion:** Results demonstrate that clients overall, but especially those receiving sickness compensation and those with a profile of interpersonal distress, significantly increase their self-perceived occupational performance following a multidisciplinary pain treatment program. **Limitations:** No control group.
Huebner, R. A., Johnson, K., Bennett, C. M., & Schneck, C. (2003)	After discharge, only 6 clients received additional OT through home health or outpatient programs. All patients demonstrated statistically significant improvements in functional ability between admission to the brain injury unit and discharge. At follow-up, only 5 of the patients were competitively employed, and 13 were unemployed. All participants had at least one activity limitation, and the most common cognitive deficits were with regard to memory and decision making while the most common emotional problems were related to depression and withdrawal. Participants also reported low scores on community integration and quality of life.	Non-RCT	25	**Conclusions:** The results of this study reflect outcomes common to patients with brain injury in other studies and show that the most significant gain in function occurred during rehabilitation. Similar to the findings of other research, FIM scores at discharge were more predictive of long-term outcomes than admission scores. **Limitations:** The retrospective data in this study were collected from charts filled out in emergency rooms and acute care, which are often prone to error and missing information.
Matuska, K., Giles-Heinz, A., Flinn, N., Neighbor, M., & Bass-Haugen, J. (2003)	Quality of life improved significantly in vitality (p<0.05), social functioning (p<0.01), and the mental health summary score (p<0.05). The average number of participants who communicated with family, friends, or support people at least 3 times per week increased from 47% to 56%. Average number of subjects participating in social or community activities increased from 56% to 66%.	Non-RCT	39	**Conclusions:** Following participation, subject scores on the vitality, social functioning, and mental health subscales of the quality of life measure significantly improved. Frequency of socialization and community participation improved post-program. **Limitations:** Potential participant selection bias because self-selection took place.
Fisher, K., & Hardie, R. J. (2002)	Statistically significant (p<0.01) improvements at discharge found for GAS and PT measures. Improvements maintained at 6 months for GAS, sit/stand, pain, OLBP, and GHQ.	Non-RCT	149	**Conclusions:** This study compares results for GAS with results of established pain impairment measures. Results indicate a correlation between goal attainment and physical mobility. **Limitations:** No control group, co-intervention not avoided (for ethical reasons).

continued

Table 3-4 (continued)

EVIDENCE OF EFFECTIVENESS OF OCCUPATIONAL THERAPY ON PARTICIPATION OUTCOMES

Author (Date)	Major Results	Study Design	Sample Size	Conclusions and Limitations
Positive Effects—Non-Randomized Controlled Trial				
Tippet, C. (2001)	All patients improved their functional ability (p<0.05) regardless of age and cognitive ability (p<0.005), although increased age and decreased cognitive ability were related to lower functional ability (p<0.005).	Non-RCT	19	***Conclusions:*** All participants improved in terms of function. A high number were able to return to their homes, and length of stay in hospital (as compared with other studies) was shorter. ***Limitations:*** Small sample size. Study does not compare discharge results with pre-fracture abilities (only admission to baseline), which would be of value.
DiFabio, R. P., Choi, T., Sodererg, J., & Hansen, C. R. (1997)	Intervention group showed improvements in 6 areas of health-related quality of life while the waitlisted group did not. Outpatient treatment was the sole predictor of positive outcome for energy/fatigue (partial R2=0.19). Treatment group was associated with a positive outcome (together with other independent variables) in the domains of social function and social support.	Non-RCT	44	***Conclusions:*** The program was beneficial to participants with MS, especially in the areas of physical health, bodily pain, energy/fatigue, social support, cognitive ability, and overall positive change in general health. ***Limitations:*** None reported in this article.
Hartman, D., Borrie, M. J., Davison, E., & Stolee, P. (1997)	Implementing the GAS provided a means of measuring achievement of functional and therapeutic recreation goals. Its use emphasized assessment of each individual's skills and identification of personal interests and goals.	Non-RCT	10	***Conclusions:*** GAS was found to be an effective means of measuring client goals, was very client-centered, and can be a valuable tool in maximizing quality of life for people with dementia. ***Limitations:*** Small sample size.
No Effect				
Egan, M., Kessler, D., Laporte, L., Metcalfe, V., & Carter, M. (2007)	There was no difference between control and intervention participants in perceived changes in occupational performance, but a clinically and statistically significant improvement was found in satisfaction with occupational performance in the intervention group. At post-test, there were no differences between groups in any of the secondary measures.	RCT	14	***Conclusions:*** Home-based OT for stroke patients shows some potential to improve participation in valued activities. A number of participants' goals were related to activities outside of leisure and self-care. ***Limitations:*** Small sample size; COPM and SF-36 may not have detected small but clinically significant changes.
Helfrich, C., Aviles, A., Badiani, C., Walens, D., & Sabol, P. (2006)	62% of participants who completed the study increased their mastery scores. No statistically significant change in the youth or adults with mental illness groups. Statistically significant change was found in the domestic violence group.	Non-RCT	73	***Conclusions:*** The intervention implementation, challenges encountered, and strategies developed for implementing shelter-based interventions are discussed. ***Limitations:*** High dropout rate.

continued

Table 3-4 (continued)
EVIDENCE OF EFFECTIVENESS OF OCCUPATIONAL THERAPY ON PARTICIPATION OUTCOMES

Author (Date)	Major Results	Study Design	Sample Size	Conclusions and Limitations
No Effect				
Wressle, E., Filipsson, V., Andersson, L., Jacobsson, B., Martinsson, K., & Engel, K. (2006)	A statistically significant proportion of the experimental group reported problems managing shopping (p=0.01). Control group had greater need for health care contact after discharge. Otherwise, no statistically significant differences were noted between groups.	RCT	41	**Conclusions:** No significant differences were found between groups indicating that a larger sample size is needed in the future. **Limitations:** No record of preventing contamination or co-intervention; outcomes measures not tested for psychometric properties; small sample size.
Horowitz, B. P., & Chang, P. F. (2004)	No statistical differences between control and experimental groups on any outcome measure.	RCT	24	**Conclusions:** The small sample size was attributed to the inability to find statistically significant differences between the participant groups. **Limitations:** Small sample size, reasons for dropouts not reported.

CIQ=Community Integration Questionnaire, COPM=Canadian Occupational Performance Measure, D-COOP-CHARTS=Dartmouth COOP Charts, FIM=Functional Independence Measure, GAS=Goal Attainment Scaling, GHQ=General Health Questionnaire, LHS=London Handicap Scale, OLBP=Oswestry Low Back Pain Disability Questionnaire, SF-36=Short Form Health Questionnaire, SWLS=Satisfaction With Life Scale, ZBI=Zarit Burden Interview.

Table 3-5

OUTCOME MEASURES USED TO CAPTURE PARTICIPATION OUTCOMES

Author (Date)	Outcome(s) Investigated	Outcome Measure(s)	Method of Administration
Yuen, H. K., Huang, P., Burik, J. K., & Smith, T. G. (2008)	Depressive symptoms Life satisfaction Self-rated health	GDS LSI-A 5-point scale rating physical health	Assessments were delivered at baseline, post-intervention, and 3-month follow-up. Assessments were delivered by research assistants blinded to the purpose of the study.
Egan, M., Kessler, D., Laporte, L., Metcalfe, V., & Carter, M. (2007)	Participation and satisfaction with valued activities Well-being Participation in everyday activities	COPM SF-36 RNLI	Evaluations were carried out at baseline (prior to randomization) and 3 months later (when treatment and control conditions were completed). All assessments were completed by a research assistant who was also an OT.
Gillen, G., Berger, S. M., Lotia, S., Morreale, J., Siber, M. I., & Trudo, W. J. (2007)	Functional ability Confidence	COPM 10-point Likert scale	Assessments were administered by an OT immediately prior to and following the community skills evaluation.
Wheeler, S. D., Lane, S. J., & McMahon, B. T. (2007)	Community integration Life satisfaction	CIQ SWLS	Assessments took place at baseline and 90-day follow-up. Data for the treatment group were collected retrospectively as treatment took place outside of the study.
Graff, M. J., Vernooij-Dassen, M. J., Thijssen, M., Dekker, J., Hoefnagels, W. H., & Rickkert, M. G. (2006)	Care-recipient ADL performance Caregiver sense of competence/ burden	Care recipients: AMPS IDDD Caregivers: SCQ	Not reported.
Helfrich, C., Aviles, A., Badiani, C., Walens, D., & Sabol, P. (2006)	Increase life skill knowledge	ACLSA	Outcomes measured at baseline and after completion of the 4-week project.
Wressle, E., Filipsson, V., Andersson, L., Jacobsson, B., Martinsson, K., & Engel, K. (2006)	Ability of older adults to manage at home after discharge	Questionnaires developed for the study to measure social network and contacts, physical and environmental resources, community assistance, transportation, perceived ADL performance, perceived mental and physical health, perceived ability to manage at home	Structured interview at baseline and follow-up.

continued

Table 3-5 (continued)

OUTCOME MEASURES USED TO CAPTURE PARTICIPATION OUTCOMES

Author (Date)	Outcome(s) Investigated	Outcome Measure(s)	Method of Administration
Austin, J., Williams, R., Ross, L., Moseley, L., & Hutchison, S. (2005)	Functional capacity: Functional status Functional performance Perceived exertion Health-related quality of life Health care utilization: Number and length of stay of hospital admissions for heart failure Prescribed heart failure medication	NYHA class I-IV 6MWT Borg RPE MLHF EuroQol	All of the following were measured at baseline and at 8 and 24 weeks: The NYHA class I-IV by the clinical nurse specialist and cardiologist. The cardiologist was blind to the group and decided on patient classification if there was a disparity in their scores. The 6 MWT and Borg RPE were administered by the clinical nurse specialist. The MHLF and EuroQol were self-completed questionnaires.
Johansson, A., & Bjorklund, A. (2005)	Independence Experienced health	IAM SF-36 FIM	Semi-structured interview.
Ng, S., Chu, M., Wu, A., & Cheung, P. (2005)	Level of functional performance Environmental risk Home isolation Self-efficacy	Modified BI CSI SEQ CEQ SAFER Telephone survey—to record subjective progress in health status, frequency of community outings, fall incidents, admissions, and relative feelings of happiness	Self-report and telephone interview.
Dooley, N. R., & Hinojosa, J. (2004)	Caregiver burden Caregiver quality of life Client's level of function Participation in daily activities	ZBI AAL-AD PSMS	Structured interview and self-report.
Horowitz, B. P., & Chang, P. F. (2004)	Health and well-being of frail older adults	MMSE FSQ SF-36 LSI-Z MOS	Self-report interview.
Persson, E., Rivano Fischer, M., & Eklund, M. (2004)	Occupational performance Psychosocial functioning Psychological general well-being	COPM MPI PGWI	COPM administered by OT interview at admission and discharge; MPI administered by social worker or psychologist at admission and discharge; PGWI administered by social worker or psychologist at admission and discharge.
Huebner, R. A., Johnson, K., Bennett, C. M., Schneck, C. (2003)	Injury status Functional ability Level of disability Community participation Quality of life Satisfaction with OT	GCS FIM ALS CIQ QOLR CSQ	Retrospective data were collected from patient's medical records along with demographic and pre-injury data. Follow-up data were collected in an interview an average of 21 months after the injury occurred.

continued

Table 3-5 (continued)

OUTCOME MEASURES USED TO CAPTURE PARTICIPATION OUTCOMES

Author (Date)	Outcome(s) Investigated	Outcome Measure(s)	Method of Administration
Matuska, K., Giles-Heinz, A., Flinn, N., Neighbor, M., & Bass-Haugen, J. (2003)	Quality of life Frequency of participation (social and community)	SF-36 Intake form	Data collection at the start of program, end of program, and at 6 months follow-up.
Dahlin Ivanoff, S., Sonn, U., & Svensson, E. (2002)	Perceived security (confidence) regarding participation in daily occupations	Perceived security (confidence) in performing daily occupations (measure developed for the study)	Interview and questionnaire.
Fisher, K., & Hardie, R. J. (2002)	Goal attainment Physical mobility Pain Impairment due to pain	GAS MPQ PINR OLBP GHQ PIRS	All measures completed at enrollment. GAS and PT measures were compared with baseline data at enrollment and at discharge 15 days later. All measures repeated at 6-month follow-up.
Clark, F., Azen, S. P., Carlson, M., Mandel, D., LaBree, L., Hay, J., et al. (2001)	Long-term effect (6-month post-treatment) of OT on overall health and psychological health	SF-36 FSQ LSI-Z CES-D MOS	Not reported.
Tippet, C. (2001).	Level of function Cognition	BI AMTS	Assessments were administered at baseline (prior to the rehabilitation course). The BI was repeated at discharge.
Gilbertson, L., & Langhorne, P. (2000)	Perceived heath status Perceived performance Satisfaction with care	D-COOP-CHARTS COPM SSQ LHS	Face-to-face interview (at 7 weeks) and mailed self-report questionnaire (at 6 months).
Liberman, R. P., Wallace, C. J., Blackwell, G., Kopelowicz, A., Vaccaro, J. V. , & Mintz, J. (1998)	Retention of skills learned in outpatient therapy	ILSS Social Activities Scale Profile of Adaptation to Life GSA Expanded BPRS Brief Symptom Inventory Rosenberg Self-Esteem Lehman Quality of Life Scale	Not reported.
Bendstrup, K. E., Ingemann Jensen, J., Holm, S., & Bengtsson, B. (1997)	Changes in ADL Quality of life Exercise tolerance Respiratory and circulatory levels	ADL score YQLQ CRDQ 6MWT FEV1 FVC	All measures completed at inclusion, 6, 12, and 24 weeks: ADL score and the YQLQ (self-administered). CRDQ, a questionnaire administered as a structured interview. 6MWT was administered by a member of the team. FEV1 and FVC were recorded by staff members at the hospital.

continued

Table 3-5 (continued)

OUTCOME MEASURES USED TO CAPTURE PARTICIPATION OUTCOMES

Author (Date)	Outcome(s) Investigated	Outcome Measure(s)	Method of Administration
Clark, F., Azen, S. P., Zemke, R., Jackson, J., Carlson, M., Mandel, D., et al. (1997)	Physical health Daily functioning Psychosocial functioning	SF-36 FSQ LSI-Z CES-D MOS	Self-administered questionnaires.
DiFabio, R. P., Choi, T., Soderberg, J., & Hansen, C. R. (1997)	Health-related quality of life Function	SF-36 MS-QOL-54 (Items added to the SF-36 to assess the disease-specific quality of life for people with multiple sclerosis)	Self-report questionnaires completed at baseline and again after 1 year.
Hartman, D., Borrie, M. J., Davison, E., & Stolee, P. (1997)	Enhancement of quality of life Setting individualized functional and recreation goals	APM GAS	APM: administered by OT or therapeutic recreation specialist by observation of performance, behavior, and level of participation. GAS: Performance of IADL and recreation activities were scored by the OT, OTA, and therapeutic recreation specialist.
Logan, P. A., Ahern, J., Gladman, J. R., & Lincoln, N. B. (1997)	Level of function in ADL and IADL Health Care provider health	Modified BI GHQ Nottingham Extended ADL Scale	Self-report and observation.
Helewa, A., Goldsmith, C. H., Lee, P., Bombardier,C., Hanes, B., Smythe, H. A., et al. (1991)	Level of function in ADL/IADL	Questionnaire (developed and validated for study) SHA BDI	Structured interview.

6MWT=6-Minute Walk Test, AAL-AD=Affect and Activity Limitation–Alzheimer's Disease Assessment, ACLSA=Ansell Casey Life Skills Assessment, ALS=Activity Limitations Survey, AMPS=Assessment of Motor and Process Skills, AMTS=Abbreviated Mental Test Score, APM=Activity Performance Measure, BDI=Beck Depression Inventory, BI=Barthel Index, Borg RPE=Borg Scale Rating of Perceived Exertion, BPRS=Brief Psychiatric Rating Scale, CEQ=Caregiver Efficacy Questionnaire, CES-D=Center for Epidemiologic Studies Depression Scale, CIQ=Community Integration Questionnaire, COPM=Canadian Occupational Performance Measure, CRDQ=Chronic Respiratory Disease Questionnaire Score, CSI=Comprehensive Severity Index, CSQ=Client Satisfaction Questionnaire, D-COOP-CHARTS=Dartmouth COOP Charts, EuroQol=European Quality of Life Instrument, FEV1=Forced expiratory volume in 1 second, FIM=Functional Independence Measure, FSQ=Functional Status Questionnaire, FVC=Forced vital capacity, GAS=Goal Attainment Scaling, GCS=Glasgow Coma Scale, GDS=Geriatric Depression Scale, GHQ=General Health Questionnaire, GSA=Global Scale Assessment, IAM=Instrumental Activity Measure, IDDD=Interview of Deterioration in Daily Activities in Dementia, ILSS=Independent Living Skills Survey, LHS=London Handicap Scale, LSI-A=Life Satisfaction Index-A, LSI-Z=Life Satisfaction Index-Z, MLHF=Minnesota Living With Heart Failure Questionnaire, MMSE=Mini Mental Status Examination, MOS=Medical Outcomes Study Health Perception Scale, MPI=Multidimensional Pain Inventory, MPQ=McGill Pain Questionnaire, MS-QOL-54=Multiple Sclerosis Quality of Life Inventory, NYHA class I-IV=New York Heart Association Scale, OLBP=Oswestry Low Back Pain Disability Questionnaire, PGWI=Psychological General Well-Being Index, PINR=Pain Intensity Numerical Rating Scale, PIRS=Pain and Impairment Relationship Scale, PSMS=Physical Self-Maintenance Scale, QOLR=Quality of Life Rating, RNLI=Reintegration to Normal Living Index, SAFER=Safety Assessment of Function and the Environment for Rehabilitation, SCQ=Sense of Competence Questionnaire, SEQ=Self-Efficacy Questionnaire, SF-36=Short Form Health Survey, SHA=Stanford Health Assessment, SSQ=Service Satisfaction Questionnaire, SWLS=Satisfaction With Life Scale, YQLQ=York Quality of Life Questionnaire Score, ZBI=Zarit Burden Interview.

Table 3-6

COMPARISON OF ICF PARTICIPATION DOMAINS AND OCCUPATIONAL PERFORMANCE AREAS

Self-Care	Productivity/Work	Leisure
General tasks and demands	Learning and applying knowledge	
Communication	Major life areas	Major life areas
Movement		
Self-care	Community, social, and civic life	
Domestic life areas		
Interpersonal interactions		

Reprinted with permission from Law, M., Baum, C., & Dunn, W. (2005). *Measuring occupational performance: Supporting best practice in occupational therapy* (2nd ed.). Thorofare, NJ: SLACK Incorporated.

Measures Used to Capture Participation Outcomes

As discussed earlier, occupational therapy focuses on enabling a person's occupational performance or participation in daily occupations (self-care, productivity, and leisure). Occupational performance is the result of complex, dynamic interactions between a person, his or her daily occupations, and the environments in which he or she lives, works, and engages in leisure. "Defined simply, successful occupational performance occurs when a person is able to complete a task or activity in a manner that achieves the goal of the task or activity, while satisfying the person" (Law & Baum, 2005).

Law and Baum (2005) have examined the measurement of participation in daily occupations in detail. According to the ICF, there are 10 categories of participation. Occupational therapy models typically organize occupational performance into three primary categories: self-care, productivity/work, and leisure (CAOT, 2002). As illustrated in Table 3-6, there is extensive overlap between the WHO participation categories and the three categories of occupational performance. During the past decade, an increasing number of measures of participation have been developed. The measures listed in this chapter fit the following criteria:

▲ Cover a broad range of participation categories within the ICF (measures specific to one area, such as self-care, are listed in other chapters)
▲ Noncategorical in nature, not focused on one diagnosis
▲ Evidence of acceptable psychometric properties
▲ Focused on the nature and experience of participation

Drawing on reviews of measures already completed within occupational therapy (Law, Baum & Dunn, 2005), we have compiled a table of measures of participation in daily occupations that are the most suitable for use in occupational therapy practice (Table 3-7).

Conclusions and Recommendations for Future Research

In summary, evidence from these systematic reviews indicates that occupational therapy intervention is effective in improving participation in daily occupations for adults across a range of diagnostic groups and in a variety of intervention settings. Furthermore, systematic reviews indicate that intervention that uses activity and occupation enhances client motivation and leads to improved functional outcomes. Areas of participation where the evidence of effectiveness is strongest include the areas of self-care, domestic life, major life areas, and community, social, and civic life. The amount of research focused on participation in a range of occupations is growing as outcomes increasingly focus on measurement at the level of participation.

The measurement of participation in daily occupations has developed a great deal during the past 10 to 15 years. With the measures that are currently available, the most reliable and valid approach to individualized measurement is to use the Canadian Occupational Performance Measure (COPM). For a group measure of participation, there remains a need to increase the availability of outcome measures in this area. Based on current evidence, the most

Table 3-7

OUTCOME MEASURES TO ASSESS PARTICIPATION INTERVENTIONS

Measure	Population	Content Domains	Reliability and Validity
Canadian Occupational Performance Measure (COPM)	All populations	Individualized assessment; client identifies occupational performance issues during interview with therapist; 5 most important issue are rated by client for performance and satisfaction.	Studies demonstrate test-retest reliability, construct validity, and responsiveness.
Community Integration Questionnaire (CIQ)	All populations (developed for acquired brain injury population)	3 scales—home integration, social integration, and productive activities. 15 items in total with each item having 3 possible response options.	Studies demonstrate internal consistency and test-retest reliability. Validated based on content, convergent, and construct (discriminative) validity.
Craig Handicap Assessment and Reporting Technique (CHART)	All populations	27 items—subscales include physical independence, mobility, occupation, social integration, and economic self-sufficiency.	Studies demonstrate test-retest reliability, construct, and criterion validity.
Life Habits Assessment (LIFE-H)	All populations	240 life habits items (69-item short version)—12 domains include nutrition, fitness, personal care, communication, housing, mobility, responsibility, interpersonal relations, community, education, employment, and recreation.	Studies demonstrate test-retest reliability, construct, and criterion validity.
London Handicap Scale (LHS)	All populations	6 domains—mobility, orientation, occupation, physical independence, social integration, and economic self-sufficiency.	Studies demonstrate internal consistency, test-retest reliability, construct, and criterion validity and responsiveness.
Occupational Performance History Interview II (OPHI-II)	All populations	42 items with 3 subscales—occupational identity, occupational competence, and occupational behavioral settings.	Validated using Rasch analysis. Studies demonstrate observer reliability and construct validity.
Occupational Self-Assessment (OSA)	All populations	2 parts—21 items for occupational performance; 8 items for environment.	Limited reliability testing to date. Validated using Rasch analysis. Studies demonstrate construct validity.
World Health Organization— Disability Schedule II (WHO-DAS II)	All populations	12- and 36-item versions—domains include communication, physical mobility, self-care, interpersonal interactions, domestic responsibilities, and work and participation in society.	Studies demonstrate internal consistency, construct, and criterion validity. Limited reliability testing to date.

promising group measures of participation are the Craig Handicap Assessment and Reporting Technique (CHART), brief version of the Life Habits Assessment (LIFE-H), and World Health Organization—Disability Schedule II (WHO-DAS II).

More research with this focus is needed. In particular, increased research focused on participation in community life would enhance our knowledge of the impact of occupational therapy services on community participation.

References

Austin, J., Williams, R., Ross, L., Moseley, L., & Hutchison, S. (2005). Randomised controlled trial of cardiac rehabilitation in elderly patients with heart failure. *European Journal of Heart Failure, 7*(3 special issue), 411-417.

Bendstrup, K. E., Ingemann Jensen, J., Holm, S., & Bengtsson, B. (1997). Out-patient rehabilitation improves activities of daily living, quality of life and exercise tolerance in chronic obstructive pulmonary disease. *European Respiratory Journal, 10*(12), 2801-2806.

Canadian Association of Occupational Therapists. (2002). *Enabling occupation: An occupational therapy perspective* (Rev. ed.). Ottawa, Ontario, Canada: CAOT Publications.

Christiansen, C., Baum, C., & Bass-Haugen, J. (2005). *Occupational therapy: Performance, participation, and well-being* (3rd ed.). Thorofare, NJ: SLACK Incorporated.

Clark, F., Azen, S. P., Carlson, M., Mandel, D., LaBree, L., Hay, J., et al. (2001). Embedding health-promoting changes into the daily lives of independent-living older adults: Long-term follow-up of occupational therapy intervention. *Journals of Gerontology. Series B: Psychological Sciences and Social Sciences, 56B*(1), P60-P63.

Clark, F., Azen, S. P., Zemke, R., Jackson, J., Carlson, M., Mandel, D., et al. (1997). Occupational therapy for independent-living older adults. A randomized controlled trial. *Journal of the American Medical Association, 278*(16), 1321-1326.

Dahlin Ivanoff, S., Sonn, U., & Svensson, E. (2002). A health education program for elderly persons with visual impairments and perceived security in the performance of daily occupations: A randomized study. *American Journal of Occupational Therapy, 56*(3), 322-330.

Deane, K. H. O., Ellis Hill, C., Playford, E. D., Ben Shlomo, Y., & Clarke, C. E. (2001). Occupational therapy for Parkinson's disease. *Cochrane Database of Systematic Reviews*, Issue 2.

DiFabio, R. P., Choi, T., Soderberg, J., & Hansen, C. R. (1997). Health-related quality of life for patients with progressive multiple sclerosis: Influence of rehabilitation. *Physical Therapy, 77*(12), 1704-1716.

Dixon, L., Duncan, D. C., Johnson, P., Kirkby, L., O'Connell, H., Taylor, H. J., et al. (2007). Occupational therapy for patients with Parkinson's disease. *Cochrane Database of Systematic Reviews*. Issue 3. Art. No.: CD002813. DOI: 10.1002/14651858.CD002813.pub2.

Dooley, N. R., & Hinojosa, J. (2004). Improving quality of life for persons with Alzheimer's disease and their family caregivers: Brief occupational therapy intervention. *American Journal of Occupational Therapy, 58*(5), 561-569.

Egan, M., Kessler, D., Laporte, L., Metcalfe, V., & Carter, M. (2007). A pilot randomized controlled trial of community-based occupational therapy in late stroke rehabilitation. *Topics in Stroke Rehabilitation, 14*(5), 37-45.

Fiorani, C., Mari, F., Bartolini, Ceravolo, M., & Provinciali, L. (1997). Occupational therapy increases ADL score and quality of life in Parkinson's disease. *Movement Disorders, 12*(Suppl 1), 135.

Fisher, K., & Hardie, R. J. (2002). Goal attainment scaling in evaluating a multidisciplinary pain management programme. *Clinical Rehabilitation, 16*(8), 871-877.

Gauthier, L., Dalziel, S., & Gauthier, S. (1987). The benefits of group occupational therapy for patients with Parkinson's disease. *American Journal of Occupational Therapy, 41*(6), 360-365.

Gilbertson, L., & Langhorne, P. (2000). Home-based occupational therapy: Stroke patients' satisfaction with occupational performance and service provision. *British Journal of Occupational Therapy, 63*(10), 464-468.

Gillen, G., Berger, S. M., Lotia, S., Morreale, J., Siber, M. I., & Trudo, W. J. (2007). Improving community skills after lower extremity joint replacement. *Physical and Occupational Therapy in Geriatrics, 25*(4), 41-54.

Graff, M. J., Vernooij-Dassen, M. J., Thijssen, M., Dekker, J., Hoefnagels, W. H., & Rikkert, M. G. (2006). Community based occupational therapy for patients with dementia and their care givers: Randomised controlled trial. *British Medical Journal, 333*(7580), 1196.

Greenhalgh, T. (2006). *How to read a paper: The basics of evidence-based medicine* (3rd ed.). London, England: Blackwell Publishing Ltd.

Hartman, D., Borrie, M. J., Davison, E., & Stolee, P. (1997). Use of goal attainment scaling in a dementia special care unit. *American Journal of Alzheimer's Disease, 12*(3), 111-116.

Hasselkus, B. R. (1992). The meaning of activity: Day care for persons with Alzheimer's disease. *American Journal of Occupational Therapy, 46*(3), 199-206.

Helewa, A., Goldsmith, C. H., Lee, P., Bombardier, C., Hanes, B., Smythe, H. A., et al. (1991). Effects of occupational therapy home service on patients with rheumatoid arthritis. *Lancet, 337*(8755), 1453-1456.

Helfrich, C., Aviles, A., Badiani, C., Walens, D., & Sabol, P. (2006). Life skill interventions with homeless youth, domestic violence victims, and adults with mental illness. *Occupational Therapy in Health Care, 20*, 189-207.

Horowitz, B. P., & Chang, P. F. (2004). Promoting well-being and engagement in life through occupational therapy lifestyle redesign: A pilot study within adult day programs. *Topics in Geriatric Rehabilitation, 20*(1), 46-58.

Huebner, R. A., Johnson, K., Bennett, C. M., & Schneck, C. (2003). Community participation and quality of life outcomes after adult traumatic brain injury. *American Journal of Occupational Therapy, 57*(2), 177-185.

Johansson, A., & Bjorklund, A. (2005). Occupational adaptation or well-tried, professional experience in rehabilitation of the disabled elderly at home. *Activities, Adaptation and Aging, 30*(1), 1-21.

Law, M., & Baum, C. (2005). Measurement in occupational therapy. In M. Law, C. Baum, & W. Dunn (Eds.), *Measuring occupational performance: Supporting best practice in occupational therapy* (2nd ed.). Thorofare, NJ: SLACK Incorporated.

Law, M., Baum, C., & Dunn, W. (2005). *Measuring occupational performance: Supporting best practice in occupational therapy* (2nd ed.). Thorofare, NJ: SLACK Incorporated.

Law, M., Steinweinder, S., & Leclair, L. (1998). Occupation, health and well-being. *Canadian Journal of Occupational Therapy, 65*(2), 81-91.

Liberman, R. P., Wallace, C. J., Blackwell, G., Kopelowicz, A., Vaccaro, J. V., & Mintz, J. (1998). Skills training versus psychosocial occupational therapy for persons with persistent schizophrenia. *American Journal of Psychiatry, 155*(8), 1087-1091.

Logan, P. A., Ahern, J., Gladman, J. R., & Lincoln, N. B. (1997). A randomized controlled trial of enhanced social service occupational therapy for stroke patients. *Clinical Rehabilitation, 11*(2), 107-113.

Matuska, K., Giles-Heinz, A., Flinn, N., Neighbor, M., & Bass-Haugen, J. (2003). Outcomes of a pilot occupational therapy wellness program for older adults. *American Journal of Occupational Therapy, 57*(2), 220-224.

McColl, M., Law, M., Stewart, D., Doubt, L., Pollock, N., & Krupa, T. (2002). *Theoretical basis of occupational therapy* (2nd ed.). Thorofare, NJ: SLACK Incorporated.

Murphy, S., & Tickle Degnen, L. (2001). The effectiveness of occupational therapy-related treatments for persons with Parkinson's disease: A meta-analytic review. *American Journal of Occupational Therapy, 55*(4), 385-392.

Ng, S., Chu, M., Wu, A., & Cheung, P. (2005). Effectiveness of home-based occupational therapy for early discharged patients with stroke. *Hong Kong Journal of Occupational Therapy, 15*, 27-36.

Persson, E., Rivano Fischer, M., & Eklund, M. (2004). Evaluation of changes in occupational performance among patients in a pain management program. *Journal of Rehabilitation Medicine, 36*(2), 85-91.

Shapero Sabari, J. (2001). Quality of life after stroke: Developing meaningful life roles through occupational therapy. *Loss Grief Care, 9*, 155-169.

Tippet, C. (2001). Broken neck of femur: Does rehabilitation improve function? *British Journal of Therapy and Rehabilitation, 8*(11), 410-417.

Trombly, C. A., & Ma, H. I. (2002). A synthesis of the effects of occupational therapy for persons with stroke, part I: Restoration of roles, tasks, and activities. *American Journal of Occupational Therapy, 56*(3), 250-259.

Wheeler, S. D., Lane, S. J., & McMahon, B. T. (2007). Community participation and life satisfaction following intensive, community-based rehabilitation using a life skills training approach. *OTJR: Occupation, Participation, and Health, 27*(1), 13-22.

Wilkins, S., Jung, B., Wishart, L., Edwards, M., & Gamble Norton, S. (2003). The effectiveness of community-based occupational therapy education and functional training programs for older adults: A critical literature review. *Canadian Journal of Occupational Therapy, 70*, 214-225.

World Health Organization. (2001). *International classification of functioning, disability, and health*. Geneva, Switzerland: Author.

Wressle, E., Filipsson, V., Andersson, L., Jacobsson, B., Martinsson, K., & Engel, K. (2006). Evaluation of occupational therapy interventions for elderly patients in Swedish acute care: A pilot study. *Scandinavian Journal of Occupational Therapy, 13*(4), 203-210.

Yarrow, S. (1999). Member's 1998 survey of the Parkinson's Disease Society of the United Kingdom. In R. Percival & P. Hobson (Eds.), *Parkinson's disease: Studies in psychological and social care* (pp. 79-92). Leicester: BPS Books.

Yuen, H. K., Huang, P., Burik, J. K., & Smith, T. G. (2008). Impact of participating in volunteer activities for residents living in long-term-care facilities. *American Journal of Occupational Therapy, 62*(1), 71.

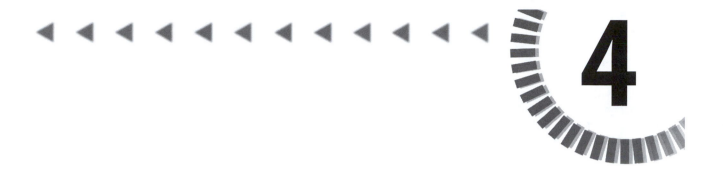

SELF-CARE OUTCOMES

Laura Bradley, MSc (OT), OT Reg. (Ont.) and
Brenda H. Vrkljan, PhD, OT Reg. (Ont.)

We hear the alarm clock, roll out of bed, hop in the shower, towel off, get dressed, and head to the kitchen. We make a cup of coffee and some breakfast, then climb into our cars or catch the nearest bus, and head off to work or school. After a long day, we stop at the bank, get some groceries, and do a few errands before heading back home. This routine exemplifies the many activities in which we engage every day that involve caring for ourselves. For many individuals, completing these self-care activities can be much more difficult. Developmental differences, aging, acute or chronic physical disabilities, mental health challenges, and other impairments may affect a person's ability to engage in everyday occupations.

Occupational therapy is concerned with facilitating people in performing their chosen occupations and overcoming environmental, social, or physical barriers by maintaining or improving abilities or compensating for decreased abilities (Lindquist & Unsworth, 1999). In fact, for some populations, daily occupational therapy consisting of self-care programs, instrumental activities of daily living (IADL) tasks, and functional and community mobility can improve functional ability (Eyres & Unsworth, 2005). Occupational therapists render a positive effect in terms of increas-ing functional abilities for many patient populations (Steultjens, Dekker, Bouter, Leemrijse, & van den Ende, 2005).

Conceptual Background

This chapter examines evidence behind occupational therapy interventions addressing self-care in three general areas: personal care, functional mobility, and community management.

Personal care is a term generally used to encompass elements of self-care that are required for a basic level of functioning, such as dressing, eating, bathing, or toileting. In certain health care fields, occupational therapy included, these activities fall under the umbrella of activities of daily living (ADL). Independence in self-care activities enables a person to maintain a level of dignity and less reliance on others, as well as offers a sense of achievement (Walker & Walker, 2001). Occupational therapists address difficulties with self-care activities to assist the individual (or caregiver) to be as independent as possible.

M. Law & M. A. McColl (Eds.)
Interventions, Effects, and Outcomes in Occupational Therapy:
Adults and Older Adults (pp. 47-118)
© 2010 SLACK Incorporated

Functional mobility refers to the ability to move from one desired location to another, either unassisted or with the assistance of therapeutic equipment or another person. The goal of occupational therapy, with regard to functional mobility, is to enhance individuals with mobility impairments to participate in their desired occupations by providing and/or adapting technological interventions (Reid, Laliberte-Rudman, & Hebert, 2002).

Community management is a term generally used to describe occupations that are more complex than traditional self-care tasks. These occupations require individuals to interact with their community environment and are sometimes referred to as IADL or extended activities of daily living (EADL) (Legg, Drummond, & Langhorne, 2006). Community management encompasses a range of occupations necessary for independent living, including preparing meals, managing finances, home maintenance, shopping, and other community-based activities (Legg et al., 2006). Another occupation identified as critical to keeping individuals active and mobile in their community is the ability to use transportation, particularly driving (Lloyd et al., 2001). However, the ability to safely manage such occupations can be significantly altered by health-related changes in sensory, cognitive, and/or motor systems due to injury, illness, aging, and/or changes in life roles (e.g., caregiver).

Occupational therapists can also be an important part of another mode of rehabilitation delivery: the multidisciplinary team. Multidisciplinary rehabilitation teams are comprised of many different health disciplines. These teams can include physical therapists/physiotherapists, occupational therapists, speech-language pathologists, dietitians, nurses, and medical doctors working together to improve the health status and functional abilities of the clients for whom they care. Multidisciplinary teams can benefit patients and caregivers in a number of ways (Trend, Kaye, Gage, Owen, & Wade, 2002). As well, they are a cost-effective option in terms of patient care (Przybylski, Dumont, Watkins, Warren, Beaulne, & Lier, 1996). Multidisciplinary teams can lead to improved ratings in health-related quality of life and social participation (Finnerty, Keeping, Bullough, & Jones, 2001; Melin & Bygren, 1992; Ryan, Enderby, & Rigby, 2006) and better health and functional outcomes (Caplan, Williams, Daly, & Abraham, 2004).

Regardless of whether an occupational therapist is working alone or as a part of a multidisciplinary team, the rehabilitation goal with regard to self-care interventions is to improve or maintain functional ability within the patient groups being treated. However, the question remains as to the effectiveness of occupational therapy with regard to achieving this goal based on the research published to date and, furthermore, what

occupational therapists can learn from this research that can further enhance clinical practice.

Search Strategy

The methodology to search the literature, identify studies, and select them based on the inclusion criteria was discussed in Chapter 2. A systematic search of health care and occupational therapy databases, as well as hand-searched relevant references, yielded critical reviews (e.g., systematic reviews or meta-analyses) and qualitative and quantitative studies that addressed occupational therapy outcomes when providing intervention related to improving areas related to the client's self-care goals. Selected studies met specific inclusion criteria, which consisted of study publication between 1980 and 2008, adult population, study intervention involving occupational therapy independently or on a multidisciplinary team, and study categorized as level of evidence 1 to 4 based on criteria by Greenhalgh (2006). For this chapter, the search terms used to capture occupational therapy sensitive outcomes are listed in Table 4-1. From this search, 57 articles met the inclusion criteria and are reviewed in this chapter in more detail in Tables 4-2 through 4-4.

Interventions Used to Improve Personal Care Outcomes

Comprehensive Occupational Therapy

In the current health care climate, health professionals often find themselves needing to do more with less and finding creative solutions to complex problems. Occupational therapists can implement several interventions with the same client with the goal of increasing functional independence. For example, clients who sustained a stroke can receive home visits from an occupational therapist to address several ADL, IADL, and leisure activities. Clients who received this treatment approach significantly improved in key areas of self-care, as measured by the Barthel Index (BI) and IADL scales (Walker, Gladman, Lincoln, Siemonsma, & Whiteley, 1999).

These interventions can be directed to the individual or to his or her caregivers. Such care can be provided in the home, hospital, or community environment. The occupational therapy interventions used can include skill development, education for the person and caregiver, task adaptation, and environmental modification. The exact nature of occupational therapy intervention depends on the setting, as well as time and institutional constraints, including financial support or equipment availability.

Table 4-1
SEARCH TERMS FOR OCCUPATIONAL THERAPY INTERVENTIONS TO IMPROVE SELF-CARE OUTCOMES

Occupation, occupational therapy (therapist), OR multidisciplinary team AND…

Primary terms: activities of daily living (ADL), driving, functional status, independent living, mobility aids, self-care, self-management, wheelchair(s).

Secondary terms: accidents, ADL disability, ambulation aids, automobile driving, automobiles, bathing, car driving, cooking, daily life activity(ies), dressing, driving ability, driving behavior, food handling, functional training, grooming, instrumental activities of daily living (IADL), mobility, mobility device, personal care, self-care skills, traffic, wheelchair fitting.

Additional terms used to focus the search included clinical effectiveness, community health services, health care delivery, health care services, health service, health services for the aged, home care, home care services, home health care, home occupational therapy, home rehabilitation, interdisciplinary education, interdisciplinary research, interdisciplinary treatment approach, intervention treatment approach, multidisciplinary care team, outcomes, outcomes assessment patient care, outcomes (health care), outcomes research, patient care team, psychotherapeutic outcomes, rehabilitation, rehabilitation care, rehabilitation centre, rehabilitation outcomes, teamwork, treatment effectiveness evaluation, treatment outcomes.

Early Supported Discharge

Post-stroke outpatient rehabilitation has long been an alternative to costly inpatient care. Outpatient treatment consisting of input from different rehabilitation professionals (i.e., occupational therapist, physical therapist, speech-language pathologist) has been associated with an improvement in functional abilities, a decrease in depression, and a decrease in subjective impairment when compared to those discharged home with no intervention (Werner & Kessler, 1996). At times, however, it is difficult for stroke survivors and their caregivers to travel to hospitals to receive treatments, and outpatient treatment often does not take into account the patient's natural environment.

Early supported discharge (ESD) is a movement that began in the mid-1990s, and its aim is to accelerate discharge home from hospital following a stroke. After a brief hospital stay, the majority of care is provided in the client's home by a team of coordinated health care professionals, including physicians; nurse practitioners; occupational, physical, and speech therapists; and/or dietitians. Studies have shown that ESD services can help people who have had a stroke regain functional skills faster than conventional discharge services (Fjærtoft, Indredavik, Johnsen, & Lydersen, 2004; Langhorne et al., 2005) and lead to a higher rate of functional ability (Alexander, Bugge, & Hagen, 2001). ESD is considered a practical alternative to outpatient hospital-based care (Gladman, Lincoln, & Barer, 1993).

Direct ADL Skill Development

As a person ages, or as a result of acute or chronic disability, individuals often find it more difficult to complete basic ADL, such as dressing, bathing, and toileting. Occupational therapists address these areas by providing rehabilitation or compensatory strategies aimed at increasing independence. Interventions could include altering the environment or providing direct training on how an activity could be performed differently to enable a person to engage in this occupation.

A review of evidence that examined the effectiveness of direct ADL retraining is promising. Corr and Bayer's (1995) randomized controlled trial looking at occupational therapy for stroke patients after hospital discharge showed that in two groups of patients discharged after stroke, those who received a home visit from an occupational therapist who taught new skills, worked on ADL, trained patients with equipment, and gave education to caregivers were re-admitted to the hospital significantly less often than those who received usual discharge care. It is also interesting to note that patients who received occupational therapy as part of their rehabilitation program were more likely to return to their home environment than those with no occupational therapy involvement (Jones, Miller, & Petrella, 2002; Landi, Cesari, Onder, Tafani, Zamboni, & Cocchi, 2006; Ostrow, Parente, Ottenbacher, & Bonder, 1989).

text continues on page 109

Table 4-2
OCCUPATIONAL THERAPY INTERVENTIONS PROMOTING SELF-CARE OUTCOMES

Author (Date)	Pop	DX	Setting	Intervention
Landi, F., Cesari, M., Onder, G., Tafani, A., Zamboni, V., & Cocchi, A. (2006)	1	3	5	OT and PT combined program for 3 hours a day. ADL such as personal hygiene, toilet use, feeding, dressing, and mobility. Setting goals to improve independence with self-care retraining, assessment for adaptive equipment, and UE splinting. ROM and strengthening exercises, musculoskeletal control, trunk and UE positioning, transfer training, postural and gait training, functional and self-care retraining, and adaptive equipment training were provided.
Ryan, T., Enderby, P., & Rigby, A. S. (2006)	1	3, 17	3	Patients were randomly assigned to a routine or augmented rehabilitation service. Both services were provided by multidisciplinary teams (OT, PT, speech-language, or therapy assistants). Maximum length of intervention was 12 weeks. *Intervention:* The augmented care group received 6 or more face-to-face contacts per week. *Control:* The routine care group received 3 or fewer face-to-face contacts per week, while the augmented care group received 6 or more.
Sanford, J. A., Griffiths, P. C., Richardson, P., Hargraves, K., Butterfield, T., & Hoenig, H. (2006)	4	18	3	*Intervention:* 4 weekly OT/PT sessions through televideo technology. Interventions targeted 3 mobility tasks and 3 transfer tasks. Interventions included individualized adaptive techniques, assistive technologies, and recommendations for home modifications to reduce environmental demands. Individualized exercise prescriptions were also included. *Control:* Same intervention but delivered by traditional home visits.
Storr, L. K., Sorensen, P. S., & Ravnborg, M. (2006)	5	5	4	*Intervention:* Inpatient rehabilitation for 3 to 5 weeks. OT, PT, psychologists, social workers, and neurologists were part of the treatment team and were not aware of the trial. OT occurred for 30 minutes 3 times per week. *Control:* Did not receive any treatment in the study, as they remained on the waiting list.
Alexander, J. A., Lichtenstein, R., Jinnet, K., Wells, R., Zazzeli, J., & Liu, D. (2005)	5	8, 12, 13, 14, 15	1	Involvement/intervention with a cross-functional multidisciplinary team. Core team included physicians, RNs, and LPNs. Other professionals when available: Social workers, psychologists, and pharmacists. Other professions sometimes involved: OTs, recreation therapy, dietitians, chaplains.
McNaughton, H., DeJong, G., Smout, R. J., Melvin, J. L., & Brandstater, M. (2005)	5	3	4	Rehabilitation after acute stroke. PT: Mobility, assessment. OT: Assessment, cognitive testing, home visits, UE function. Speech-language pathology: Cognition, assessment swallowing, comprehension, expression.
Thorsen, A., Widen Holmqvist, L., de Pedro-Cuesta, J., & von Koch, L. (2005)	--	3	2, 3	Patients were randomized to either a home rehabilitation group through early supportive discharge or a conventional rehabilitation group. *Intervention:* The home rehabilitation group received services from OT, PT, and speech-language pathology. Mean number of home visits were 12 over a mean of 14 weeks. Duration and treatment were individual, but common focuses included speech and communication activities, ADL work, and ambulation. Both groups first received medical and rehabilitation treatment in the stroke unit. If required, those in the conventional rehabilitation group received further treatment in the geriatrics or rehabilitation departments.
Unsworth, C. A., & Duncombe, D. (2005)	4	18	2	Clients received OT interventions as well as PT, speech-language pathology, physician, nurse, dietitian, and neuropsychologist. OT interventions included motor relearning and both remedial and compensatory techniques.

continued

Table 4-2 (continued)
OCCUPATIONAL THERAPY INTERVENTIONS PROMOTING SELF-CARE OUTCOMES

Author (Date)	Pop	DX	Setting	Intervention
Yagura, H., Miyai, I., Suzuki, T., & Yanagihara, T. (2005)	--	3	4	Patients were either given inpatient rehab in a stroke rehabilitation unit or general rehabilitation ward. Both groups had 40-minute sessions of OT, PT, and speech therapy as needed, 5 days a week. Patients received standard rehabilitation nursing care. The only difference between the 2 wards was the existence of weekly interdisciplinary rehabilitation team conferences. The stroke rehabilitation unit had these weekly meetings. The general rehabilitation ward did not have weekly meetings. Instead meetings were held irregularly, as needed, particularly for patients with severe disabilities. Discharge planning was provided by social workers. Patients were also seen by physicians.
Bode, R. K., Heinemann, A. W., Semik, P., & Mallinson, T. (2004)	5	3	2, 4	Speech-language pathology, PT, and OT interventions. Analyses were conducted on therapeutic activities, which were classified as function-focused activities or impairment-focused activities. Function-focused activities in OT: Dressing, toileting, functional communication, community integration, tub/toilet/shower transfers, etc. Function-focused activities in PT: Walking stairclimbing, tub/toilet/shower transfers, etc. Function-focused activities in speech-language pathology: Auditory comprehension, money management, alternative/augmentative communication, chewing, swallowing, oral expression, etc. Impairment-focused activities in OT: Sensory/perceptual/motor, cognitive problem solving, therapeutic adaptation/equipment, etc. Impairment-focused activities in PT: Positioning, casting, splinting, balance training, etc. Impairment-focused activities in speech-language pathology: Memory, orientation, alertness, concentration, etc.
Caplan, G. A., Williams, A. J., Daly, B., & Abraham, K. (2004)	1	18	3	OT, PT, geriatrician or geriatric registrar, and nurses. ***Intervention:*** Comprehensive geriatric assessment team: A nurse would develop a care plan and initiate a process for any referrals. The patient was then presented at weekly multidisciplinary rounds. The multidisciplinary team performed appropriate intervention for a maximum of 4 weeks, and those still in need of care were referred to appropriate services. ***Control:*** The usual care group was discharged from the emergency department with the plan provided by the "medical officer" there.
Fleming, S. A., Blake, H., Gladman, J. R. F., Hart, E., Lymbery, M., Dewey, M. E., et al. (2004)	1	21	1	***Intervention:*** Inpatient rehabilitation (called care home rehabilitation services) was largely provided by OTs and also some social services staff. PTs, general practitioners, and nurses were not considered part of the intervention, as they were provided by referral/community services. ***Control:*** Usual health and social care.
Hastings, J., Gowans, S., & Watson, D. E. (2004)	2	18	2	2 or more hours of OT consultation. Patients were typically also referred to PT. 11 OT interventions, 4 focused on improving function during hospital stay. The interventions were ADL assessment and training, pre-discharge safety assessment and recommendations, education on energy conservation, transfer training, equipment recommendations, UE and LE strengthening, psychosocial, splinting, cognitive assessment, community support recommendations, and information on funding for home modifications.

continued

Table 4-2 (continued)

OCCUPATIONAL THERAPY INTERVENTIONS PROMOTING SELF-CARE OUTCOMES

Author (Date)	Pop	DX	Setting	Intervention
Jousset, N., Fanello, S., Bontoux, L., Dubus, V., Billabert, C., Vielle, B., et al. (2004)	2	20	3, 4	Patients participated in either a functional restoration program or active individual therapy for 5 weeks. Functional restoration program: Consisted of group, sport-like activities, which were adjusted for individual capacity. It took place for 6 hours a day, 5 days a week. Activities included warm-ups, stretching, strengthening and proprioceptive exercises, aerobic activities, OT, balneotherapy, endurance training, and individual interventions with a psychiatrist and psychologist. Active individual therapy: Consisted of 1-hour treatment sessions with a PT, 3 times per week. Patients were taught exercises, which they were instructed to do 50 minutes per day, on the 2 days that they did not see the PT. Activities included pain coping strategies, range of motion, strengthening, and functional training activities, etc.
Keren, O., Motin, M., Heinemann, A. W., O'Reilly, C. M., Bode, R. K., Semik, P., et al. (2004)	4	3	4	Inpatient rehabilitation involving OT, PT, and speech-language therapy. Studied the relationship between intensity of OT and outcomes.
Lincoln, N. B., Walker, M. F., Dixon, A., & Knights P. (2004)	5	3	3	Patients were randomly assigned to either the conventional care group or the community stroke team. ***Intervention:*** Stroke team: Patients were initially assessed by 2 members of the stroke team, and services were allocated based on individual need following a team meeting. Patients received services in their homes for as long as it was deemed to be beneficial. Examples of service include OT, PT, and speech therapies and time with a mental health nurse and rehabilitation support worker. ***Control:*** Conventional rehabilitation group: Patients were free to attend programs, which they chose. These included services at day hospitals, outpatient departments, social services, and OT.
Liu, K. P., Chan, C. C., Lee, T. M., & Hui-Chan, C. W. (2004)	4	3	4	Patients were randomly assigned to a mental imagery group or a functional retraining group. Different OTs led each group. Training for both groups involved 5 1-hour a week sessions for 3 weeks. Patients in both groups also received 1-hour sessions of PT 5 days a week. This focused on muscle strengthening and walking. ***Intervention:*** In the mental imagery group, participants were taught to practice specific tasks. ***Control:*** In the retraining group, a demonstration-then-practice model was used, but unlike in the mental imagery group, therapists assisted patients when problems were encountered (i.e., decreased motor control).
MacPhee, A. H., Kirby, R. L., Coolen, A. L., Smith, C., MacLeod, D. A., & Dupuis, D. J. (2004)	5	18	4	Participants were randomly assigned to the control group or the wheelchair skills training program group. Both groups received typical treatment received during a rehabilitation stay. ***Intervention:*** The wheelchair skills training program group took part in the training, which consisted of a maximum of 6 30-minute sessions where they were taught proper wheelchair skills techniques and then practiced a series of skills learned. Participants were given feedback if they were not able to perform a skill, and encouraging feedback was given when they performed a skill correctly.

continued

Table 4-2 (continued)

OCCUPATIONAL THERAPY INTERVENTIONS PROMOTING SELF-CARE OUTCOMES

Author (Date)	Pop	DX	Setting	Intervention
Pankow, L., Luchins, D., Studebaker, J., & Chettleburgh, D. (2004)	1	18	3	**Intervention:** Vision rehabilitation: Specific intervention depended on goals established by participants. Orientation and mobility training was provided by a trainer with a master's degree in orientation and mobility instruction. Blind rehabilitation training was provided by an instructor with a master's degree in blind rehabilitation teaching and involved activities such as identifying clothes using tactile methods and identifying and sorting money using tactical methods. OT services were largely targeted at those with hemianopsia and involved provision of prism training. Driving instruction was provided by a certified driving rehabilitation specialist. **Control:** The control group received education about ocular disease and demonstration of functional aids (optical and non-optical). They were contacted by phone to discuss when rehabilitation would begin, as they were on a waiting list. Intervention was a minimum of 4 weeks.
Weiss, Z., Snir, D., Klein, B., Avraham, I., Shani, R., Zetler, H., et al. (2004)	4	3	3, 4, 5	Patients chose either home rehabilitation or inpatient rehabilitation at a hospital, referred to as institutional rehabilitation. **Intervention 1:** The home rehabilitation group received home visits from an OT, PT, nurse, and physician, with frequency and time of visit based on individual need. On average, OT visited once a week, and PT twice weekly. Intervention taught exercises to patients and provided instruction to family members. Nurses and doctors followed patients' general health. Average duration of home rehabilitation was 56.8 days, and cost was an average of $442 per patient. **Intervention 2:** The institutional rehabilitation group received inpatient rehabilitation in either a rehabilitation unit of a general hospital or a geriatric hospital. Patients were treated according to usual protocol of the particular unit, which generally included individual OT and PT, for 45-minute sessions 4 to 5 times a week. Average duration of treatment was 59.82 days, at a cost of $320 per patient a day.
Bohannon, R. W., Ahlquist, M., Lee, N., & Maljanian, R. (2003)	4	3	2	OT, PT, and speech therapy (measured in therapy units of 15 minutes). Analysis focused on relationship between therapy intensity and functional outcome.
Wade, D. T., Gage, H., Owen, C., Trend, P., Grossmith, C., & Kaye, J. (2003)	4	4	4	**Intervention:** 6 weeks of intervention in a day hospital program involving a Parkinson's disease specialist nurse, OT, PT, and speech-language therapist. Each patient received 2 hours of individualized treatment in the morning and then participated in group activities in the afternoon. **Control:** No intervention.
Alvund, K., Jepsen, E., Vass, M., & Lundemark, H. (2002)	4	18	3	**Intervention:** Received home visit from interdisciplinary team made up of home nurse and PT or OT. General practitioners were consulted regarding medical concerns, but did not actually visit the clients' home. **Control:** Received standard discharge plans (more limited coordination but no details provided).
Jones, G. R., Miller, T. A., & Petrella, R. J. (2002)	1	22	4	Inpatient rehabilitation on a rehabilitation unit at an acute care hospital. The team consisted of a chief physician, social worker, OT, PT, and nursing staff. OT: Approximately 1 hour a day, 5 days a week for 3 to 6 weeks. PT: Approximately 1.5 hours a day, 5 days a week for 3 to 6 weeks.

continued

Table 4-2 (continued)

OCCUPATIONAL THERAPY INTERVENTIONS PROMOTING SELF-CARE OUTCOMES

Author (Date)	Pop	DX	Setting	Intervention
Naglie, G., Tansey, C., Kirkland, J. L., Ogilvie-Harris, D. J., Detsky, A. S., Etchells, E., et al. (2002)	1	17	4	Patients were randomly assigned to either care from an interdisciplinary care team or typical inpatient care services. Both groups received post-operative surgical care, but only the interdisciplinary group received daily medical care from a senior medical resident. **Intervention:** Interdisciplinary care consisted of a nurse specialist, social worker, PT, and OT. **Control:** The patients in the usual care group had access to allied health professionals through consultation, but had limited access to OT and clinical nurse specialists.
Saltvedt, I., Opdahl Mo, E. S., Fayers, P., Kaasa, S., & Sletvold, O. (2002)	1	18	2, 5	Patients were randomized to either a general medical ward or the geriatric evaluation and management unit (GEMU). **Intervention:** The GEMU took an interdisciplinary approach to care, and team members included a geriatrician, residents, nurses, 2 OTs, 1 PT, and a research-type nurse for the duration of the study. Other disciplines such as dentistry and social work were involved as necessary. Patients on the unit were encouraged to participate in ADL and communal meals and to engage in "early mobilization." Upon discharge, those in the GEMU and medical wards were cared for by general practitioners in the community. In the GEMU group, discharge was discussed in a meeting with the patient, team members, and families. As necessary, an OT would also do a home visit. **Control:** Patients on the medical wards were given routine treatment, as determined by the department of internal medicine. Internal medicine residents and those from other subspecialties were responsible for patient care. OT and PT involvement occurred when prescribed by a doctor. Discharge planning for those on the medical wards involved hospital staff calling home care nurses to make arrangements, when necessary.
Trend, P., Kaye, J., Gage, H., Owen, C., & Wade, D. (2002)	4	4	1	**Intervention:** 6 weeks of intervention, based on individual needs of patients, as assessed at the first session. 6 sessions total, and each patient received 2 hours of individual attention. Team members included OT, PT, speech-language therapist, and nurse. Group activities included relaxation and educational sessions on Parkinson's disease from various professions. Caregivers also took part in aspects of the intervention.
Alexander, H., Bugge, C., & Hagen S. (2001)	4	3	4	OT, PT, dietitians, community nursing, podiatry, speech-language therapy. Analysis focused on relationship between intensity of rehabilitation services and functional outcome.
Finnerty, J. P., Keeping, I., Bullough, R. G. N., & Jones, J. (2001)	4	18	4, 5	**Intervention:** 6-week, outpatient pulmonary rehabilitation for patients with COPD involving OT, PT, respiratory specialist nurse, and dietitian. Patients received 2 visits per week (1 exercise, 2 education). OT provided referrals to social services and other agencies, as appropriate, gave advice on coping with low activity levels and loss of interest in leisure activities, due to breathlessness. **Control:** Routine outpatient care.

continued

Table 4-2 (continued)
Occupational Therapy Interventions Promoting Self-Care Outcomes

Author (Date)	Pop	DX	Setting	Intervention
Von Koch, L., de Pedro-Cuesta, J., Kostulas, V., Almazan, J., & Holmqvist, L. W. (2001)	--	3	3, 4	Patients were randomized (1:1) to a home rehabilitation group or routine rehabilitation group. **Intervention:** The home rehabilitation group program took place within the context of early discharge (when the patient was independent in toileting, according to the Katz ADL Index). This group was based on individual needs of patients, but duration of therapy did not exceed 4 months, post-discharge from hospital. **Control:** The routine rehabilitation group received rehabilitation in a stroke unit. Upon discharge, if deemed necessary by a specialist, participants received additional service from geriatric or rehabilitation departments, as inpatients or through day care.
Lin, J. H., Chang, C. M., Liu, C. K., Huang, M. H., & Lin, Y. T. (2000)	--	3	4	Comprehensive inpatient rehabilitation was multidisciplinary and involved medical doctors, PT, OTs, speech therapists, rehabilitation nurses, social workers, and psychologists.
Mayo, N. E., Wood-Dauphinee, S., Cote, R., Gayton, D., Carlton, J., Buttery, J., et al. (2000)	4	3	2, 3, 4	Participants were randomized to 1 of 2 groups. **Intervention:** Home care: Prompt discharge from acute care to home, with immediate follow-up from a multidisciplinary team, which involved nursing, OT, PT, speech therapy, and dietary consults. Intervention was 4 weeks, with services provided based on individual need. **Control:** Usual care group: Patients in this group experienced typical discharge planning and follow-up procedures. Patients accessed various services (OT, PT, speech therapy) through either extended acute care hospital stays, outpatient rehab, home care through community agencies, or private care (as arranged by patient).
McCabe, P., Nason, F., Turco, P. D., Friedman, D., & Seddon, J. M. (2000)	5	18	4	Optometry, OT, and social work. All patients participated in the standard vision rehabilitation program from the Massachusetts Eye and Ear Infirmary's Vision Rehabilitation Service. The program is aimed at helping patients use remaining vision to the fullest capacity. This included adjustment counseling and training in the use of optical and non-optical devices and adaptive techniques. Patients were randomly assigned to either family-focused or individual-focused intervention. In the family-focused intervention, family was included as much as possible in all aspects and was provided with additional educational opportunities. In the individual-focused intervention, the individual progressed through intervention without family involvement. OT role: Prescription of adaptive devices and teaching of techniques, energy conservation, and joint protection, etc.
Sulch, D., Perez, I., Melbourne, A., & Kalra, L. (2000)	4	3	3, 4	Patients were randomized to either a conventional multidisciplinary care or integrated care pathway group in a stroke rehabilitation unit. Integrated care pathway coordination was overseen by an experienced nurse. Both groups had access to an interdisciplinary team, which consisted of nurses, doctors, OT, PT, social work, and speech therapy. **Intervention:** Patients in the integrated care pathway group had their care managed using integrated care pathway principles of organization and care (i.e., coordination of therapeutic activities in a parallel, time-sensitive manner).

continued

Table 4-2 (continued)
Occupational Therapy Interventions Promoting Self-Care Outcomes

Author (Date)	Pop	DX	Setting	Intervention
Freeman, J. A., Langdon, D. W., Hobart, J. C., & Thompson, A. J. (1999)	4	5	4	Individualized, goal-oriented, inpatient, multidisciplinary, rehabilitation program.
Nikolaus, T., Specht-Leible, N., Bach, M., Oster, P., & Schlierf, G. (1999)	1	18	1, 3	Patients were randomly assigned to 1 of 3 groups: *Intervention:* Comprehensive geriatric assessment and further in-hospital and post-discharge follow-up by an interdisciplinary home intervention team. The home intervention team consisted of nurses, a PT, OT, social worker, and secretary. This team worked closely with hospital staff and the primary care doctor. *Control 1:* Comprehensive geriatric assessment with recommendation followed by usual care at home. *Control 2:* Assessment of ADL and cognition followed by usual hospital and home care.
DiFabio, R. P., Soderberg, J., Choi, T., Hansen, C. R., & Schapiro, R. T. (1998)	2	5	4	Multidisciplinary/extended outpatient rehabilitation program (5 hours, 1 day a week for 1 year) involving OT, PT, social work, chaplaincy-led support group, therapeutic recreation, and nutritional education. OT aimed to help clients maintain UE function for ADL and to enhance communication and attention span.
Mathiowetz, V., & Matuska, K. M. (1998)	2	5	4	A total rehabilitation program including OT, PT, nursing, nutrition, and pharmacological interventions. OT interventions included compensatory strategy training for self-care, home management, work and leisure activities, fatigue management education, activities and/or exercises to remediate decreased strength, endurance, range of motion, and coordination of UE. PT interventions included ambulation training with aids, stretching exercises to increase range of motion, and aerobic exercises to increase endurance and strength. Nursing taught self-management strategies for medication, bowel and bladder function, and encouraged independence. Neurologist adjusted medications. Speech- language pathology, nutritionist, and neuropsychologist provided services when required.
Widen Holmqvist, L. W., von Koch, L., Kostulas, V., Holm, M., Widsell, G., Tegler, H., et al. (1998)	4	3	3, 4	Patients were randomly assigned to either an early supported discharge program with rehabilitation at home or routine rehabilitation, which consisted of service in hospital, day care, and/or outpatient rehabilitation. *Intervention:* Home rehabilitation team consisted of 2 OTs, 2 PTs, 1 speech therapist, and a social worker, who worked in a consulting capacity. 1 therapist was assigned to act as case manager for the patient. Home rehab lasted for 3 to 4 months, and the program was individualized through consultation with team members, patient, and patient's family. Activities were task oriented and functionally based. If required, patients in the routine rehabilitation gorup were transferred to inpatient rehab or day care. *Control:* Routine rehab refers to "heterogeneous" intervention, which included best practice of hospital or outpatient care or that established during the study (i.e., electrical nerve stimulation or home-based rehabilitation initiated by the department of geriatrics).
Brosseau, L., Philippe, P., Potvin, L., & Boulanger, Y. L. (1996)	5	3	4	Acute inpatient rehabilitation involving OT and PT, as well as speech therapy. Rehabilitation sessions lasted 1 hour in length per session.

continued

Table 4-2 (continued)

OCCUPATIONAL THERAPY INTERVENTIONS PROMOTING SELF-CARE OUTCOMES

Author (Date)	Pop	DX	Setting	Intervention
Drummond, A. E., Miller, N., Colquohoun, M., & Logan, P. C. (1996)	--	3	4	Patients were randomly assigned to either a stroke unit or conventional ward, where they received OT. Nurses helped with washing and dressing intervention on the stroke unit.
Patti, F., Reggio, A., Nicoletti, F., Sellaroli, T., Deinite, G., & Nicoletti, F. (1996)	4	4	4	OT, PT, speech therapy. All patients in the first study and 12 patients in the second study were given inpatient physical rehabilitation for 4 weeks. 8 patients from the second study were used as controls. Thus, they received drug treatment only. The programs were individualized. Patients were assessed on function, and some were given programs similar to those of a "healthy individual." In contrast, lower functioning patients were given programs focused on assistive devices, movements to control rigidity, etc. The OT taught compensatory techniques related to self-care management, educated on assistive devices, and conducted a home visit at discharge. Patients were given anti-Parkinson drugs.
Przybylski, B. R., Dumont, E. D., Watkins, M. E., Warren, S. A., Beaulne, A. P., & Lier, D. A. (1996)	4	21	1	OT and PT, with OTA/PTA involvement as well. ***Intervention:*** The "enhanced" group received more hours of care, based on a 1 full-time equivalent OT and 1 full-time equivalent PT/50-bed ratio. Thus, this group had ongoing care, follow-up, and restorative intervention. ***Control:*** The control group received fewer hours of OT/PT, based on a 1 full-time equivalent OT and 1 full-time equivalent PT/200 bed ratio. Thus, this group received primarily consultative services.
Werner, R. A., & Kessler, S.(1996)	--	3	4	***Intervention:*** 12 weeks of outpatient rehabilitation. This consisted of 1 hour of OT and 1 hour of PT 4 times per week. Individual goals were established in team meetings, following an evaluation by OT, PT, and physiatrist. Goals were functionally based and aimed at walking, feeding, etc. Therapy included muscle retraining/facilitation, strengthening, and mobilization. ***Control:*** Did not receive any outpatient therapy.
Heinemann, A. W., Hamilton, B., Linacre, J. M., Wright, B. D., & Granger, C. (1995)	--	6, 7	4	Patients were involved in inpatient medical rehabilitation. OT, PT, psychology, vocational rehabilitation, social services, therapeutic recreation, speech therapy. (*Only speech, OT, PT, and psychology were included in analyses.)
Hui, E., Lum, C. M., Woo, J., Or, K. H., & Kay, R. L. (1995)	1	3	2, 4	***Control:*** Conventional inpatient rehab under the care of a neurologist or care under a team of geriatricians. Under the conventional care, patients received inpatient rehabilitation until a neurologist determined that they had reached their full potential, at which point they were discharged. ***Intervention:*** Patients who received care from the geriatric team were treated on the same rehabilitation ward, but were discharged as soon as they were considered capable of coping at home. They then continued rehabilitation in a day hospital. On the medical ward, both groups had equal access to PT and OT, and family and social services were arranged at discharge for both groups
Comella, C. L., Stebbins, G. T., Brown-Toms, N., & Goetz, C. G. (1994)	4	4	4	A physical rehabilitation/intervention program involving OT and PT. Intervention consisted of 69 repetitive exercises aimed at improving range of motion, endurance, balance, gait, and fine motor dexterity. The program was 1 hour per day, 3 times per week for 4 weeks. There were 2 intervention programs separated by 6 months. A cross-over design allowed participants not in the intervention to act as a control group. Participants were randomly assigned to the first or second intervention group. All patients were given anti-Parkinson medication.

continued

Table 4-2 (continued)

OCCUPATIONAL THERAPY INTERVENTIONS PROMOTING SELF-CARE OUTCOMES

Author (Date)	Pop	DX	Setting	Intervention
Kalra, L. (1994)	1	3	2, 4	Patients were randomly assigned to either a stroke unit or general wards. Regardless of setting, patients had access to OT and PT with OTA/PTA, as well as nursing. Other services that were available (as required) to patients included speech therapy, social work, and nursing home placement officers.
Dam, M., Tonin, P., Ermani, M., Pizzolato, G., Iaia, V., & Battistin, L. (1993)	4	3	4	Long-term rehabilitation (OT, PT, sometimes speech therapy). The OT intervention consisted of individual and group activities. Group activities were aimed at helping patients use learned skills in various environments as well as to promote socialization.
Gladman, J. R., Lincoln, N. B., & Barer, D. H. (1993)	4	3	3, 4	Patients discharged from the hospital were randomly assigned to either a home rehabilitation or conventional rehabilitation (hospital) group. *Intervention:* Home rehabilitation involved assessment and treatment by OTs and PTs, as well as arrangement of "other relevant help." Home rehabilitation was provided, in this context, for 6 months at which time those requiring further services were referred back to conventional care. *Control:* Group received conventional care through outpatient hospital-based rehabilitation. Patients who were discharged from health care of the elderly wards were generally referred to day hospitals. Those patients discharged from medical wards received outpatient PT and OT.
Johansson, K., Lindgren, I., Widner, H., & Wiklund, I. (1993)	--	3	4	Both groups received standard inpatient stroke rehabilitation, which involved daily OT and PT. *Intervention:* In addition, the acupuncture group received acupuncture treatment, which was started 4 to 10 days after stroke. Acupuncture was given for 10 weeks, twice a week to the affected and unaffected side using manual and electrical stimulation.
Melin, A. L., & Bygren, L. O. (1992)	4	18	3, 4, 5	*Intervention:* Patients were discharged as soon as home care was arranged through primary care and home assistance services. A few days after discharge, team and project physicians visited patients in their homes to assess medical and functional needs and to develop a treatment plan. The team had weekly interdisciplinary meetings to discuss patients' care, and patients had access to assistance 24 hours a day through a telephone service. Team members: Physicians, district nurses, OT, PT, home service assistants, geriatric psychiatrist (unclear if he or she saw patients). *Control:* Followed typical discharge and services. This included the possibility of various services including rehabilitation at a long-stay hospital, followed by home care or immediate home care after discharge, which did not involve the intervention program or 24-hour telephone line.
Montgomery Orr, P., & Bratton, G. N. (1992)	--	19	4	OT, PT, social work, rehabilitation nursing, rheumatologist. Patients took part in a 6-day inpatient program that involved education, exercise and mobility, achievement of independence in ADL, counseling, OT, and PT. Patients received 60 to 90 minutes of individual OT per day. The general goal of OT was to increase functional abilities in daily activities. Intervention included hand therapy, joint protection, energy conservation, exercise, adaptive equipment, and splinting.
Indredavik, B., Bakke, F., Solberg, R., Rokseth, R., Lund Haaheim, L., & Holme, I. (1991)	4	3	2	6 weeks of post-stroke OT and PT treatment. *Intervention:* A stroke unit. *Control:* General medical ward.

continued

Table 4-2 (continued)

OCCUPATIONAL THERAPY INTERVENTIONS PROMOTING SELF-CARE OUTCOMES

Author (Date)	Pop	DX	Setting	Intervention
Jongbloed, L., Stacey, S., & Brighton, C. (1989)	4	3, 16, 17	2	Upon admission to hospital, participants with CVA and a resulting weakness in the extremities on one side of their body were assigned to 1 of 2 OT treatment groups. The functional treatment group or the sensorimotor integrative treatment group. The intervention was 8 weeks long. Participants received 40 minutes of OT per day, 5 days per week during this time. They received help with self-care activities such as dressing their affected side and transfers using their unaffected side. Once the OT routine was established by the OT, a nurse's aide carried it out. Participants were also receiving medical care, nursing care, and PT during the study intervention period.
Ostrow, P., Parente, R., Ottenbacher, K. J., & Bonder, B. (1989)	4	3, 18	2	Hospital patients who were receiving rehabilitation services that included OT were compared to patients receiving rehabilitation without OT. Other rehabilitation services included PT, speech therapy, and vocational therapy. **Intervention:** Patients in the OT treatment group received at least 1.5 hours of OT over a period of 3 days during their hospital stay. **Control:** No OT.
Carlton, R. S. (1987)	5	21	3	Food service workers randomly assigned to intervention or control group. **Intervention:** Received body mechanics instruction taught by OT that was given 2 weeks before data were collected. Participants were videotaped practicing the techniques, and video was used to provide them with feedback. **Control:** Received no instruction.

Population: 1=geriatric (65+); 2=adult (25 to 64); 3=young adult (18 to 24); 4=adult and geriatric; 5=young adult, adult, and geriatric.

Diagnosis: 3=stroke; 4=Parkinson's disease; 5=multiple sclerosis; 6=spinal cord injury; 7=acquired brain injury; 8=dementia or Alzheimer's disease; 12=depression; 13=bipolar; 14=schizophrenia; 15=addiction/substance abuse; 16=upper extremity injury; 17=lower extremity injury; 18=other; 19=arthritis; 20=chronic pain; 21=no diagnosis; 22=joint replacement.

Setting: 1=long-term care; 2=acute care; 3=home care; 4=rehabilitation; 5=primary care.

Table 4-3

EVIDENCE OF EFFECTIVENESS OF OCCUPATIONAL THERAPY ON SELF-CARE OUTCOMES

Author (Date)	Major Results	Study Design	Sample Size	Conclusions and Limitations
Positive Effects—Randomized Controlled Trial				
Landi, F., Cesari, M., Onder, G., Tafani, A., Zamboni, V., & Cocchi, A. (2006)	No differences in the prevalence of clinical problems. Significant differences in transfers, locomotion, dressing, and personal hygiene p=0.005. OT should not be only considered for home interventions.	RCT	50	**Conclusions:** Older adults who had strokes fared better in their level of independence in ADL after receiving OT intervention that those who did not. **Limitations:** Small sample size; therapists involved were not blinded; outcomes after discharge were not examined.
Ryan, T., Enderby, P., & Rigby, A. S. (2006)	Results at the 3-month follow-up suggested that the stroke subgroup, receiving more intensive therapy, had more positive outcomes on both health-related quality of life and social participation compared to those stroke patients who received less intense intervention. When adjustments were made due to missing data, those stroke patients experiencing more intense therapy again had more positive outcomes on the anxiety and depression outcome measure compared to those with stroke in the control group. Upon adjustment, those in the intense therapy group with hip fracture also demonstrated more positive outcomes on the depression measure compared to those with hip fracture in the less intense group. No other significant differences were found between the two hip fracture subgroups.	RCT	160	**Conclusions:** Researchers suggest that therapists in the community focus more on therapy aimed at changing activity and social participation of patients and less on impairment. This focus may also lead to decreased depression; this reasoning may help to explain the results found in the study. **Limitations:** The researchers were unable to achieve a 2:1 (intensive/non-intensive therapy) ratio that they originally sought, small sample size/unable to obtain desired sample size, the nature of the intervention provided by therapists is not known.
Sanford, J. A., Griffiths, P. C., Richardson, P., Hargraves, K., Butterfield, T., & Hoenig, H. (2006)	Statistically significant increase in overall self-efficacy for treatment group (mean change 8.8, 95% CI 3.8 to 13.7). Televideo "just missed" statistical significance. Concluded that multi-factorial, individualized, home-based OT/PT improves self-efficacy in mobility-impaired adults.	RCT	65	**Conclusions:** The study indicates that OT/PT interventions increased overall self-efficacy for the treatment group. **Limitations:** Small and heterogeneous samples, limited statistical power, 20% dropout rate.

continued

Table 4-3 (continued)

EVIDENCE OF EFFECTIVENESS OF OCCUPATIONAL THERAPY ON SELF-CARE OUTCOMES

Author (Date)	Major Results	Study Design	Sample Size	Conclusions and Limitations
Positive Effects—Randomized Controlled Trial				
Thorsen, A., Widen Holmqvist, L., de Pedro-Cuesta, J., & von Koch, L. (2005)	SOC and MMSE scores were not significantly different between groups at 5-year follow-up and were similar to results obtained at baseline for each group. At 5 years, more patients were independent in ADL within the home rehabilitation group (HRG) compared to the conventional rehabilitation group (CRG) and showed more improvement in motor capacity. Both groups were similar in social activities as measured by the FAI, but the HRG was significantly more involved in activities such as washing dishes and reading books. In both groups, motor capacity scores were lower at 5 years than 1 year, compared to group baselines (p<0.001). In both groups, the number of patients becoming independent in ADL as measured by the Katz Extended ADL Index increased in the first 12 months post-stroke, but then decreased significantly (p=0.003 HRG, p=0.008 CRG) in both groups between 12 months and 5 years post-stroke. The HRG group showed better outcomes in manual dexterity, personal ADL function, 10-meter timed walking, and subjective dysfunction, although these results were not significant. Between 46 and 53 months, significantly more people survived in the HRG than the CRG (p=0.022).	RCT	54	***Conclusions:*** Early supported discharge, with pre-discharge care in an acute stroke unit and post-discharge treatment at home, has positive results on extended ADL function of patients up to 5 years after stroke. ***Limitations:*** Long length of follow-up (5 years) may mean that results are impacted by confounding variables and not just those of rehabilitation.

continued

Table 4-3 (continued)

EVIDENCE OF EFFECTIVENESS OF OCCUPATIONAL THERAPY ON SELF-CARE OUTCOMES

Author (Date)	Major Results	Study Design	Sample Size	Conclusions and Limitations
Positive Effects—Randomized Controlled Trial				
Caplan, G. A., Williams, A. J., Daly, B., & Abraham, K. (2004)	There was an insignificant trend to increased visits to general practitioner, emergency department, and outpatient clinics in the intervention group, during the first month. However, in the first 30 days after the emergency department visit, there were significantly fewer total admissions (emergency and elective) in the intervention vs. control group ($p=0.048$). However, there were no differences between groups in terms of emergency admissions in the first 30 days. There was a significant decrease in the number of intervention group patients admitted to the hospital as emergencies during the 18 months of follow-up ($p=0.0072$). There were no between-group differences in terms of nursing home admissions, and, at the end of the study, there were no differences in mortality rates. Those in the intervention group experienced better physical function, as measured by the BI, from baseline to 6 months compared to the control group ($p<0.001$). In terms of cognition, the control group demonstrated cognitive decline at 6 and 12 months, but the treatment group did not show cognitive decline until the 18-month follow-up.	RCT	739	***Conclusions:*** This study demonstrates that comprehensive geriatric assessment team with an interdisciplinary team can lead to better health and functional outcomes for geriatric patients discharged from the emergency department. ***Limitations:*** Risk of contamination because those in the control group may have been receiving comprehensive geriatric assessment-type services from other sources, follow-up assessors were not blinded to group membership.

continued

Table 4-3 (continued)

EVIDENCE OF EFFECTIVENESS OF OCCUPATIONAL THERAPY ON SELF-CARE OUTCOMES

Author (Date)	Major Results	Study Design	Sample Size	Conclusions and Limitations
Positive Effects—Randomized Controlled Trial				
Jousset, N., Fanello, S., Bontoux, L., Dubus, V., Billabert, C., Vielle, B., et al. (2004)	The functional restoration program (FRP) treatment group showed a non-significant trend toward fewer sick days at 6 month, compared to the active individual therapy (AIT) group (p=0.12). However, sick days did become significantly different between groups when "adjusted on the variable" related to ergonomic programs in the workplace. AIT participants worked more frequently in places that were enrolled in the regional ergonomics program. The FRP group had more involvement in sport and leisure activities than the AIT group at 6 months (p=0.02). As well, they had better physical capacity. At 6 months, job restrictions were more common in the FRP group than in the AIT group (p=0.03). Both groups reported improvement in self-confidence. However, improvements in physical capacity awareness (p=0.01) and body image were reported more often in the FRP group. When comparing baseline and 6-month outcomes within groups, it is evident that all "parameters" were significantly improved in the FRP group at 6 months. However, in the AIT group, social interest, endurance, anxiety-depression, and pain intensity were not significantly different from baseline. In both groups, there were decreases in the need for pain treatment, as well as decreased contact with family doctors (p<0.001) and specialists (p<0.01).	RCT	86	**Conclusions:** FRP had more of an impact on reducing sick days when adjustments for enrollment in an ergonomic workplace program were made. FRP participants also showed improved physical capacities in most dimensions compared to AIT patients. However, they did not differ in terms of flexibility and weight-lifting ability. **Limitations:** At the 6-month evaluation, PTs and the psychiatrist were not blind to the treatment groups to which participants belonged.

continued

Table 4-3 (continued)

EVIDENCE OF EFFECTIVENESS OF OCCUPATIONAL THERAPY ON SELF-CARE OUTCOMES

Author (Date)	Major Results	Study Design	Sample Size	Conclusions and Limitations
Positive Effects—Randomized Controlled Trial				
Lincoln, N. B., Walker, M. F., Dixon, A., & Knights P. (2004)	Comparison between groups at 6 months showed no significant differences in independence related to ADL or IADL function. There were also no significant between-group differences in mood, knowledge of stroke, or available stroke-related resources. In terms of satisfaction with services, the only significant difference was that those in the community stroke group were more satisfied with the emotional support they received compared to their conventional-group counterparts (p=0.02). When comparing between groups, in terms of caregiver outcomes, those caregivers with a patient in the community stroke team group were significantly more satisfied with overall services (p=0.01) as well as knowledge regarding stroke (p=0.03). The caregivers in the community stroke group also reported significantly less caregiver strain than those in the conventional group (p=0.03).	RCT	421	**Conclusions:** Rehabilitation provided by community stroke teams provide particular benefits to caregivers, in terms of reduction of strain and being more satisfied with services received. **Limitations:** Limited information was collected in terms of specific types of interventions received, self-report follow-up by mail led to some missing information and the possibility that those least satisfied with service would not reply, follow-up was limited to 6 months.
Liu, K. P., Chan, C. C., Lee, T. M., & Hui-Chan, C. W. (2004)	After completing the second and third weeks of training, the mental imagery group had significantly higher levels of performance than the retraining group (p=0.011, week 2). The mental imagery group also demonstrated higher levels of performance on the untrained tasks at the end of training (p<0.001) and on the tasks performed at 1-month following the intervention (p<0.001). In terms of cognitive and sensorimotor abilities, there were no significant between-group differences, as measured by the CTT and FMA subscales. However, the mental imagery group showed significantly greater improvement in CTT subscale scores over time than compared to the retraining group.	RCT	46	**Conclusions:** The results indicate a significant impact of mental imagery on improving task performance of "trained" as well as new tasks compared to patients in a control group. **Limitations:** The site of patients' brain lesions were not controlled for, small sample size, short follow-up period after intervention, previous experience and patient preference may have acted as a confounding variable, the degree to which patients engaged (actively) in the imagery processes was not controlled for.

continued

Table 4-3 (continued)

EVIDENCE OF EFFECTIVENESS OF OCCUPATIONAL THERAPY ON SELF-CARE OUTCOMES

Author (Date)	Major Results	Study Design	Sample Size	Conclusions and Limitations
Positive Effects—Randomized Controlled Trial				
MacPhee, A. H., Kirby, R. L., Coolen, A. L., Smith, C., MacLeod, D. A., & Dupuis, D. J. (2004)	"The control group's mean percentage score ± SD increased from 60.1% ± 14.4% to 64.9% ± 13.3%, an 8% improvement of the post-test relative to the pretest (p=0.01). The wheelchair skills training program (WSTP) group's mean score increased from 64.9% ± 9.4% to 80.9% ± 5.6%, a 25% improvement of the post-test relative to the pretest (p<0.000). The WSTP group showed significantly greater improvements than the control group (p<0.000). Among the specific skills, significantly greater improvements were seen in the WSTP group for the gravel and high-curb descent skills (p<0.001)."	RCT	35	***Conclusions:*** The WSTP is safe and practical and has a clinically significant effect on the independent wheeled mobility of new wheelchair users. ***Limitations:*** Small sample size; non-random sample; age-related factors may have contributed to difficulty performing a full wheelie; wheelchairs may have created skill limitations or affected some skill retention.
Pankow, L., Luchins, D., Studebaker, J., & Chettleburgh, D. (2004)	Following intervention, the treatment group had significantly better scores on the FIMBA living skills portion of the inventory and on the NAS2 compared to the control group (p=0.027, p=0.045, respectively). There was no significant post-intervention between group differences on the FIMBA motor and orientation section. Goal attainment for the treatment group was 29 of 30 and 1 of 30 for the control group (p<0.01). 30=number of goals per group.	RCT	20	***Conclusions:*** Results support previous literature, which suggests that independence in functional activities is not possible without rehabilitation. ***Limitations:*** Evaluators and participants were not blind to their group status, lack of significant difference between groups in terms FIMBA orientation and mobility may be a result of the inability to use the FIMBA to evaluate driving, which was a goal of some participants, participants in the control group had a pre-test/post-test gap of 2+ months.

continued

Table 4-3 (continued)
EVIDENCE OF EFFECTIVENESS OF OCCUPATIONAL THERAPY ON SELF-CARE OUTCOMES

Author (Date)	Major Results	Study Design	Sample Size	Conclusions and Limitations
Positive Effects—Randomized Controlled Trial				
Wade, D. T., Gage, H., Owen, C., Trend, P., Grossmith, C., & Kaye, J. (2003)	At both evaluation points, those in the treatment group performed faster on the Stand-Walk-Sit test compared to controls (p=0.044). At 24 weeks, the control group showed some decrease on this assessment compared to baseline. When looking at the SF-36 at "cross-over" point, the mental component summary scores and the general health and mental health subscales showed decreased scores for the intervention group while controls showed improvement. Results of the Caregiver Strain Index at the 24-week point showed that caregivers in the treatment group were experiencing more strain than those of control patients. At 6 months after the study began, deterioration was seen to be significant on the PD, the SF-36 physical component summary, and the general health subscale, as well as the EuroQol.	RCT	144	**Conclusions:** All patients showed deterioration across time, which was statistically significant at 6 months after treatment, and outcomes were largely not impacted by rehabilitation. However, some patients may have experienced small benefits in mobility due to treatment. **Limitations:** Cross-over design may have led to bias against treatment effects, patient awareness of disease progression may have led to increased depression that impacts significant findings on psychological and well-being measures, patient data lost during follow-up may have led to biased results and also impacted the statistical power of the study.
Saltvedt, I., Opdahl Mo, E. S., Fayers, P., Kaasa, S., & Sletvold, O. (2002)	Patients in the geriatric management and evaluation unit (GEMU) had a significantly longer length of hospitalization after inclusion, compared to the medical ward group (p<0.001). Groups did not differ in terms of diagnoses at discharge, with the exception of psychiatric diagnoses. The GEMU had significantly more psychiatric diagnoses than the medical ward group (p<0.001). Also, at discharge, the GEMU had a median of 3 diagnoses, whereas the medical ward group had 2 diagnoses. Mortality rates in the first year of follow-up were significantly lower for the GEMU group than the medical ward group (p=0.004 at 3 months; p=0.02 at 6 months; and p=0.06 at 12 months). Reduction in mortality was the greatest during the first 3 months. At 2-year follow-up, 50% of patients were dead in each group. In terms of causes of death, heart disease was the most common cause of death in both groups at 3 and 12 months. At 12 months, infectious disease was a more common cause of death in the GEMU group (p=0.04).	RCT	254	**Conclusions:** The researchers suggest that the reduction in mortality, seen in the GEMU group, is attributable to the treatment and assessment, as well as the organizational structure of care within the unit, which recognizes the potential of multiple difficulties/diagnoses in geriatric patients. **Limitations:** Death certificates may not be the most reliable way to obtain information about cause of death, sudden death without a known cause was registered (for the study) as cardiac death (n=7). This may have impacted the results.

continued

Table 4-3 (continued)

EVIDENCE OF EFFECTIVENESS OF OCCUPATIONAL THERAPY ON SELF-CARE OUTCOMES

Author (Date)	Major Results	Study Design	Sample Size	Conclusions and Limitations
Positive Effects—Randomized Controlled Trial				
Finnerty, J. P., Keeping, I., Bullough, R. G. N., & Jones, J. (2001)	The control group showed no significant difference in scores for symptoms, impacts on daily life, or integrated total scores on the SGRQ, as measured across the 6-month study period. The treatment group showed a significant reduction in total SGRQ scores at 12 weeks, compared to baseline ($p<0.001$). At 24 weeks, the treatment group also demonstrated a significant difference in mean total SGRQ scores, compared to baseline ($p<0.001$). Comparing changes from baseline scores to those at 12 weeks, between the active and control groups, there was a significant mean reduction in total scores, in favor of the treatment group ($p<0.01$). A similar significant difference was seen when comparing between-group scores at baseline to those at 24 weeks; the mean difference was a reduction in scores in favor of the active group ($p<0.02$). For the treatment group, there were significant reductions in all 3 components (symptoms, impacts on daily living, activity scores) of the SGRQ ($p<0.01$). After 12 weeks, a mean increase in walking distance for the active group was significantly greater than observed change in mean distance for the control group ($p<0.02$).	RCT	65	**Conclusions:** 6-week outpatient pulmonary rehabilitation program significantly increased patients' quality of life and was maintained for 6 months. Exercise tolerance was also increased and was maintained for at least 3 months. **Limitations:** The nature of pulmonary rehabilitation that should be offered was not fully addressed (i.e., which type and intensity of exercise is required to sustain improvement).

continued

Table 4-3 (continued)

Evidence of Effectiveness of Occupational Therapy on Self-Care Outcomes

Author (Date)	Major Results	Study Design	Sample Size	Conclusions and Limitations
Positive Effects—Randomized Controlled Trial				
Mayo, N. E., Wood-Dauphinee, S., Cote, R., Gayton, D., Carlton, J., Buttery, J., et al. (2000)	Results on the impact of physical health indicated a significant group effect, in that the home group had significantly higher scores than the usual care group across assessment points. Although physical health results were similar between groups at 1 month, at the 3-month evaluation, the home group's mean score was 5 points higher than the usual care group, and this was seen as a clinically important difference. There was no significant effect of group or time, when looking at the impact on mental health. In terms of the secondary health-related quality of life, the only between-group difference occurred on the Physical Role subscale, where the home group had significantly better results (p=0.0186). A time X group interaction indicated both groups improved over time, but the home group showed significantly more improvement(p<0.001). Both groups showed significant improvement across time on the measures of impairment (STREAM and TUG), as well as on the basic ADL measure. In terms of evaluating reintegration, the home group showed significantly more improvement from 1- to 3-month evaluations than the usual care group. The significance remained when adjustments were made for multiple comparisons (p<0.05).	RCT	114	***Conclusions:*** Researchers concluded that "prompt and supported discharge" led to better physical health and greater satisfaction with community reintegration following stroke. ***Limitations:*** Patients could not be blinded to the treatment that they were receiving, small sample size, patients without a caregiver were excluded.

continued

Table 4-3 (continued)

EVIDENCE OF EFFECTIVENESS OF OCCUPATIONAL THERAPY ON SELF-CARE OUTCOMES

Author (Date)	Major Results	Study Design	Sample Size	Conclusions and Limitations
Positive Effects—Randomized Controlled Trial				
Nikolaus, T., Specht-Leible, N., Bach, M., Oster, P., & Schlierf, G. (1999)	There was no significant difference between groups, in terms of mortality rate of new admissions to nursing homes or rate of hospital re-admissions. Fewer individuals in the treatment group needed assistance with IADL compared to those in the assessment and control groups. The intervention group had better functional abilities (p=0.03), higher scores on perceived health (p=0.04), and higher life satisfaction (p=0.04). They used more community resources compared to the other 2 groups (p<0.05). However, the intervention group demonstrated a mean net saving of approximately $4,000 per subject (per year) in the group, in part because of the decreased number of days spent in hospital.	RCT	545	**Conclusions:** Researchers concluded that length of hospital stay could be shortened by home intervention and that this intervention may also delay, but not prevent, admission to nursing homes. **Limitations:** Interviewers were not blinded to patients' treatment groups, patients and their "proxies" may have provided different information.
Widen Holmqvist, L. W., von Koch, L., Kostulas, V., Holm, M., Widsell, G., Tegler, H., et al. (1998)	At 3 months, patients in the home rehabilitation group (HRG) reported more dysfunction in communication (p=0.0150) and emotional behavior (p=0.0233) compared to the routine rehabilitation group (RRG) patients. At discharge, most patients were dependent, in terms of IADL function and to a greater extent (non-significant) for the HRG than RRG. At 3 months, patients in both groups demonstrated moderate to "almost complete" recovery of personal ADL function, total motor capacity, manual dexterity, walking, and linguistic ability. Overall, there was an 18% decrease in frequency of activities at 3 months compared to before stroke. With the exception of aphasic scores, the HRG demonstrated, non-significantly, better performance on the above-mentioned outcomes. Those in the HRG group experienced more frequent falls; however, the difference was not significant. The HRG spent significantly fewer days in hospital than the RRG (p=0.0008).	RCT	81	**Conclusions:** Home rehabilitation with early supported discharge reduced days spent in hospital but was not associated with significant differences in many functional outcomes compared to traditional rehabilitation. Non-significant between-group differences favored the home rehabilitation group, in terms of better outcomes. **Limitations:** Small sample size.

continued

Table 4-3 (continued)

EVIDENCE OF EFFECTIVENESS OF OCCUPATIONAL THERAPY ON SELF-CARE OUTCOMES

Author (Date)	Major Results	Study Design	Sample Size	Conclusions and Limitations
Positive Effects—Randomized Controlled Trial				
Drummond, A. E. R., Miller, N., Colquohoun, M., & Logan, P. C. (1996)	Total scores for the BI demonstrated significant between-group differences at 3 (p=0.02) and 6 months (p=0.01) but not at 12 months. Also, at 3 months, those in the stroke unit were more independent in feeding, dressing, grooming, and urinary continence. At 6 months, those in the stroke unit were more independent in grooming, feeding, and dressing compared to those on conventional wards, and at 12 months, the stroke unit group continued to be significantly more independent in dressing. Total scores on the self-care section of the Rivermead ADL Scale showed significant between-group differences in total score at 3 (p=0.03) and 6 (p=0.02) but not 12 months. In terms of subscales, the stroke unit group was more independent in eating, tooth brushing, dressing, and undressing at 3 months and more independent in tooth brushing 6 months. On the Rivermead ADL Scale (household section), there were significant between-group differences at 3 (p<0.001) and 6 months (p=0.01) but not at 12 months. Again, at 3 months, the stroke unit group was more independent than those on conventional wards in such things as making a snack and meal preparation, using money, and performing car transfers. At 6 months, the stroke group was significantly more independent in washing clothes and using money, and at 12 months, they were more independent in such things as preparing a meal and hot drink. The Extended ADL Scale revealed significant between-group differences in total scores at 6 (p=0.07) and 12 (p=0.03) but not at 3 months.	RCT	315	***Conclusions:*** Participants in the stroke unit consistently demonstrated more independence in ADL such as feeding, dressing, using money, and making a hot drink. However, some significant effects appeared to decrease over time. Researchers suggested that it is unclear what elements of the stroke unit led to a better outcome, but that it may be related to the involvement of OT. ***Limitations:*** No data on whether patients who were unavailable at each follow-up were different, in some regard, from those who we evaluated.

continued

Table 4-3 (continued)

EVIDENCE OF EFFECTIVENESS OF OCCUPATIONAL THERAPY ON SELF-CARE OUTCOMES

Author (Date)	Major Results	Study Design	Sample Size	Conclusions and Limitations
Positive Effects—Randomized Controlled Trial				
Patti, F., Reggio, A., Nicoletti, F., Sellaroli, T., Deinite, G., & Nicoletti, F. (1996)	In the first study, participants (all of whom had rehab) showed decreased UPDRS scores and increased FIM and BI scores between baseline and follow-up at the end of treatment (p<0.05). Patients also demonstrated a significant increase in walking speed. At the follow-up months after treatment had stopped, there was a tendency (not significant) toward deterioration, as seen by decreasing BI and FIM scores and increasing UPDRS, NUDS, WRS scores and mean ambulation times. In the second study, patients receiving rehabilitation performed better than controls in terms of ADL function between baseline and the first follow-up (p=0.048 FIM and 0.05 BI). The intervention group maintained these improvements across the study period. Over time, the control group had decreases in UPDRS and NUDS scores; there were also significant reductions in mean amplitude and step speed at the final evaluation (p<0.05). The treated group showed a decrease in UPDRS scores between baseline and the first follow-up (p<0.05), which lasted to 6 months. WRS and NUDS scores also showed a decrease for the treatment group, when comparing baseline to scores at the 6-month follow-up.	(1) RCT (2) Non-RCT	(1) 8 (2) 20	**Conclusions:** Researchers concluded that treatment in a rehabilitation program showed potential to increase functional independence and decrease Parkinson's disease disability. However, as per the first study, stopping treatment caused deterioration and a return to baseline scores. Results of the second study suggested similar results. **Limitations:** Small sample size, especially in creation of treatment and control groups.
Przybylski, B. R., Dumont, E. D., Watkins, M. E., Warren, S. A., Beaulne, A. P., & Lier, D. A. (1996)	Significant results suggest that enhanced care vs. routine care (OT/PT) is more effective in maintaining, promoting, or limiting decline in functional activities, as measured by the FIM and FAM (at 18 months F=0.062, 24 months F=0.074). The results of the COVS also suggest that the enhanced group had better mobility performance than the controls, with significance at 18 and 24 months (F=0.086, F=0.084, respectively). Results also indicate a net savings of $16,973 in nursing staff dollars, in terms of providing enhanced care to 30 nursing home residents at a 1:30 ratio compared to a 1:200 ratio over 2 years.	RCT	115	**Conclusions:** The treatment group, which received more OT/PT services, had better functional status, both overall as well as on many functional components, compared to the control group. Additionally, cost analysis revealed a cost savings in the enhanced care group compared to routine care. **Limitations:** Some or all of the calculated cost savings of enhanced care may be due to sampling error, the level of significance seen as acceptable appears to be adjusted, based on limited power.

continued

Table 4-3 (continued)

EVIDENCE OF EFFECTIVENESS OF OCCUPATIONAL THERAPY ON SELF-CARE OUTCOMES

Author (Date)	Major Results	Study Design	Sample Size	Conclusions and Limitations
Positive Effects—Randomized Controlled Trial				
Werner, R. A., & Kessler, S. (1996)	During the 3-month treatment period, the intervention group showed significant improvement in corrected motor scores, but the control group did not (p=0.03). After the initial change, further change was not seen in either group (3 to 9 months). Patients in the intervention group showed significant improvement in eating, bathing, dressing, tub and shower transfers, and stair climbing. The largest improvements were seen in bathing (p=0.03) and dressing UE (p=0.003) and dressing LE (p=0.004). The intervention group also showed improvement on the SIP, compared to controls (p=0.39, 0 to 3 months). During the first 3 months, the treatment group change in SIP was significant but the improvement from 3 to 9 months was not significant. Controls demonstrated non-significant improvement across time in SIP scores. There was a non-significant trend toward decreased depression in the intervention group and no change in the controls. When examining Brunnstrom's motor recovery ratings, the treatment group showed a significant improvement within the first 3 months and no significant improvement thereafter. The controls showed no change on Brunnstrom during the 9-month period.	RCT	49	***Conclusions:*** Researchers concluded that intervention for those who have experienced stroke can result in functional gains, which may be maintained for up to 6 months post-intervention. ***Limitations:*** Lack of intervention in the control group, high dropout rate in both groups (especially in controls).

continued

Table 4-3 (continued)

EVIDENCE OF EFFECTIVENESS OF OCCUPATIONAL THERAPY ON SELF-CARE OUTCOMES

Author (Date)	Major Results	Study Design	Sample Size	Conclusions and Limitations
Positive Effects—Randomized Controlled Trial				
Kalra, L. (1994)	At discharge, BI scores were significantly higher for the stroke unit (SU) group than the general ward (GW) group. Although median BI scores were similar at baseline, when measured across time (weekly), they were higher for the SU than GW group. During the "linear phase," the rate of functional change was slower in the GW than the SU group. Those in the SU had significantly shorter lengths of stay in the hospital compared to GW patients (p<0.001). Those in the GW group received significantly more PT than those in the SU group (p<0.05). There were no between-group differences in amount of OT received.	RCT	141	**Conclusions:** Researchers concluded that there was a more significant, faster functional recovery in those who received treatment in the SU compared to the GW group. **Limitations:** OTs were not blind to patient treatment group.
Johansson, K., Lindgren, I., Widner, H., & Wiklund, I. (1993)	Patients in both groups showed significant improvement up to 3 months in balance, mobility, and ADL function (p<0.0001). Those receiving acupuncture improved faster and more than controls (p<0.02 mobility at 1 and 3 months). They also showed more significant and rapid improvement in walking and balance, and faster improvement in ADL function—a difference that remained up to 12 months (p<0.0001, 12 months). Controls spent more time in geriatric rehabilitation and nursing homes compared to those in the acupuncture group. The acupuncture group also had better outcomes on several aspects of the QLI compared to controls at 3, 6, and 12 months (p=0.01 emotion at 3 months, p=0.003 mobility at 6 months).	RCT	78	**Conclusions:** The results revealed that those in the acupuncture group had faster and greater improvements in balance, mobility, ADL function, and quality of life compared to controls. **Limitations:** Lost participants at 12 months may have contributed to the inability to find significance in the quality of life scores, specifically related to social isolation and energy at 12 months.

continued

Table 4-3 (continued)

Evidence of Effectiveness of Occupational Therapy on Self-Care Outcomes

Author (Date)	Major Results	Study Design	Sample Size	Conclusions and Limitations
Positive Effects—Randomized Controlled Trial				
Melin, A. L., & Bygren, L. O. (1992)	Both groups showed significant improvement in personal ADL, IADL, cognition, social activities, and indoor and outdoor walking from baseline to follow-up (p<0.001). Social contacts increased for the team group (p=0.01) but did not change in the control group from baseline to follow-up. There were no between-group differences in terms of personal ADL, walking indoors, cognition, and social activities between baseline and follow-up. However, the intervention group showed significant improvement in IADL (p=0.04) and walking outdoors (p=0.03) from baseline to follow-up, compared to the control group. A between-group difference was seen in the number of diagnoses at 6 months, in that the control group displayed an increase, and the intervention group showed a decrease compared to baseline (p<0.001). It was also found that controls took more drugs at 6 months compared to those in the team group (p=0.05). It was found that hospitalized patients used more drugs than discharged patients at 6 months. At 6 months, a greater proportion of controls were in the hospital than those in the treatment group (p=0.03).	RCT	249	**Conclusions:** Results indicated the home-care program did appear to be significantly related to better medical and functional outcomes compared to typical care experienced by controls. Specifically, those in the treatment group had better IADL function and fewer medical diagnoses than controls at 6 months. **Limitations:** OT conducting follow-up assessments was aware of patients' status as either a control or treatment subject. Patients were also aware of their group assignment, and this may have created bias when completing follow-up evaluations.
Indredavik, B., Bakke, F., Solberg, R., Rokseth, R., Lund Haaheim, L., & Holme, I. (1991)	At the 6-week assessment: Morality rates were higher in the group treated on general medical wards compared to those in stoke units (p=0.02). Stroke unit treatment group had significantly higher mean scores on the BI (p=0.0014), and results showed a similar significant pattern at 52 weeks (p=0.001). Neurological scores were significantly higher for those treated in the stroke units compared to medical wards at both 6 (p=0.007) and 52 weeks (p=0.004). Those receiving treatment in the stroke unit spent significantly less time in institutions during the first year after stroke compared to the group treated in medical wards (p=0.004).	RCT	220	**Conclusions:** Researchers concluded that treatment in a stroke unit improves functional outcomes and reduces early mortality rates and need for institutionalization. **Limitations:** The researchers were not blinded to the patients' group membership.

continued

Table 4-3 (continued)

EVIDENCE OF EFFECTIVENESS OF OCCUPATIONAL THERAPY ON SELF-CARE OUTCOMES

Author (Date)	Major Results	Study Design	Sample Size	Conclusions and Limitations
Positive Effects—Randomized Controlled Trial				
Carlton, R. S. (1987)	The intervention group performed significantly better (p<0.001) than the control group on a novel task (during the body mechanics evaluation), but no differences were observed in the workplace.	RCT	30	***Conclusions:*** Participants who received body mechanics testing performed better than those who received no training during lab testing but this did not translate to their work environment. ***Limitations:*** Small sample size.
Positive Effects—Non-Randomized Controlled Trial				
Alexander, J. A., Lichtenstein, R., Jinnet, K., Wells, R., Zazzeli, J., & Liu, D. (2005)	The older the patient and the more days spent as an inpatient, the greater the ADL impairment at baseline (p<0.01 for number of days as an inpatient). Team size was not significantly correlated with ADL function at any point in time. Greater individual participation on cross-functional teams was significantly correlated with less ADL-related impairment at baseline, as well as decreased impairment across time for patients treated by a team (p<0.05). Higher team functioning was associated with higher ADL function at baseline (p<0.05) but not with improvement across time. Cross-functional team participation was positively correlated with ADL function across time. This result suggested that level of participation on a cross-functional team may aid or hinder ADL progress of clients and may impact client functioning more than team functioning.	Non-RCT	1638	***Conclusions:*** Patients with the poorest health status received the greatest amount of rehabilitation. Additionally, some types of rehab (OT, community nursing) are correlated with specific health outcomes. ***Limitations:*** Limited generalizability, study design: not possible to match organizational and patient characteristics across the duration of the study.
Unsworth, C. A., & Duncombe, D. (2005)	OTs at one hospital had more contact with clients to cause a statistically significant difference (p<0.001) in self-care. Length of stay and younger age did not significantly affect scores. Clients in both sites improved significantly between admission and discharge in all AusTOMs-OT domains (p<0.05). The AusTOMs-OT can be used to provide data for benchmarking purposes.	Non-RCT	82	***Conclusions:*** More client contact resulted in better self-care scores. AusTOMs-OT can be used to establish clinical benchmarks when comparing client outcomes. ***Limitations:*** Data collected on "number of OT contacts" did not include the nature or length of contact. There were many other health professionals involved so increased scores cannot be fully attributed to OT interventions.

continued

Table 4-3 (continued)

Evidence of Effectiveness of Occupational Therapy on Self-Care Outcomes

Author (Date)	Major Results	Study Design	Sample Size	Conclusions and Limitations
Positive Effects—Non-Randomized Controlled Trial				
Bode, R. K., Heinemann, A. W., Semik, P., & Mallinson, T. (2004)	When controlling for severity of stroke, longer hospital stays and more intense function-focused therapy was associated with greater-than-expected gains in mobility and self-care. However, when variables related to therapy were added to the model for cognition, results were not significant (p=0.06). Patients who improved more than expected in the area of self-care were less impaired at baseline, had longer hospital stays, and received higher average intensity of OT. In terms of mobility, variables that predict residual change scores are different for men and women. Men who had greater than expected gains in functional mobility had longer hospital admissions (t=3.93) and received more function-focused PT (t=3.23). In contrast, women who had greater than expected gains in mobility were less impaired at admission (as a significant predictor).	Non-RCT	198	***Conclusions:*** When controlling for severity of stroke, longer hospital stays and more intense function-focused therapy was associated with greater-than-expected gains in mobility and self-care. ***Limitations:*** Selection bias, measure of impact of speech-language pathology may not have been sensitive enough, therapy services addressed in the study may not be representative of national rehabilitation programs, residual change scores are relative and not as reliable as estimates at specific points in time.
Hastings, J., Gowans, S., & Watson, D. E. (2004)	Statistically significant results for all tests were set at p<0.05. Functional independence was significantly improved. Significant negative relationship between initial FIM scores and OT treatment intensity. Significant positive correlation between changes in FIM scores and OT time or OT attendances (but with outliers, OT time with FIM was p=0.10). Both OT (p=0.062) and PT (p=0.055) predicted FIM scores.	Non-RCT	23	***Conclusions:*** FIM scores improved significantly with positive correlation with OT attendances and time spent with OT. Individuals with lower function received more OT. ***Limitations:*** Because OT and PT occurred concurrently, it is hard to distinguish how each played a role in affecting FIM scores; small sample size; uncontrolled pre-test/post-test; no control group.

continued

Table 4-3 (continued)

EVIDENCE OF EFFECTIVENESS OF OCCUPATIONAL THERAPY ON SELF-CARE OUTCOMES

Author (Date)	Major Results	Study Design	Sample Size	Conclusions and Limitations
Positive Effects—Non-Randomized Controlled Trial				
Keren, O., Motin, M., Heinemann, A. W., O'Reilly, C. M., Bode, R. K., Semik, P., et al. (2004)	Impairment improved significantly between admission and discharge (p<0.001). However, there was no significant correlation between therapy intensity and improvement in impairment severity. This is true for all types of therapy. Function as measured by both OT and PT "therapy-measured function" improved between admission and discharge. Equivalent gains were made in both types of therapy, when comparing therapy-measured function at baseline and discharge for each therapy. This type of analysis was not conducted for speech therapy as the group receiving this therapy was considered to be too small. More intense OT was associated with greater motor (p=0.044) and cognitive gains (p=0.001). The other 2 therapies were not significantly correlated with any measure of gain.	Non-RCT	50	**Conclusions:** There was a significant reduction of impairment between admission and discharge. Functional abilities, as measured by the FIM, were also improved. Specifically relevant to OT was the fact that intensity of this therapy was positively correlated with motor and cognitive functions. **Limitations:** Limited generalizability (1 rehab center only), small sample size, co-linearity of predictors (i.e., motor and cognitive status) at admission places limitations on an "unambiguous" interpretation of outcomes.
Weiss, Z., Snir, D., Klein, B., Avraham, I., Shani, R., Zetler, H., et al. (2004)	Pre- and post-intervention results for the home rehabilitation group indicated improvement in some areas of mobility (bed position p=0.003; walking up stairs p=0.022), and ADL (function in kitchen p=0.001; drinking p=0.013). Improvements were also seen in some areas of range of motion (shoulder p=0.021, active elbow p=0.001). At 14 months post-stroke, the FAI scores were "slightly" higher for the home rehabilitation group than the institutional rehabilitation group (p=0.000). In a regression analysis, FAI scores were also significantly negatively correlated with hospitalization during follow-up (p=0.34).	Non-RCT	191	**Conclusions:** Home rehabilitation was an effective method in term of improving outcomes following stroke, as well as in terms of cost effectiveness, for the population studied. **Limitations:** Some limitations with the outcome measures, numerous differences between groups at baseline, selection bias, many participants lost to follow-up.

continued

Table 4-3 (continued)

EVIDENCE OF EFFECTIVENESS OF OCCUPATIONAL THERAPY ON SELF-CARE OUTCOMES

Author (Date)	Major Results	Study Design	Sample Size	Conclusions and Limitations
Positive Effects—Non-Randomized Controlled Trial				
Bohannon, R. W., Ahlquist, M., Lee, N., & Maljanian, R. (2003)	All selected independent variables were significantly correlated with function at discharge (p<0.001). However, the strongest predictor was function at admission; this relationship was positive and accounted for 78.8% of the variance of discharge function. In contrast, all other variables (age, stroke severity, therapy units, and longer stay) formed significant, inverse relationships function at discharge. However, patients with higher FIM scores at admission demonstrated less improvement over time of hospitalization. There was a weakly significant, positive relationship between number of therapy units (regardless of therapy type) and changes in function over time of hospital stay.	Non-RCT	451	**Conclusions:** Relatively short, acute hospitalization (M=5.5 days) can be associated with some increases in functional independence; this illustrates the value of rehabilitation services. **Limitations:** Correlational results only, specific interventions within disciplines were not described, and this could impact ability to replicate findings.
Jones, G. R., Miller, T. A., & Petrella, R. J. (2002)	85% of patients who were admitted to hospital from their homes were able to return home after inpatient rehabilitation. FIM discharged scores improved significantly during inpatient rehabilitation (p<0.001). This improvement was largely due to a significant improvement in motor FIM scores (p<0.001). Differences between admission and discharge scores of the cognitive FIM scale were not significantly different. Functional gains on the motor subscale of the FIM were supported by improved efficacy (p<0.001) and efficiency (p<0.001) as measured by MRFS. At discharge, mean scores for transfers and locomotion were significantly lower than those for self-care and sphincter control. The interview at 6-weeks post-discharge indicated that patients did not demonstrate further improvement in motor function at that point. Patients with shorter hospitalizations (less than 4 weeks) showed better response to rehabilitation in terms of MRFS efficacy and efficiency scores.	Non-RCT	100	**Conclusions:** Although FIM scores improved over the course of rehabilitation, patients were still dependent in areas of transfer mobility and locomotion. Thus, rehabilitation programs need to improve in order to address these areas more appropriately. **Limitations:** Follow-up information was only obtained from 44% of the study participants.

continued

Table 4-3 (continued)

EVIDENCE OF EFFECTIVENESS OF OCCUPATIONAL THERAPY ON SELF-CARE OUTCOMES

Author (Date)	Major Results	Study Design	Sample Size	Conclusions and Limitations
Positive Effects—Non-Randomized Controlled Trial				
Trend, P., Kaye, J., Gage, H., Owen, C., & Wade, D. (2002)	Significant benefits post-treatment were seen in health-related quality of life (p=0.001), patient-reported depression (p=0.029), mobility (timed walk; p=0.023), gait (p=0.031), voice (p<0.001), and articulation (p=0.007). Caregivers reported higher quality of life and less depression and anxiety than patients. However, caregivers did not show significant changes in these measures over the course of the study. A majority of patients and caregivers reported that they had increased knowledge of Parkinson's disease at the end of the program.	Non-RCT	118	**Conclusions:** The multidisciplinary program provided benefits to patients as well as caregivers, despite caregivers not demonstrating significant change in response to the outcomes measured. **Limitations:** Lack of control group, short-term nature of the study, and lack of follow-up.
Alexander, H., Bugge, C., & Hagen S. (2001)	All 6 types of rehabilitation were associated with decreased disability scores (BI) in the first 3 months (p<0.01 for PT, OT, speech-language therapy, dietitian) post-stroke. Only some of the items on the Medical Outcome Study SF-36 were significantly correlated with types of rehabilitation utilized. For example, community nursing was associated with improved mental health (p=0.011 at 1 month) and social functioning (p=0.133 at 1 month) between 1 and 3 months post-stroke.	Non-RCT	152	**Conclusions:** OT was significantly correlated with decreased body pain and with improved physical functioning between 1- and 3-month assessments. Patients rated as most disabled, with poorest social and physical functioning, received the most rehabilitation (OT, PT, dietitian, speech-language therapy). **Limitations:** Study design did not allow for causation to be established, small sample size, smaller sample size in some intervention groups than others (i.e., podiatry).

continued

Table 4-3 (continued)
EVIDENCE OF EFFECTIVENESS OF OCCUPATIONAL THERAPY ON SELF-CARE OUTCOMES

Author (Date)	Major Results	Study Design	Sample Size	Conclusions and Limitations
Positive Effects—Non-Randomized Controlled Trial				
Lin, J. H., Chang, C. M., Liu, C. K., Huang, M. H., & Lin, Y. T. (2000)	Results demonstrated a significant difference between admission and discharge scores on FIM subscales (i.e., self-care, transfer, sphincter control, social cognition, total $p<0.0001$, for all). Only rehabilitation stay and motor recovery stages of the affected limb were significant predictors of rehabilitation efficiency ($p<0.05$). However, significant correlations with rehabilitation effectiveness included age, motor recovery stage of the affected limb, FIM admission scores on self-care sphincter control, and transfers ($p<0.05$). Better rehabilitation efficiency was predicted by shorter stay and higher arm motor recovery stages. Higher arm motor recovery stage and younger age was associated with better rehabilitation effectiveness and explained 24% of the variance of effectiveness. In terms of nominal variables evaluated, sensory impairment was the only one significantly correlated with both rehab efficiency and effectiveness ($p<0.05$). Given the variance that remained unaccounted for, the researchers suggest that factors unassociated with medical, rehabilitation, or demographics (as examined in this study) are associated with rehabilitation efficiency and effectiveness. Personal and socio-cultural factors may be among the unexplored factors associated with unaccounted for variance.	Non-RCT	110	**Conclusions:** Shorter inpatient stay and higher arm motor recovery stage predicted better rehabilitation efficiency, although a large amount of variance remained unaccounted for. Younger age and higher arm motor recovery stage was associated with better rehabilitation effectiveness. **Limitations:** Assessing function (with the FIM) 48 hours after discharge may not have been associated with a "plateau" in recovery status (related to fixed insurance reimbursement).

continued

Table 4-3 (continued)

EVIDENCE OF EFFECTIVENESS OF OCCUPATIONAL THERAPY ON SELF-CARE OUTCOMES

Author (Date)	Major Results	Study Design	Sample Size	Conclusions and Limitations
Positive Effects—Non-Randomized Controlled Trial				
McCabe, P., Nason, F., Turco, P. D., Friedman, D., & Seddon, J. M. (2000)	Looking at the entire population, there were significant gains across assessment times in terms of visual capacity (p=0.0001), as measured by the FVPT. There were significant decreases across time in terms of dependency (p=0.01, FAQ) and in difficulty performing tasks (p=0.03) as measured by self-report. Baseline vision did not significantly predict ability to improve level of function. There was no significant difference between the family and individual-focused groups in terms of functional change scores. There was a non-significant trend toward higher FVPT scores in the family-focused group, relative to the individual group.	Non-RCT	97	**Conclusions:** The intervention program using optometry, OT, and social work has benefits for patients' functional outcomes, when measured both subjectively and objectively. Although involvement of family did not statistically significantly impact patient outcomes, the experiences from a clinical perspective were reportedly beneficial. **Limitations:** Limited power, related to sample size, a key outcome measure was a new tool with limited prior use, dropouts were less educated than those who completed the program, making generalizations more difficult.
Freeman, J. A., Langdon, D. W., Hobart, J. C., & Thompson, A. J. (1999)	Improvements were seen in all measures during inpatient rehab, except EDSS and FS scores, which deteriorated over the course of 12 months. LHS and FIM scores, which measured handicap and disability, respectively, declined after discharge from inpatient rehab and remained only slightly above baseline at 9- and 12-month assessments. 51% of patients who increased in FIM scores peaked at discharge. Over 12 months, 10 of these patients showed a marked deterioration in function, as classified as a loss of 15 or more points on the FIM (n=41). Improvements in the physical component scores of the health-related quality of life lasted for at least 10 months after discharge. GHQ scores demonstrated sustained improvement across the 12-month study period. For example, 74% of patients reported emotional disturbance (>5 GHQ points) at admission, while this number had decreased to 47% at 12 months. SF-36 scores showed the greatest improvement at 3 months when examining the physical dimension and the greatest improvement at 6 months when looking at the mental dimension. Wide CIs (95%) suggest that estimates of duration and carry-over of treatment are imprecise and indicate variation between individual results.	Non-RCT	50	**Conclusions:** Researchers concluded that there needs to be continuity of care to ensure that benefits seen in rehabilitation are carried over to community. **Limitations:** Selection bias, deterioration in scores after discharge may be due to the fact that it is difficult to transfer skills/benefits of the inpatient rehabilitation environment to the community/home. The FIM measures performance (what the patient did). It does not accurately reflect abilities the patient possessed. Design made it impossible to exclude extraneous variables, which may have impacted results.

continued

Table 4-3 (continued)

EVIDENCE OF EFFECTIVENESS OF OCCUPATIONAL THERAPY ON SELF-CARE OUTCOMES

Author (Date)	Major Results	Study Design	Sample Size	Conclusions and Limitations
Positive Effects—Non-Randomized Controlled Trial				
DiFabio, R. P., Soderberg, J., Choi, T., Hansen, C. R., & Schapiro, R. T. (1998)	Patients who participated in this outpatient rehabilitation program had fewer symptoms, less fatigue (p=0.004), and a lower rate of decline in physical function compared to participants on the waiting list.	Non-RCT	50	**Conclusions:** Improvements seen within the treatment group may be attributable not only to the intervention's focus on maintenance of physical function, but also to the social and environmental support provided. **Limitations:** Patients not randomly assigned to treatment or control, significant attrition rates, small sample size, changes that occurred in each group between baseline and 1 year were not accounted for.
Mathiowetz, V., & Matuska, K. M. (1998)	Participants who were in the rehabilitation program improved significantly between admission and discharge for self-care activities and continued to improve significantly up to 6 weeks post-discharge. 85% of the equipment prescribed by OTs was used, and 94% was found to be effective. 100% of the participants were satisfied with OT services (p<0.05).	Non-RCT	30	**Conclusions:** Those who received the rehabilitation program improved significantly between discharge and 6 weeks post-discharge for most self-care activities. 100% of participants were satisfied with OT services and felt the equipment was effective. **Limitations:** No control group; raters were not blinded; dropouts were not reported.

continued

Table 4-3 (continued)

EVIDENCE OF EFFECTIVENESS OF OCCUPATIONAL THERAPY ON SELF-CARE OUTCOMES

Author (Date)	Major Results	Study Design	Sample Size	Conclusions and Limitations
Positive Effects—Non-Randomized Controlled Trial				
Brosseau, L., Philippe, P., Potvin, L., & Boulanger, Y. L. (1996)	Results suggested that age (B=0.59, alpha=0.05) was a significant predictor of length of stay in that older patients had longer lengths of stay. Also functional scores (B=−0.30) and balance status (B=−0.13), as assessed 1 week after admission to the rehabilitation unit, significantly predicted length of stay. Those with better functional scores and balance at follow-up tended to have significantly shorter stays in the rehab unit. Patients with perceptual problems (B=0.19) had longer lengths of stay, compared to those without perceptual difficulties. These 4 aforementioned variables account for 44% of the variance, when examining the length of stay outcome. The following were indirect predictors of length of stay: Rehabilitation program predicted functional scores at the 1-week assessment, in that a more intense program contributed to better functional outcomes. Functional and motor scores at admission impacted functional ability at 1 week. Those with better functional and motor ability had shorter lengths of stay. However, the rehab program was a relatively weak predictor of length of stay. Functional status at admission contributed to 68.7% of the total variance. Communication problems had the most significant impact on the rehabilitation program. Those with communication problems received more intense rehabilitation compared to older patients or those with medical complications. Researchers suggest that, based on these results, patients with functional, balance, and/or perceptual problems should receive more intense rehabilitation in order to reduce length of stay.	Non-RCT	152	**Conclusions:** Better functional status 1-week after admission to rehabilitation and balance status were associated with shorter lengths of stay. Additionally, perceptual status was a significant contributor to length of stay. Those with perceptual problems had longer stays than those with higher perceptual abilities. **Limitations:** Study design does not allow for use of a control group; relatively short time between initial assessment and follow-up.

continued

Table 4-3 (continued)
EVIDENCE OF EFFECTIVENESS OF OCCUPATIONAL THERAPY ON SELF-CARE OUTCOMES

Author (Date)	Major Results	Study Design	Sample Size	Conclusions and Limitations
Positive Effects—Non-Randomized Controlled Trial				
Comella, C. L., Stebbins, G. T., Brown-Toms, N., & Goetz, C. G. (1994)	Results indicated that, after rehabilitation, participants showed improvement in total UPDRS scores (p=0.002). Motor and ADL sub-sections of the UPDRS also showed improvement when assessed immediately following intervention (p=0.007, p=0.005, respectively). Specifically within the motor section, the factors associated with rigidity and bradykinesia were significantly improved after rehabilitation. Timed finger tapping as well as GDS scores were not significantly different from baseline to the post-intervention assessment. At the 6-month evaluation, scores for UPDRS (total), motor, and ADL had returned to baseline.	Non-RCT	16	***Conclusions:*** Benefits to "active" rehabilitative therapy were seen; however, when this therapy ceased, patients returned to baseline function. ***Limitations:*** Small sample size, limited discussion of results as related to outcomes of control group.

continued

Table 4-3 (continued)

EVIDENCE OF EFFECTIVENESS OF OCCUPATIONAL THERAPY ON SELF-CARE OUTCOMES

Author (Date)	Major Results	Study Design	Sample Size	Conclusions and Limitations
Positive Effects—Non-Randomized Controlled Trial				
Dam, M., Tonin, P., Ermani, M., Pizzolato, G., Iaia, V., & Battistin, L. (1993)	At the end of the first year of study, significant improvements were seen in mean BI and HSS scores compared to mean scores at entry. These results were expressed as a 65% improvement in mean BI scores and a 42% improvement in mean HSS scores. No similar improvement was seen in these mean scores thereafter. Functional improvement: 25% of patients reached a "good level" of independence at the 6-month evaluation, as indicated by a score of more than 70 on the BI. 43% of patients reached this "good level" of independence at the 9-month evaluation, and, by the 24-month evaluation, 79% of patients had a score of more than 70 on the BI. Ability to walk: At the 6-month evaluation, 18% of patients regained their ability to walk, as measured by the HSS gait scores. At the 24-month evaluation, 74% of patients had regained the ability to walk. Approximately 10% of patients obtained the ability to walk (HSS gait) and a "good level of functional independence" (BI) in the second year of therapy. At 3- and 12-month assessments, patients who had suffered a hemorrhagic stroke were less compromised than those with ischemic stroke. By the end of the study, this significant difference did not exist. Sphincter control was also significantly inversely correlated with outcome measures.	Non-RCT	51	***Conclusions:*** Patients with severe disabilities at 3 months post-stroke may attain functional independence in response to long-term rehabilitation (results not significant). Functional improvement was greater than neurological improvement. ***Limitations:*** Correlational results only.

continued

Table 4-3 (continued)

EVIDENCE OF EFFECTIVENESS OF OCCUPATIONAL THERAPY ON SELF-CARE OUTCOMES

Author (Date)	Major Results	Study Design	Sample Size	Conclusions and Limitations
Positive Effects—Non-Randomized Controlled Trial				
Montgomery Orr, P., & Bratton, G. N. (1992)	The disability index was significantly lower at the discharge assessment than at baseline (p=0.005). Disability index scores were also lower at final follow-up than at discharge (p=0.025). Self-assessed pain severity also decreased over the course of intervention (p=0.005). Pain severity was also lower at the 5- to 10-week follow-up than it was at discharge, but the difference was not significant. Between admission (baseline assessment) and discharge, patients also reported needing significantly less help from others, in all evaluated tasks, except for errands/chores (i.e., p=0.0000 grooming, p=0.0000 arising, p=0.0192 eating, p=0.0000 gripping, p=0.0013 hygiene, p=0.0009 reaching). Decreased number of participants at follow-up did not allow for any correlations to be "sufficiently established" in terms of examining assistance.	Non-RCT	36	***Conclusions:*** Based on patients' self-assessments, there were significant increases in functional ability following the rehabilitation program. Patients also reported significant decreases in pain and the need for assistance in daily activities, as assessed at the time of discharge. ***Limitations:*** No control group, high attrition rate for follow-up, limited time for follow-up.
No Effect				
Storr, L. K., Sorensen, P. S., & Ravnborg, M. (2006)	There were no significant differences between groups on any of the outcome measures. However, there was a trend in terms of bodily pain, with benefit seen for the control group. In terms of 9HPT (right arm) and EDSS results, a non-significant benefit was seen for intervention vs. control group. The EDSS result may suggest some improvement in terms of ambulation.	RCT	233	***Conclusions:*** There was no significant impact of multidisciplinary rehabilitation. ***Limitations:*** Large difference between number of participants in the 2 groups, low recruitment level/ insufficient statistical power, limited time period for study.

continued

Table 4-3 (continued)

EVIDENCE OF EFFECTIVENESS OF OCCUPATIONAL THERAPY ON SELF-CARE OUTCOMES

Author (Date)	Major Results	Study Design	Sample Size	Conclusions and Limitations
No Effect				
McNaughton, H., DeJong, G., Smout, R. J., Melvin, J. L., & Brandstater, M. (2005)	The New Zealand population was older and prior to stroke was more dependent in ADL and mobility functions than the US population. The US population was significantly more likely to be diagnosed with a mental health disorder and/or depression (p<0.001, in both cases). At the time of admission to rehabilitation facilities, the US group showed a non-significant trend toward lower mean FIM scores and significantly poorer scores on the CSI (p<0.001). Length of stay in the rehabilitation facility was significantly shorter for US patients, compared to NZ patients. However, during the stay, US patients spent significantly more time with a PT and OT (p<0.001, for OT and PT) compared to the NZ group. In terms of intervention, NZ physiotherapists spent more time in assessment and lower level mobility activities, whereas US therapists spent a greater amount of time in higher level mobility activities, such as transfers. NZ OTs spent more time in assessment (also home assessment). US OTs spent more time than NZ counterparts on upper limb activities. Overall, NZ therapists (all 3 disciplines) spent more time on assessment and non-functional activities compared to US therapists. At the time of discharge, more NZ patients were going to institutional care (p=0.006). US patients showed greater improvement in FIM (p<0.001) and CSI scores during admission. However, mean FIM scores at the time of discharge were similar across groups (US M=87.2, NZ M=85.6).	Non-RCT	NZ n=130 US n=1161	**Conclusions:** Results suggest that rehabilitation practices vary in a number of ways between the 2 countries and that intervention activities, as well as intensity of intervention, may impact outcomes. **Limitations:** Differences in age between the US and NZ populations may have had a confounding influence, unclear whether the rehabilitation facilities assessed in this study were representative of rehabilitation practices within each respective country, more NZ patients lived alone before onset of stroke, which may explain why NZ patients were more likely to proceed to institutionalized care, compared to US patients.

continued

Table 4-3 (continued)
EVIDENCE OF EFFECTIVENESS OF OCCUPATIONAL THERAPY ON SELF-CARE OUTCOMES

Author (Date)	Major Results	Study Design	Sample Size	Conclusions and Limitations
No Effect				
Yagura, H., Miyai, I., Suzuki, T., & Yanagihara, T. (2005)	At baseline, there were no significant differences between groups in terms of FIM or SIAS scores. There were also no differences between groups after rehabilitation based on discharge FIM and SIAS evaluations. Length of stay, cost of hospitalization per day, and discharges to home did not differ significantly between groups. When examining outcomes based on baseline level of disability, those with severe disabilities in the general rehabilitation ward (GRW) were more likely than their counterparts in the stroke rehabilitation unit (SRU) to go to chronic care or nursing homes (p<0.001). In fact, all those with severe disability in the GRW were transferred to chronic care hospitals or nursing homes. However, there was no significant difference in FIM or SIAS scores. For those with mild or moderate disability, there were no between-group differences (SRU or GRW) in length of stay, FIM, SIAS, or discharge location.	Non-RCT	178	**Conclusions:** Researchers suggest that those with severe disability require more preparation in terms of discharge. Thus, these patients benefit from weekly interdisciplinary conferences of the SRU, as it appears to play an important role in facilitating discharges home. **Limitations:** Patients were assigned to SRU or GRW groups, based on bed availability; thus, they were not completely randomly assigned.
Fleming, S. A., Blake, H., Gladman, J. R. F., Hart, E., Lymbery, M., Dewey, M. E., et al. (2004)	No significant differences between groups in terms of survival and rates of residential or nursing care or living at home at either 3 or 12 months. No significant difference between groups on the BI, Nottingham Extended ADL Scale, or GHQ-12 scores. Those in the treatment group (care home rehabilitation services [CHRS]) spent fewer days in the hospital (mean number of hospital bed days saved at 3 months was 21.1 and by 12 months was 27.6). However, the treatment group took significantly longer to return to their homes after admission and by 12 months had spent a mean of 19.1 more days in the hospital or CHRS than controls.	RCT	165	**Conclusions:** Researchers concluded that CHRS involvement did not reduce rates of placement in long-term or nursing residence. Nor did it have significant impacts on psychological well-being or activity levels. Although the treatment group had decreased hospital stays, they had more days in CHRS. Thus, demand for services was shifted from institution to other social services. **Limitations:** The study did not meet the predetermined sample size, which was seen as necessary to ensure sufficient statistical power, CHRS did not consist of "true" multidisciplinary teams, the amount/level of rehabilitation services provided may have been too low to significantly impact health outcomes in the treatment group.

continued

Table 4-3 (continued)

EVIDENCE OF EFFECTIVENESS OF OCCUPATIONAL THERAPY ON SELF-CARE OUTCOMES

Author (Date)	Major Results	Study Design	Sample Size	Conclusions and Limitations
No Effect				
Alvund, K., Jepsen, E., Vass, M., & Lundemark, H. (2002)	Baseline measures indicated that control and intervention groups were similar, but at follow-up, those in the intervention group showed more improvement, as measured by the BI, although the difference was not significant. A significant effect was found for the intervention group when analyses were restricted to those discharged from medical wards. Also, fewer patients in the intervention group demonstrated a decline in function, as compared to controls. Those discharged from geriatric wards did not show similar significant results. There was no difference between re-admission status for those receiving intervention vs. controls. Patients from medical wards, who had intervention, were less likely to be re-admitted compared to medical ward controls. However, the difference was not significant.	RCT	149	**Conclusions:** Although many results failed to reach significance, the researchers suggest that the study highlights many important trends, which warrant further investigation with larger samples. **Limitations:** Small sample size, a sizable number of patients were excluded because they were considered too high functioning, researchers do not know the length of stay in the group of those excluded vs. those included.
Naglie, G., Tansey, C., Kirkland, J. L., Ogilvie-Harris, D. J., Detsky, A. S., Etchells, E., et al. (2002)	A greater proportion of patients in the treatment group were alive, had no change in residence, and had no decline in ambulation or transfer status at both 3 and 6 months, compared to controls. However, analyses indicated that these were not significant differences at either time point. Those in the treatment group received significantly more PT than the control group (p<0.001), and more treatment group patients received OT, dietitian, or social work services than compared to the control group. The treatment group also had a significantly longer length of stay in the facility than controls (p<0.001). A subgroup analysis involving elderly with cognitive impairment showed a non-significant trend toward improvement of outcome measures for those receiving interdisciplinary care.	RCT	279	**Conclusions:** This randomized controlled trial failed to find significant differences between interdisciplinary and typical care, in terms of mortality rates, residential change, mobility, transfers, and ADL function at 3 and 6 months postoperatively. **Limitations:** Limited statistical power, heterogeneous sample.

continued

Table 4-3 (continued)

EVIDENCE OF EFFECTIVENESS OF OCCUPATIONAL THERAPY ON SELF-CARE OUTCOMES

Author (Date)	Major Results	Study Design	Sample Size	Conclusions and Limitations
No Effect				
Von Koch, L., de Pedro-Cuesta, J., Kostulas, V., Almazan, J., & Holmqvist, L. W. (2001)	At the 1-year follow-up, there were no significant differences in any of the patient outcome measures or in self-reported number of falls. Number of deaths or "dependencies" was non-significantly lower in the home rehabilitation group (HRG) (25%) than in the routine rehabilitation group (RRG) (44%) (p=0.074). In terms of resource use, there was a significant difference in number of days spent during the initial hospitalization; total number of "bed days" during the first year were significantly lower for the HRG group vs. the RRG group (p=0.002). There were also significant differences in where the groups obtained various services. The HRG had more visits to outpatient primary care nurses (p=0.03) and home rehabilitation (p<0.001) compared to the RRG. In contrast, the RRG had higher attendance at the day hospital (p<0.001), hospital-based OT (p=0.02), and private practice PT (p=0.03). Cost comparison of health and rehabilitative care after 1 year indicated a between-group difference of approximately 2,300 Euros per patient, with the cost being less for the HRG. There were no significant between-group differences in terms of the need for home adaptation.	RCT	83	***Conclusions:*** Results suggest that early supported discharge and home rehabilitation are as effective as routine care for patients with moderate post-stroke impairment. ***Limitations:*** The number of variables being evaluated, relative to the sample size, may have limited the potential for finding significant results, detail on intervention limited.

continued

Table 4-3 (continued)

EVIDENCE OF EFFECTIVENESS OF OCCUPATIONAL THERAPY ON SELF-CARE OUTCOMES

Author (Date)	Major Results	Study Design	Sample Size	Conclusions and Limitations
No Effect				
Sulch, D., Perez, I., Melbourne, A., & Kalra, L. (2000)	Although the difference was not significant, the integrated care pathway (ICP) group spent an average of 5 more days in the hospital compared to the rehabilitation group. Also, more ICP patients died compared to those in the conventional group (most after discharge); however, the difference was not significant. More patients in the conventional group were institutionalized compared to the ICP group, but not significantly so. The conventional group demonstrated significantly "faster" functional improvement between the 4- and 12-week assessments than the ICP group (p<0.01). Both groups demonstrated a decline in depression and anxiety scores over the course of the study. Both groups showed a significant improvement in quality of life as measured between the 4th and 26th week (p<0.005). In the conventional care group, patients had higher quality of life scores compared to the ICP group by the 26th week.	RCT	152	***Conclusions:*** No significant benefit to ICP over conventional care was demonstrated. Both groups showed decreased anxiety and quality of life over the course of study. Those in the conventional group demonstrated higher quality of life scores and faster functional improvements at some time points in the study. ***Limitations:*** Measures may have lacked necessary degree of sensitivity to detect change.

continued

Table 4-3 (continued)
EVIDENCE OF EFFECTIVENESS OF OCCUPATIONAL THERAPY ON SELF-CARE OUTCOMES

Author (Date)	Major Results	Study Design	Sample Size	Conclusions and Limitations
No Effect				
Heinemann, A. W., Hamilton, B., Linacre, J. M., Wright, B. D., & Granger, C. (1995)	Patients who had greater motor abilities at admission received more intense psychology (B=0.57) and speech therapy (B=0.49), but not OT. Those with greater cognitive impairment at admission received more intense speech therapy (B=−0.42). Greater intensity of all therapy was associated with greater motor function at admission, younger age, uninterrupted program, and longer onset-admission interval. OT, PT, and speech intensity were not related to any outcomes in patients with TBI. However, intensity of psychology intervention was related to cognitive outcomes in patients with TBI, in the sense that those receiving more intense intervention had greater cognitive function at discharge (B=016); they also made more efficient gains in cognition (B=0.22) and achieved more of the potential gain (B=0.23). Longer length of stay was only significantly associated with achievement of more of the calculated potential cognitive gain (B=0.31). Interruption of rehabilitation was correlated with poorer outcomes for all measures, except for achievement of potential motor gains. Speech therapy, OT, and PT were not significant in predicting any outcomes in the TBI or SCI group.	Non-RCT	246	**Conclusions:** Improvement without significant correlation to therapy may be related to concepts of spontaneous recovery. **Limitations:** No cross-validation with a sample of other hospitals; therapy may not have reflected activities measured by the FIM.
Hui, E., Lum, C. M., Woo, J., Or, K. H., & Kay, R. L. (1995)	At both assessment periods, there was no significant difference between overall BI means between groups. Both groups showed improved BI scores at 3 months. An analysis of the group with BI scores of 15+ demonstrated a significantly higher BI score in the day hospital group than in the conventional group (p=0.04) at 3 months but not at 6 months. At 6 months, there was no significant difference in mean costs between the two treatment groups. No significant group differences for well-being, use of community resources, financial support, patient or caregiver satisfaction. At 6 months, those in the geriatric day hospital had significantly fewer outpatient visits compared to the group receiving conventional treatment (p=0.03).	RCT	120	**Conclusions:** Functional improvement, as measured by the BI was seen in both treatment groups; however, a more marked improvement was seen at the earlier 3-month assessment for those treated by the geriatricians, and especially those within the geriatric group who were more disabled at baseline (BI subgroups).

continued

Table 4-3 (continued)

EVIDENCE OF EFFECTIVENESS OF OCCUPATIONAL THERAPY ON SELF-CARE OUTCOMES

Author (Date)	Major Results	Study Design	Sample Size	Conclusions and Limitations
No Effect				
Gladman, J. R., Lincoln, N. B., & Barer, D. H. (1993)	At discharge from hospital, BI scores were higher for those in the hospital-based services group (p<0.05). Those in the home rehabilitation group were more likely than those in the hospital group to receive rehabilitation services after discharge (p<0.05). However, for those receiving treatment, number of attendances in the first 6 months was higher for those in the hospital-based services group (p<0.05). There were no significant differences between groups in terms of total extended ADL scores at 3 and 6 months. However, those in the domiciliary group who had been discharged from a stroke unit had better scores than those in the hospital-based group (p<0.05 household and leisure components). There were no significant differences between groups in the BI score obtained at 6 months. However, those who had been discharged from a stroke unit and were receiving home-based rehabilitation showed significantly more improvement in BI scores from baseline to 6 months. There were also no significant differences between groups in terms of perceived health status. Caregiver assessments also failed to yield any significant differences between groups. Those in the elderly subgroup and receiving home care were more likely than elders in the hospital-based group to have a "bad" outcome, such as death or institutionalization, at 6 months.	RCT	327	***Conclusions:*** Overall, there were no significant differences between groups who received home-based rehabilitation vs. hospital-based services, in terms of functional recovery or perceived health status; one exception to this was the sub-group of patients discharged from the stroke unit to home care. There were also no significant differences between groups on any of the care-giving measures. ***Limitations:*** Limited generalizability.

continued

Table 4-3 (continued)

EVIDENCE OF EFFECTIVENESS OF OCCUPATIONAL THERAPY ON SELF-CARE OUTCOMES

Author (Date)	Major Results	Study Design	Sample Size	Conclusions and Limitations
No Effect				
Jongbloed, L., Stacey, S., & Brighton, C. (1989)	No statistically significant differences were found between the groups on the 3 outcome measures.	Non-RCT	90	***Conclusions:*** No statistically significant differences. ***Limitations:*** Did not include a group of subjects that did not receive OT (spontaneous recovery=confounding factor); All subjects received physical therapy based on the Bobath neurodevelopmental approach. Thus, subjects in the functional treatment group, though not exposed to neurodevelopmental techniques in OT, experienced these treatment techniques in PT. All subjects received similar treatment in self-care. It would have been preferable to implement sensorimotor integrative and functional treatment in self-care. Subjects discharged from hospital less than 8 weeks after admission could not be included in analyses. Self-care, mobility, and meal preparation were not measured in relation to the patient's environment, motivation, or role requirements (newly recognized way that occupational performance should be measured as per Health and Welfare Canada, 1987).

continued

Table 4-3 (continued)

EVIDENCE OF EFFECTIVENESS OF OCCUPATIONAL THERAPY ON SELF-CARE OUTCOMES

Author (Date)	Major Results	Study Design	Sample Size	Conclusions and Limitations
No Effect				
Ostrow, P., Parente, R., Ottenbacher, K. J. & Bonder, B. (1989)	No significant differences were found for functional status (BI) between those patients whose rehabilitation program included OT vs. those whose program did not include OT. However, "patients who received OT as part of their rehabilitation program were more likely to be discharged to home environments. This result occurred despite the fact that patients receiving OT were rated as more severely impaired than patients who did not receive OT as part of their rehabilitation program."	Non-RCT	193	***Conclusions:*** While no differences in function were found between the groups, participants who received OT as part of their rehabilitation program were more often discharged to their homes. ***Limitations:*** Field study, no control group, possibility of complex treatment interactions and multiple treatment interactions could not be eliminated, BI may not be sensitive enough to change in functional performance over a short period of time, other factors not considered in the study may have influenced the relationship between intervention and functional outcome.

9HPT=Nine-Hole Peg Test, AusTOMs-OT=Australian Therapy Outcome Measure for Occupational Therapy, BI=Barthel Index, COVS=Clinical Outcome Variables Scale, CSI=Comprehensive Severity Index, CTT=Colour Trials Test, EDSS=Expanded Disability Status Scale, EuroQol=European Quality of Life Instrument, FAI=Frenchay Activities Index, FAM=Functional Assessment Measure, FAQ=Functional Assessment Questionnaire, FIM=Functional Independence Measure, FIMBA=Functional Independence Measure for Blind Adults, FMA=Fugl-Meyer Assessment, FS=Functional Systems, FVPT=Functional Vision Performance Test, GDS=Geriatric Depression Scale, GHQ=General Health Questionnaire, HSS= Hemiplegic Stroke Scale, LHS=London Handicap Scale, MMSE=Mini Mental Status Examination, MRFS=Montabello Rehabilitation Factor Score, NUDS=Northwestern University Disability Scale, PD=Parkinson's Disease Disability Questionnaire, QLI=Quality of Life Index, SF-36=Short Form Health Survey, SGRQ=St. George Respiratory Questionnaire, SIAS=Stroke Impairment Assessment Set, SIP=Sickness Impact Profile, SOC=Sense of Coherence Scale, STREAM=Stroke Rehabilitation Assessment of Movement, TUG=Timed Up and Go Test, UPDRS=Unified Parkinson's Disease Rating Scale, WRS=Webster Rating Scale.

Table 4-4

OUTCOME MEASURES USED TO CAPTURE SELF-CARE OUTCOMES

Author (Date)	Outcome(s) Investigated	Outcome Measure(s)	Method of Administration
Landi, F., Cesari, M., Onder, G., Tafani, A., Zamboni, V., & Cocchi, A. (2006)	Functional outcomes	MDS-PAC	Administered at admission and every 2 weeks afterwards by therapists or trained staff (nurses or medical doctors) who were blinded to group allocation.
Ryan, T., Enderby, P., & Rigby, A. S. (2006)	Health-related quality of life Social participation Psychological variables (anxiety and depression) Functional ability Impairment	BI FAI HADS EQ-5D and EQ-VAS Therapy Outcome Measure	Follow-up occurred at 3 months (all intervention was completed) by therapy assistants who were blinded to group assignment and not involved in intervention. Follow-up occurred in patients' homes.
Sanford, J. A., Griffiths, P. C., Richardson, P., Hargraves, K., Butterfield, T., & Hoenig, H. (2006)	Increased mobility self-efficacy through changes in confidence Perceived ability in mobility and transfers inside the home	Modified FES	Trained research staff collected data via telephone interviews with all subjects at week 1 (baseline) and week 6 (1 week after completing 4-week intervention). Data collected include subject characteristics and outcome measures.
Storr, L. K., Sorensen, P. S., & Ravnborg, M. (2006)	Quality of life Activity	VAS MSIS EDSS FAMS LASQ GNDS 9HPT TW10	Patients in the intervention group were assessed 2 to 3 weeks before and after admission to rehabilitation unit. The control group was examined twice within this same time period, both before admission. Examination was conducted by a neurologist who was blinded to group affiliation. Evaluations were conducted in the patients' homes. VAS and the quality of life measures were completed as self-reports.
Alexander, J. A., Lichtenstein, R., Jinnet, K., Wells, R., Zazzeli, J., & Liu, D. (2005)	ADL function	Basic ADL Scale	ADL assessment was performed by appropriate professional. Measures taken at program entry (baseline), every 6 months for 2 years and every year thereafter for a period of 2 years.
McNaughton, H., DeJong, G., Smout, R. J., Melvin, J. L., & Brandstater, M. (2005)	Discharge location Functional change	FIM CSI	Assessments were completed by therapists. Unclear timeline, but it seems that assessment occurred at entry to the rehab facility and at discharge.

continued

Table 4-4 (continued)

Outcome Measures Used to Capture Self-Care Outcomes

Author (Date)	Outcome(s) Investigated	Outcome Measure(s)	Method of Administration
Thorsen, A., Widen Holmqvist, L., de Pedro-Cuesta, J., & von Koch, L. (2005)	Body functions-physiological Activity/ADL function Motor capacity Survival Falls Social involvement Cognitive function	MMSE LMCA 9HPT TW10 BI Katz ADL Index Katz Extended ADL Index FAI SOC SIP Reinvang Aphasia Test	The assessments were completed at baseline 3, 6, and 12 months and 5 years into the study. Assessments were conducted by an "external" assessor and purpose-trained PT and speech-language pathologist.
Unsworth, C. A., & Duncombe, D. (2005)	Outcomes of clients with neurological problems.	AusTOMs-OT	OTs were trained in the administration of the AusTOMs-OT at admission and discharge.
Yagura, H., Miyai, I., Suzuki, T., & Yanagihara, T. (2005)	Functional ability, disability Impairment Length of stay Cost of hospitalization per day Discharge disposition	FIM Motor subscale of the SIAS	FIM and SIAS data were collected at admission and discharge. Follow-up assessments were conducted by assessors who were blinded to the study conditions.
Bode, R. K., Heinemann, A. W., Semik, P., & Mallinson, T. (2004)	Functional gains after first stroke	FIM Residual change scores=The difference between actual and predicted discharge status	FIM was administered by therapist in appropriate discipline at admission and discharge.
Caplan, G. A., Williams, A. J., Daly, B., & Abraham, K. (2004)	Admissions to hospital within 30 days of the first emergency department visit Mortality Emergency and elective admissions to hospital Admissions to nursing homes Cognitive function Physical function IADL function	MSQ BI Modified IADL Index Information about admissions was collected through patient questionnaires as well as by examining electronic hospital admission data	Baseline information was collected from patients while in the emergency department. Those discharged "after hours" were visited by a team member (usually by a nurse) within 24 hours of discharge, and an assessment was conducted. Follow-up occurred at 3, 6, 12, and 18 months, through a telephone interview. Follow-up interviews were conducted by a research assistant or by various members of the interdisciplinary team.
Fleming, S. A., Blake, H., Gladman, J. R. F., Hart, E., Lymbery, M., Dewey, M. E., et al. (2004)	Place of residence Personal ADL IADL Psychological well-being Hospital and care home rehabilitation service bed days Use of day bed and hospital outpatient departments Contact with general practitioners Use of social services	BI Nottingham Extended ADL Scale Health Questionnaire (12-point version): Psychological well-being	Health outcomes were assessed through self-report via mailings at 3 and 12 months after randomization. Use of health and social services identified through use of "routinely held service data" by a researcher was independent of clinical services and blinded to group membership.

continued

Table 4-4 (continued)
OUTCOME MEASURES USED TO CAPTURE SELF-CARE OUTCOMES

Author (Date)	Outcome(s) Investigated	Outcome Measure(s)	Method of Administration
Hastings, J., Gowans, S., & Watson, D. E. (2004)	Functional status	FIM	Administered by therapist during surgical admission or subsequent medical admission from an organ transplant. At admission and before discharge.
Jousset, N., Fanello, S., Bontoux, L., Dubus, V., Billabert, C., Vielle, B., et al. (2004)	Number of sick-leave days Satisfaction at work Physical parameters (trunk strength and flexibility, endurance, lifting capacity) Level of pain in past 48 hours Impacts on activities Psychological status	Trunk flexibility—fingertip-floor distance Trunk strength—estimated by the duration of isometric contractions of flexors and extensors Lifting capacity—Progressive isoinertial lifting evaluation, with results expressed as percentage of body weight Endurance measured through use of bicycle ergometers Level of pain (48 hours)—10 cm horizontal VAS French version of the Dallas Pain Questionnaire Quebec Back Pain Disability Scale HADS	Self-reports: Number of sick days, work satisfaction, HADS, pain scale. Measures were taken at baseline and 6 months into the study. At 6 months, PT performed the physical portions of the evaluation at the rehabilitation center. A psychiatrist oversaw the testing procedures and the completion of the questionnaires by patients.
Keren, O., Motin, M., Heinemann, A. W., O'Reilly, C. M., Bode, R. K., Semik, P., et al. (2004)	Impairment Functional ability	MMSE SIAS National Institutes of Health Stroke Scale FIM Items from the RIC-FAS	Impairment measures were administered at admission and discharge. FIM scores were assessed at admission, discharge, and weekly during patient stays. Discipline-specific measures assessed admission, discharge status, and functional goals.
Lincoln, N. B., Walker, M. F., Dixon, A., & Knights, P. (2004)	Mood Quality of life Functional abilities Knowledge of stroke and satisfaction with services 6 months after recruitment Burden of care-caregiver	BI Extended Activities of Daily Living Scale General Health Questionnaire Carer Strain Index EuroQol	Outcomes were patient-completed at 6 months after recruitment to study. At this 6-month point, caregivers also completed the GHQ-12, Carer Strain Index, satisfaction with care, knowledge of stroke questionnaire. Missing information was sought through telephone calls and home visits where possible.

continued

Table 4-4 (continued)

Outcome Measures Used to Capture Self-Care Outcomes

Author (Date)	Outcome(s) Investigated	Outcome Measure(s)	Method of Administration
Liu, K. P., Chan, C. C., Lee, T. M., & Hui-Chan, C. W. (2004)	Task performance/relearning	15 trained and 5 new (not seen during training) tasks (rating performance on a 7-point Likert scale from complete dependence to complete independence) CTT Three subtests of the FMA: UE motor function, LE motor function, and sensation.	The CTT and FMA were completed before and after intervention. Task performance was measured before and after intervention. At 1-month post-intervention, 5 most difficult tasks were used to assess performance. Assessments were carried out by OTs, who were blinded to group affiliation.
MacPhee, A. H., Kirby, R. L., Coolen, A. L., Smith, C., MacLeod, D. A., & Dupuis, D. J. (2004)	Wheelchair skills Quality of life	WST, version 2.4 PIADS	The WST and PIADS were completed within 10 days of admission to the program and before the training program began. The WST was completed again post-training session. (For the control group, it was completed 4 weeks after the pre-training WST or prior to discharge—whichever came first; for the intervention group, it was completed 1 week after program completion.) The WST is administered by a tester (rehab professional) who records success or failure on a number of wheelchair skills. The PIADS is a self-administered questionnaire that was completed by the participant.
Pankow, L., Luchins, D., Studebaker, J., & Chettleburgh, D. (2004)	Function independence Psychological well-being	FIMBA NAS2 Goal attainment of participant	NAS2: Self-report measure, given orally by an optometrist/ psychiatric social worker/rehabilitation specialist prior to intervention. A vision evaluation was also administered at baseline. The blind rehabilitation/orientation and mobility instructor administered the living skills, mobility, and orientation portions of the FIMBA. Pre-intervention test occurred at least 4 weeks before intervention, and post-intervention assessment occurred at 4 to 6 weeks after intervention.

continued

Table 4-4 (continued)
OUTCOME MEASURES USED TO CAPTURE SELF-CARE OUTCOMES

Author (Date)	Outcome(s) Investigated	Outcome Measure(s)	Method of Administration
Weiss, Z., Snir, D., Klein, B., Avraham, I., Shani, R., Zetler, H., et al. (2004)	Physical components (range of motion, coordination sensation, etc.) Mobility ADL function Activities/social participation	BI FAI	Patients in the home rehabilitation group had a physical assessment and ADL assessment at the beginning of intervention. These assessments were conducted by an OT and PT. Approximately 14 months after stroke, the BI and FAI were administered through a phone interview with the patient or family member to patients in both groups.
Bohannon, R. W., Ahlquist, M., Lee, N., & Maljanian, R. (2003)	Functional independence at discharge Changes in functional independence between admission and discharge	5 items from the FIM: Bed, chair, wheelchair transfers Eating Walking Expression Memory	FIM scores assessed by therapist(s) at admission and discharge. A research nurse then obtained this information from either therapy notes or the therapist, for purposes of the study.
Wade, D. T., Gage, H., Owen, C., Trend, P., Grossmith, C., & Kaye, J. (2003)	Caregiver strain Disability level Functional abilities Mobility Speech Anxiety and depression Dexterity	Caregiver Strain Index EQ-5D PD PDQ-39 SF-36 9HPT Stand-Walk-Sit Test HADS Speech-related items from the UPDRS	Main outcome assessment was conducted at 24 weeks, which was about 4 months after the treatment group had completed the intervention program. Assessments were conducted by an independent assessor, who was not involved in the study and was blinded to group affiliation. Baseline assessments occurred after randomization, and the final follow-up assessment took place at 48 weeks.
Alvund, K., Jepsen, E., Vass, M., & Lundemark, H. (2002)	Functional status/ability Re-admissions	Revised BI Re-admissions to hospital	Interview conducted, with patient, by research OT and research nurse. Baseline interview regarding functional ability was conducted a few days before discharge and follow-up was 3 months post-discharge in the client's home/nursing home.
Jones, G. R., Miller, T. A., & Petrella, R. J. (2002)	Degree of disability Functional change Rehabilitation efficacy	FIM Motor FIM subscale—13 items—focus on physical ability MRFS	Patients were assessed using the FIM within 48 hours of admission to hospital and re-assessed the day before discharge. A subgroup of patients were contacted by telephone, and a FIM was conducted by a trained interviewer at 6 weeks after discharge. All 18 FIM items were included in this telephone FIM.

continued

Table 4-4 (continued)

OUTCOME MEASURES USED TO CAPTURE SELF-CARE OUTCOMES

Author (Date)	Outcome(s) Investigated	Outcome Measure(s)	Method of Administration
Naglie, G., Tansey, C., Kirkland, J. L., Ogilvie-Harris, D. J., Detsky, A. S., Etchells, E., et al. (2002)	Mortality rates Ambulation and transfers (bed/chair) Place of residence	Modified BI Residential status was assessed on a 1 to 3 scale: 1=Own home 2=Relative's home or retirement home 3=Nursing home, acute or chronic care hospital, rehabilitation hospital Other measures included IADL scores, health care utilization information taken from medical records, and workload time measurement sat 6 months	Baseline (pre-fracture) assessment, 3 and 6 month follow-ups after surgery. Follow-up assessments were conducted by research assistants who were blinded to group belonging. Interviews were conducted with both patient and caregiver where possible.
Saltvedt, I., Opdahl Mo, E. S., Fayers, P., Kaasa, S., & Sletvold, O. (2002)	Mortality Causes of death	N/A	Baseline data were collected prior to randomization. Demographic information was obtained through interview with patient and caregiver. Information about length of stay and diagnoses was obtained from the hospital. Information about targeting was retrieved from patient and caregiver interview and from nurses on the patients' ward. Death and cause of death were taken from medical certificates.
Trend, P., Kaye, J., Gage, H., Owen, C., & Wade, D. (2002)	Mobility Gait Speech Caregiver strain Psychological well-being Social service needs Health-related quality of life Perceptions of the intervention program	Abridged Emerson and Enderby Measures BI HADS EQ-5D Mobility was assessed using TW10	BI was administered by a Parkinson's disease nurse specialist during the first treatment. HADS and EuroQol were administered by an independent research assistant in the first and last week of intervention, but were self-report measures. Speech therapist tested patients on aspects of speech before and after intervention. A PT assessed gait and mobility.
Alexander, H., Bugge, C., & Hagen S. (2001)	Level of disability Health status	BI Medical Outcomes Study SF-36	Baseline data obtained from patients' physicians. Subsequent data were obtained from rehab professionals.
Finnerty, J. P., Keeping, I., Bullough, R. G. N., & Jones, J. (2001)	Change in quality of life	SGRQ 6MWT	Self-administered, but under the supervision of a blinded observer at baseline, 12, and 24 weeks into the study.

continued

Table 4-4 (continued)
OUTCOME MEASURES USED TO CAPTURE SELF-CARE OUTCOMES

Author (Date)	Outcome(s) Investigated	Outcome Measure(s)	Method of Administration
Von Koch, L., de Pedro-Cuesta, J., Kostulas, V., Almazan, J., & Holmqvist, L. W. (2001)	ADL function IADL function Frequency of social interactions Manual dexterity Motor capacity Perceived dysfunction Coping ability Spouses' health-related quality of life Severity of dysphasia Mortality Number and outcome of falls and dependency	BI Katz ADL Index Katz Extended ADL Index FAI SIP SOC	Follow-up evaluation occurred at 6 months and 1 year after stroke. The 1-year follow-up occurred in patients' homes, and assessments were conducted by an external assessor who was blinded to group belonging, as well as being uninvolved in the randomization processes and implementation of rehabilitation.
Lin, J. H., Chang, C. M., Liu, C. K., Huang, M. H., & Lin, Y. T. (2000)	Functional recovery Rehabilitation efficiency and effectiveness Neurological "status"	FIM Brunnstrom Motor Recovery Scales Efficiency and effectiveness of rehabilitation were measured using various calculations related to FIM scores (i.e., actual vs. potential rehabilitation gains)	Initial assessments were conducted within 3 days of patient's referral to the rehabilitation unit. Patients were also assessed within 48 hours of discharge from inpatient rehabilitation unit. Patients were assessed by a senior PT, who was trained in administration of the FIM.
Mayo, N. E., Wood-Dauphinee, S., Cote, R., Gayton, D., Carlton, J., Buttery, J., et al. (2000)	Functional abilities Reintegration Health-related quality of life	Physical Component Summary of the SF-36 CNS STREAM TUG BI Older Americans Resource Scale for IADL RNLI	Assessment occurred before randomization, at 4 weeks (at the end of intervention), at 2 months, and at 3 months. Assessments were conducted by OTs and PTs who were not involved in intervention and were blinded to group assignment.
McCabe, P., Nason, F., Turco, P. D., Friedman, D., & Seddon, J. M. (2000)	Functional abilities within the rehabilitation setting and within the patient's daily environment	FAQ FVPT	Assessment was done at time of enrollment in study, prior to group assignment. Follow-up occurred at the end of the intervention. The FAQ was administered over the phone by research assistants who were blind to intervention groups. The FVPT was given by the OT or technician.

continued

Table 4-4 (continued)

OUTCOME MEASURES USED TO CAPTURE SELF-CARE OUTCOMES

Author (Date)	Outcome(s) Investigated	Outcome Measure(s)	Method of Administration
Sulch, D., Perez, I., Melbourne, A., & Kalra, L. (2000)	Length of hospital stay Quality of life Anxiety and depression Functional abilities	Length of hospital stay BI HADS	BI was administered at weeks 1, 4, 12, and 26 of the study. HADS was administered at 4, 12, and 26 weeks. Rankin scores and the EuroQol Quality of Life Scores were assessed at 12 and 26 weeks. Total time of OT and PT were documented daily, while discharge location and mortality were noted up until week 26. Two observers who were not directly involved in the study completed the assessments, independently of each other.
Freeman, J., A., Langdon, D. W., Hobart, J. C., & Thompson, A. J. (1999)	Disability (functional change) Handicap (socioeconomic limitations) Emotional well-being Health-related quality of life	Motor portion of the FIM LHS SF-36 GHQ	LHS—self-report. FIM—therapist report/completed, although not explicitly stated. SF-36 and GHQ were self-report. Patients were assessed at admission, at discharge, and at 3-month intervals for 1 year after discharge.
Nikolaus, T., Specht-Leible, N., Bach, M., Oster, P., & Schlierf, G. (1999)	Functional abilities Survival Direct costs of care over 12 months Hospital re-admissions Nursing home placement	BI Lawton-Brody Questionnaire MMSE Economic and housing conditions were assessed using a standardized questionnaire Social support info collected by looking at social contact and activities	At 1 year after randomization, follow-up assessments were conducted by a trained interviewer who was not associated with the intervention team. Assessment was conducted through telephone interviews or mailed surveys, and information was verified through home visit and from patients' general practitioner. During initial assessment, assessors were blinded to group assignment of patients.
DiFabio, R. P., Soderberg, J., Choi, T., Hansen, C. R., & Schapiro, R. T. (1998)	Symptom frequency Fatigue Functional status	MS Symptom-Related Checklist—26 Part of the RIC-FAS	MS Symptom-Related Checklist—patient completed, at baseline and at 1 year after admission to study. RIC-FAS items—completed at baseline and 1 year after admission to study.

continued

Table 4-4 (continued)

OUTCOME MEASURES USED TO CAPTURE SELF-CARE OUTCOMES

Author (Date)	Outcome(s) Investigated	Outcome Measure(s)	Method of Administration
Mathiowetz, V., & Matuska, K. M. (1998)	Frequency of use and effectiveness of equipment prescribed by OT satisfaction with OT services Self-care ability	RIC-FAS	Participants were evaluated upon admission (based on therapist observation, client report, and caregiver report), at discharge (another therapist would administer the outcome measure), and 6 weeks post-discharge (using telephone interviews). During the telephone interview, participants also rated the frequency of use and effectiveness of equipment. At 4 weeks post-discharge, participants were mailed a satisfaction with OT services questionnaire.
Widen Holmqvist, L. W., von Koch, L., Kostulas, V., Holm, M., Widsell, G., Tegler, H., et al. (1998)	Self-reported falls IADL/ADL function Social activities Manual dexterity Motor function Subjective disability/impairment Walking Coping skills Patient satisfaction with program Speech-related variables	FAI Extended Katz Index BI Lindmark Motor Capacity Assessment 9HPT SIP TW10 SOC (short version)	Follow-up occurred at 3, 6, and 12 months after stroke. Patients were interviewed in their homes by a research PT who was not associated with the study. Patients with dysphasia were also assessed by a research speech therapist. Self-report measures included falls and satisfaction with study.
Brosseau, L., Philippe, P., Potvin, L., & Boulanger, Y. L. (1996)	Length of stay: Defined as the number of days from first day of admission to the department of physical rehabilitation to the last day of treatment	FIM FMA	Patients were assessed twice, in order to determine functional status. The FIM and FMA was administered within 72 hours of admission to rehab program and again 1 week later. Patients were assessed through observation of a physiotherapist who was independent of patients' treatment.
Drummond, A. E. R., Miller, N., Colquohoun, M., & Logan, P. C. (1996)	ADL independence (personal and instrumental)	BI Rivermead ADL Scale Extended ADL Scale	Patients were assessed at baseline, prior to randomization. Follow-up assessments occurred at 3, 6, and 12 months after randomization, by an assessor who was blinded to group allocation. Patients were either evaluated in their homes or the hospital outpatient department, depending on whether or not they had been discharged.

continued

Table 4-4 (continued)

OUTCOME MEASURES USED TO CAPTURE SELF-CARE OUTCOMES

Author (Date)	Outcome(s) Investigated	Outcome Measure(s)	Method of Administration
Patti, F., Reggio, A., Nicoletti, F., Sellaroli, T., Deinite, G., & Nicoletti, F. (1996)	Disability and impairment Functional abilities in ADL	UPDRS WRS NUDS FIM BI Timed tests for UE and LE were used to evaluate disability secondary to Parkinson's disease	In the first study, baseline measures were taken within 4 days of admission. Follow-up occurred at the end of the rehab program and at 3 months after the rehabilitation program. In the second study, an additional follow-up occurred at 6 months after the start of the study. Testing was completed by a neurologist.
Przybylski, B. R., Dumont, E. D., Watkins, M. E., Warren, S. A., Beaulne, A. P., & Lier, D. A. (1996)	Cost of care Functional status and mobility	FAM FIM COVS	The COVS was administered by a PT, who did not treat patients and was blinded to their group belonging. A nurse, also blinded to participants' groups and not involved in their care, administered the FIM/FAM. Patients were tested every 6 months over a 2-year period.
Werner, R. A., & Kessler, S. (1996)	Functional abilities/independence Depression Subjective impairment (physical and psychosocial)	SIP FIM JHFT Brunnstrom's Motor Rating Timed evaluations of transfers, stair climbing, and walking speed BDI	Evaluations were conducted at baseline and 3 and 9 months into the study. Patients completed self-reports on the psychological measures, as well as self-esteem. An OT not involved in the study and blinded to group belonging completed the other assessments.
Heinemann, A. W., Hamilton, B., Linacre, J. M., Wright, B. D., & Granger, C. (1995)	Functional abilities/change Achievement of motor and cognitive potential Length of stay Efficiency of motor and cognitive change	FIM	The FIM was administered at admission and discharge.
Hui, E., Lum, C. M., Woo, J., Or, K. H., & Kay, R. L. (1995)	Hospital services received/cost Functional state Well-being Patient/caregiver satisfaction Mood	BI Self-report health scale Self-reports (1 to 4 scale) regarding satisfaction GDS	Follow-up information was collected after ictus (a sudden attack—blow, seizure, or stroke).

continued

Table 4-4 (continued)
OUTCOME MEASURES USED TO CAPTURE SELF-CARE OUTCOMES

Author (Date)	Outcome(s) Investigated	Outcome Measure(s)	Method of Administration
Comella, C. L., Stebbins, G. T., Brown-Toms, N., & Goetz, C. G. (1994)	Disability ADL function Motor function Depression	UPDRS GDS Timed finger taps	Assessments were conducted by a neurologist at baseline, the end of the treatment program, and 6 months after the end of each intervention phase. Controls were evaluated at these times as well. Neurologist was blinded to participants' group belonging.
Kalra, L. (1994)	Functional abilities/change Length of stay Amount and duration of therapy across admission	BI	BI scores were assessed weekly by OTs. Although OTs were not blinded to group affiliation and were involved in treatment, they were unaware that scores would be used for comparison with another group. Patients released prior to 12 weeks had a post-discharge visit, at which a therapist administered a functional assessment.
Dam, M., Tonin, P., Ermani, M., Pizzolato, G., Iaia, V., & Battistin, L. (1993)	Neurological recovery following stroke Functional recovery following stroke	HSS BI	HSS and BI administered at entry to study (3 months post-stroke) and every 3 months after this point until end of study (24 months post-stroke).
Gladman, J. R., Lincoln, N. B., & Barer, D. H. (1993)	Perceived health Functional change (personal and instrumental ADL) Caregiver involvement Life satisfaction	Nottingham Health Profile Extended ADL Scale BI Brief Assessment of Social Engagement Nottingham version of the Life Satisfaction Index	The Extended Activities of Daily Living Scale was given to participants at 3 and 6 months after randomization, through a mailed survey. At 6 months, an independent and blinded observer administered the BI and Nottingham Health Profile by way of an interview. The Nottingham version of the Life Satisfaction Index was administered to caregivers at 6 months.
Johansson, K., Lindgren, I., Widner, H., & Wiklund, I. (1993)	ADL function Motor function and balance Quality of life Length of stay (institutionalization)	BI Nottingham Health Profile The motor assessment examined 31 different movements including walking, sit, stand, balance	Motor, balance, and ADL function were assessed before beginning the intervention and, at 1 and 3 months after stroke. ADL function was assessed again at 12 months. The Nottingham Health Profile was administered at 3, 6, and 12 months post-stroke.

continued

Table 4-4 (continued)

OUTCOME MEASURES USED TO CAPTURE SELF-CARE OUTCOMES

Author (Date)	Outcome(s) Investigated	Outcome Measure(s)	Method of Administration
Melin, A. L., & Bygren, L. O. (1992)	Functional abilities Use of long-stay hospital services Aspects of medical well-being (diagnoses, drugs used)	Modified Katz Index Instrumental ADL MMSE Self-report social activities and contacts of the preceding week were used as a measure of social function	Initial assessment (after randomization) was conducted by an assistant nurse who was blinded to group belonging. Follow-up assessment was at 6-months after randomization. It was conducted by a team OT who was not blinded to patients' group. Medical charts were read by project and team physicians in order to obtain information about medical conditions, diagnoses, and drugs. Self-report: Social function/ activities. Information such as length of stay was obtained from medical records and records of the Stockholm County Council.
Montgomery Orr, P., & Bratton, G. N. (1992)	Self-assessed pain Functional abilities Need for assistance	HAQ VAS for pain Written form stating whether patient needed help (from another individual) with daily activities on each disability question	The questionnaire was self-administered prior to the start of the program, at discharge from the program, and at follow-up, 5 to 10 weeks after discharge from the program.
Indredavik, B., Bakke, F., Solberg, R., Rokseth, R., Lund Haaheim, L., & Holme, I. (1991)	Proportion of patients at home Proportion of patients in an institution Mortality Functional state	BI Neurological Score (by the Scandinavian Stroke Study Group)	Prognostic and neurological scores established at admission were assessed by an on-call doctor. A specialized team involving a doctor, PT, and nurse conducted additional assessments. Evaluation at 6 weeks marked the end of the stay in the stroke unit. A secondary assessment took place at 52 weeks. The BI was administered 24 to 48 hours after randomization, at days 21 and 42 (±2 days), at discharge, at 90 days (±7 days), and 365 days (±14). The prognostic and neurological scores were assessed at day 0, before randomization. Then, the neurological score was assessed on the same schedule as the BI.
Jongbloed, L., Stacey, S., & Brighton, C. (1989)	Performance in self-care and mobility Functional abilities via meal preparation Sensorimotor performance	BI Meal Preparation Test Eight subtests of the Sensorimotor Integration Test Battery	Outcome measures were administered by an independent evaluator before the treatment began and again after 8 weeks of treatment. The BI and Meal Preparation Test were also re-administered after 4 weeks of treatment (3 times total).

continued

Table 4-4 (continued)
OUTCOME MEASURES USED TO CAPTURE SELF-CARE OUTCOMES

Author (Date)	Outcome(s) Investigated	Outcome Measure(s)	Method of Administration
Ostrow, P., Parente, R., Ottenbacher, K. J., & Bonder, B. (1989)	Function Severity of condition Discharge destination status and destination change	BI Discharge data sheet and hospital chart	Blind examiners administered the BI. It was administered as soon as possible (when medical condition permitted it) and then again immediately prior to discharge. Patient status was monitored throughout hospital stay (chart information—recorded by data coordinators at hospital). The discharge data sheet was completed at discharge by data coordinators. Follow-up phone calls were made at 1 month and 3 months after hospital discharge to determine any changes in discharge status.
Carlton, R. S. (1987)	Body mechanics when lifting and lowering	WEST 2 WCED Modified WEST 2 BME WRBME	At 2 weeks (body mechanics evaluation) and 3 weeks (workplace observation) after the intervention, group received their educational session. Completed by assessor who was blind to treatment group.

6MWT=6-Minute Walking Test, 9HPT=Nine-Hole Peg Test, AusTOMs-OT=Australian Therapy Outcome Measure for Occupational Therapy, BDI=Beck Depression Inventory, BI=Barthel Index, CNS=Canadian Neurological Scale, COVS=Clinical Outcome Variables Scale, CSI=Comprehensive Severity Index, CTT=Colour Trials Test, EDSS=Expanded Disability Status Scale, EQ-5D=EuroQol 5D, EQ-VAS=EuroQol Visual Analog Scale, EuroQol=European Quality of Life Instrument, FAI=Frenchay Activities Index, FAM=Functional Assessment Measure, FAMS=Functional Assessment in Multiple Sclerosis, FAQ=Functional Assessment Questionnaire, FES=Falls Efficacy Scale, FIM=Functional Independence Measure, FIMBA=Functional Independence Measure for Blind Adults, FMA=Fugl-Meyer Assessment, FVPT=Functional Vision Performance Test, GDS=Geriatric Depression Scale, GHQ=General Health Questionnaire, GNDS=Guy's Neurological Disability Scale, HADS=Hospital Anxiety and Depression Scale, HAQ=Health Assessment Questionnaire-Modified, HSS=Hemiplegic Stroke Scale, JHFT=Jebsen's Hand Function Test, LASQ=Life Appreciation and Satisfaction Questionnaire, LHS=London Handicap Scale, LMCA=Lindmark Motor Capacity Assessment, MDS-PAC=Minimum Data Set—Post-Acute Care, MMSE=Mini Mental Status Examination, MRFS=Montabello Rehabilitation Factor Score, MSIS=Multiple Sclerosis Impairment Scale, MSQ=Mental Status Questionnaire, NAS2=Nottingham Adjustment Scale 2, NUDS=Northwestern University Disability Scale, PD=Parkinson's Disease Disability Questionnaire, PDQ-39=Parkinson's Disease Questionnaire, PIADS=Psychosocial Impact of Assistive Devices Scale, RIC-FAS=Rehabilitation Institute of Chicago-Functional Assessment Scale, RNLI=Reintegration to Normal Living Index, SF-36=Short Form Health Survey, SGRQ=St. George Respiratory Questionnaire, SIAS=Stroke Impairment Assessment Set, SIP=Sickness Impact Profile, SOC=Sense of Coherence Scale, STREAM=Stroke Rehabilitation Assessment of Movement, TUG=Timed Up and Go Test, TW10=Timed 10-Meter Walking, UPDRS=Unified Parkinson's Disease Rating Scale, VAS=Visual Analog Scale, WRS=Webster Rating Scale, WST=Wheelchair Skills Test.

A recent Cochrane Review has shown that people recovering from stroke living at home who receive occupational therapy intervention are less likely to deteriorate and more likely to be independent in their ability to complete ADL than those who receive no occupational therapy interventions or usual care in hospitals (Legg et al., 2006). Similarly, those who receive post-stroke care in a dedicated stroke ward including occupational therapy intervention consistently demonstrate more independence in ADL than those treated in a conventional care ward (Drummond, Miller, Colquohoun, & Logan, 1996).

Development of Self-Care Occupations

What occupational therapists can do is only half of the equation. The other half speaks to how occupational therapists approach their interventions. These interventions are, as the profession title suggests, often occupation based. This means that occupational therapists focus not only on the movements and components of tasks, but will try to place these elements into a framework that respects the larger occupation in which the client is trying to participate. With respect to elements of a person's function, research examining self-care activities is promising. Evidence suggests that function-focused activities can improve functional outcomes more than impairment-focused interventions (Bode, Heinemann, Semik, & Mallinson, 2004).

Effects of Occupational Therapy in Promoting Personal Care Outcomes

Comprehensive Occupational Therapy

Empirical Studies

Meta-analysis results indicate that stroke patients who received community occupational therapy intervention were significantly better able to complete self-care activities and had a reduction of activity limitation than those who received no therapy or leisure therapy (Walker et al., 2004). Steultjens and colleagues (2003) found that occupational therapy intervention for acute stroke patients shows a small, but significant, positive effect for comprehensive occupational therapy (training or sensory-motor functions, cognitive functions, dressing or cooking skills, education regarding assistive devices, provision of splints and slings, and education of caregivers) on primary ADL, EADL, and social participation. According to Walker, Hawkins, Gladman, and Lincoln (2001), stroke patients who received post-discharge home visits by an occupational therapist 1 to 15 times during a 6-month period showed a significant increase in ADL and IADL abilities and an improved quality of life at 6 and 12 months compared to those with no intervention. Finally, comprehensive occupational therapy treatment (including direct patient intervention, staff training, and environmental assessment) for patients with stroke showed significantly less deterioration in ADL as measured by the Barthel Index (BI) at 0, 3, and 6 months post-intervention compared with those receiving conventional ward treatment (Sackley et al., 2006).

With individuals with rheumatoid arthritis, comprehensive occupational therapy (defined as training of motor function, training of skills, instruction on joint protection, counseling, advice and instruction on assistive devices, provision of splints) and instruction on joint protection resulted in a non-significant, but positive increase in functional ability (Steultjens, Dekker, Bouter, van Schaardenberg, Van, & van den Ende, 2002). In another study examining rheumatoid arthritis, one-on-one intervention was compared with a group intervention program. Both groups offered occupational therapy education, joint protection, PT, splinting, social services, and home modifications. No significant differences were found between groups at 0, 12, and 24 months; however, the individual occupational therapy group had a significant improvement in perceived self-management (Hammond, Young & Kidao, 2004). These studies indicate that comprehensive occupational therapy intervention offered in a group or on a one-on-one basis can be effective in improving functional ability; however, clients receiving one-on-one intervention may feel better able to cope with their disability than those in a group setting.

Involvement in a total rehabilitation program including occupational therapy, physical therapy/physiotherapy, nursing, nutrition, and pharmacological interventions was shown to have significant improvement in self-care activities for a group of individuals with multiple sclerosis. These gains were maintained at 6 weeks post-discharge. Occupational therapy intervention included compensatory strategies, home management and fatigue management education, and strength and range of motion activities; however, due to the nature of the intervention, it is difficult to determine which aspect of the program was responsible for the higher rate in functional ability (Mathiowetz & Matuska, 1998). Similarly, in a second study, patients with multiple sclerosis who participated in a multidisciplinary program with occupational therapy, physical therapy, social work, chaplaincy, and therapeutic recreation had fewer multiple sclerosis-related symptoms and less fatigue than those patients on a waiting list (DiFabio, Soderberg, Choi, Hansen, & Schapiro, 1998).

In a study examining people with arthritis, involvement in a multidisciplinary team (occupational therapy, physical therapy, social work, nursing, and rheumatology) was associated with improved function, decreased need for assistance, and decreased pain. Occupational therapy involvement with these patients involved joint protection education, energy conservation, adaptive equipment, and splinting interventions (Montgomery Orr & Bratton, 1992). Despite these positive findings, it should be noted that with certain populations (e.g., Parkinson's disease) gains are always held in tandem with degeneration, and cessation of programs can be associated with return to baseline scores (Comella, Stebbins, Brown-Toms, & Goetz, 1994; Patti, Reggio, Nicoletti, Sellaroli, Deinite, & Nicoletti, 1996).

The primary focus of hospital-based, occupational therapy intervention is to optimize occupational performance with regard to ADL functioning, thereby encouraging clients to return to their previous level of functioning (Hagsten, Svensson, & Gardulf, 2004). Recent evidence suggests that occupational therapy training provided in a hospital setting can positively impact the performance of ADL and IADL following discharge.

A randomized trial of the effects of occupational therapy intervention following joint replacement found a significant difference in ADL and IADL functioning for individuals who received occupational therapy-specific interventions (e.g., technical aids, ADL training, pre-discharge home assessment) as compared to those who received only general attention from staff on a hospital ward (Hagsten, Svensson, & Gardulf, 2006). Occupational therapy training improved patient recovery with regard to dressing, toileting, and bathing/hygiene. Two months after discharge, clients who received occupational therapy training reported they regained their ADL and IADL abilities, although some required assistive devices and other home adaptations to facilitate occupational performance.

Multidisciplinary teams that include occupational therapists have also been shown to be effective on a number of functional mobility outcomes. For example, a study that included multidisciplinary intervention (occupational, physical, and speech therapists) for clients with stroke showed increases in functional independence at discharge as measured by five items from the functional independence measure (Bohannon, Ahlquist, Lee, & Maljanian, 2003). In another randomized controlled trial, three or four face-to-face weekly occupational and physical therapy sessions were seen to significantly improve functional mobility and self-efficacy with household tasks compared with visits through teleconference (Sanford, Griffiths, Richardson, Hargraves, Butterfield, & Hoenig, 2006).

These results show promise that involvement in a multidisciplinary program can be associated with functional gains. However, these findings must be interpreted with care given that benefits cannot be attributed to occupational therapy per se and perceived or actual gains may be affected by level of decline associated with diagnosis.

Early Supported Discharge
Empirical Studies
In a 2000 randomized controlled trial, researchers concluded that "prompt and supported discharge" from a multidisciplinary team (occupational therapy, physical therapy, nursing, speech-language pathology, and dietary consultants) led to better physical health and greater satisfaction with community re-integration after stroke than a control group receiving typical discharge protocol as measured by the General Health Questionnaire, Short Form 36 (SF-36), Timed Up and Go Test (TUG), Barthel Index (BI), and Reintegration to Normal Living Index (RNLI), among others (Mayo et al., 2000). Another randomized controlled trial completed in 2005 showed that ESD had positive results on extended ADL function, which was maintained up to 5 years after stroke (Thorsen, Widen Holmqvist, de Pedro-Cuesta, & von Koch, 2005). Weiss and colleagues (2004) found in their non-randomized controlled trial that not only was ESD an effective method for improving outcomes after stroke, as measured by the BI and Frenchay Activities Index (FAI), but ESD could also be considered a cost-effective method of service delivery compared to institutional rehabilitation.

Widen Holmqvist and colleagues (1998) completed a randomized controlled trial that showed non-significant but positive trends toward ESD (consisting of occupational therapy, physical therapy, speech-language pathology, and social work) in terms of better functional ADL outcomes. Interesting to note, however, was that the reduction of falls and subjective disability measures favored institutional care.

Early research into supported geriatric discharge, in which geriatric patients received in-home intervention from physical therapy, occupational therapy, and social work, showed that this service delivery method was associated with reduction in length of hospital stays and increased independence with IADL. In addition, researchers suggest that this type of intervention may delay (but not prevent) admission to nursing home care and can be associated with a significant net savings per year due to reduction of hospital stays (Nikolaus, Specht-Leible, Bach, Oster, & Schlierf, 1999).

Although these results are promising, caution must be used in interpreting these results, as ESD interventions are not always uniform, and team demographics may shift from one hospital team to another. Studies that compare similar ESD programs over several geographic environments are necessary. Despite this, these studies show that an ESD program after stroke can have a positive impact on functional abilities and community re-integration, as well as being considered a cost-effective alternative to conventional discharge programs.

Direct ADL Skill Development

Empirical Studies

A number of empirical articles regarding direct retraining of ADL point toward a positive functional change for participants. The largest body of empirical evidence was found in the population of those recovering from stroke. In an occupational therapy intervention focused on compensatory strategies (self-talk, writing, sequence strips) for apraxia impairment in stroke, significant improvements were seen in ADL and functional abilities as measured by the Barthel Index (BI) (Donkervoort, Dekker, Stehmann Saris, & Deelman 2001). In another study, stroke patients involved in direct occupational therapy interventions to address ADL ability showed significant improvement in ADL and patient-reported quality of life as measured by the Functional Independence Measure (FIM) and Quality of Life Index (QLI) (Unsworth & Cunningham, 2002). These interventions resulted in a significant improvement in the test of motor functioning, significant reduction of ADL disability, and significant improvement in ADL activities as measured by the BI and direct ADL observations (van Heugten, Dekker, Deelman, van Dijk, Stehmann Saris, & Kinebanian, 1998). In the second phase of their trial, van Heugten and colleagues (2000) found significant improvements in ADL ability after occupational therapy group intervention targeting post-stroke apraxia, although the degree of improvement was directly related to pre-stroke level of ability and post-stroke level of impairment. In a cross-over trial, stroke patients receiving home occupational therapy intervention for dressing and energy conservation showed significant improvements in dressing. Improvements were maintained during the "off" phase of the trial (Walker, Drummond, & Lincoln, 1996).

In a group occupational therapy intervention (twice per week for 5 weeks) that focused on mobility, dexterity, and ADL for people with Parkinson's disease, a significant increase in functional abilities over 1 year was seen compared with those who received no intervention. However, in this study, educational portions were also provided by physical therapy/physiotherapy, speech pathology, social work, and dietitians, so it is difficult to determine if the positive change was as a result of occupational therapy alone (Gauthier, Dalziel, & Gauthier, 1987).

Significant positive changes after direct occupational therapy ADL retraining have also been seen in those recovering from total joint replacement. For example, early individualized post-joint replacement operative training was seen to significantly improve ADL and IADL abilities as measured by the Klein-Bell and direct observation of tasks. These gains were maintained at a 2-month follow-up (Hagsten et al., 2004). In a clinical trial by Hagsten and Soderback (1994), occupational therapy intervention, including patient ADL training, equipment training, and home visits, showed a significant increase in dressing, hygiene, and mobility abilities compared with those with conventional ward treatment.

Studies examining those individuals in long-term care or geriatric settings have also determined that occupational therapy interventions have a significant positive effect. For example, sensory-based occupational therapy activities (45 minutes a day, 5 days a week for 8 weeks) to address feeding concerns in a long-term care setting showed significant increase in feeding abilities compared with regularly scheduled activities (Hames-Hahn & Llorens, 1988). In the population of older clients with upper and lower extremity injuries, a full occupational therapy assessment, referral, and home equipment and pre-discharge training showed significant increase in a patient's functional abilities at discharge and at 7 days follow-up when compared with regular care. However, no significant changes were found in self-reported anxiety levels (Hendriksen & Harrison, 2001). Finally, in a medical ward, patients receiving ADL training from an occupational therapist showed significantly increased skills in bathing and hygiene and a positive trend toward improvement in eating and mobility as measured by Klein Bell, compared with those without occupational therapy intervention (Soderback & Guidetti, 1992).

In each of these studies, occupational therapy intervention direct retraining of ADL abilities can result in a significant positive change for individuals with stroke, Parkinson's disease, joint replacements, and for those in long-term care facilities or on medical wards. Occupational therapy intervention can also affect discharge location and decrease re-admissions as a result of ADL dependency.

Development of Self-Care Occupations

Empirical Studies

In a study that compared an occupational therapy biomechanical approach with an occupational adaptation frame of reference for patients recovering from arthroplasty, those who were in the occupational adaptation group engaging in occupation-based interventions showed a significantly greater improvement in their chosen task as measured by the FIM. In other words, directing treatment in an occupation framework rather than a physical or biomedical component approach is associated with greater functional gains (Buddenberg & Schkade, 1998). In the population of people post-stroke, an occupational therapy intervention that focused on occupation and patient-specific role activities showed a significant increase in independence, and patients were more often discharged to a less restrictive environment than a group focusing on biomechanical range of motion, ADL training, and outings, as measured by clinical SOAP notes (Ward-Gibson & Schkade, 1997). These results show the promising possibilities of incorporating rehabilitation programs with occupations meaningful to the participant to impact functional change.

Interventions Used to Improve Functional Mobility Outcomes

Environmental Modification

Wheelchairs (both power and manual) and other wheeled devices such as scooters have impacted individuals' abilities to access their immediate and external environments. Life stories related by wheelchair users in the 1950s, 1960s, and 1970s indicated some wheelchair users who were previously bedridden were able to access universities, jobs, leisure pursuits, and the community at large (Tremblay, Campbell, & Hudson, 2005).

Wheeled seating interventions are typically selected to impact on the person, in terms of pain relief and pressure management, their environment, in terms of access, and their occupation, in terms of increasing opportunities for participation (Reid et al., 2002). Users of wheeled mobility to access their community have two realities to face. First, they are offered better opportunities to participate and interact with their social communities within their abilities (Devitt, Chau, & Jutai, 2003). Coupled with this, however, is the fact that their opportunities are only as great as the environmental accessibility surrounding them (Reid et al., 2002). Occupational therapists, as part of their role, can help individuals achieve a balance between functional mobility and environmental accessibility and can offer specific training and testing programs to help their clients use their wheeled mobility systems more effectively (Buning, Angelo, & Schmeler, 2001; Davies, De Souza, & Frank, 2003; MacPhee, Kirby, Coolen, Smith, MacLeod, & Dupuis, 2004).

For the occupational therapist, wheeled or adaptive wheeled devices can also include adapted public transportation. A randomized controlled trial showed occupational therapy treatment to address community mobility in the post-stroke population led to clients making more outdoor journeys and rendered clients more likely to get out of the house than a control group. Benefits were greater with those who had a decreased perception of their own mobility abilities (Logan, Gladman, Avery, Walker, Dyas, & Groom, 2004).

Effects of Occupational Therapy in Promoting Functional Mobility Outcomes

Environmental Modification

Empirical Studies

In a randomized clinical trial, it was suggested that wheelchair users were not necessarily able to predict the need for adjustment, repair, or exchange of their wheelchairs, possibly leading to risk of pressure sores, accidents, or near accidents. It was found that the intervention group, in which an occupational therapist would schedule follow-up for wheelchair maintenance, significantly decreased the incidence of accidents compared to a control group of no follow-up after initial prescription. In addition, it was found that 99% of inspected wheelchairs required some form of maintenance work at the scheduled check-up (Hansen, Tresse, & Gunnarsson, 2004).

Trefler, Fitzgerald, Hobson, Bursick, and Joseph (2004) found that participants with an individually fitted wheelchair (fitted by an occupational therapist) had less difficulty propelling the system, showed an increase in forward reach to reach desired objects, increased their quality of life via social functions, and had an increase in satisfaction with their equipment.

A study by Amos and colleagues (2001) showed a statistically significant increase in functional reach when a patient is sitting on an occupational therapist-recommended wedge cushion with a solid seat insert when compared with conventional sling seats. This can lead to greater ability to reach desired items and complete functional tasks when the participant is in the wheelchair.

These results indicate occupational therapists have an important role to play in wheelchair prescription, and those patients who have wheeled mobility systems fitted by an occupational therapist have been seen to have fewer accidents, increased functional reach, increased satisfaction, and greater potential for social involvement than people with no occupational therapy involvement.

Occupational therapy intervention to assist those returning to public transit use has enabled participants to access bus services with confidence (McInerney & McInerney, 1992). Although limited in both quantity and scope, with these results, it can be said that occupational therapy involvement in the selection and use of adapted transportation options can lead to decreased isolation, increased independence, and more community engagement. More research in this area is needed.

Interventions Used to Improve Community Management Outcomes

For occupational therapists, determining interventions that support independence and enable community involvement and participation at a level with which individuals are satisfied is a critical element of clinical practice. Preliminary evidence on EADL training suggests that such interventions have a positive effect on a person's level of functioning. For example, individuals who participated in a community-based occupational therapy intervention program after their stroke showed a non-significant, but positive change in EADL scores as measured by the Barthel Index (BI) and greater satisfaction with services received than those patients receiving routine inpatient services (Gilbertson, Langhorne, Walker, Allen, & Murray, 2000). Evidence for interventions that specifically target occupations associated with community management (e.g., meal preparation, driving, etc.) is promising, but limited in its scope.

Skill Development for Meal Preparation

An IADL that is often the focus of occupational therapy intervention is meal preparation. Enhancing cooking skills can help clients return to independent living, as well as encourage leisure and paid occupations and provide an opportunity for social interaction (Haley & McKay, 2004). The client's age, ability, and life roles should be considered when determining whether this occupational performance area should be targeted for intervention. Few studies have evaluated the effects of occupational therapy intervention on meal preparation, with most of this research focusing on people with cognitive-related dysfunctions (e.g., schizophrenia, acquired brain injury [ABI]) and improvements in underlying skills (e.g., memory recall, fine-motor skills), rather than on the effectiveness of occupational therapy intervention per se.

Training for Driving

In North America, driving an automobile is closely linked with independence. The mobility afforded by accessing an automobile is recognized as a means to having choice and control over one's daily routine. However, problems with vision, cognition, and/or physical mobility that result from health conditions (e.g., stroke, macular degeneration, dementia, etc.) can affect driving safety. As individuals age, they are more likely to experience health-related changes that compromise driving safety (Stav, Hunt, & Arbesman, 2006).

As noted by Lloyd and colleagues (2001), occupational therapists have specialized clinical training in "physical, psychological, visual perceptual and cognitive assessment, which is advantageous when examining driving capability" (p. 154). Much research has focused on assessing cognitive, sensory, and motor function with regard to driving safety, and early research suggests that independence in functional activities, such as driving, is not possible without rehabilitation (Hunt & Arbesman, 2008; Pankow, Luchins, Studebaker, & Chettleburgh, 2004). In addition to this research, preliminary evidence for occupational therapy-based interventions that facilitate safe operation of a motor vehicle is promising, but limited in scope.

Effects of Occupational Therapy in Promoting Community Management Outcomes

Skill Development for Meal Preparation

Empirical Studies

For individuals with chronic schizophrenia, significant improvements in meal preparation were noted in both home- and clinic-based cooking groups (Duncombe, 2004). Greatest gains were made by individuals who had limited cooking experience. However, there were no context-specific differences between groups. Given that both groups were facilitated by an occupational therapist, attributing gains directly to occupational therapy-specific strategies requires further investigation. Nonetheless, this evidence indicates that such interventions can lead to improvements in performance.

Eakman and Nelson (2001), in a study of individuals with ABI, found that hands-on, occupation-based training (i.e., learning a cooking task) facilitated memory recall abilities. The term *hands-on* is used to describe a teaching technique in which individuals engage in the occupation, rather than passively watching a demonstration. Results suggested that using hands-on techniques can facilitate memory recall for clients with ABI. These results differ from those of another study that compared how individuals with ABI could prepare a simple meal after two different interventions, namely a hands-on technique versus parquetry block assembly task. No significant differences between groups were found post-intervention in the ability to prepare a simple meal; however, the perceptual skills parquetry group showed a significant improvement in constructional abilities (Neistadt, 1992). Evidence to support occupational therapy interventions that use active learning approaches is limited. Studies that employ more rigorous research designs are necessary.

Training for Driving

Empirical Studies

Most research on driving in the field of occupational therapy has focused on the use of remediation strategies (i.e., computer-based retraining programs) with individuals with stroke (Mazer, Sofer, Korner-Bitensky, Gelinas, Hanley, & Wood-Dauphinee, 2003). Mazer and colleagues (2003) conducted a randomized controlled trial to compare the effectiveness of the Useful Field of View (UFOV) computer-based program and traditional computerized visuoperception retraining programs on driving performance of clients with stroke (see Mazer et al., 2003, for protocol). Other outcome measures included visuoperception tests (i.e., Complex Reaction Time, Motor-Free Visual Perception Test [MVPT], Single and Double Letter Cancellation Test, Money Road Map Test of Direction Sense, Trail Making Test [TMT] Parts A and B, Bells Test, Charron Test) and the Test of Everyday Attention. Results indicated there were no significant differences between groups on any of the outcome measures, including the on-road driving evaluation. However, results suggested that improvements were experienced by individuals with right-sided lesions after UFOV training with regard to their on-road performance, which suggests that training should target specific visuoperceptual skills (e.g., divided attention). The use of driving simulators for driver training offers another potential intervention tool for occupational therapists to use with clients. However, most research has focused on its utility as an assessment tool (Stern & Schold Davis, 2006) rather than as a means for driver training. The use of driving simulators as well as other virtual reality-based software in clinical practice must be evaluated to determine their effectiveness as an occupational therapy intervention, particularly with regard to whether virtual training translates to actual changes in real-world performance.

Occupational therapists provide opportunities for driver retraining, particularly if their clinical practice is in the area of driver rehabilitation. A systematic review of the effectiveness of older driver retraining reported that current evidence is limited but sufficiently positive (Kua, Korner-Bitensky, Desrosiers, Man-Son-Hing, & Marshall, 2007). Retraining programs included in the review were physical retraining (one study), visual perceptual-based interventions (one study), education-based interventions (five studies), and a combination of all three, including traffic engineering improvements (one study). There is limited evidence to suggest that physical retraining and visual perception retraining improve driving-related skills in older drivers. There is moderate evidence that educational interventions improve driver awareness and on-road driving behavior of older drivers, but do not reduce crashes. Given the relationship between mobility, health, and independence in their community for this growing segment of the driving population, the merit of such retraining programs warrants further investigation.

Measures Used to Capture Self-Care Outcomes

When examining outcomes that are sensitive to occupational therapy intervention to impact self-care, it is useful to characterize the typical outcomes measured in these studies. In the empirical articles selected, several outcome measures were used. Some studies used up to six separate measures, and nearly one quarter of the studies used modified or home-made versions of existing measures. Standardized tools should be selected more frequently when conducting research to investigate occupational therapy interventions. The increased use of standardized outcome measures will make comparison across studies easier for clinicians and researchers. The studies that did use standardized outcome measures showed a preference for using certain tools. The Barthel Index (BI), Nottingham Scale, Functional Independence Measure (FIM), and Canadian Occupational Performance Measure (COPM) were selected most frequently as outcome measures.

Drawing on reviews of measures already completed within occupational therapy (Law, Baum, & Dunn, 2005) and the measures used in studies reviewed for this project, we have compiled a table of measures most suitable for use in occupational therapy to assess outcomes of productivity intervention. As indicated by the majority of research in this area, the outcomes focus on assessment at the levels of body function or participation. These outcome measures are reviewed in Table 4-5.

Table 4-5
Outcome Measures to Assess Self-Care Interventions

Measure	Population	Content Domains	Reliability and Validity
Barthel Index (BI)	Adults	10 checklist items on a 2- or 3-point ordinal scale. Administration can take up to 1 hour of observation. Scoring will take between 2 and 5 minutes.	Studies show excellent intra-rater, inter-rater reliability, some predictive validity.
Canadian Occupational Performance Measure (COPM)	All populations	Semi-structured interview focusing on problem identification in 3 areas: Self-care, productivity, and leisure; 5 most important issues are rated by client for performance and satisfaction.	Studies demonstrate internal consistency, test-retest reliability, and content, construct, and criterion validity.
Functional Independence Measure (FIM)	Rehabilitation clients aged 7 and over	18 items scored on a 7-point scale in self-care, mobility, communication, cognition, and toileting domains.	Excellent inter-rater, intra-rater reliability and internal consistency, good validity.
Nottingham Extended Activities of Daily Living Scale	Adults and older adults	22 items measuring IADL at home and in the community. Uses a self-rated 4-point scale assessing what the person actually does, from not doing an activity at all to doing it on their own.	Studies demonstrate excellent internal consistency, good test-retest reliability, and excellent construct validity.

Conclusions and Recommendations for Future Research

The nature of certain interventions as well as the role of occupational therapists across teams varied across these studies. In the examples of early supported discharge and stroke rehabilitation, it was concluded that differences in service delivery led to difficulty generalizing results. Study designs that compare similar programs and intervention methods are needed.

Within the selected body of literature, occupational therapists were most commonly working with people who have sustained a stroke, ABI, or geriatrics. Within selected studies, there were three areas most commonly addressed by occupational therapy self-care interventions. The first, targeting ADL retraining, includes direct retraining of activities such as bathing, toileting, feeding, and dressing. The second, interventions targeting IADL retraining, includes occupations such as driving, shopping, home management, and cooking. Finally, provision of and training in cognitive compensation strategies was the third most common area of intervention. This includes interventions such as memory retraining and energy conservation.

References

Alexander, H., Bugge, C., & Hagen, S. (2001). What is the association between the different components of stroke rehabilitation and health outcomes? *Clinical Rehabilitation, 15,* 207-215.

Alexander, J. A., Lichtenstein, R., Jinnet, K., Wells, R., Zazzeli, J., & Liu, D. (2005). Cross-functional team processes and patient functional improvement. *Health Services Research, 40,* 1335-1355.

Alvund, K., Jepsen, E., Vass, M., & Lundemark, H. (2002). Effects of comprehensive follow-up home visits after hospitalization on functional ability and readmissions in older people. A randomized controlled study. *Scandinavian Journal of Occupational Therapy, 9,* 17-22.

Amos, L., Brimner, A., Dierckman, H., Easton, H., Grimes, H., Kain, J., et al. (2001). Effects of positioning on functional reach. *Physical and Occupational Therapy in Geriatrics, 20*(1), 59-72.

Bode, R. K., Heinemann, A. W., Semik, P., & Mallinson, T. (2004). Relative importance of rehabilitation therapy characteristics on functional outcomes for persons with stroke. *Stroke, 35*(11), 2537-2542.

Bohannon, R. W., Ahlquist, M., Lee, N., & Maljanian, R. (2003). Functional gains during acute hospitalization for stroke. *Neurorehabilitation and Neural Repair, 17*(3), 192-195.

Brosseau, L., Philippe, P., Potvin, L., & Boulanger, Y. L. (1996). Post-stroke inpatient rehabilitation. I. predicting length of stay. *American Journal of Physical Medicine and Rehabilitation, 75,* 422-430.

Buddenberg, L. A., & Schkade, J. K. (1998). Special feature: A comparison of occupational therapy intervention approaches for older patients after hip fracture. *Topics in Geriatric Rehabilitation, 13*(4), 52-68.

Buning, M. E., Angelo, J. A., & Schmeler, M. R. (2001). Occupational performance and the transition to powered mobility: A pilot study. *American Journal of Occupational Therapy, 55*(3), 339-344.

Caplan, G. A., Williams A. J., Daly, B., & Abraham, K. (2004). A randomized controlled trial of comprehensive geriatric assessment and multidisciplinary intervention after discharge of elderly from the emergency department: The DEED II study. *Journal of the American Geriatrics Society, 52,* 1417-1423.

Carlton, R. S. (1987). The effects of body mechanics instruction on work performance. *American Journal of Occupational Therapy, 41*(1), 16-20.

Comella, C. L., Stebbins, G. T., Brown-Toms, N., & Goetz, C. G. (1994). Physical therapy and Parkinson's disease: A controlled clinical trial. *Neurology, 44* (3 Pt 1), 376-378.

Corr, S., & Bayer, A. (1995). Occupational therapy for stroke patients after hospital discharge: A randomized controlled trial. *Clinical Rehabilitation, 9*(4), 291-296.

Dam, M., Tonin, P., Ermani, M., Pizzolato, G., Iaia, V., & Battistin, L. (1993). The effects of long-term rehabilitation therapy on post-stroke hemiplegic patients. *Stroke, 24*, 1186-1191.

Davies, A., De Souza, L. H., & Frank, A. O. (2003). Changes in the quality of life in severely disabled people following provision of powered indoor/outdoor chairs. *Disability and Rehabilitation, 25*(6), 286-290.

Devitt, R., Chau, B., & Jutai, J. W. (2003). The effect of wheelchair use on the quality of life of persons with multiple sclerosis. *Occupational Therapy in Health Care, 17*(3-4), 63-79.

DiFabio, R. P., Soderberg, J., Choi, T., Hansen, C. R., & Schapiro, R. T. (1998). Extended outpatient rehabilitation: Its influence on symptom frequency, fatigue and functional status for persons with progressive multiple sclerosis. *Archives of Physical Medicine and Rehabilitation, 79*, 141-146.

Donkervoort, M., Dekker, J., Stehmann Saris, F. C., & Deelman, B. G. (2001). Efficacy of strategy training in left hemisphere stroke patients with apraxia: A randomised clinical trial. *Neuropsychological Rehabilitation, 11*(5), 549-566.

Drummond, A. E., Miller, N., Colquohoun, M., & Logan, P. C. (1996). The effects of a stroke unit on activities of daily living. *Clinical Rehabilitation, 10*, 12-22.

Duncombe, L. W. (2004). Comparing learning of cooking in home and clinic for people with schizophrenia. *American Journal of Occupational Therapy, 58*(3), 272-278.

Eakman, A. M., & Nelson, D. L. (2001). The effect of hands-on occupation on recall memory in men with traumatic brain injuries. *Occupational Therapy Journal of Research, 21*(2), 109-114.

Eyres, L., & Unsworth, C. A. (2005). Occupational therapy in acute hospitals: The effectiveness of a pilot program to maintain occupational performance in older clients. *Australian Occupational Therapy Journal, 52*(3), 218-224.

Finnerty, J. P., Keeping, I., Bullough, R. G. N., & Jones, J. (2001). The effectiveness of outpatient pulmonary rehabilitation in chronic lung disease: A randomized control trial. *Chest, 119*, 1705-1710.

Fjærtoft, H., Indredavik, B., Johnsen, R., & Lydersen, S. (2004). Acute stroke unit care combined with early supported discharge. Long term effects on quality of life: A randomized controlled trial. *Clinical Rehabilitation, 18*, 580-586.

Fleming, S. A., Blake, H., Gladman, J. R. F., Hart, E., Lymbery, M., Dewey, M. E., et al. (2004). A randomised controlled trial of care home rehabilitation service to reduce long-term institutionalisation for elderly people. *Age and Ageing, 33*, 384-390.

Freeman, J. A., Langdon, D. W., Hobart, J. C., & Thompson, A. J. (1999). Inpatient rehabilitation in multiple sclerosis: Do the benefits carry over into the community? *Neurology, 52*, 50-56.

Gauthier, L., Dalziel, S., & Gauthier, S. (1987). The benefits of group occupational therapy for patients with Parkinson's disease. *American Journal of Occupational Therapy, 41*(6), 360-365.

Gilbertson, L., Langhorne, P., Walker, A., Allen, A., & Murray, G. D. (2000). Domiciliary occupational therapy for patients with stroke discharged from hospital: Randomised controlled trial. *BMJ, 320*(7235), 603-606.

Gladman, J. R., Lincoln, N. B., & Barer, D. H. (1993). A randomized controlled trial of domiciliary and hospital-based rehabilitation for stroke patients after discharge from hospital. *Journal of Neurology, Neurosurgery and Psychiatry, 56*, 960-966.

Greenhalgh, T. (2006). *How to read a paper: The basics of evidence-based medicine* (3rd ed.). London, England: Blackwell Publishing Ltd.

Hagsten, B. E., & Soderback, I. (1994). Occupational therapy after hip fracture: A pilot study of the clients, the care and the costs. *Clinical Rehabilitation, 8*(2), 142-148.

Hagsten, B., Svensson, O., & Gardulf, A. (2004). Early individualized postoperative occupational therapy training in 100 patients improves ADL after hip fracture: A randomized trial. *Acta Orthopaedica Scandinavica, 75*(2), 177-183.

Hagsten, B., Svensson, O., & Gardulf, A. (2006). Health-related quality of life and self-reported ability concerning ADL and IADL after hip fracture: A randomized trial. *Acta Orthopaedica Scandinavica, 77*(1), 114-119.

Haley, L., & McKay, E. A. (2004). Baking gives you confidence: Users' views of engaging in the occupation of baking. *British Journal of Occupational Therapy, 67*(3), 125-128.

Hames-Hahn, C. S., & Llorens, L. A. (1988). Impact of a multisensory occupational therapy program on components of self-feeding behavior in the elderly. *Physical and Occupational Therapy in Geriatrics, 6*(3-4), 63-86.

Hammond, A., Young, A., & Kidao, R. (2004). A randomised controlled trial of occupational therapy for people with early rheumatoid arthritis. *Annals of the Rheumatic Diseases, 63*(1), 23-30.

Hansen, R., Tresse, S., & Gunnarsson, R. K. (2004). Fewer accidents and better maintenance with active wheelchair check-ups: A randomized controlled clinical trial. *Clinical Rehabilitation, 18*(6), 631-639.

Hastings, J., Gowans, S., & Watson, D. E. (2004). Effectiveness of occupational therapy following organ transplantation. *Canadian Journal of Occupational Therapy, 71*(4), 238-242.

Heinemann, A. W., Hamilton, B., Linacre, J. M., Wright, B. D., & Granger, C. (1995). Status and therapeutic intensity during inpatient rehabilitation. *American Journal of Physical Medicine and Rehabilitation, 74*, 315-326.

Hendriksen, H., & Harrison, R. A. (2001). Occupational therapy in accident and emergency departments: A randomized controlled trial. *Journal of Advanced Nursing, 36*(6), 727-732.

Hui, E., Lum, C. M., Woo, J., Or, K. H., & Kay, R. L. (1995). Outcomes of elderly stroke patients: Day hospital versus conventional medical management. *Stroke, 22*, 1616-1619.

Hunt, L. A., & Arbesman, M. (2008). Evidence-based and occupational perspective of effective interventions for older clients that remediate or support improved driving performance. *American Journal of Occupational Therapy, 62*(2), 136-148.

Indredavik, B., Bakke, F., Solberg, R., Rokseth, R., Lund Haaheim, L., & Holme, I. (1991). Benefit of a stroke unit: A randomized control trial. *Stroke, 22*, 1026-1031.

Johansson, K., Lindgren, I., Widner, H., & Wiklund, I. (1993). Can sensory stimulation improve the functional outcome in stroke patients? *Neurology, 43*, 2189-2192.

Jones, G. R., Miller, T. A., & Petrella, R. J. (2002). Evaluation of rehabilitation outcomes in older patients with hip fractures. *American Journal of Physical Medicine and Rehabilitation, 81*(7), 489-497.

Jongbloed, L., Stacey, S., & Brighton, C. (1989). Stroke rehabilitation: Sensorimotor integrative treatment versus functional treatment. *American Journal of Occupational Therapy, 43*(6), 391-397.

Jousset, N., Fanello, S., Bontoux, L., Dubus, V., Billabert, C., Vielle, B., et al. (2004). Effects of functional restoration versus 3 hours physical therapy: A randomized control trial. *Spine, 29*, 487-494.

Kalra, L. (1994). The influence of stroke unit rehabilitation on functional recovery from stroke. *Stroke, 25*, 821-825.

Keren, O., Motin, M., Heinemann, A. W., O'Reilly, C. M., Bode, R. K., Semik, P., et al. (2004). Relationship between rehabilitation therapies and outcome of stroke patients in Israel: A preliminary study. *Israel Medical Association Journal, 6*, 736-741.

Kua, I., Korner-Bitensky, N., Desrosiers, J., Man-Son-Hing, M., & Marshall, S. (2007). Older driver retraining: A systematic review of evidence of effectiveness. *Journal of Safety Research, 38*, 81-90.

Landi, F., Cesari, M., Onder, G., Tafani, A., Zamboni, V., & Cocchi, A. (2006). Effects of an occupational therapy program on functional outcomes in older stroke patients. *Gerontology, 52*(2), 85-91.

Langhorne, P., Taylor, G., Murray, G., Dennis, M., Anderson, C., Bautz-Holter, E., Dey, P., Indredavik, B., Mayo, N., Power, M., Rodgers, H., Ronning, OM., Rudd, A., Suwanwela, N., Widen-Holmqvist, L., & Wolfe C. (2005). Early supported discharge services for stroke patients: Meta-analysis of individual patients' data. *Lancet, 365*, 501-506.

Law, M., Baum, C., & Dunn, W. (2005). *Measuring occupational performance: Supporting best practice in occupational therapy* (2nd ed.). Thorofare, NJ: SLACK Incorporated.

Legg, L. A., Drummond, A. E., & Langhorne, P. (2006). Occupational therapy for patients with problems in activities of daily living after stroke. *Cochrane Database of Systematic Reviews*, Issue 4.

Lin, J. H., Chang, C. M., Liu, C. K., Huang, M. H., & Lin, Y. T. (2000). Efficiency and effectiveness of stroke rehabilitation after first stroke. *Journal of the Formosan Medical Association, 99*, 483-490.

Lincoln, N. B., Walker, M. F., Dixon, A., & Knights P. (2004). Evaluation of a multiprofessional community stroke team: A randomized controlled trial. *Clinical Rehabilitation, 18*, 40-47.

Lindquist, B., & Unsworth, C. (1999). Occupational therapy—Reflections on the state of the art. *World Federation of Occupational Therapy—Bulletin, 39*, 26-30.

Liu, K. P., Chan, C. C., Lee, T. M., & Hui-Chan, C. W. (2004). Mental imagery for promoting relearning for people after stroke. *Archives of Physical Medicine and Rehabilitation, 85*, 1403-1408.

Lloyd, S., Cormack, C. N., Blais, K., Messeri, G., McCallum, M. A., Spicer, K., et al. (2001). Driving and dementia: A review of the literature. *Canadian Journal of Occupational Therapy, 68*(3), 149-156.

Logan, P. A., Gladman, J. R. F., Avery, A., Walker, M. F., Dyas, J., & Groom, L. (2004). Randomised controlled trial of an occupational therapy intervention to increase outdoor mobility after stroke. *British Medical Journal, 329*(7479), 1372-1374.

MacPhee, A. H., Kirby, R. L., Coolen, A. L., Smith, C., MacLeod, D. A., & Dupuis, D. J. (2004). Wheelchair skills training program: A randomized clinical trial of wheelchair users undergoing initial rehabilitation. *Archives of Physical Medicine and Rehabilitation, 85*(1), 41-50.

Mathiowetz, V., & Matuska, K. M. (1998). Effectiveness of inpatient rehabilitation on self-care abilities of individuals with multiple sclerosis. *Neurorehabilitation, 11*(2), 141-151.

Mayo, N. E., Wood-Dauphinee, S., Cote, R., Gayton, D., Carlton, J., Buttery, J., et al. (2000). There's no place like home: An evaluation of early supported discharge for stroke. *Stroke, 31*, 1016-1023.

Mazer, B. L., Sofer, S., Korner-Bitensky, N., Gelinas, I., Hanley, J., & Wood-Dauphinee, S. (2003). Effectiveness of a visual attention retraining program on the driving performance of clients with stroke. *Archives of Physical Medicine and Rehabilitation, 84*(4), 541-550.

McCabe, P., Nason, F., Turco, P. D., Friedman, D., & Seddon, J. M. (2000). Evaluating the effectiveness of a vision rehabilitation intervention using an objective and subjective measure of functional performance. *Ophthalmic Epidemiology, 7*, 259-270.

McInerney, C. A., & McInerney, M. (1992). A mobility skills training program for adults with developmental disabilities. *American Journal of Occupational Therapy, 46*(3), 233-239.

McNaughton, H., DeJong, G., Smout, R. J., Melvin, J. L., & Brandstater, M. (2005). A comparison of stroke rehabilitation practice and outcomes between New Zealand and United States facilities. *Archives of Physical Medicine and Rehabilitation, 86*(12 Suppl), S115-S120.

Melin, A. L., & Bygren, L. O. (1992). Efficacy of the rehabilitation of elderly primary health care after short-stay hospital treatment. *Medical Care, 30*, 1004-1015.

Montgomery Orr, P., & Bratton, G. N. (1992). The effect of an inpatient arthritis program on self-assessed functional ability. *Rehabilitation Nursing, 17*, 306-310.

Naglie, G., Tansey, C., Kirkland, J. L., Ogilvie-Harris, D. J., Detsky, A. S., Etchells, E., et al. (2002). Interdisciplinary inpatient care for elderly people with hip fracture: A randomized controlled trial. *Canadian Medical Association Journal, 167*, 25-32.

Neistadt, M. E. (1992). Occupational therapy treatments for constructional deficits. *American Journal of Occupational Therapy, 46*(2), 141-148.

Nikolaus, T., Specht-Leible, N., Bach, M., Oster, P., & Schlierf, G. (1999). A randomized trial of comprehensive geriatric assessment and home intervention in the care of hospitalized patients. *Age and Ageing, 28*(6), 543-550.

Ostrow, P., Parente, R., Ottenbacher, K. J., & Bonder, B. (1989). Functional outcomes and rehabilitation: An acute care field study. *Journal of Rehabilitation Research and Development, 26*(3), 17-26.

Pankow, L., Luchins, D., Studebaker, J., & Chettleburgh, D. (2004). Evaluation of a vision rehabilitation program for older adults with visual impairment. *Topics in Geriatric Rehabilitation, Vision Rehabilitation, 20*(3), 223-232.

Patti, F., Reggio, A., Nicoletti, F., Sellaroli, T., Deinite, G., & Nicoletti, F. (1996). Effects of rehabilitation therapy on Parkinson's disability and functional independence. *Journal of Neurologic Rehabilitation, 10*, 223-231.

Przybylski, B. R., Dumont, E. D., Watkins, M. E., Warren, S. A., Beaulne, A. P., & Lier, D. A. (1996). Outcomes of enhanced physical and occupational therapy service in a nursing home setting. *Archives of Physical Medicine and Rehabilitation, 77*, 554-561.

Reid, D., Laliberte-Rudman, D., & Hebert, D. (2002). Impact of wheeled seating mobility devices on adult users' occupational performance: A critical literature review. *Canadian Journal of Occupational Therapy, 69*(5), 261-280.

Ryan, T., Enderby, P., & Rigby, A. S. (2006). A randomized controlled trial to evaluate intensity of community-based rehabilitation provision following stroke or hip fracture in old age. *Clinical Rehabilitation, 20*, 123-131.

Sackley, C., Wade, D. T., Mant, D., Atkinson, J. C., Yudkin, P., Cardoso, K., et al. (2006). Cluster randomized pilot controlled trial of an occupational therapy intervention for residents with stroke in UK care homes. *Stroke, 37*(9), 2336-2341.

Sanford, J. A., Griffiths, P. C., Richardson, P., Hargraves, K., Butterfield, T., & Hoenig, H. (2006). The effects of in-home rehabilitation on task self-efficacy in mobility-impaired adults: A randomized clinical trial. *Journal of the American Geriatrics Society, 54*(11), 1641-1648.

Saltvedt, I., Opdahl Mo, E. S., Fayers, P., Kaasa, S., & Sletvold, O. (2002). Reduced mortality in treating acutely sick, frail older patients in a geriatric evaluation and management unit. A prospective randomized trial. *Journal of the American Geriatrics Society, 50*, 792-798.

Soderback, I., & Guidetti, S. (1992). The effect of personal care training at a medical department: A study in occupational therapy. *Clinical Rehabilitation, 6*(3), 203-208.

Stav, W. B., Hunt, L. A., & Arbesman, M. (2006). *Occupational therapy practice guidelines for driving and community mobility.* Bethesda, MD: American Occupational Therapy Association.

Stern, E. B., & Schold Davis, E. (2006). Driving simulators. In J. M. Pellerito, Jr. (Ed.), *Driver rehabilitation and community mobility.* St. Louis, MO: Elsevier Mosby.

Steultjens, E. M., Dekker, J., Bouter, L. M., Leemrijse, C. J., & van den Ende, C. H. (2005). Evidence of the efficacy of occupational therapy in different conditions: An overview of systematic reviews. *Clinical Rehabilitation, 19*(3), 247-254.

Steultjens, E. M., Dekker, J., Bouter, L. M., van de Nes, J. C., Cup, E. H., & van den Ende, C. H. (2003). Occupational therapy for stroke patients: A systematic review. *Stroke, 34*(3), 676-687.

Steultjens, E. M., Dekker, J., Bouter, L. M., van Schaardenberg, D., Van, K., & van den Ende, C. H. (2002). Occupational therapy for rheumatoid arthritis: A systematic review. *Arthritis Care and Research, 47*(6), 672-685.

Storr, L. K., Sorensen, P. S., & Ravnborg, M. (2006). The efficacy of multidisciplinary rehabilitation in stable multiple sclerosis patients. *Multiple Sclerosis, 12*, 235-242.

Sulch, D., Perez, I., Melbourne, A., & Kalra, L. (2000). Randomized control trial of integrated (managed) care pathway for stroke rehabilitation. *Stroke, 31*, 1929-1934.

Thorsen, A., Widen Holmqvist, L., de Pedro-Cuesta, J., & von Koch, L. (2005). A randomized controlled trial of early supported discharge after stroke: Five year follow up of patient outcome. *Stroke, 36*, 297-302.

Trefler, E., Fitzgerald, S. G., Hobson, D. A., Bursick, T., & Joseph, R. (2004). Outcomes of wheelchair systems intervention with residents of long-term care facilities. *Assistive Technology, 16*(1), 18-21.

Tremblay, M., Campbell, A., & Hudson, L. (2005). When elevators were for pianos: An oral history account of the civilian experience of using wheelchairs in Canadian society, the first twenty-five years: 1945-1970. *Disability and Society, 20*(2), 103-116.

Trend, P., Kaye, J., Gage, H., Owen, C., & Wade, D. (2002). Short term effectiveness of intensive multidisciplinary rehabilitation for carers. *Clinical Rehabilitation, 16*, 717-725.

Unsworth, C. A., & Cunningham, D. T. (2002). Examining the evidence base for occupational therapy with clients following stroke. *British Journal of Occupational Therapy, 65*(1), 21-29.

Unsworth, C. A., & Duncombe, D. (2005). A comparison of client outcomes from two acute care neurological services using self-care data from the Australian therapy outcome measures for occupational therapy (AusTOMs-OT). *British Journal of Occupational Therapy, 68*(10), 477-482.

van Heugten, C. M., Dekker, J., Deelman, B. G., Stehmann Saris, J. C., & Kinebanian, A. (2000). Rehabilitation of stroke patients with apraxia: The role of additional cognitive and motor impairments. *Disability and Rehabilitation, 22*(12), 547-554.

van Heugten, C. M., Dekker, J., Deelman, B. G., van Dijk, A. J., Stehmann Saris, J. C., & Kinebanian, A. (1998). Outcome of strategy training in stroke patients with apraxia: A phase II study. *Clinical Rehabilitation, 12*(4), 294-303.

Von Koch, L., de Pedro-Cuesta, J., Kostulas, V., Almazan, J., & Holmqvist, L. W. (2001). Randomized controlled trial of rehabilitation at home after stroke: One-year follow-up of patient outcome, resource use and cost. *Cerebrovascular Diseases, 12*, 131-138.

Wade, D. T., Gage, H., Owen, C., Trend, P., Grossmith, C., & Kaye, J. (2003). Multidisciplinary rehabilitation for people with Parkinson's disease: A randomised controlled study. *Journal of Neurology, Neurosurgery and Psychiatry, 74*, 158-162.

Walker, M. F., Drummond, A. E. R., & Lincoln, N. B. (1996). Evaluation of dressing practice for stroke patients after discharge from hospital: A crossover design study. *Clinical Rehabilitation, 10*(1), 23-31.

Walker, M. F., Gladman, J. R. F., Lincoln, N. B., Siemonsma, P., & Whiteley, T. (1999). Occupational therapy for stroke patients not admitted to hospital: A randomized controlled trial. *Lancet, 354*(9175), 278-280.

Walker, M. F., Hawkins, K., Gladman, J. R., & Lincoln, N. B. (2001). Randomized controlled trial of occupational therapy at home: Results at 1 year. *Journal of Neurology, Neurosurgery and Psychiatry, 70*(2), 267.

Walker, M. F., Leonardi-Bee, J., Bath, P., Langhorne, P., Dewey, M., Corr, S., et al. (2004). Individual patient data meta-analysis of randomized controlled trials of community occupational therapy for stroke patients. *Stroke, 35*(9), 2226-2232.

Walker, C. M., & Walker, M. F. (2001). Dressing ability after stroke: A review of the literature. *British Journal of Occupational Therapy, 64*(9), 449-454.

Ward-Gibson, J., & Schkade, J. (1997). Occupational adaptation intervention with patients with cerebrovascular accident: A clinical study. *American Journal of Occupational Therapy, 51*(7), 523-529.

Weiss, Z., Snir, D., Klein, B., Avraham, I., Shani, R., Zetler, H., et al. (2004). Effectiveness of home rehabilitation after stroke in Israel. *International Journal of Rehabilitation Research, 27*(2), 119-125.

Werner, R. A., & Kessler, S. (1996). Effectiveness of an intensive outpatient rehabilitation program for post-acute stroke patients. *Rehabilitation/Association of Academic Physiatrists, 75*, 114-120.

Widen Holmqvist, L. W., von Koch, L., Kostulas, V., Holm, M., Widsell, G., Tegler, H., et al. (1998). A randomized controlled trial of rehabilitation at home after stroke in Southwest Stockholm. *Stroke, 29*, 591-597.

Yagura, H., Miyai, I., Suzuki, T., & Yanagihara, T. (2005). Patients with severe stroke benefit most by interdisciplinary rehabilitation team approach. *Cerebrovascular Diseases, 20*, 258-263.

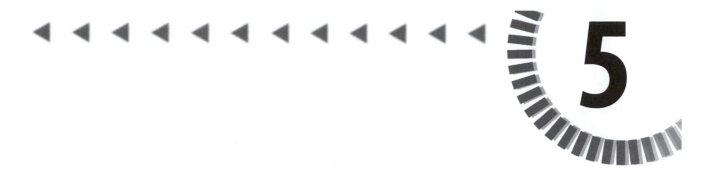

PRODUCTIVITY—
WORK AND VOLUNTEER WORK
OUTCOMES

Mary Law, PhD, FCAOT and Rebecca Gewurtz, MSc (OT), OT Reg. (Ont.)

An outcome of importance for occupational therapy is a person's productivity. As defined within the discipline, productivity refers to the "activities that customarily fill the bulk of one's day and which contribute to economic preservation, home and family maintenance, and service or personal development" (McColl, Law, Stewart, Doubt, Pollock, & Krupa, 2002). Examples of productivity outcomes include paid or unpaid work, household management, and school. In this book, household management, also called instrumental activities of daily living (IADL), is discussed in Chapters 3 and 4. Thus, this chapter focuses on occupational therapy interventions, effects, and outcomes for the areas of work and volunteer work.

Conceptual Background

Occupational therapists provide intervention for people to participate in the productivity-based occupations of work and volunteer work. Rehabilitation programs can provide education and instruction to promote healthy work habits or can be in the form of preparing the worker to return to work through retraining/hardening, modifying duties, and/or redefining job position. Occupational therapists also provide education and functional training to help people to learn the safest way to carry out their jobs and prevent injury or re-injury.

Occupational therapists have a long history of providing interventions focused on improving participation in work and/or volunteer work. Vocational rehabilitation and work-related rehabilitation has been at the core of the profession since the beginning (Canadian Association of Occupational Therapists [CAOT], 1993; Harvey-Krefting, 1985). Today, there continues to be a focus on providing interventions for people to participate in work in all areas of practice including people with mental illnesses, acquired brain injuries, physical disabilities, and developmental disabilities. Occupational therapists are involved in creating and developing work opportunities for people who are interested in entering the workplace, as well as helping individuals return to work or school after the onset of an illness or injury.

A great deal of attention within the occupational therapy literature has focused on the meaning of work and other productive occupations for individuals. Productive occupations are an important component

M. Law & M. A. McColl (Eds.)
Interventions, Effects, and Outcomes in Occupational Therapy:
Adults and Older Adults (pp. 119-143)
© 2010 SLACK Incorporated

of adult life and are associated with improved access to social determinants of health. For example, paid and unpaid work often provides opportunities to participate in community life and contribute to society. Most individuals spend a considerable amount of their time devoted to work and often organize their daily routine around their roles and responsibilities in this area. Productive occupations are often central to one's identity and can provide opportunities to connect with others in meaningful ways. Many productive occupations are associated with access to financial resources either through direct remuneration or, in the case of education, through access to future employment or career opportunities. Opportunities to engage in productive occupations that offer the right balance of challenge and predictability seem to be associated with health, well-being, and self-actualization.

The importance of work is no less relevant for people with disabilities. Individuals with disabilities have repeatedly expressed the importance of work in their recovery (Jiranek & Kirby, 1990; Lord, Schnarr, & Hutchison, 1987; Rogers, 1995). Equal opportunity for work is an essential component of various human rights and disability legislation in many jurisdictions. Most individuals, regardless of their disability status, enjoy work and seek opportunities to be challenged through work.

The holistic perspective of occupational therapy is well-suited to the study of work and work-related interventions. The Person-Environment-Occupation (PEO) framework (Law, Cooper, Strong, Stewart, Rigby, & Letts, 1996), when applied to work, can be thought of as Work-Workplace-Worker (Cockburn, Kirsh, Krupa, & Gewurtz, 2004). This framework allows for a unique way of viewing and intervening around productivity that distinguishes occupational therapists from other professionals who have expertise in this area. Occupational therapy assessments in this area often consider how the worker in the particular workplace is able to carry out the essential components of his or her work role and responsibilities (Sandqvist & Henriksson, 2004). Interventions can focus on the level of the worker (skill development, work hardening, work conditioning), the workplace (modified workstations, flexible schedules, support from others), or the work (modified duties, restructuring non-essential components). This broad perspective focuses interventions on improving the fit between the worker, the workplace, and the work and allows for an individualized approach according to the unique circumstances of each client.

Given the importance of productive occupations, occupational therapists have focused on assessing work capacity and assisting individuals to engage or re-engage in productive occupations. For example,

many occupational therapy services are directly organized around productive occupations. Workplace disability and insurance, vocational rehabilitation services, and disability management are major industries for the profession of occupational therapy (CAOT, 2004a, 2004b). Many occupational therapists are involved in helping individuals resume their career development by returning to paid or unpaid work or school.

Occupational therapists working in this area often use different approaches depending on the individual's connection to the workplace. For individuals with a pre-existing connection to the workplace, the focus in this area of practice is often to minimize disability by assisting employees to stay in the workplace or to facilitate a return to work for those who are on leave. Occupational therapists in this area work with workers, supervisors/managers, and sometimes co-workers to improve the fit between the worker, the workplace, and the work.

However, occupational therapists also work with individuals who are disconnected from work and other productive occupations. For example, the onset of several mental illnesses often occurs during critical periods of career development and can interrupt education pursuits. In these cases, occupational therapists must develop and create opportunities for individuals to engage in meaningful productive occupations. Examples include creating alternative businesses or community-based enterprises (Krupa, Lagarde, & Carmichael, 2003; Rebeiro, Day, Semeniuk, O'Brian, & Wilson, 2001) or providing ongoing and individualized support as individuals pursue their employment or education goals (Kirsh, Cockburn, & Gewurtz, 2005).

Search Strategy

The methodology to search the literature, identify studies, and select them based on the inclusion criteria was discussed in Chapter 2. A systematic search of health care and occupational therapy databases, as well as hand-searched relevant references, yielded critical reviews (e.g., systematic reviews or meta-analyses) and qualitative and quantitative studies that addressed occupational therapy outcomes when providing intervention related to improving areas related to the client's productivity. Selected studies met specific inclusion criteria, which consisted of study publication between 1980 and 2008, adult population, study intervention involving occupational therapist independently or on a multidisciplinary team, and study categorized as level of evidence 1 to 4 based on criteria by Greenhalgh (2006). For this chapter, the search terms used to capture occupational therapy-sensitive outcomes are listed in Table 5-1. A total of

Table 5-1

SEARCH TERMS FOR OCCUPATIONAL THERAPY INTERVENTIONS TO IMPROVE PRODUCTIVITY OUTCOMES

Occupation, occupational therapy (therapist), OR multidisciplinary team AND...

Primary terms: child rearing, education, employee productivity, employment, home-making, job, job performance, parenting, productivity, re-employment, vocation, volunteer, work.

Secondary terms: job re-entry, return to work, vocational rehabilitation.

Additional terms used to focus the search included health care services, health service, health services for the aged, home care, home care services, home health care, home occupational therapy, home rehabilitation, interdisciplinary education, interdisciplinary research, interdisciplinary treatment approach, intervention treatment approach, multidisciplinary care team, outcomes, outcomes assessment patient care, outcomes (health care), outcomes research, patient care team, rehabilitation, rehabilitation care, rehabilitation centre, rehabilitation outcomes, teamwork, treatment effectiveness evaluation, treatment outcomes.

22 empirical studies met the inclusion criteria and are reviewed in this chapter in more detail in Tables 5-2 through 5-4.

Interventions Used to Improve Productivity Outcomes

Findings from the review have been organized according to area of intervention indicated in the literature appraised for this project. Further research regarding interventions and outcomes is needed before any firm conclusions can be drawn about occupational therapy-sensitive outcomes in those areas. However, this review provides an overview of occupational therapy interventions directed at productive occupations that have been studied to date. It provides a glimpse into what occupational therapists are doing in this area and where further research is needed.

Education and Provision of Information to Clients

Occupational therapists are experts in activity analysis and so are able to identify the types of movements and body mechanics that are best suited to a work situation to minimize injury. These interventions typically center on body mechanics and focus on the worker and how he or she can learn to adjust to meet the demands of the work. Such interventions would be particularly relevant for individuals returning to work following an injury to prevent further injury. Furthermore, sectors where certain injuries

seem particularly prevalent could benefit from investing in body mechanic education to prevent injury among workers and the associated disability costs.

Modification of Work Tasks and Activities

Occupational therapy intervention has also focused on improving knowledge, activity levels, and work participation through modification of work-related tasks and activities (can also be called *ergonomics*). These types of interventions would also be useful for preventing injury in vulnerable sectors or for individuals trying to re-engage in their productive occupations after the onset of a disability or illness. Proactive workplaces could implement these strategies to improve productivity and reduce strain and injury among workers.

Comprehensive Programs to Improve Work Skills and Participation

Occupational therapists often provide opportunities for individuals to try out various work-related tasks and develop and improve their skills through practice and education. Interventions in this area can be distinguished between those where individuals practice and learn in simulated settings versus those provided to individuals on the job. In the mental health sector, accumulating evidence is suggesting that rapid job placement with the provision of on-the-job support and accommodations rather than long assessments or prevocational training periods are associated with improved vocational outcomes (Kirsh, Krupa, Cockburn, & Gewurtz, 2006). Furthermore, workplace

text continues on page 137

Table 5-2

OCCUPATIONAL THERAPY INTERVENTIONS PROMOTING PRODUCTIVITY OUTCOMES

Author (Date)	Pop	DX	Setting	Intervention
Darragh, A., Harrison, H., & Kenny, S. (2008)	5	21	3	**Intervention:** Microscope workers were divided by workstation into 2 separate groups, education-only and education-training, and both completed pretest assessments of their working conditions. The education-only group received an informational handout that covered topics such as an ergonomics overview, workstation risk factors, the symptoms of repetitive strain, goals of ergonomics program, and guidelines to follow for injury prevention. The education-training group received the same informational handout along with a 1-hour lecture that included a discussion of the results of their workplace assessments. Immediately after the lecture, workers in this group also received one-on-one hands-on training to implement the principles they had learned in the lecture. **Control:** Workers in this group completed the workplace assessment but received no other intervention.
Kielhofner, G., Braveman, B., Fogg, L., & Levin, M. (2008)	5	18	1	**Intervention:** The program was developed and delivered by OTs and was based on principles from the Model of Human Occupation and the social model of disability. The program consisted of 8 weekly 1-hour group sessions that were led by an OT and peer mentors and were designed to educate clients about topics relevant to the employment process and encourage them to learn from others' experiences. OTs and peer mentors were also available for office hours throughout the duration of the study (9 months) where participants could receive individual attention. Participants were not required to attend all group sessions and could make as much or as little use of the OTs and peer mentors as they wished. **Control:** Participants were offered a series of educational groups 1 hour a week for 8 weeks and monthly presentations on topics related to employment for the following 9 months that were all delivered by an experienced OT. Participants were also provided with written materials related to employment and productivity and could meet individually with an OT on request. The program was designed to be similar to standard care received in supported living facilities.
Kool, J., Bachmann, S., Oesch, P., Knuesel, O., Ambergen, T., de Bie, R., et al. (2007)	2	20	4	**Intervention:** 3-week intervention comparing functional-centered vs. pain-centered treatment. **Control 1:** Functional-centered treatment—activity despite pain by using work stimulation, strength, endurance, and cardiovascular training. Conducted by OT, PT, sports therapist, social worker, nurse, and rheumatologist. **Control 2:** Pain-centered treatment—emphasized pain reduction and included passive and active mobilization, stretching, strength training, and education. (No OT.)
Schene, A., Koeter, M., Kikkert, M., Swinkels, J., & McCrone, P. (2007)	5	12	3	**Intervention:** Patients received usual outpatient treatment for depression, which included anti-depressants and home visits from psychiatric residents. They also received a year-long OT program that consisted of 3 phases: a diagnostic phase, therapeutic phase, and follow-up phase. In the diagnostic phase, the OT worked with the patient and his or her employer and physician to develop a treatment and work reintegration plan. During therapy, the patients attended weekly group sessions and had individual sessions every other week, and during follow-up, they received up to 3 individual visits from an OT. **Control:** Patients received the usual outpatient treatment for depression that included treatment with anti-depressants and home visits from psychiatry residents.

continued

Table 5-2 (continued)
OCCUPATIONAL THERAPY INTERVENTIONS PROMOTING PRODUCTIVITY OUTCOMES

Author (Date)	Pop	DX	Setting	Intervention
Lee, H., Tan, H., Ma, H., Tsai, C., & Liu, Y. (2006)	2	14	1	**Intervention:** Participants attended 1-hour sessions once a week for 12 weeks that focused on a variety of topics, including the impact of stress on cognition, self-awareness of negative emotions, techniques to handle negative emotions, emotional intelligence, communication skills, assertiveness training, and problem-solving skills. Each session began with a warm-up to increase motivation and participation followed by a short lecture and then role play to apply the skills learned in the lecture. Participants also received homework to continue reinforcing their skills.
Li, E., Li-Tsang, C., Lam, C., Hui, K., & Chan, C. (2006)	5	16, 18	3	**Intervention:** A multidisciplinary team composed of a vocational rehabilitation counselor, OTs, and social workers developed and administered a 3-week work readiness training program that was focused on changing injured workers' attitudes regarding return to work. Participants in the program received 1-hour individual counseling sessions once a week and participated in daily group training sessions that lasted 2 to 3 hours. **Control:** Patients received advice on job placement from social workers in a community work health center.
Nordmark, B., Blomqvist, P., Andersson, B., Hagerstrom, M., Nordh-Grate, K., Ronnqvist, R., et al. (2006)	5	19	5	**Intervention:** Combination of vocational rehabilitation and pharmacological treatment. Multidisciplinary team met with the group once every 3 months for the first year and once every 6 months for the second year. Vocational rehabilitation included worksite inspections and recommendations for ergonomic adjustments, assessment for technical aid need (OT role).
de Buck, P., Le Cessie, S., van den Hout, W. B., Peeters, A., Ronday, H., Westedt, M., et al. (2005)	5	18, 19	4	**Intervention:** A multidisciplinary job retention vocational rehabilitation program that lasted between 4 and 12 weeks. Team included a rheumatologist, social worker, PT, OT, and psychologist. The intervention included an assessment, education, vocational counseling, guidance (e.g., identification of resources), and medical/non-medical treatment.
Sang, L. S., & Ying Eria, L. P. (2005)	5	23	4	**Intervention:** 12-week OT work program with 3 to 4 training activities worked on at each session. Training activities based on the physical demands and nature of the clients' previous job before the work injury. The training level of the work program was based on the overload training principle to train the clients' functional strength level.
Sarajuuri, J., Kaipio, M., Koskinen, S., Niemela, M., Servo, A., & Vilkki, J. (2005)	5	7	4	**Intervention:** Subjects participated in an intensive 6-week multidisciplinary rehabilitation program at a rehabilitation center for neurologic patients. The program focused on neuropsychologic rehabilitation and psychotherapy, with vocational interventions and follow-up support. Treatment takes place in individual and group settings, and while the program is standardized, accommodations can be made to suit individual patient's needs. **Control:** Subjects in the control group received conventional care in the local health care system and any rehabilitation services they were referred to by their primary care physician.

continued

Table 5-2 (continued)

OCCUPATIONAL THERAPY INTERVENTIONS PROMOTING PRODUCTIVITY OUTCOMES

Author (Date)	Pop	DX	Setting	Intervention
Kielhofner, G., Braveman, B., Finlyason, M., Paul-Ward, A., Goldbaum, L., & Goldstein, K. (2004)	5	18	4	**Intervention:** Vocational OT program for people with AIDS interested in employment (4 phases). **Phase 1:** Weekly groups learning about self-assessment, vocational planning, job search, and skills development. **Phase 2:** Volunteering, internships, and temporary work experiences that included assessment and feedback regarding job performance and job coaching. **Phase 3:** Participants were placed in paid work or were assisted to apply for and carry out secure employment. **Phase 4:** Ongoing contact and support to help maintain employment.
McDermott, C., Richards, S. C. M., Ankers, S., Harmer, J., & Moran, C. J. (2004)	5	18	4	**Intervention:** OT was involved in a lifestyle management program "to empower patients to gain greater control over symptoms by explaining and exploring some of the complex interactions within the condition." Pacing techniques, intended to lessen symptoms and stabilize energy, were shown.
Nieuwenhuijsen, E. R. (2004)	5	21	4	**Intervention:** Multicomponent intervention to staff for 1 year. Intervention included education, adding a wellness ergonomics team, and analysis of selected workstations. OT and PT worked on all components and did job analysis.
Bendix, T., Bendix, A., Labriola, M., Haestrup, C., & Ebbehoj, N. (2000)	2	23	4	**Intervention:** Participants with lower back pain took part in 1 of 2 outpatient groups—functional restoration group (multidisciplinary treatment including OT and PT) or physical training only. **Control 1:** 3-week functional restoration program (8 total hours including exercises, OT work hardening, group therapy [psychology], stretching, and theory). **Control 2:** Outpatient intensive physical training for 1.5 hours, 3 times a week for 8 weeks (aerobics and strengthening exercises with fitness machines).
Braverman, S., Spector, J., Warden, D., Wilson, B., Ellis, T., Bamdad, M., et al. (1999)	5	7	4	**Intervention:** Interprofessional rehabilitation program with individual and group therapy focused on inpatient milieu-oriented neuropsychology and modified to be military relevant (10 hours a day for 8 weeks). OT groups included cognitive and work skills, community re-entry outings, and planning and organization groups. Individual therapy included neuropsychology, work therapy, OT, and speech-language pathology (OT sessions focused on individual goals).
Lindh, M., Lurie, M., & Sanne, H. (1997)	5	20	4	**Intervention:** Multidisciplinary team completed an evaluation and then set goals for individual programs. Programs were carried out until a client was able to return to work, a client was recommended to remain not working, client showed no compliance, or the client contacted a work evaluation unit. OT was involved in vocational training, contacting potential employers, and recommending further vocational process.
Pratt, J., McFadyen, A., Hall, G., Campbell, M., & McLay, D. (1997)	2	21	4	**Intervention:** Injured police officers involved in return-to-work program. One OT addressed physical conditioning and job stimulation. Another OT addressed related psychosocial issues. Participants are encouraged to build endurance and work tolerance slowly and gradually increase the time they spend on the activity program. OTs completed worksite visits to assess the specific job requirements, tasks, and demands of policing and helping inform interventions.

continued

Table 5-2 (continued)

OCCUPATIONAL THERAPY INTERVENTIONS PROMOTING PRODUCTIVITY OUTCOMES

Author (Date)	Pop	DX	Setting	Intervention
Corey, D., Koepfler, L., Etlin, D., & Day, H. (1996)	5	23	4	**Intervention:** Compared multidisciplinary treatment (including OT) with usual care for patients with soft tissue injuries. **Control 1:** "Usual care"—treatment by usual physician with assessment and recommendations from Worker's Compensation Board medical consultant (no rehabilitation therapy). **Control 2:** Interdisciplinary program—functional restoration approach (active physical treatment, work hardening, education, counseling for job satisfaction, medication reduction, anxiety and anger, sleep disruption, pain management).
Gruwsved, A., Soderback, I., & Fernholm, C. (1996)	2	20	4	**Intervention:** Individualized, vocational OT training program based on the Model of Human Occupation, rehabilitative model, biomechanical model, and occupational adaptive frames of reference.
Furth, H. J., Holm, M. B., & James, A. (1994)	5	16	4	**Intervention:** Participants receiving OT at a hand therapy clinic were given an educational session about preventing re-injury. They practiced techniques learned and were given a handout with written recommendations by OT, such as ergonomic equipment, therapeutic maintenance techniques, body mechanics, and work simplification techniques.
Dortch, H. L., & Trombly, C. A. (1990)	2	21	4	**Intervention:** Participants were randomly assigned to 1 of 2 intervention groups or control group. Both groups received education about undesirable hand movements, hand anatomy, and physiology provided by an OT. **Group 1:** Given job-specific handouts to outline problems occurring from repetitive hand movement and given positions to reduce incidence. **Group 2:** Given same handout but OT instructor discussed it in detail. Workstations to practice simulated job. **Group 3:** Served as a control group.
Carlton, R. S. (1987)	5	21	3	**Intervention:** Received body mechanics instruction taught by OT that was given 2 weeks before data were collected. Participants were videotaped practicing the techniques, and video was used to provide them with feedback. **Control:** Received no instruction.

Population: 1=geriatric (65+); 2=adult (25 to 64); 3=young adult (18 to 24); 4=adult and geriatric; 5=young adult, adult, and geriatric.

Diagnosis: 7=acquired brain injury; 12=depression; 14=schizophrenia; 16=upper extremity; 18=other; 19=arthritis; 20=chronic pain; 21=no diagnosis; 23=back pain.

Setting: 1=long-term care; 2=acute care; 3=home care; 4=rehabilitation; 5=primary care.

Table 5-3
Evidence of Effectiveness of Occupational Therapy on Productivity Outcomes

Author (Date)	Major Results	Study Design	Sample Size	Conclusions and Limitations
Positive Effects—Randomized Controlled Trial				
Darragh, A., Harrison, H., & Kenny, S. (2008)	All 3 groups had baseline scores on the LAC that did not show a statistically significant difference between them. Post-test scores showed that both the education-only and education-training groups had significant improvements while the control group's scores decreased. Further analysis showed that the education-training group had the highest score, and it was significantly higher than both the education-only and control groups. The education-only group also had a significantly higher score than control.	RCT	51	***Conclusions:*** Results of this study show that an ergonomic workplace intervention grounded in principles of OT was effective in promoting positive environmental change and behavioral change in microscope workers. The intervention was also highly efficient as it only required a 1-hour training session and 7 to 10 minutes of individual work with each employee to produce results. ***Limitations:*** This study did not demonstrate blinding of participants and investigators. The same researchers completed the assessments and delivered the training. Subjects were also aware they were being studied.
Kielhofner, G., Braveman, B., Fogg, L., & Levin, M. (2008)	Participants involved in the intervention were significantly more likely to be involved in productive activity at all 3 time points. Odds ratios indicate a large effect size; participants who received the intervention were twice as likely to be productively engaged compared to the control. At the 9-month time point, all participants in the control group except one were productively engaged in employment while only half of those who received the intervention were productively engaged in 2 or more roles indicating greater intensity of participation. Conservative intention-to-treat analysis also showed that participants in the intervention were approximately twice as likely to engage in productive activity at all 3 time points.	Non-RCT	46	***Conclusions:*** This study supports the effectiveness of a program based on principles from the Model of Human Occupation and the social model of disability in promoting sustained productive engagement in a population of adults living with HIV/AIDS. ***Limitations:*** Lack of randomization, the individualized nature of the intervention, and attrition rate of 29.3% limit the interpretation of these results.
Kool, J., Bachmann, S., Oesch, P., Knuesel, O., Ambergen, T., de Bie, R., et al. (2007)	After 1 year: Functional-centered treatment group had significantly more workdays than the patient-centered treatment group, p=0.011. The odds ratio of returning to work in the functional-centered treatment group relative to the patient-centered treatment group was 2.1, CI (1.1, 3.9). The differences in unemployment rates and in the numbers of patients receiving compensation for permanent disability were not statistically significant. (3-month results presented in different paper.)	RCT	174	***Conclusions:*** Functional-centered treatment is more effective than patient-centered treatment in terms of increasing workdays. ***Limitations:*** Intervention teams were not similar, unable to blind subjects and treatment teams.

continued

Table 5-3 (continued)

EVIDENCE OF EFFECTIVENESS OF OCCUPATIONAL THERAPY ON PRODUCTIVITY OUTCOMES

Author (Date)	Major Results	Study Design	Sample Size	Conclusions and Limitations
Positive Effects—Randomized Controlled Trial				
Li, E., Li-Tsang, C., Lam, C., Hui, K., & Chan, C. (2006)	C-LASER scores show that subjects in the intervention group showed significant positive progress from pre-contemplating a return to work to taking action toward return to work while patients in the control group showed a deterioration in scores and little progress. Subjects in the intervention group also had significantly higher total scores (p=0.028) on the SF-36 and significantly lower scores on the C-STAI (p=0.036). Significant within-group changes were also found in the intervention group when comparing pre- and post-test scores in these 3 assessments. No significant changes between intervention and control groups or between pre- and post-test scores were found on measures of physical ability.	RCT	64	**Conclusions:** Results show that the work readiness training program was effective in reducing stress and anxiety in injured workers, improved their self-perception of health status, and created positive behavioral changes toward work readiness. **Limitations:** Due to ethical obligations, all subjects in the control group received the intervention once the study was complete so long-term employment outcomes could not be studied. Possible sampling bias, because subjects were recruited from the same rehabilitation center. Services provided to control group were not comparable in intensity or duration to the intervention.
Bendix, T., Bendix, A., Labriola, M., Haestrup, C., & Ebbehoj, N. (2000)	Work capability, health care contact, absent days, back pain, leg pain, and ADL were not significantly different. Overall assessment question showed significant improvement (p=0.03). No results found as clinically important.	RCT	115	**Conclusions:** The functional restoration program was superior to a comparatively short time-consuming outpatient physical training program only with respect to overall assessment questions. **Limitations:** The outcome measures were not described in detail and lacked psychometric properties, recall bias is possible with self-report tools, there was a high dropout rate (14% and 19%), the outpatient physical training program was not described in enough detail to be reproduced, and the timing of interventions was different.
Lindh, M., Lurie, M., & Sanne, H. (1997)	Group receiving multidisciplinary outpatient rehabilitation improved work stability. In the immigration subgroup, there was no difference between control and rehabilitation groups. No difference in the frequency of work returnees between rehabilitation group and control group.	RCT	157	**Conclusions:** There was some indication of improvement for workers who received early rehabilitation. **Limitations:** High attrition rate, no clinical outcome measures, intervention not well described and, therefore, difficult to reproduce, weak statistical analysis.

continued

Table 5-3 (continued)
Evidence of Effectiveness of Occupational Therapy on Productivity Outcomes

Author (Date)	Major Results	Study Design	Sample Size	Conclusions and Limitations
Positive Effects—Randomized Controlled Trial				
Corey, D., Koepfler, L., Etlin, D., & Day, H. (1996)	Significant increase in return to work and work readiness for intervention group (p=0.02), intervention group reported significantly less pain (p=0.008), intervention group reported better sleep (p=0.002). No significance in medication use, quality of life, active pain management strategies, or frequency of medical visits.	RCT	138	**Conclusions:** The functional restoration program was associated with greater improvements with sleep, increased probability of return to work, and lower level of pain than was usual care. **Limitations:** Outcome measures were not described in detail nor did they demonstrate psychometric properties, no clear description of OT in intervention, brief description of intervention, which is difficult to reproduce, follow-up assessments varied with time and possibility for recall bias, high dropout rate.
Dortch, H. L., & Trombly, C. A. (1990)	Groups showed similar levels of hand use at the beginning of the study (H=4.24, df=2, p=0.2). Participants who received the educational intervention significantly decreased the number of traumatic hand movements performed compared to the control group; however, no significant differences were found between the two educational groups (H=4.99, df=2, p=0.1).	RCT	18	**Conclusions:** Employees performed fewer at-risk repetitive motions immediately after the preventative education program. **Limitations:** None stated.
Carlton, R. S. (1987)	The intervention group performed significantly better (p<0.001) than the control group on a novel task (during the body mechanics evaluation) but no differences were observed in the workplace.	RCT	30	**Conclusions:** Participants who received body mechanics testing performed better than those who received no training during lab testing but this did not translate to their work environment. **Limitations:** Small sample size.
Positive Effects—Non-Randomized Controlled Trial				
Lee, H., Tan, H., Ma, H., Tsai, C., & Liu, Y. (2006)	WSQP scores showed a significant and clinically relevant decrease in stress (p=0.039), while groups receiving the intervention showed a non-significant but noticeable increase in stress levels. Further analysis of WSPQ scores showed that most improvements were found in domains relating to intrinsic job factors (p=0.0131), organizational structure and climate (p=0.0001), and career and achievement (p=0.0394).	Non-RCT	29	**Conclusions:** This study shows that the intervention was effective at reducing work-related stress in patients with schizophrenia; however, the effects of treatment were short lived and were not sustained over a 12-week period. **Limitations:** Lack of a control group and the lead researcher delivering the intervention limits the interpretation and validity of results. The use of multiple t-tests to analyze data also increases the chances of a type I error.

continued

Table 5-3 (continued)

EVIDENCE OF EFFECTIVENESS OF OCCUPATIONAL THERAPY ON PRODUCTIVITY OUTCOMES

Author (Date)	Major Results	Study Design	Sample Size	Conclusions and Limitations
Positive Effects—Non-Randomized Controlled Trial				
Nordmark, B., Blomqvist, P., Andersson, B., Hagerstrom, M., Nordh-Grate, K., Ronnqvist, R., Svensson, H., & Klareskog, L. (2006)	14% increase in full-time work. Full-time work disability decreased 65% and increased in part-time work (65%).	Non-RCT	110	*Conclusions:* A trend toward improvement (continued work or improved work status) for people with RA was seen for participants who received a combination of vocational and pharmacological treatment. *Limitations:* Weak statistical analysis, only used assessment tools at baseline, no comparison group, intervention not well described, outcome measures and baseline measures not well described, dropouts not reported.
Sang, L. S., & Ying Eria, L. P. (2005)	Significant before and after differences for physical demand characteristic levels of participants who completed the work hardening program (p<0.05). 75% of participants who took part resumed employment (62.5% resumed previous job, 25% resumed previous job with modifications, and 12.5% returned to work with alternate job). Comparable to the rate of return to work found in previous studies (50% to 85%).	Non-RCT	32	*Conclusions:* The rate of returning to work for back injured workers in this study was comparable to that of other studies. *Limitations:* Small sample size, other influential factors were not measured systematically in work hardening program.
Sarajuuri, J., Kaipio, M., Koskinen, S., Niemela, M., Servo, A., & Vilkki, J. (2005)	At the end of follow-up, the intervention group showed significantly more improvement (p=0.017; 95% CI 1.26-38.44) than control with 89% of patients in the intervention group engaged in productive activity compared to 55% of those in control. The only potentially confounding variable that was found to be significantly associated with the outcome was pre-injury employment status as subjects who were unemployed at the time of injury were less likely than others to be productive at follow-up.	Non-RCT	39	*Conclusions:* Results of this study support the proposition that neuropsychologically oriented rehabilitation programs with adequate post-discharge maintenance therapy can improve productivity in patients with significant traumatic brain injury. *Limitations:* The results of this study are weakened by the lack of randomization, a control group that was not well matched to the treatment group, and a small sample size.

continued

Table 5-3 (continued)
EVIDENCE OF EFFECTIVENESS OF OCCUPATIONAL THERAPY ON PRODUCTIVITY OUTCOMES

Author (Date)	Major Results	Study Design	Sample Size	Conclusions and Limitations
Positive Effects—Non-Randomized Controlled Trial				
Kielhofner, G., Braveman, B., Finlyason, M., Paul-Ward, A., Goldbaum, L., & Goldstein, K. (2004)	67% of the 90 participants who completed the program achieved employment (n=50), returned to school (n=2), or began a volunteer position or internship (n=8). Consequently, the overall success rate was 46.5%, and the success rate for program completers was 66.7%. "The occupational narrative, which participants told in their initial assessment interview, was closely associated with both program completion and successful outcomes."	Non-RCT	90	**Conclusions:** Program completion led to positive outcomes for participants. The use of narratives was associated with program completion. **Limitations:** No control group, other factors, such as the client's health status, may have affected the outcomes of participants, high dropout rate.
McDermott, C., Richards, S. C. M., Ankers, S., Harmer, J., & Moran, C. J. (2004)	42% of participants reported new part-time or full-time employment, voluntary work, or training. 82% of participants' overall condition improved. Baseline measures were compared for the treated patients reporting new activity (improvers) and no new activity (non-improvers). The median duration of illness was not significantly different between improvers and non-improvers. The median score for mental fatigue was significantly lower for improvers than non-improvers (non-improvers had worse mental fatigue pre-group [p=0.005]). No significance with improvement for anxiety (p=0.66), depression (p=0.94), or physical fatigue (p=0.35).	Non-RCT	98	**Conclusions:** Lifestyle management programs may be beneficial; however, further research is required. **Limitations:** No control group, selection bias (non-random survey).
Nieuwenhuijsen, E. R. (2004)	62.5% of participants changed behavior pattern in a positive direction from baseline to year-end intervention; 87.5% showed positive behavior changes after wellness ergonomic team or mini-workshop. No change in reported pain, some decrease in reported difficulty sitting (15% to 10% from baseline to end of intervention).	Non-RCT	40	**Conclusions:** A theoretical path model of factors that affect health-related change for repetitive stress injuries was devised. **Limitations:** Outcome measures were not described and lacked psychometric properties, survey used as outcome measure not well described, small sample size, weak statistical analysis.

continued

Table 5-3 (continued)
EVIDENCE OF EFFECTIVENESS OF OCCUPATIONAL THERAPY ON PRODUCTIVITY OUTCOMES

Author (Date)	Major Results	Study Design	Sample Size	Conclusions and Limitations
Positive Effects—Non-Randomized Controlled Trial				
Pratt, J., McFadyen, A., Hall, G., Campbell, M., & McLay, D. (1997)	Preliminary results are based on the 15 of 42 clients who had completed the return-to-work program in the first 8 months. A significant improvement in pre- to post-intervention scores was found for lifting capacity (t=2.27, p<0.05) and grip strength (t=3.51, p<0.01). No correlation was found between "clients' age, amount of time since injury or medical diagnoses (the mean time was 7 months) or number of sessions attended." 12 out of the 15 participants were able to resume work within the police force, 9 were fully operational, and 3 were placed on light duties.	Non-RCT	15	**Conclusions:** No correlations were found between length of time since diagnosis, age, or number of sessions attended and return to work. **Limitations:** Small sample size, no control group, non-randomized, incomplete data since preliminary study, possible volunteer bias, short-term outcomes only, all patients received therapy (inpatient and outpatient) prior to entering program, which may influence outcomes, and intervention and outcome measures were not well described.
Gruwsved, A., Soderback, I., & Fernholm, C. (1996)	Post-treatment: 2 subjects decreased resting time, 3 subjects performed activities formerly avoided due to pain, 2 subjects showed decrease in degree of assessed pain, and 3 patients attained their individual OT goals (T>50).	Non-RCT	4	**Conclusions:** 50% of participants decreased their resting time, and 75% performed activities that they had previously avoided because of pain. **Limitations:** Inclusion criteria of subjects were not clearly defined, no record of psychometric properties of the outcomes measures, no account for impact of co-intervention on treatment outcomes, only a small sample from subject population tested with outcome measures.
No Effects				
Schene, A., Koeter, M., Kikkert, M., Swinkels, J., & McCrone, P. (2007)	Percentage of patients in the study diagnosed with major depression dropped significantly in the first 6 months of the study but not at any time after that. There was no difference between intervention and control regarding the percentage of patients without depression. Total BDI scores dropped significantly for both intervention and control groups over the course of the study. A significant interaction between time and condition was found in the period between the 13th and 42nd months of the study. Subjects in the intervention group had significantly faster rates of return to work (p=0.01) and also worked significantly more hours during the first 18 months of the study than control. In the last 18 months of the study, the difference between intervention and control ceased to be significant, but both groups continued to show significant improvement in amount of work. In those patients who were working during the study, no changes were found in work-related stress at any time point.	RCT	48	**Conclusions:** This study showed that OT in conjunction with usual treatment for depression had no impact on symptom severity nor did it speed up recovery but it did initiate faster and more intensive return to work. **Limitations:** The results of this study should be interpreted with caution as it had a small sample size and limited amount of data. Not all outcomes could be evaluated in every patient (i.e., work-related stress) as they did not apply.

continued

Table 5-3 (continued)
EVIDENCE OF EFFECTIVENESS OF OCCUPATIONAL THERAPY ON PRODUCTIVITY OUTCOMES

Author (Date)	Major Results	Study Design	Sample Size	Conclusions and Limitations
No Effects				
de Buck, P., Le Cessie, S., van den Hout, W. B., Peeters, A., Ronday, H., Westedt, M., et al. (2005)	No significant difference in occurrence of job loss over full follow-up period. No significant differences in pain, job satisfaction, quality of life, or physical health between 2 groups. Experimental group had significantly less fatigue (p=0.04), less anxiety (p=0.01), less depression (p=0.04), and mental health subscale (p=0.01) than control group over 24-month period (p=0.01).	RCT	62	**Conclusions:** No significant differences were found between the treatment group and usual care after 24 months. **Limitations:** High dropout rate of participants, some outcome measures not validated by psychometric properties, no description of roles of different professions.
Braverman, S., Spector, J., Warden, D., Wilson, B., Ellis, T., Bamdad, M., et al. (1999)	At 12-month follow-up, 96% of population returned to work in military, and 66% returned to active duty.	RCT	67	**Conclusions:** Results were not significant, but 96% of participants did return to work (66% of these to active duty). **Limitations:** Only one arm of randomized controlled trial described (in great detail) and did not really compare intervention with previous therapy, weak statistical analysis, minimal description of outcome measures and battery tests used, psychometric properties were not described.
Furth, H. J., Holm, M. B., & James, A. (1994)	"A significantly lower degree was found of absolute completion of recommendations at T1 and T2 than had been anticipated (p<0.002). No significant difference between T1 and T2 was found, indicating that cuing at T1 had little effect on subjects' actual follow-through rate."	Non-RCT	15	**Conclusions:** Participants did not follow through with OT recommendations as much as was expected. **Limitations:** Volunteer bias demonstrated in the sample, small sample size.

BDI=Beck Depression Inventory, C-LASER=Chinese Lam Assessment on Stages of Employment Readiness, C-STAI=Chinese State Trait and Anxiety Inventory, LAC=Laboratory Assessment Checklist, SF-36=Short Form Health Survey, WSQP=Work-Related Stress Questionnaire for Chronic Psychiatric Patient.

Table 5-4
OUTCOME MEASURES USED TO CAPTURE PRODUCTIVITY OUTCOMES

Author (Date)	Outcome(s) Investigated	Outcome Measure(s)	Method of Administration
Darragh, A., Harrison, H., & Kenny, S. (2008)	Evaluation of the worker's habits and workstation Self-perceived comfort while working	LAC ECS	The LAC was administered by OT grad students at baseline and 2 weeks later once the intervention was complete. The ECS was completed by study subjects at baseline only.
Kielhofner, G., Braveman, B., Fogg, L., & Levin, M. (2008)	Amount of productive social participation	N/A	Data on productive participation (i.e., employment, volunteering, involved in training or schooling) were collected by researchers either by phone or directly from participants at 3, 6, and 9 months.
Kool, J., Bachmann, S., Oesch, P., Knuesel, O., Ambergen, T., de Bie, R., et al. (2007)	Work days Return to work Rate of patients receiving financial compensation for permanent disability Unemployment rate	Work days Return to work Rate of patients receiving financial compensation for permanent disability Unemployment rate	Baseline, 3 months, and 1 year follow-up.
Schene, A., Koeter, M., Kikkert, M., Swinkels, J., & McCrone, P. (2007)	Depressive symptoms Hours of work Work-related stress	Structured interview for the diagnosis of DSM-IV mood disorders BDI QOS—Psychic Strains section	All outcomes data were collected at baseline and 3-, 6-, 12-, and 42-month follow-up.
Lee, H., Tan, H., Ma, H., Tsai, C., & Liu, Y. (2006)	Work-related stress	WSQP	The WSQP was administered by researchers at baseline, week 12, and week 24.
Li, E., Li-Tsang, C., Lam, C., Hui, K., & Chan, C. (2006)	Self-perceived physical ability Overall health status Pain coping ability Stress and anxiety levels	SFS LLUMC SF-36 C-LASER C-STAI	Assessments were completed by research assistants blinded to participant allocation at baseline and 3 weeks later once the intervention was complete.
Nordmark, B., Blomqvist, P., Andersson, B., Hagerstrom, M., Nordh-Grate, K., Ronnqvist, R., Svensson, H., & Klareskog, L. (2006)	Changes in work status (working, full-time/part-time) Drawing from sick benefit Disease activity/work ability RA activity by joint (28 joint count) Rheumatoid factor by x-rays of hands and feet, erythrocyte sedimentation rate Functional status	Self-report of current ability to work and disease status were given Swedish version of HAQ, C-reactive protein, and pain using VAS	Self-report at baseline, 3, 6, 9, 12, 18, and 24 months. At baseline, RA activity by joint (28 joint count), rheumatoid factor by x-rays of hands and feet, erythrocyte sedimentation rate, functional status.

continued

Table 5-4 (continued)
OUTCOME MEASURES USED TO CAPTURE PRODUCTIVITY OUTCOMES

Author (Date)	Outcome(s) Investigated	Outcome Measure(s)	Method of Administration
de Buck, P., Le Cessie, S., van den Hout, W. B., Peeters, A., Ronday, H., Westedt, M., et al. (2005)	Job loss (unemployment/work disability) Job satisfaction Pain Physical functioning Anxiety/depression Quality of life	Report of receiving full work disability pension or unem- ployment HVAS VAS HAQ HADS SF-36 CI Job categorized by physical and mental demands	Clinical assessment by trained research nurse (blind). Assessment at baseline, 6-, 12-, 18-, and 24-month follow-up.
Sang, L. S., & Ying Eria, L. P. (2005)	Quantify job demand level Physical demand characteristics/ physical strength Work status/return to work	Handbook for Analyzing Jobs and Dictionary of Occupational Titles VCWS 19 Telephone follow-up ques- tions to determine work status	Self-report questions about job demands administered/analyzed by the OT at baseline. VCWS 19 was given before and after the work hardening program. The OT provided and rated simulated job tasks that assessed a range of physical components to come up with an overall physical strength rating. Telephone questionnaire given 3 months post-program to see if client returned to work.
Sarajuuri, J., Kaipio, M., Koskinen, S., Niemela, M., Servo, A., & Vilkki, J. (2005)	Engagement in productive activ- ity (work, study, or volunteer- ing)	Questionnaire developed by researchers	Assessments were mailed to patients and their caregivers 2 years after they had completed the neurorehabilitation program. If questionnaires were not returned or did not have adequate information, subjects were inter- viewed by telephone.
Kielhofner, G., Braveman, B., Finlyason, M., Paul- Ward, A., Goldbaum, L., & Goldstein, K. (2004)	Initial participant characteristics that best predict program com- pletion and successful program outcomes Rate of program completion Rate of successful outcomes for clients who complete the program	OPHI-II WRI OSA Open-ended interviews about perceptions of progress and experiences in the program, work status, factors that influenced outcomes	The OPHI-II, WRI, and OSA were given at baseline, and the open- ended interview occurred at 6, 12, 18, and 24 months. The WRI and OSA are self-report questionnaires while the OPHI-II is a semi-structured interview.
McDermott, C., Richards, S. C. M., Ankers, S., Harmer, J., & Moran, C. J. (2004)	Client's ability to return to paid or volunteer work after the pro- gram Relationship between return to work and baseline variables (duration and severity of illness, anxiety/depression, age)	CFS HADS Audit (questionnaire to evalu- ate work status, change in condition)	CFS and HADS administered at baseline. The audit questionnaire was mailed out 1 year after the last patient entered the program (median follow-up duration 1.5 years, range 1 to 2 years). Self- report questionnaires

continued

Table 5-4 (continued)

OUTCOME MEASURES USED TO CAPTURE PRODUCTIVITY OUTCOMES

Author (Date)	Outcome(s) Investigated	Outcome Measure(s)	Method of Administration
Nieuwenhuijsen, E. R. (2004)	Changes in health behavior patterns (posture, breaks, stretching, etc.) and changes in pain	Survey (designed by team, included Likert-type scales and Karasek occupational stress scale), 156-item assessment instrument to measure work and occupational informational knowledge	Self-report, baseline, and 6 weeks pre-intervention (survey), 1 year later at end of intervention.
Bendix, T., Bendix, A., Labriola, M., Haestrup, C., & Ebbehoj, N. (2000)	Quality of life Back and leg pain Days off work and work capability Change in ADL performance	Overall quality of life assessment: 5-point scale to question "How much has treatment influenced your quality of life?" Coded scale measured work capability, count of days off, count for health care contacts Scale to measure back and leg pain MRS Questionnaire to measure programs	Self-report. Measures at baseline and 1 year follow-up after intervention.
Braverman, S., Spector, J., Warden, D., Wilson, B., Ellis, T., Bamdad, M., et al. (1999)	Successful return to work and return to duty in the military	MRI EEG Assessments in neuropsychology, psychiatry, neurology, speech-language pathology, and OT (evaluations to establish goals) Cognitive testing used to determine if could return to work	Battery of tests at baseline, post-program, and 6, 12, and 24 months follow-up. Baseline: Magnetic resonance imaging, EEG, assessments in neuropsychology, psychiatry, neurology, speech-language pathology, and OT. Post: Cognitive testing. Study does not identify how they are administered.
Lindh, M., Lurie, M., & Sanne, H. (1997)	Work stability Return to work	At work during follow-up contact to determine stability and return to work	Self-report, baseline, followed for 5 years at 3-month intervals.
Pratt, J., McFadyen, A., Hall, G., Campbell, M., & McLay, D. (1997)	Change in grip strength Lifting capacity/work-related performance Psychological adjustment to illness/pain Stress management strategies Perceived form and function of social support Change in grip strength	MV VCWS MPQ HUS SOS	Does not specify methods of administration or at which times measures are administered.

continued

Table 5-4 (continued)

OUTCOME MEASURES USED TO CAPTURE PRODUCTIVITY OUTCOMES

Author (Date)	Outcome(s) Investigated	Outcome Measure(s)	Method of Administration
Corey, D., Koepfler, L., Etlin, D., & Day, H. (1996)	Decrease in chronic pain Improved quality of sleep Ability to return to work Change in medication use Change in device use	Non-VAS (0 to 10) for pain levels Screen questionnaire for pain medication use, use of braces, and devices 3-point scale for quality of sleep Follow-up call repeats above plus adds questions on inquiry of depression, enjoyment of life, perception of quality of life, work status, and visit to doctors	Baseline screening and follow-up telephone call (varied from 9 to 27 months after intake) and self-report.
Gruwsved, A., Soderback, I., & Fernholm, C. (1996)	Experience of pain Goal achievement Pattern of engagement Work capacity analysis	Symtrack instrument GAS Activity logs Video observation	GAS and activity logs once a week over 3 months.
Furth, H. J., Holm, M. B., & James, A. (1994)	Injury prevention (clients remaining uninjured) Participant follow-through in using ergonomic equipment, therapeutic maintenance techniques, body mechanics, work simplification techniques	Re-injury prevention checklists Follow-through checklists	Checklists were completed via telephone interview between the researcher and participant 2 weeks and 4 weeks after education session.
Dortch, H. L., & Trombly, C. A. (1990)	Number of movements identified with cumulative trauma disorder in participants' jobs	Checklist (for live interval recording) adapted from Armstrong, Fonkle, Joseph, and Goldstein (1982)	Randomly chosen observation session took place 1 week prior to the educational intervention session and 1 week after the intervention session. Investigator recorded the number of cumulative trauma disorder movements seen at set 30-second intervals as the participant performed regular job.
Carlton, R. S. (1987)	Body mechanics when lifting and lowering	WEST 2 WCED Modified WEST 2 BME WRBME	At 2 weeks (body mechanics evaluation) and 3 weeks (workplace observation) after the intervention, group received their educational session. Completed by assessor who was blind to treatment group.

BDI=Beck Depression Inventory, BME=Body Mechanics Evaluation, CFS=Chalder Fatigue Scale, CI=Charlson Index, C-LASER=Chinese Lam Assessment on Stages of Employment Readiness, C-STAI=Chinese State Trait and Anxiety Inventory, ECS=Employee Comfort Survey, GAS=Goal Attainment Scaling, HADS=Hospital Anxiety and Depression Scale, HAQ=Health Assessment Questionnaire, HUS=Hassles and Uplift Scales, HVAS=Horizontal Visual Analog Scale, LAC=Laboratory Assessment Checklist, LLUMC=Loma Linda University Medical Centre Activity Sort, MPQ=McGill Pain Questionnaire, MRS=Manniches Rating Scale, MV=Martin Vigorimeter, OPHI-II=Occupational Performance History Interview, OSA=Occupational Self-Assessment, QOS=Questionnaire Organization Stress, SF-36=Short Form Health Survey, SFS=Spinal Function Sort, SOS=Significant Other Scale, VAS=Visual Analog Scale, VCWS 19=Valpar Component Work Sample 19, WCED=Work Capacity Evaluation Device, WEST 2=Work Evaluation Systems Technology, WRBME=Work-Related Body Mechanics Evaluation, WRI=Worker Role Interview, WSQP=Work-Related Stress Questionnaire for Chronic Psychiatric Patient.

insurance boards are increasingly implementing early return-to-work policies (Eakin, MacEachen, & Clarke, 2003). Such policies encourage return to work with modified duties and accommodations prior to full recovery. However, such approaches require support and understanding from employers, supervisors, and co-workers.

Work hardening, job simulation, and various approaches to education and skill development are commonly used interventions by occupational therapists working in this area. However, such approaches are time limited. Eventually, individuals should be given opportunities to try out their skills and capabilities and discover their strengths and weaknesses in real settings. Furthermore, there can be challenges in transferring skills assessed and learned in simulated or clinical settings to the actual workplace environment. For example, simulated settings cannot account for the organizational culture or the availability of support at work, which are known to be key factors in the experiences of people with disabilities in the workplace (Gewurtz & Kirsh, in press; Harlan & Robert, 1998).

Effects of Occupational Therapy in Promoting Productivity Outcomes

In this section, we examine the research evidence that has studied occupational therapy interventions whose purpose is to impact a client's work productivity. The studies are reviewed and summarized, providing information on the strength of evidence linking occupational therapy interventions to client productivity outcomes. The interventions are in three areas—prevention through education and provision of information to clients, modification of work tasks and activities, and comprehensive programs to improve work skills and participation. The results of our empirical reviews are organized by these areas of intervention. The section concludes with recommendations on how clinical treatment can proceed and/or where future research directions rest.

Education and Provision of Information to Clients

Three empirical studies (two randomized trials and one small before-and-after study) have evaluated the effect of client education strategies to improve use of proper body mechanics to prevent injury. These studies have been conducted with food services workers (Carlton, 1987), industrial workers (Dortch & Trombly, 1990), and office workers (Nieuwenhuijsen,

2004). Findings from these two trials indicate that occupational therapy interventions led to significant improvements in knowledge and use of appropriate body mechanics and postures. Carlton (1987) found that changes in performance during the study did not generalize to changes in the work situation, while the results from the study by Dortch and Trombly (1990) did indicate carryover to work. A fourth empirical study by Kielhofner and colleagues (2008) reported a non-randomized two-group design of an education-based program to increase productive participation of people living with HIV/AIDS within supportive living facilities. The results of this study indicated that participants involved in the program were significantly more likely to be involved in productive activity at each time of evaluation.

Modification of Work Tasks and Activities

Three before-and-after studies of occupational therapy intervention using task and activity modification have been conducted (Furth, Holm, & James, 1994; McDermott, Richards, Ankers, Harmer, & Moran, 2004; Nieuwenhuijsen, 2004). Furth, Holm, and James (1994) studied people with hand injury after an educational session where participants practiced skills in body mechanics and work simplification techniques and learned about ergonomic equipment. Findings from this study indicated that participants increased their knowledge and use of these behaviors in the workplace. A lifestyle management program to assist people with chronic fatigue to gain control over symptoms through pacing techniques demonstrated an increase in participation in work or volunteer work (McDermott et al., 2004). Nieuwenhuijsen (2004), in a study of 40 office workers, reported that 87.5% showed positive behavior changes after wellness ergonomic team or mini-workshop. Evidence to support this type of intervention is weak, and larger studies using more rigorous research designs are needed.

Comprehensive Programs to Improve Work Skills and Participation

The majority of empirical studies and three systematic reviews found in this scoping review focused on studies examining comprehensive programs to improve outcomes in productivity.

Systematic Reviews

Occupational therapy can provide treatment to help people return to their workplace after injury. A systematic review about the effectiveness of workplace rehabilitation intervention for treatment of work-related upper extremity disorders reported a positive impact of worksite interventions to enable injured workers to carry out their employment duties. These interventions included ergonomic modifications in keyboard designs, rest-exercise breaks, case manager's training on accommodations, and exercise programs (Williams, Westmorland, Schmuck, & MacDermid, 2004). The evidence to support this finding was not extensive.

Some interventions include therapy programs that involve work conditioning, work hardening, and environmental modification interventions to return to work duties. Specific physical conditioning programs to improve aerobic performance, muscle strength, endurance, and coordination for people with chronic back pain were determined to be effective interventions when compared to usual care (Schonstein, Kenny, Keating, & Koes, 2003).

Two systematic reviews of comprehensive, multidisciplinary interventions for productivity have been reported (Scheer, Watanabe, & Radack, 1997; Twamley, Jeste, & Lehman, 2003). Scheer and colleagues (1997) examined the effect of interventions for people with subacute/chronic lower back pain on return-to-work outcomes. Twelve studies involving a variety of interventions such as multidisciplinary pain clinics, exercise, and cognitive-behavioral strategies were reviewed. Results indicate that the majority of prospective studies investigating return to work after experiencing chronic lower back pain have methodological limitations. More research is needed to provide more confidence in determining effective multidisciplinary interventions to help improve work capacity for this population.

A second systematic review conducted a meta-analysis of the randomized controlled trials of vocational rehabilitation intervention for people with mental illness (Twamley et al., 2003). The interventions included assertive community treatment (ACT) teams, supported employment, transitional employment programs, paid work placement, case management, and social skill training. Analysis of 11 studies indicated that these programs led to significant improvements in the percentage of participants who worked at any point during the research.

Empirical Studies

Sixteen empirical studies examined the effects of comprehensive programs involving occupational therapy to improve productivity. From this sample, four before-and-after studies (Gruwsved, Soderback, & Fernholm, 1996; Kielhofner, Braveman, Finlayson, Paul-Ward, Goldbaum, & Goldstein, 2004; Pratt, McFadyen, Hall, Campbell, & McLay, 1997; Sang & Ying Eria, 2005), one randomized cross-over design (Lee, Tan, Ma, Tsai, & Liu, 2006), and two randomized controlled trials (Darragh, Harrison, & Kenny, 2008;

Schene, Koeter, Kikkert, Swinkels, & McCrone, 2007) involved interventions that are implemented solely by occupational therapists. Occupational therapy involvement within multidisciplinary programs makes up the remaining studies—six randomized controlled trials (Bendix, Bendix, Labriola, Haestrup, & Ebbehoj, 2000; Corey, Koepfler, Etlin, & Day, 1996; de Buck et al., 2005; Kool et al., 2007; Li, Li-Tsang, Lam, Hui, & Chan, 2006; Lindh, Lurie, & Sanne, 1997), one non-randomized controlled trial (Sarajuuri, Kaipio, Koskinen, Niemela, Servo, & Vilkki, 2005), and two before-and-after study designs (Braverman et al., 1999; Nordmark et al., 2006). While the interventions differed slightly, these studies typically included the following components in their programs:

▲ Participation in work or volunteer work (through worksite placements, work hardening programs, job simulation)
▲ Provision of education/information about vocational resources
▲ Skills development (vocational planning, job search strategies, job interviews)
▲ Job coaching
▲ Career counseling about work or volunteer work
▲ Vocational rehabilitation groups

Results from the four before-and-after occupational therapy only studies found that work participation and activity levels increased significantly after intervention. The program evaluated in the study by Kielhofner and colleagues (2004) was the most comprehensive. The study participants had HIV/AIDS and were interested in employment. The program that was studied had four phases:

▲ Phase 1: Weekly groups learning about self-assessment, vocational planning, job search, and skills development
▲ Phase 2: Volunteering, internships, and temporary work experiences to provide assessment and feedback regarding job performance
▲ Phase 3: Placement in paid work or assistance to apply for and carry out secure employment
▲ Phase 4: Ongoing contact and support to help maintain employment

Sixty-seven percent of the 90 participants who completed the program achieved employment (n=50), returned to school (n=2), or began a volunteer position or internship (n=8). Outcomes from the other three studies (Gruwsved et al., 1996; Pratt et al., 1997; Sang & Ying Eria, 2005) also indicated a positive effect of intervention on work tolerance and physical work demands for people with chronic pain or work injury. Only one quasi-experimental randomized controlled trial was conducted to compare an education-training with no intervention (Darragh et al., 2008). The results of this study showed that an occupational therapy-based ergonomic workplace intervention was effective in promoting environmental change and behavioral change in microscope workers.

Moreover, two before-and-after multidisciplinary studies of people with chronic pain or arthritis were also conducted (Braverman et al., 1999; Nordmark et al., 2006). The results from these multidisciplinary studies mirror the occupational therapy-only studies, indicating that a comprehensive program to improve work participation led to increases in return to work and participation in full-time work. Because these six studies did not include comparative groups, or the design methods were not rigorous, these results must be interpreted with caution.

There are, however, six randomized controlled trials involving occupational therapy independently and within a multidisciplinary program to improve work participation (Bendix et al., 2000; Corey et al., 1996; de Buck et al., 2005; Kool et al., 2007; Li et al., 2006; Lindh et al., 1997). Participants in these studies had chronic pain (three studies), soft tissue injury (two studies), or arthritis. Each trial focused on slightly different outcomes.

Bendix and colleagues (2000) compared a functional restoration program that was 8 hours in length (exercise, occupational therapy work hardening, group therapy, stretching, and theory) to an outpatient intensive physical training program (aerobics, strengthening) for 1.5 hours, three times a week (36 hours total). There were no significant differences between these two different programs and treatment doses on outcomes of work capability, health care contact, absent days, back pain, leg pain, and activities of daily living (ADL). The only difference was a significant improvement in overall assessment scores for the functional restoration group.

Corey and colleagues (1996) compared usual care through recommendation from a medical workers' compensation board consultant (no rehabilitation) to a multidisciplinary functional restoration approach (active physical treatment, work hardening, education, counseling for job satisfaction, medication reduction, anxiety and anger, sleep disruption, pain management). The functional restoration program led to significant increases in return to work and work readiness, less pain, and improved sleep. De Buck and colleagues (2005) found that a multidisciplinary program did not change rates of job loss but led to significant improvements in fatigue, anxiety, depression, and mental health.

The impact of occupational therapy in having positive effects on affective (or psycho-emotional) components of return to work was also evident when addressing the impact of psycho-emotional affects of work on adults with schizophrenia (Lee et al., 2006) and depression (Schene et al., 2007). Lee and colleagues (2006) reported in their randomized cross-over design that occupational therapy intervention was effective in reducing work-related stress for adults with schizophrenia living in a long-term care facility over a short follow-up period. In the randomized controlled trial by Schene and colleagues (2007), occupational therapy intervention did not speed up recovery; however, it did initiate faster and more intensive return to work. A third study with a weaker study design (non-randomized controlled design) for a population of adults with a traumatic brain injury demonstrated an improvement in productivity with neuro-psychologically oriented multidisciplinary rehabilitation (Sarajuuri et al., 2005).

The final study by Lindh, Lurie, and Sanne (1997) found that a multidisciplinary program led to improved rates of work stability. However, this study had many limitations in its design and demonstrated weak methods of outcome evaluation.

Although these studies are promising, there remains a need for more research in this area. In particular, there is a need to better understand how skills learned in simulated or clinical settings are transferred into the work environment and how effective interventions are in terms of preventing disability or injury. Furthermore, the interventions included in this review do not represent all occupational therapy interventions directed at improving productive outcomes. There is a need to better understand the range of approaches that occupational therapists are using in this area in order to highlight specific gaps in the research literature.

Measures Used to Capture Productivity Outcomes

When examining outcomes that are sensitive to occupational therapy intervention to impact productivity, it is useful to characterize the typical outcomes measured in these studies. Using the World Health Organization's International Classification of Functioning, Disability, and Health (ICF) (2001) classification, the outcomes assessed in these studies cross the three areas of body function/structure, activity, and participation. Under body function/structure, outcomes include strength, physical capacity, pain, fatigues, anxiety, and depression. In the area of simple activity, outcomes include lifting and psychological coping. Under participation, outcomes center on rates of participation in work and/or volunteer work. The majority of outcomes reported in these studies are in the body function and participation areas.

Based on the scoping reviews completed for this chapter, there is evidence to support the impact of occupational therapy intervention focused on productivity on the following outcomes:

▲ Body function/structure
 △ Knowledge of ergonomics and body mechanics
 △ Use of proper movements and posture(s)
 △ Symptoms of anxiety and depression
 △ Strength, physical demand capacity
 △ Pain
 △ Fatigue
▲ Activity
 △ General activity levels
 △ Lifting ability
▲ Participation
 △ Work/return to work
 △ Volunteer work
 △ Sleep patterns

Drawing on reviews of measures already completed within occupational therapy (Law, Baum, & Dunn, 2005) and the measures used in studies reviewed for this project, we have compiled a table of measures most suitable for use in occupational therapy to assess outcomes of productivity intervention. As indicated by the majority of research in this area, the outcomes focus on assessment at the levels of body function or participation. These outcome measures are reviewed in Table 5-5.

Conclusions and Recommendations for Future Research

Occupational therapy interventions to impact productivity outcomes for clients have focused mostly on the worker and the work tasks. Given the costs associated with workplace injury and disability compensation, proactive workplaces are beginning to invest in developing healthy workplace policies and practices that would benefit all workers and reduce the incidence and impact of the disability. However, less research has been directed at examining the impact of such interventions and the contributions that occupational therapists can make to the creation of healthy workplaces.

There is growing agreement that basic body functions are poor indicators of an individual's ability to perform at work or school (Sandqvist & Henriksson, 2004). Rather, many occupational therapists are advocating for holistic approaches to consider how the worker is able to manage the demands of his or her particular work in the actual workplace environment. More research should be conducted on examining such context-specific interventions to identify the outcomes and challenges.

A recent review of work initiatives for people with mental illnesses in Canada highlights some of the innovative practices that occupational therapists are currently involved in to improve participation in productive occupations (Kirsh et al., 2006). However, to date, not all approaches have been subjected to rigorous evaluation. For example, we know that occupational therapists are involved in affirmative/alternative businesses, but have less empirical evidence about the outcomes of such initiatives. We also know that occupational therapists are not alone in their involvement in such initiatives, and there is little understanding about what occupational therapists, as opposed to other professionals or paraprofessionals, might offer.

Furthermore, there is growing support for the effectiveness of models of supported employment (Kirsh, Cockburn, & Gewurtz, 2004; Moll, Huff, & Detwiler, 2003). Although many occupational therapists have adopted the principles of supported employment in their work with clients around productive occupations, it is unclear if outcomes are improved when occupational therapists work as part of supported employment or supported education programs. More research should be directed at understanding how occupational therapists can contribute to this approach to employment.

Table 5-5
OUTCOME MEASURES TO ASSESS PRODUCTIVITY INTERVENTIONS

Measure	Population	Content Domains	Reliability and Validity
Canadian Occupational Performance Measure (COPM)	All populations	Semi-structured interview focusing on problem identification in 3 areas: self-care, productivity, and leisure; 5 most important issues are rated by client for performance and satisfaction.	Studies demonstrate internal consistency, test-retest reliability, and content, construct, and criterion validity.
Chalder Fatigue Scale (CFS)	All populations	14-item instrument that uses a 4-choice response format to measure both mental and physical fatigue intensity.	Studies demonstrate internal consistency, reliability, good face validity, and reasonable discriminant validity.
Health Assessment Questionnaire (HAQ)	All populations with some adaptations (originally for use with RA patients)	Self-report questionnaire that assesses 5 dimensions of health: disability, discomfort, drug side effects, dollar costs, and death.	Studies demonstrate test-retest reliability, face and content validity, construct validity, criterion validity, and responsiveness to change.
McGill Pain Questionnaire (MPQ)	All populations	Interview or self-administered tool with 3 sections: 20 sets of adjectives that describe the experience of pain, a diagram of the body on which people indicate where their pain is, plus a 1-item pain intensity scale.	Studies demonstrate content, construct, and criterion validity and adequate overall reliability.
Occupational Performance History Interview (OPHI)	All populations as long as able to participate in an in-depth interview	Semi-structured interview covering occupational roles, daily routine, activity/occupational choices, critical life events, occupational behavior settings. 3 rating scales (occupational identity, occupational competence, occupational behavior settings) and a life history narrative.	Studies demonstrate observer reliability, construct, and content validity.
Valpar Component Work Samples (VCWS)	Adolescents and adults	Assesses task performance on simulated work tasks. Skills and attitudes needed for each task are analyzed and scores on characteristics such as time to complete task are given.	Studies demonstrate test-retest reliability, content, and construct validity.
Visual Analog Scale (VAS)	All populations	A measurement tool to assess characteristics that range across a continuum (like pain). A VAS consists of a 10-cm line that has 2 opposite word descriptions at either end (no pain _____ severe pain). The participant puts a mark on the line to indicate where he or she falls on the continuum with respect to the characteristic in question.	Studies demonstrate good overall validity and test-retest and inter-rater reliability.

continued

Table 5-5 (continued)
OUTCOME MEASURES TO ASSESS PRODUCTIVITY INTERVENTIONS

Measure	Population	Content Domains	Reliability and Validity
Work Environment Impact Scale	Adults experiencing job difficulties due to illness or injury	17 items—categorized as environmental qualities facilitating return to work, environmental qualities inhibiting return to work, recommended reasonable accommodations, worker's goals, request for OT involvement.	Studies demonstrate internal consistency, content, and construct validity.
Worker Role Interview (WRI)	Injured workers	Therapist rates client on 17 factors that support or hinder successful return to work on a 4-point scale (1=strongly interferes with returning to work; 4=strongly supports client returning to work). 6 content areas: Personal causation, values, interests, roles, habits, environment.	Studies demonstrate internal consistency and test-retest reliability.

References

Bendix, T., Bendix, A., Labriola, M., Haestrup, C., & Ebbehoj, N. (2000). Functional restoration versus outpatient physical training in chronic low back pain: A randomized comparative study. *Spine, 25*(19), 2494-2500.

Braverman, S., Spector, J., Warden, D., Wilson, B., Ellis, T., Bamdad, M., et al. (1999). A multidisciplinary TBI inpatient rehabilitation programme for active duty service members as part of a randomized clinical trial. *Brain Injury, 13*(6), 405-415.

Canadian Association of Occupational Therapists. (1993). *Occupational therapy guidelines for client-centred mental health practice.* Ottawa, Ontario, Canada: Author.

Canadian Association of Occupational Therapists. (2004a). Health occupation and disability management services. *Canadian Journal of Occupational Therapy, 71*(2), 116-117.

Canadian Association of Occupational Therapists. (2004b). Workplace health and occupational therapy. *Canadian Journal of Occupational Therapy, 71*(3), 186-187.

Carlton, R. S. (1987). The effects of body mechanics instruction on work performance. *American Journal of Occupational Therapy, 41*(1), 16-20.

Cockburn, L., Kirsh, B., Krupa, T., & Gewurtz, R. (2004). Mental health and mental illness in the workplace: Occupational therapy solutions for complex problems. *Occupational Therapy Now, 6*(5), 7-14.

Corey, D., Koepfler, L., Etlin, D., & Day, H. (1996). A limited functional restoration program for injured workers: A randomized trial. *Journal of Occupational Rehabilitation, 6*(4), 239-249.

Darragh, A., Harrison, H., & Kenny, S. (2008). Effect of an ergonomics intervention on workstations of microscope workers. *American Journal of Occupational Therapy, 62*(1), 61-69.

de Buck, P., Le Cessie, S., van den Hout, W. B., Peeters, A., Ronday, H., Westedt, M., et al. (2005). Randomized comparison of a multidisciplinary job-retention vocational rehabilitation program with usual outpatient care in patients with chronic arthritis at risk for job loss. *Arthritis and Rheumatism: Arthritis Care and Research, 53*(5), 682-690.

Dortch, H. L., & Trombly, C. A. (1990). The effects of education on hand use with industrial workers in repetitive jobs. *American Journal of Occupational Therapy, 44*(9), 777-782.

Eakin, J. M., MacEachen, E., & Clarke, J. (2003). "Playing it smart" with return to work: Small workplace experience under Ontario's policy of self-reliance and early return. *Policy and Practice in Health and Safety, 1*(2), 19-40.

Furth, H. J., Holm, M. B., & James, A. (1994). Reinjury prevention follow-through for clients with cumulative trauma disorders. *American Journal of Occupational Therapy, 48*(10), 890-898.

Gewurtz, R., & Kirsh, B. (in press). Disruption, disbelief, and resistance: A meta-synthesis of disability in the workplace. *Work: A Journal of Prevention, Assessment, and Rehabilitation.*

Greenhalgh, T. (2006). *How to read a paper: The basics of evidence-based medicine* (3rd ed.). London, England: Blackwell Publishing Ltd.

Gruwsved, A., Soderback, I., & Fernholm, C. (1996). Evaluation of a vocational training programme in primary health care rehabilitation: A case study. *Work, 7*(1), 47-61.

Harlan, S., & Robert, P. (1998). The social construction of disability in organizations: Why employers resist reasonable accommodation. *Work and Occupations, 25*(4), 397-435.

Harvey-Krefting, L. (1985). The concept of work in occupational therapy: A historical review. *American Journal of Occupational Therapy, 39*, 301-307.

Jiranek, D., & Kirby, N. (1990). The job satisfaction and/or psychological well being of young adults with an intellectual disability and non-disabled young adults in either sheltered employment, competitive employment or unemployment. *Australia and New Zealand Journal of Developmental Disabilities, 16*, 133-148.

Kielhofner, G., Braveman, B., Finlayson, M., Paul-Ward, A., Goldbaum, L., & Goldstein, K. (2004). Outcomes of a vocational program for persons with AIDS. *American Journal of Occupational Therapy, 58*(1), 64-72.

Kielhofner, G., Braveman, B., Fogg, L., & Levin, M. (2008). A controlled study of services to enhance productive participation among people with HIV/AIDS. *American Journal of Occupational Therapy, 62*(1), 36-45.

Kirsh, B., Cockburn, L., & Gewurtz, R. (2004). Doing work well: Preserving and promoting mental health in the workplace. *Occupational Therapy Now, 6*(5), 25-27.

Kirsh, B., Cockburn, L., & Gewurtz, R. (2005). Best practice in occupational therapy: Program characteristics that influence vocational outcomes for people with serious mental illnesses. *Canadian Journal of Community Mental Health, 25*(2), 173-191.

Kirsh, B., Krupa, T., Cockburn, L., & Gewurtz, R. (2006). Work initiatives in Canada: A decade of development. *Canadian Journal of Community Mental Health, 25*(2), 173-191.

Kool, J., Bachmann, S., Oesch, P., Knuesel, O., Ambergen, T., de Bie, R., et al. (2007). Function-centered rehabilitation increases work days in patients with nonacute nonspecific low back pain: 1-year results from a randomized controlled trial. *Archives of Physical Medicine and Rehabilitation, 88*(9), 1089-1094.

Krupa, T., Lagarde, M., & Carmichael, K. (2003). Transforming sheltered workshops into affirmative businesses: An outcome evaluation. *Psychiatric Rehabilitation Journal, 26*(4), 359-367.

Law, M., Baum, C., & Dunn, W. (2005). *Measuring occupational performance: Supporting best practice in occupational therapy* (2nd ed.). Thorofare, NJ: SLACK Incorporated.

Law, M., Cooper, B., Strong, S., Stewart, D., Rigby, P., & Letts, L. (1996). The person-environment-occupation model: A transactive approach to occupational performance. *Canadian Journal of Occupational Therapy, 63*(1), 9-23.

Lee, H., Tan, H., Ma, H., Tsai, C., & Liu, Y. (2006). Effectiveness of a work-related stress management program in patients with chronic schizophrenia. *American Journal of Occupational Therapy, 60*(4), 435-441.

Li, E., Li-Tsang, C., Lam, C., Hui, K., & Chan, C. (2006). The effect of a "training on work readiness" program for workers with musculoskeletal injuries: A randomized control trial (RCT) study. *Journal of Occupational Rehabilitation, 16*(4), 529-541.

Lindh, M., Lurie, M., & Sanne, H. (1997). A randomized prospective study of vocational outcome in rehabilitation of patients with non-specific musculoskeletal pain: A multidisciplinary approach to patients identified after 90 days of sick-leave. *Scandinavian Journal of Rehabilitative Medicine, 29*(2), 103-112.

Lord, J., Schnarr, A., & Hutchison, P. (1987). The voice of the people: Qualitative research and the needs of consumers. *Canadian Journal of Community Mental Health, 6*(2), 25-36.

McColl, M., Law, M., Stewart, D., Doubt, L., Pollock, N., & Krupa, T. (2002). *Theoretical basis of occupational therapy* (2nd ed.). Thorofare, NJ: SLACK Incorporated.

McDermott, C., Richards, S. C. M., Ankers, S., Harmer, J., & Moran, C. J. (2004). An evaluation of a chronic fatigue lifestyle management programme focusing on the outcome of return to work or training. *British Journal of Occupational Therapy, 67*(6), 269-273.

Moll, S., Huff, J., & Detwiler, L. (2003). Supported employment: Evidence for a best practice model in psychosocial rehabilitation. *Canadian Journal of Occupational Therapy, 70*(5), 298-310.

Nieuwenhuijsen, E. R. (2004). Health behavior change among office workers: An exploratory study to prevent repetitive strain injuries. *Work, 23*(3), 215-224.

Nordmark, B., Blomqvist, P., Andersson, B., Hagerstrom, M., Nordh-Grate, K., Ronnqvist, R., Svensson, H., & Klareskog, L. (2006). A two-year follow-up of work capacity in early rheumatoid arthritis: A study of multidisciplinary team care with emphasis on vocational support. *Scandinavian Journal of Rheumatology, 35*(1), 7-14.

Pratt, J., McFadyen, A., Hall, G., Campbell, M., & McLay, D. (1997). A review of the initial outcomes of a return-to-work programme for police officers following injury or illness. *British Journal of Occupational Therapy, 60*(6), 253-258.

Rebeiro, K., Day, D. G., Semeniuk, B., O'Brian, M. C., & Wilson, B. (2001). Northern Initiative for social action: An occupation-based mental health program. *American Journal of Occupational Therapy, 55*(5), 493-500.

Rogers, J. A. (1995). Work is key to recovery. *Psychosocial Rehabilitation Journal, 18*(4), 5-10.

Sandqvist, J. L., & Henriksson, C. M. (2004). Work functioning: A conceptual framework. *Work, 23*(2), 147-157.

Sang, L. S., & Ying Eria, L. P. (2005). Outcome evaluation of work hardening program for manual workers with work-related back injury. *Work, 25*(4), 297-305.

Sarajuuri, J., Kaipio, M., Koskinen, S., Niemela, M., Servo, A., & Vilkki, J. (2005). Outcome of a comprehensive neurorehabilitation program for patients with traumatic brain injury. *Archives of Physical Medicine and Rehabilitation, 86*(12), 2296-2302.

Scheer, S. J., Watanabe, T. K., & Radack, K. L. (1997). Randomized controlled trials in industrial low back pain. Part 3. Subacute/chronic pain interventions. *Archives of Physical Medicine Rehabilitation, 78*, 414-423.

Schene, A., Koeter, M., Kikkert, M., Swinkels, J., & McCrone, P. (2007). Adjuvant occupational therapy for work-related major depression works: Randomized trial including economic evaluation. *Psychological Medicine, 37*(3), 351-362.

Schonstein, E., Kenny, D. T., Keating, J., & Koes, B. W. (2003). Work conditioning, work hardening, and functional restoration for workers with back and neck pain. *Cochrane Database of Systematic Reviews*, Issue 3.

Twamley, E. W., Jeste, D. V., & Lehman, A. F. (2003). Vocational rehabilitation in schizophrenia and other psychotic disorders: A literature review and meta-analysis of randomized controlled trials. *Journal of Nervous and Mental Disease, 19*(8), 515-523.

Williams, R. M., Westmorland, M. G., Schmuck, G., & MacDermid, J. C. (2004). Effectiveness of workplace rehabilitation interventions in the treatment of work-related upper extremity disorders: A systematic review. *Journal of Hand Therapy, 17*, 267-273.

World Health Organization. (2001). *International classification of functioning, disability, and health*. Geneva, Switzerland: Author.

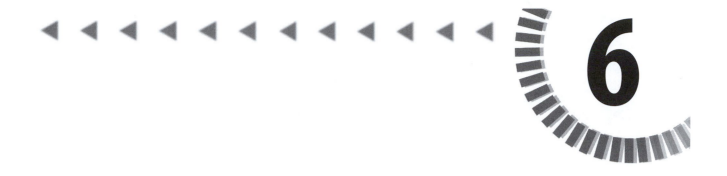

LEISURE OUTCOMES

Mary Ann McColl, PhD, MTS

This chapter explores leisure outcomes that may be affected by occupational therapy interventions. Leisure is one of the three key elements of occupation (self-care and productivity being the other two). Despite its strong links with the origins of the profession, leisure is almost always listed last among the three elements. Leisure is sometimes construed as a luxury, only to be indulged in when one's obligations have been fully discharged. Several authors note the historical tension associated with crafts and diversionary activities and ask if leisure is appropriately valued by occupational therapists or if it is considered by some to be less important than work and self-care (Bundy, 2005; Friedland, 1988).

Conceptual Background

Although there is no consensus in the literature on the definition of leisure (Christiansen, Baum, & Bass-Haugen, 2005), for the sake of this book, leisure will be defined as the activities in which one engages when one is freed from obligation to be productive (McColl, Law, Doubt, Pollock, & Stewart, 2002). Numerous authors have attempted definitions of leisure, and many take the form of the one above—defining leisure in terms of

what it is not, rather than what it is (Primeau, 2003). The Canadian Occupational Performance Measure (COPM) (Law, Baptiste, Carswell, McColl, Polatajko, & Pollock, 2005) defines leisure as consisting of quiet recreation, active recreation, and socialization. Most definitions include a subset of the characteristics of leisure listed in Table 6-1.

Primeau (2003) identifies four major categories of leisure definitions:

▲ Leisure as the use of discretionary time
▲ Leisure as the activities that take place when the context is free, safe, and comfortable
▲ Leisure as a specific set of observable behaviors associated with hobbies, games, sports, social activities, etc.
▲ Leisure as an experience that is characterized by positive affect

Each of these suggests a different approach to the characterization of leisure. This lack of consensus of what constitutes leisure, or what parameters define it, contributes to both the possible breadth of leisure, but also the difficulty of studying it when there is no agreement on what it is or how to measure it.

M. Law & M. A. McColl (Eds.)
Interventions, Effects, and Outcomes in Occupational Therapy:
Adults and Older Adults (pp. 145-154)
© 2010 SLACK Incorporated

Table 6-1

DEFINITIONS AND CHARACTERISTICS OF LEISURE

Characteristics of leisure	Non-obligatory Freely chosen Discretionary	Intrinsically rewarding Fun, pleasurable Playful	Relaxing Satisfying Voluntary
Related concepts	Entertainment Diversion Socialization	Passing time Relaxation Fandom	Amusement Play Hobby
Leisure as an opportunity for	Experimentation Exploration Self-expression Cognitive stimulation Creativity	Competition Imagination Relaxation Sensual enjoyment Service	Skill development Mastery Competence Vicarious competition Agency
Benefits of leisure	Belonging Community engagement Personal fulfillment	Acculturation Self-concept Social relationships	Meaning—personal, social, spiritual

Not surprisingly, there is relatively little occupational therapy theory associated with leisure. Classical occupational therapy theory tells us that leisure is on a continuum with work, that both work and leisure entail a similar set of skills and aptitudes, and that work and leisure are related to one another in terms of the preferences, skills, aptitudes, and opportunities (Bundy, 2005; Christiansen et al., 2005). Accordingly, individuals choose leisure activities that prepare them for work and that dovetail with other choices of lifestyle (Christiansen & Townsend, 2004). Prost (1992) notes that underemployment, a condition common among people with disabilities, has negative impacts on leisure participation and satisfaction. Leisure may be the medium through which issues and conflicts are resolved and reconciled (Fine, 2001; Frances, 2006). Leisure is sometimes considered a "hallmark of functioning," and it serves as a medium for aiding re-entry into everyday functioning and community involvement (Butin, 1996; Lloyd, King, McCarthy, & Scanlan, 2007).

Leisure by definition takes place during a person's free time, and thus it is in a temporal relationship with the other two elements of occupation—self-care and work (Christiansen et al., 2005). Cross-sectionally, focusing on a particular point in time, time use can be plotted to account for allocations to self-care, productivity, and leisure. Whereas self-care prepares the individual for other occupations, productivity typically occupies a fixed part of each day, and leisure occupies those hours reserved for recreation, restoration, and recharging.

According to Kielhofner (1988) and Shannon (1970, 1972), leisure is also related to work and self-care in a longitudinal way (i.e., over time). Across the lifespan, the balance of productivity and leisure changes as the developmental demands of the life cycle change. In childhood and older age, leisure dominates the main part of a person's day, whereas in adulthood, work dominates, and only small allocations of time to leisure are permitted. These two occupations, work and leisure, are perceived to be in a kind of dynamic tension with one another.

The literature suggests that there are at least five different types of leisure activity:

▲ Diversionary leisure, aimed at providing a change from usual activities
▲ Playful leisure, characterized by an affective tone of joyfulness and humor
▲ Serious leisure, where one is learning something or practicing a highly skilled occupation
▲ Hobbies, where one participates in an activity of interest with some continuity and expertise
▲ Fandom, where leisure participation is passive and vicarious

Play and leisure are related concepts. Play is sometimes considered the childhood version of leisure, but play has a unique meaning in terms of its developmental role among children. Play has been shown to be related to self-concept, social adaptation, and even survival (Kielhofner & Miyake, 1981). The development from solitary to parallel to cooperative play in childhood is an analogue of the development of social relationships in adulthood (Christiansen et al., 2005).

Occupational therapists use leisure both as an outcome (end) and as a therapeutic tool (means). As means, leisure activities may be a treatment tool to help improve specific occupational outcomes. As ends, leisure is an occupational outcome that occupational therapists seek to promote in order to enhance health and well-being. This chapter focuses on leisure as an outcome and the occupational therapy interventions that appear most successful in promoting positive leisure outcomes.

Historically, occupational therapists have used activity analysis to understand how leisure activities could be analyzed for their skill requirements, prescribed and used therapeutically to develop skills—that is, as a means to remediate occupation. For example, weaving was often employed as a therapeutic medium, because it required upper extremity range of motion and coordination, relatively little strength, precision of movement, repetition, and mobilization. Cognitively, weaving required the ability to count, follow a pattern, and engage in problem solving. Emotionally, it offered a quiet, neutral activity that makes few emotional demands beyond a minor requirement for patience and attention. Creatively, it offers an opportunity for expression through pattern and texture.

There are several examples in the literature of leisure as means in occupational therapy. Leisure activities, such as toy-making (Esdaile, 1996) and table-top games (Hoppes, 1997), are sometimes used by occupational therapists for the opportunities they afford to work toward occupational goals. Leisure activities are valued for their potential to promote "flow" and to make participants lose track of time, thereby extending their tolerance for occupational activities. Outdoor activities, such as kayaking (Fines & Nichols, 1994) and hiking (Frances, 2006), have also been explored for their beneficial effects. A review article by Fine (2001) uncovered nine articles that provided consistent evidence that leisure activity has a significant effect on depression and self-esteem in the elderly. Hodgson and Lloyd (2002), in a qualitative study, found that leisure activity was an important factor in preventing relapse in substance abuse rehabilitation.

Leisure activities are often sought by occupational therapists for the benefits they confer in terms of offsetting the effects of stress, promoting mastery, reinforcing identity, and ultimately promoting well-being. Leisure activities have been shown to be important in recovery from mental illness (Lloyd et al., 2007). Leisure activities are sometimes considered for the potential to add meaning. Personal meaning may be added through leisure activities chosen to reinforce the individual's identity and sense of value. Social meaning may be achieved by engaging in leisure activities that bring with them opportunities for social interaction and social validation of worth. Spiritual meaning may be encountered in leisure activities that bring one into contact with sacred and existential ideas or that transcend boundaries of time and place.

Search Strategy

This literature review focuses on leisure as an outcome in occupational therapy; that is, leisure as an end to be pursued in therapy. The search strategy sought intervention studies aimed at improving leisure participation and satisfaction and was guided by the keywords listed in Table 6-2. A systematic search of health care and occupational therapy databases, as well as hand-searched relevant references, yielded both review and empirical (qualitative and quantitative) papers that addressed the occupational therapy outcomes when providing interventions related to leisure goals. Selected studies met specific inclusion criteria, which consisted of study publication between 1980 and 2008, adult population, study intervention involving occupational therapist independently or on a multidisciplinary team, and being categorized as level of evidence 1 to 4 based on criteria by Greenhalgh (2006). A total of nine empirical studies qualified for inclusion and are reviewed in this chapter.

Tables 6-3 through 6-5 provide detailed information on the interventions used, the conclusions drawn about the effectiveness of occupational therapy for enhancing leisure, and the outcome measures applied.

Interventions Used to Improve Leisure Outcomes

Table 6-3 shows the nine studies describing seven interventions that qualified for this study. Interventions used to promote leisure participation or satisfaction tended to consist of a mixture of almost all nine of the intervention categories mentioned in Chapter 1. The main emphasis appeared to be on skills teaching and equipment prescription, with a secondary emphasis on task adaptation and support provision/enhancement.

The least intensive of the five interventions involved two to three home visits to explore leisure interests and prescribe and try adaptive devices to enhance leisure participation (Schweitzer, Mann, Nochajski, & Tomita, 1999). Another relatively low-intensity program (Jongbloed, 1993; Jongbloed & Morgan, 1991) offered five home visits to assess leisure interests, teach new skills, offer support, and provide opportunities to try new activities. Five inpatient group

Table 6-2
SEARCH TERMS FOR OCCUPATIONAL THERAPY INTERVENTIONS TO IMPROVE LEISURE OUTCOMES

Occupation, occupational therapy (therapist), OR multidisciplinary team AND...

Primary terms: hobby (ies), leisure, leisure activities, play, recreation.

Secondary terms: activity, leisure participation, leisure time, play and playthings, playful, playfulness, play participation, play therapy.

Additional terms used to focus the search included clinical effectiveness, community health services, health care delivery, health care services, health service, health services for the aged, home care, home care services, home health care, home occupational therapy, home rehabilitation, interdisciplinary education, interdisciplinary research, interdisciplinary treatment approach, intervention treatment approach, multidisciplinary care team, outcomes, outcomes assessment patient care, outcomes (health care), outcomes research, patient care team, psychotherapeutic outcomes, rehabilitation, rehabilitation care, rehabilitation centre, rehabilitation outcomes, teamwork, therapy effect, treatment effectiveness evaluation, treatment outcomes.

sessions were offered by Daniel and Manigandan (2005), aimed at promoting a positive attitude toward leisure and solving problems associated with leisure participation. The remaining four programs were more intensive, again focusing on a mix of skills teaching, support enhancement, and task adaptation. A multidisciplinary weekly intervention including occupational therapy was offered as a home program over 8 to 12 weeks (Desrosiers et al., 2007). Another occupational therapy home program was offered as 18 half-hour sessions over 6 months (Drummond & Walker, 1995). Logan and colleagues (2004) offered an occupational therapy home program over eight visits focused on removing barriers to leisure participation. Finally, Hartman-Maeir and associates (2007) offered a multidisciplinary outpatient program to stroke survivors on a weekly basis.

Four of the five interventions identified focused on seniors, and one focused on adults. In older age groups, the work-play balance tends to favor leisure, and leisure is expected to account for a large proportion of time allocations. Five of the seven programs involved stroke patients, one was a mixed group with motor and sensory disabilities, and one involved adults with spinal cord injuries. Five of the programs involved home care with visiting therapists, one was an inpatient rehabilitation program, and one was an outpatient leisure rehabilitation program. Attention to leisure might often be delayed during hospitalization and postponed until productivity and self-care goals are well in hand. Occupational therapy programs focusing on leisure outcomes appear to be relatively low-intensity programs, with infrequent visits and short duration. Programs varied from as brief as 3 hours to as long as several weeks or months.

Effects of Occupational Therapy in Promoting Leisure Outcomes

Table 6-4 shows that brief, consultation-type interventions, like those used by Jongbloed (1993), Jongbloed and Morgan (1991), and Schweitzer et al. (1999), are unlikely to be successful. The more intensive programs, such as those offered by Drummond and Walker (1995, 1996), Daniel and Manigandan (2005), Logan and colleagues (2004), Hartman-Maier and colleagues (2007), and Desrosiers and associates (2007), were more likely to result in positive leisure outcomes. There appear to be clear benefits of well-designed programs with a clear theoretical rationale for their expected effects and well-designed studies with measurement of appropriate outcomes. The most consistent messages about effectiveness from these seven programs were that more is better and that brief, superficial interventions are not effective.

Measures Used to Capture Leisure Outcomes

There was no consensus in Table 6-5 on the measures used to assess leisure participation among the nine studies cited. The Nottingham Leisure

text continues on page 153

Table 6-3

Occupational Therapy Interventions Promoting Leisure Outcomes

Author (Date)	Pop	DX	Setting	Intervention
Desrosiers, J., Noreau, L., Rochette, A., Carbonneau, H., Fontaine, L., Viscogliosi, C., et al. (2007)	5	3	3	**Intervention:** Weekly visits for 8 to 12 weeks from OT and recreational therapist; focusing on leisure awareness, self-awareness, and skill development, OT as consultant to recreational therapist. **Control:** Weekly home visits for conventional therapy.
Hartman-Maeir, A., Eliad, Y., Kizoni, R., Nahaloni, I., Kelberman, H., & Katz, N. (2007)	5	3	4	**Intervention:** Community-dwelling stroke patients who were at least 1-year post-onset participated in a multidisciplinary outpatient rehabilitation program. The program was designed to meet the long-term needs of severely disabled stroke survivors and consisted of group treatments conducted by rehabilitation professionals (OT, PT, speech therapy, social workers, nurses) and volunteers from the community 2 to 4 times per week. **Control:** Participants were community-dwelling stroke survivors 1-year post-onset who were not participating in any rehabilitation program.
Daniel, A., & Manigandan, C. (2005)	2	6	4	**Intervention:** 5 1-hour sessions; discussion group focused on leisure participation and problem solving. **Control:** No group sessions.
Logan, P. A., Gladman, J., Avery, A., Walker, M. F., Dyas, J., & Groom, L. (2004)	5	3	3	**Intervention:** Participants received a home visit from an OT who assessed barriers to outdoor mobility, negotiated mobility goals with the client, and created a treatment plan to meet those goals. The treatment plan was delivered over 7 more home visits lasting 3 months. **Control:** Participants received 1 home visit from an OT that included advice and encouragement regarding outdoor activity and written information on improving mobility.
Parker, C. J., Gladman, C. R. F., Drummond, A. E. R., Dewey, M. E., Lincoln, N. B., Barer, D., et al. (2001)	4	3	3	**Intervention:** 18 30-minute sessions over 6 months; including skills training, equipment prescription and trial, adaptation of activity, logistical support, liaison with community organizations. **Control 1:** Same frequency and duration (9 hours over 6 months) of conventional OT, focusing on ADL and perceptual training. **Control 2:** No OT.
Schweitzer, J. A., Mann, W. C., Nochajski, S., & Tomita, M. (1999)	4	18	3	**Intervention:** 2 to 3 visits for assessment of home-based leisure activity and prescription and trial of assistive device.
Drummond, A., & Walker, M. (1995)	4	3	3	**Intervention:** 18 30-minute sessions over 6 months; including skills training, equipment prescription and trial, adaptation of activity, logistical support, liaison with community organizations. **Control 1:** Same frequency and duration (9 hours over 6 months) of conventional OT, focusing on ADL and perceptual training. **Control 2:** No OT.
Jongbloed (1993); Jongbloed, L., & Morgan, D. (1991)	4	3	3	**Intervention:** 5 weekly visits from OT of 1 hour each; includes assessment of pre-morbid and current leisure interests, linking with leisure opportunities, skill teaching, equipment prescription and trial, support for activities. **Control:** Same amount of time with OT, but only discussion of leisure activities and no active facilitation.

Population: 1=geriatric (65+); 2=adult (25 to 64); 3=young adult (18 to 24); 4=adult and geriatric; 5=young adult, adult, and geriatric.

Diagnosis: 3=stroke; 6=spinal cord injury; 18=other.

Setting: 1=long-term care; 2=acute care; 3=home care; 4=rehabilitation; 5=primary care.

Table 6-4

EVIDENCE OF EFFECTIVENESS OF OCCUPATIONAL THERAPY ON LEISURE OUTCOMES

Author (Date)	Major Results	Study Design	Sample Size	Conclusions and Limitations
Positive Effects—Randomized Controlled Trial				
Desrosiers, J., Noreau, L., Rochette, A., Carbonneau, H., Fontaine, L., Viscogliosi, C., et al. (2007)	Leisure group participation showed significant effects on number, duration, and satisfaction with active leisure. No significant difference for passive leisure. No significant differences between groups for depression, well-being, or health-related quality of life.	RCT	29, 27	Weekly leisure education programming for 3 to 4 months post-discharge from stroke can be successful in promoting active leisure.
Daniel, A., & Manigandan, C. (2005)	Significant improvement in leisure participation by intervention group.	RCT	25, 25	Attitude change around leisure enhances leisure participation, which in turn enhances quality of life.
Logan, P. A., Gladman, J. R., Avery, A., Walker, M. F., Dyas, J., & Groom, L. (2004)	At both follow-ups, more participants in the intervention group responded that they were getting out of the house in the previous month than control. At 4 months, mobility scores were significantly higher in the intervention group. At 10 months, there were no significant differences on any outcome between groups.	RCT	168	The outdoor mobility program was effective in increasing mobility after stroke in both the long and short term. The small sample size may have prevented some smaller treatment effects from being noticed.
Drummond, A., & Walker, M. (1995)	Leisure scores increased significantly for the leisure rehabilitation group (intervention) over both controls groups (ADL and no treatment groups) at 3 and 6 months. No significant differences between the groups on either motor performance or functional performance.	RCT	21, 21, 23	A more sustained input of 6 months' duration can be successful in impacting leisure participation among stroke survivors.
Positive Effects—Non-Randomized Controlled Trial				
Hartman-Maeir, A., Eliad, Y., Kizoni, R., Nahaloni, I., Kelberman, H., & Katz, N. (2007)	There was significant improvement in all areas in the intervention group after participation in the rehabilitation program. Life satisfaction scores showed that the intervention group had significantly higher levels of satisfaction with "life as a whole" (p=0.01) and "leisure situation" (p=0.03).	Non-RCT	83	The community rehabilitation program had a significant positive effect on activity level and life satisfaction. These results provide support for the value of ongoing community-based programs for stroke survivors living in the community.
No Effect				
Jongbloed, L. (1993); Jongbloed, L., & Morgan, D. (1991)	Main effect of time on number of activities. No statistically significant effect of intervention—i.e., no significant difference between the intervention and control group for activity involvement or satisfaction.	RCT	20, 20	5 1-hour leisure facilitation sessions immediately post-discharge from stroke not effective in altering leisure participation immediately or 5 months later.

continued

Table 6-4 (continued)

Evidence of Effectiveness of Occupational Therapy on Leisure Outcomes

Author (Date)	Major Results	Study Design	Sample Size	Conclusions and Limitations
No Effect				
Parker, C. J., Gladman, J. R. F., Drummond, A. E. R., Dewey, M. E., Lincoln, N. B., Barer, D., et al. (2001)	No significant effects of program on mood, leisure participation, or ADL independence.	RCT	20, 20	This elaborate 5-site trial showed no short- or long-term benefits of leisure-oriented OT or ADL-oriented OT.
Schweitzer, J. A., Mann, W. C., Nochajski, S., & Tomita, M. (1999)	No statistical evaluation of Leisure Satisfaction Questionnaire reported.	RCT	153, 156, 157	Anecdotal reports of increased utilization and satisfaction with leisure adaptive devices.

Table 6-5
OUTCOME MEASURES USED TO CAPTURE LEISURE OUTCOMES

Author (Date)	Outcome(s) Investigated	Outcome Measure(s)	Method of Administration
Desrosiers, J., Noreau, L., Rochette, A., Carbonneau, H., Fontaine, L., Viscogliosi, C., et al. (2007)	Participation in leisure Satisfaction with leisure Perceived well-being Depressive symptoms Health-related quality of life	Duration and number of leisure activities per day LSS General well-being scale CES-D SIP	Participants were measured pre- and post-program by a blinded assessor.
Hartman-Maeir, A., Eliad, Y., Kizoni, R., Nahaloni, I., Kelberman, H., & Katz, N. (2007)	Functional ability Performance of ADL Leisure participation Life satisfaction Health status	FIM IADLq ACS LiSat-9 SIS	Subjects in the intervention were assessed before and after entering the community rehabilitation program, and subjects in the control were only assessed 1-year post-stroke. All assessments were completed by an OT who had no other involvement in the study.
Daniel, A., & Manigandan, C. (2005)	Satisfaction with leisure activities Quality of life	LSS WHO QOL—BREF	Assessments were delivered at baseline and 2 weeks later once the study was completed.
Logan, P. A., Gladman, J. R., Avery, A., Walker, M. F., Dyas, J., & Groom, L. (2004)	Amount of time spent out-doors Functional performance Leisure activity General health status	Questionnaire developed by researchers Nottingham Extended ADL Scale Nottingham Leisure Questionnaire GHQ	Outcomes were evaluated by independent blinded assessors at baseline and 4- and 10-month follow-up.
Parker, C. J., Gladman, C. R. F., Drummond, A. E. R., Dewey, M. E., Lincoln, N. B., Barer, D., et al. (2001)	Leisure participation Mood ADL	Nottingham Leisure Questionnaire GHQ Nottingham Extended ADL Scale	Self-report questionnaires (with the help of caregiver if necessary); 6 months and 12 months post-program.
Schweitzer, J. A., Mann, W. C., Nochajski, S., & Tomita, M. (1999)	Leisure participation Pattern of assistive device use Satisfaction with leisure activity	Leisure Study Interview Follow-up questionnaire	Interview—face-to-face or telephone; 1 month after receipt of assistive device.
Drummond, A., & Walker, M. (1995)	Number of leisure activities Functional performance Motor performance	Nottingham Leisure Questionnaire Rivermead ADL Scale Rivermead Motor Function Assessment	Baseline at discharge, 3 months, 6 months—midway and end of intervention. Interviewer administered.
Jongbloed, L. (1993); Jongbloed, L., & Morgan, D. (1991)	Involvement in leisure activities Satisfaction with leisure activities Cognitive function ADL Depression	Katz Adjustment Index (Free Time Activities and Satisfaction with Free Time Activities subscales) MMSE BI Zung Depression Scale	At end of program—5 weeks post-discharge, 18 weeks post-discharge. Interview-administered. Confirmation from significant other.

ACS=Activity Card Sort, BI=Barthel Index, CES-D=Center for Epidemiologic Studies Depression Scale, FIM=Functional Independence Measure, IADLq=Lawton Instrumental Activities of Daily Living Questionnaire, LiSat-9=Life Satisfaction Questionnaire, LSS=Leisure Satisfaction Scale, MMSE=Mini Mental Status Examination, SIP=Sickness Impact Profile, SIS=Stroke Impact Scale, WHO QOL—BREF=World Health Organization Quality of Life Scale—Brief.

Table 6-6

OUTCOME MEASURES TO ASSESS LEISURE INTERVENTIONS

Measure	Population	Content Domains	Reliability and Validity
Activity Card Sort (ACS)	Adults	4 domains: Instrumental activities, low-demand leisure, high-demand leisure, social activities	Test-retest 0.90 Internal consistency 0.61 to 0.82 Moderate correlation with Occupational Questionnaire
Interest Checklist	General population	5 categories: Manual skills, physical sports, social recreation, ADL, cultural/educational	Multiple studies based on factor analysis and independence of subscales
Leisure Competence Measure (LCM)	Adults and seniors	8 subscales: Leisure awareness, leisure attitudes, leisure skills, social behaviors, interpersonal skills, community integration, social contact, community participation	Inter-rater reliability: 0.71 to 0.91 Internal consistency 0.92 Moderate correlations with Geriatric Depression Scale and Mini Mental Status Examination
Leisure Diagnostic Battery (LDB)	Individuals without significant cognitive impairment	Leisure attitude measure, leisure interest measure, leisure motivation scale, leisure satisfaction measure	Internal consistency 0.87-0.93 Some evidence of validity for individual subscales
Leisure Satisfaction Scale (LSS)	General population	Short form—6 subscales: Psychological, social, educational, relaxation, physiological, aesthetic	Internal consistency 0.93 Content validity affirmed by expert panel

Questionnaire was used in three of the studies. It is safe to say that there appear to be no psychometrically strong, sensitive measures of leisure participation for this area of research. A review by Connolly and colleagues (2005) suggests five additional measures that should be considered by occupational therapy researchers wishing to capture outcomes in this area (Table 6-6). These measures have sound development and acceptable psychometric properties: Activity Card Sort (ACS), Interest Checklist, Leisure Competence Measure (LCM), Leisure Diagnostic Battery (LDB), and Leisure Satisfaction Scale (LSS).

In some of these studies, evaluators have done their programs a disservice by evaluating them on the basis of variables like depression and well-being. It would be surprising indeed if a relatively minor intervention like leisure counseling would have a significant effect on such pervasive, multifactorial outcomes as these.

Conclusions and Recommendations for Further Research

In conclusion, despite its status as one of the three core concepts of occupational therapy, leisure has received relatively little attention, either in practice or in research, as evidenced by the fact that only nine articles could be found that met the search criteria. Furthermore, three of the programs examined offered only 3 to 5 hours of occupational therapy on leisure. It is clear that relative to self-care and productivity, leisure has not been a priority. While there are good and obvious reasons for this, it does call into question our conception of a balance of self-care, productivity, and leisure. It requires us to look again at the research on balance in occupational therapy and to explore the basis upon which this balance might be founded.

The focus of leisure interventions appears to be on skills and tools, rather than on values, attitudes, or motivation for leisure. The assumption must, therefore, be that the true barriers to successful and satisfying leisure performance are inadequate skills or the need for adaptive equipment. It seems conceivable that a deeper focus on underlying feelings and perceptions toward leisure might produce more satisfactory outcomes.

References

Bundy, A. C. (2005). Measuring play performance. In M. Law, C. Baum, & W. Dunn (Eds.), *Measuring occupational performance: Supporting best practice in occupational therapy* (2nd ed.). Thorofare, NJ: SLACK Incorporated.

Butin, D. (1996). Psychosocial and psychological components. In K. Larson, R. Stevens-Ratchford, L. Pedretti, & J. Crabtree (Eds.), *ROTE: The role of OT with the elderly* (pp. 610-629). Bethesda, MD: American Occupational Therapy Association.

Christiansen, C., Baum, C., & Bass-Haugen, J. (2005). *Occupational therapy: Performance, participation and well-being* (3rd ed.). Thorofare, NJ: SLACK Incorporated.

Christiansen, C. H., & Townsend, E. A. (2004). *Introduction to occupation: The art and science of living.* Upper Saddle River, NJ: Prentice Hall.

Connolly, K., Law, M., & MacGuire, B. (2005). Measuring leisure performance. In M. Law, C. M. Baum, & W. Dunn (Eds.), *Measuring occupational performance: Supporting best practice in occupational therapy* (2nd ed., pp. 249-275). Thorofare, NJ: SLACK Incorporated.

Daniel, A., & Manigandan, C. (2005). Efficacy of leisure intervention groups and their impact on quality of life among people with spinal cord injury. *International Journal of Rehabilitation Research, 28*(1), 43-48.

Desrosiers, J., Noreau, L., Rochette, A., Carbonneau, H., Fontaine, L., Viscogliosi, C., et al. (2007). Effect of a home leisure education program after stroke: A randomized controlled trial. *Archives of Physical Medicine and Rehabilitation, 88*(9), 1095-1100.

Drummond, A., & Walker, M. (1995). A randomized controlled trial of leisure rehabilitation after stroke. *Clinical Rehabilitation, 9*(4), 283-290.

Drummond, A., & Walker, M. (1996). Generalisation of the effects of leisure rehabilitation for stroke patients. *British Journal of Occupational Therapy, 59*(7), 330-334.

Esdaile, S. A. (1996). A play-focused intervention involving mothers of preschoolers. *American Journal of Occupational Therapy, 50*(2), 113-123.

Fine, J. (2001). The effect of leisure activity on depression in the elderly: Implications for the field of occupational therapy. *Occupational Therapy in Health Care, 13*(1), 45-59.

Fines, L., & Nichols, D. (1994). An evaluation of a twelve week recreational kayak program: Effects on self-concept, leisure satisfaction, and leisure attitude of adults with traumatic brain injuries. *Journal of Cognitive Rehabilitation,* September/October, 10-15.

Frances, K. (2006). Outdoor recreation as an occupation to improve quality of life for people with enduring mental health problems. *British Journal of Occupational Therapy, 69*(4), 182-186.

Friedland, J. (1988). Diversional activity: Does it deserve its bad name? *American Journal of Occupational Therapy, 42,* 603-608.

Greenhalgh, T. (2006). *How to read a paper: The basics of evidence-based medicine* (3rd ed.). London, England: Blackwell Publishing Ltd.

Hartman-Maeir, A., Eliad, Y., Kizoni, R., Nahaloni, I., Kelberman, H., & Katz, N. (2007). Evaluation of a long-term community based rehabilitation program for adult stroke survivors. *Neurorehabilitation, 22*(4), 295-301.

Hodgson, S., & Lloyd, C. (2002). Leisure as a relapse prevention strategy. *British Journal of Therapy and Rehabilitation, 9*(3), 86-91.

Hoppes, S. (1997). Can play increase standing tolerance? A pilot-study. *Physical and Occupational Therapy in Geriatrics, 15*(1), 65-73.

Jongbloed, L. (1993). Evaluating the efficacy of OT intervention related to leisure activities. *Canadian Journal of Rehabilitation, 7*(1), 19-20.

Jongbloed, L., & Morgan, D. (1991). An investigation of involvement in leisure activities after a stroke. *American Journal of Occupational Therapy, 45*(5), 420-427.

Kielhofner, G. (1988). Model of human occupation. In S. Robinson (Ed.), *Mental health focus.* Rockville, MD: American Occupational Therapy Association.

Kielhofner, G., & Miyake, S. (1981). The therapeutic use of games with mentally retarded adults. *American Journal of Occupational Therapy, 35*(6), 375-382.

Law, M., Baptiste, S., Carswell, A., McColl, M. A, Polatajko, H., & Pollock, N. (2005). *Canadian Occupational Performance Measure* (4th ed.). Ottawa, Ontario, Canada: CAOT Publications.

Lloyd, C., King, R., McCarthy, M., & Scanlan, M. (2007). The association between leisure motivation and recovery: A pilot study. *Australian Occupational Therapy Journal, 54,* 33-41.

Logan, P. A., Gladman, J., Avery, A., Walker, M. F., Dyas, J., & Groom, L. (2004). Randomised controlled trial of an occupational therapy intervention to increase outdoor mobility after stroke. *BMJ, 329*(7479), 1372-1375.

McColl, M. A., Law, M. C., Stewart, D., Doubt, L., Pollock, N., & Krupa, T. (2002). *Theoretical basis of occupational therapy* (2nd ed.). Thorofare, NJ: SLACK Incorporated.

Parker, C. J., Gladman, C. R. F., Drummond, A. E. R., Dewey, M. E., Lincoln, N. B., Barer, D., et al. (2001). A multicentre randomized controlled trial of leisure therapy and conventional occupational therapy after stroke. *Clinical Rehabilitation, 15,* 42-52.

Primeau, L. A. (2003). Play and leisure. In E. B. Crepeau, E. S. Cohn, & B. A. B. Schell (Eds.), *Willard & Spackman's occupational therapy* (10th ed., pp. 567-569). Philadelphia, PA: Lippincott Williams & Wilkins.

Prost, A. (1992). Leisure and disability: A contradiction in terms. *World of Leisure and Recreation, 34,* 8-9.

Schweitzer, J. A., Mann, W. C., Nochajski, S., & Tomita, M. (1999). Patterns of engagement in leisure activity by older adults using assistive devices. *Technology and Disability, 11*(1-2), 103-117.

Shannon, P. D. (1970). The work-play model: A basis for occupational therapy programming in psychiatry. *American Journal of Occupational Therapy, 24,* 215-218.

Shannon, P. (1972). Work-play theory and the occupational therapy process. *American Journal of Occupational Therapy, 26,* 169-172.

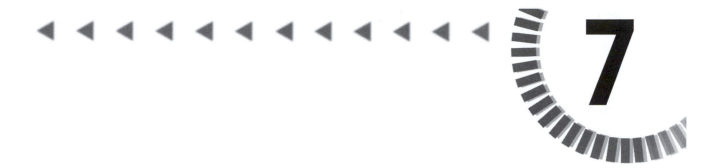

ENVIRONMENTAL CHANGE TO IMPROVE OUTCOMES

Mary Law, PhD, FCAOT; Briano Di Rezze, MSc (OT), OT Reg. (Ont.); and Laura Bradley, MSc (OT), OT Reg. (Ont.)

Occupational therapy intervention focuses on removing environmental barriers and increasing supports in order to maximize an individual's occupational performance or participation. Prevalent strategies in occupational therapy practice address the individual, his or her occupations, and immediate physical and social environments (in terms of safety, accessibility, and social supports) (O'Brien, Dyck, Caron, & Mortenson, 2002).

Conceptual Background

Many environmental influences can affect disability outcomes (Jongbloed & Crichton, 1990). Occupational therapists view disability as a problem highly influenced by barriers in the environment that cannot always be remedied by changing the individual's capabilities (Law, 1991). Environmental factors influence the daily activities of all people, not just those with disabilities. For example, older adults at risk for decreased activity and falls can be helped through community social supports and physical accessibility measures.

Environmental factors are a part of the World Health Organization's International Classification of Functioning, Disability, and Health (ICF) (2001). Within this classification, five categories of environmental factors are listed. These factors include the following:

▲ "Products and technology—natural or human-made products or systems of products, equipment, and technology in an individual's immediate environment

▲ Natural environment and human-made changes to the environment—animate and inanimate elements of the natural or physical environment

▲ Support and relationships—people or animals that provide practical physical or emotional support, nurturing, protection, assistance, and relationships to other persons, in their home, place of work, school, or at play or in other aspects of their daily activities

▲ Attitudes—attitudes that are the observable consequences of customs, practices, ideologies, values, norms, factual beliefs, and religious beliefs

▲ Services, systems, and policies—services that provide benefits, structured programs, and operations, in various sectors of society, designed to

M. Law & M. A. McColl (Eds.)
*Interventions, Effects, and Outcomes in Occupational Therapy:
Adults and Older Adults* (pp. 155-182)
© 2010 SLACK Incorporated

meet the needs of individuals. Systems that are administrative control and organizational mechanisms and are established by governments at the local, regional, national, and international levels, or by other recognized authorities. Policies constituted by rules, regulations, conventions, and standards established by governments at the local, regional, national, and international levels, or by other recognized authorities." (WHO, 2007)

As outlined in Chapter 1, occupational therapy intervention often focuses on removing/modifying environmental barriers and increasing environmental supports in order to maximize an individual's participation in daily occupations (O'Brien et al., 2002). Occupational therapy aims to increase clients' functional independence for daily activities, social participation, and quality of life (Steultjens, Dekker, Bouter, Jellema, Bakker, & van den Ende, 2004).

The ultimate outcome of occupational therapy intervention strategies is increased participation in daily occupations. Intermediate outcomes relative to the environment center on changes to the physical, cultural, social, or institutional environment. These interventions and outcomes include the following:

▲ Physical environment—safety, accessibility, and social supports

▲ Social environment—family supports, role expectations, education, and training

▲ Cultural-institutional environment—facilitators and barriers created by cultural beliefs, attitudes and values, organizational and institutional policies, and expectations

In relation to the ICF environmental factors categories, the physical environment corresponds to the ICF categories of products and technology and natural environment and human-made changes. The social environment encompasses the ICF categories of support and relationships while the cultural-institutional environment focuses on the ICF categories of societal attitudes and services, systems, and policies.

Occupational therapy interventions with respect to the environment center on changes to the client's environment in order to improve participation in daily occupations. Such interventions include advocacy to change environmental conditions, using adaptations in physical and social environments, or analyzing and improving caregiver competence and skills as well as helping caregivers to understand client behavior and assist with change in the caregiver's role.

The reviews completed for this project indicate that the majority of empirical research about environmental interventions and outcomes in occupational therapy are in two areas: (1) physical environment (modifications of home/community and the use of assistive devices/adaptive equipment) and (2) social environment.

Findings from the review have been organized according to these two categories. Further research regarding interventions and outcomes within the cultural and institutional environments is needed before any firm conclusions can be drawn about occupational therapy sensitive-outcomes in that area.

Search Strategy

The methodology to search the literature, identify studies, and select them based on the inclusion criteria was discussed in Chapter 2. A systematic search of health care and occupational therapy databases, as well as hand-searched relevant references, yielded critical reviews (e.g., systematic reviews or meta-analyses), as well as qualitative and quantitative studies that addressed occupational therapy outcomes when providing intervention related to the client's environment. Selected studies met specific inclusion criteria, which consisted of study publication between 1980 and 2008, adult population, study intervention involving occupational therapist independently or on a multidisciplinary team, and study categorized as level of evidence 1 to 4 based on criteria by Greenhalgh (2006). For this chapter, the search terms used to capture occupational therapy-sensitive outcomes are listed in Table 7-1. A total of 34 articles met the inclusion criteria, are reviewed in this chapter, and are provided in more detail in Tables 7-2 through 7-4.

Interventions Used to Improve Environmental Outcomes

In the next sections, we discuss the nature of interventions to change environmental outcomes and examine the research evidence that has studied occupational therapy interventions focused on changing environmental outcomes. The results of our empirical summaries are organized by the nature of the intervention and the environmental factor that is the target of the intervention. The section concludes with recommendations on how clinical treatment can proceed and/or where future research directions rest.

Intervention to Improve the Physical Environment

Occupational therapists often focus on modifications of the physical environment and provision of assistive devices/adaptive equipment. These interventions aim to improve and/or maintain the client's activities of daily living (ADL) functioning and prevent falls and injuries. Physical modifications can entail changes to specific areas of the home or other environments, as well as following the principles of

Table 7-1

SEARCH TERMS FOR OCCUPATIONAL THERAPY INTERVENTIONS TO IMPROVE ENVIRONMENTAL OUTCOMES

Occupation, occupational therapy (therapist), OR multidisciplinary team AND...

Primary terms: accessibility, accident, aids, design, devices, environment, equipment, falls, prevention, safety, technology.

Secondary terms: accidental falls, accident prevention, accident proneness, accidents home, architectural accessibility, assistive technology, assistive technology devices, community program, disability aids, environment design, equipment, equipment design, facility environment, falling, health care equipment, home accident, home environment, home safety, household equipment, institutional environment, medical technology, occupational accident, occupational safety, orthopaedic equipment, orthopaedic equipment supplies, patient safety, person environment fit, preventative health care, psychosocial environment, safety behavior: home physical environment, safety management, safety status: falls occurrence, self-help devices, self-help equipment, social environment, technical aid, work environment.

Additional terms used to focus the search included clinical effectiveness, interdisciplinary education, interdisciplinary research, interdisciplinary treatment approach, outcomes, outcomes assessment, outcomes (health care), outcomes research, patient care, patient care team, rehabilitation outcomes, treatment effectiveness evaluation, treatment outcomes.

universal design. Typically, intervention centers on identification and removal of hazards and the addition of environmental modifications and supports.

A review of the literature by Tse in 2005 indicated that occupational therapy intervention often seeks to reduce risk of falls and injury by identifying and eliminating the environmental hazards and increasing safety features within that environment. From this review, the frequent environmental modifications by occupational therapy within the community/home setting include grab rails, removal of rugs and obstacles, contrast edge added to steps, shower seats, elevated toilet seats, bathroom floors made non-slip, and stair rails installed. The most frequent occupational therapy recommendations from environmental assessments in institutional settings include increasing lighting, lowering bed heights, using or removing carpeting, non-slip floor surfaces, bed alarms, individual seating, wheelchair safety, bed stabilizers, bedside commodes at night, and safer use of electronic devices.

As well, occupational therapists often prescribe assistive devices to be used in the home and community to maintain independent functioning. In a qualitative study describing a training apartment for clients with acquired brain injury (ABI), Erikson and colleagues (2004) demonstrated how occupational therapy environmental intervention to help clients use assistive devices and equipment improved independence for daily activities and an overall increased perception of self-confidence and sense of control. In an article that described adaptive equipment prescribed by occupational therapists to 121 families, the most frequently issued devices were for bathing and grooming difficulties (37%), while 20% were prescribed for general safety concerns, 16% for incontinence, 12% for mobility difficulties, 4% to assist with eating problems, and 4% for difficulties engaging in meaningful activities (Gitlin & Chee, 2006).

Through environmental modifications, occupational therapy can increase initiative, autonomy, pleasure in doing daily activities, and improve quality of life through adaptation of the physical environment (Graff, Vernooij-Dassen, Thijssen, Dekker, Hoefnagels, & Rikkert, 2006). Environmental modifications are often teamed with provision of information and education in the use of these modifications. Occupational therapy is most often a part of a multidisciplinary intervention aimed at addressing safety issues. Interventions used by these teams include a variety of environmental strategies, client and caregiver training and education, devices, and education (Tse, 2005), and these are often combined with a drug, vision, and blood pressure assessment (Chang et al., 2004).

Intervention to Improve the Social Environment

For people with disability and/or chronic disease, occupational therapy can focus on providing interventions for family members and caregivers. In these situations, the role of the therapist is to mobilize and develop the client's social support system to enable the client to maintain/improve participation in daily occupations. In this intervention, change is not expected within the client, but in his or her support system (Friedland & McColl, 1989). With additional supports in place, client functioning can be maintained or, in some situations, improve.

Occupational therapy intervention with caregivers centers on methods to adapt the physical environment for the client and reinforce strategies for engaging him or her in daily occupations. The goal of intervention is to maintain/improve daily performance of ADL and quality of life of the client and to contribute to improvements in sense of competence and quality of life for primary caregivers (Graff et al., 2006). Through occupational therapy intervention, caregivers receive education as well as training in assisting with independence, supervision skills, and in dealing with caregiver role changes (Graff et al., 2006).

Effects of Occupational Therapy in Promoting Environmental Outcomes

Physical Environment

Systematic Reviews

Two Cochrane Collaborations publications have systematically reviewed intervention focused on modification of the home environment as part of systematic reviews of interventions to decrease falls (Gillespie, Gillespie, Robertson, Lamb, Cumming, & Rowe, 2003; Lyons et al., 2006). Gillespie and colleagues (2003) examined 62 studies to review the evidence about the effectiveness of programs to decrease the incidence of falls in both community-dwelling older adults and for those living in institutional settings. Most of the studies were multidisciplinary in nature, and many did not specify the health professionals involved, although the interventions are consistent with what occupational therapy provides to change the physical environment. The multidisciplinary interventions generally consisted of assessment, referral, and treatment protocols to address multifactorial health/environment risk factors for falls. Occupational therapy intervention typically occurred if treatment was labeled a home hazard modification. This review concluded that home hazard assessment and modification that is professionally prescribed for older adults with a history of falls leads to changes in the physical home environment and that these outcomes were associated with a significant reduction in the incidence of falls during the study period.

Lyons and colleagues (2006) reviewed 14 studies to determine whether modification of the home environment decreases injuries occurring in the home

for older adults (>65 years) who are at risk for falls. Occupational therapy was involved in eight of these studies. Outcomes assessed in these studies included incidence of falls and/or injuries and hazard reduction (including safety knowledge, possession, use of and compliance with safety equipment). The interventions, carried out by multidisciplinary teams, provided multifactorial injury prevention strategies to prevent falls and to identify home hazards and provide information and education to change hazards. Within some of these studies, occupational therapists also performed assessment and home modifications in addition to the prevention and education programs. For example, assessment and identification of environmental hazards led to home modifications, such as removal of mats and electrical cords; installation of non-slip mats, night lights, stair rails, and grab bars in bathrooms; and advice on footwear and activities. In some studies, an exercise program was implemented as well. The results of this review indicate that significant effects were only evident when the outcomes of home hazard reduction were achieved along with other outcome changes. Specifically, the largest effects to rates of falls were seen when programs combined home modifications, exercise, and vision correction.

Empirical Studies

As part of this project, we reviewed 22 quantitative studies of occupational therapy intervention and eight multidisciplinary interventions whose purpose was to change physical environments. The intervention in most of the studies centered on environmental safety assessments of the home followed by changes in the physical environment through the provision of assistive devices/equipment and home modifications.

Many of the studies also simultaneously included an education and training program for clients and their family members (Buri, 1997; Campbell et al., 2005; Chamberlain, Thornley, Stow, & Wright, 1981; Chiu & Man, 2004; Corcoran & Gitlin, 2001; Gitlin, Corcoran, Winter, Boyce, & Hauck, 2001; Gitlin, Hauck, Dennis, & Winter, 2005; Gitlin, Miller, & Boyce, 1999; Gitlin, Winter, Corcoran, Dennis, Schinfeld, & Hauck, 2003; Gitlin, Winter, Dennis, Corcoran, Schinfeld, & Hauck, 2006; Haines, Bennell, Osborne, & Hill, 2004; Hendriks, van Haastregt, Diederiks, Evers, Crebolder, & van Eijk, 2005; Mann, Ottenbacher, Fraas, Tomita, & Granger, 1999; Shaw et al., 2003; Stark, 2004; Tolley & Atwal, 2003; Weatherall, 2004; Yang, Mann, Nochajski, & Tomita, 1997). Results of these studies indicate that the provision of assistive devices/equipment and home modifications when combined with education and training leads to increased use of devices over time, changes in the physical home environment, and associated increases in ADL and reductions in falls

text continues on page 178

Table 7-2

OCCUPATIONAL THERAPY INTERVENTIONS PROMOTING ENVIRONMENTAL OUTCOMES

Author (Date)	Pop	DX	Setting	Intervention
Gentry, T. (2008)	5	5	3	***Intervention:*** Subjects received training in the use of a personal digital assistant (PDA) as a cognitive aid over 4 home visits from an OT. Participants were also allowed to contact the OT with questions regarding the use of the PDA during an 8-week post-training period.
Petersson, I., Lilja, M., Hammel, J., & Kottorp, A. (2008)	1	18	3	***Intervention:*** Community-dwelling elders who had applied for a home modification through the local Agency for Home Modification and were approved to receive the modification. ***Control:*** Community-dwelling elders who had applied for home modification through the same agency but whose request had not been approved yet (waitlist control group).
DeCraen, A., Gussekloo, J., Blauw, G. J., Willems, C. G., & Westendorp, R. (2006)	1	24	3	***Intervention:*** Received a home visit by an OT who assessed subjects and provided necessary interventions. Interventions included education and training on existing assistive devices, recommendations for new assistive devices or community-based services when necessary, and aiding subjects to acquire the recommended devices or services. ***Control:*** Received no visits from OT.
Gitlin, L. N., Winter, L., Dennis, M. P., Corcoran, M., Schinfeld, S., & Hauck, W. W. (2006)	1	24	3	***Intervention:*** 6-month intervention consisted of 4 90-minute visits and 1 20-minute telephone call (by OT) and 1 90-minute visit (by PT). Education and problem solving (OT), home modification (OT), energy conserving techniques (not mentioned who administered), balance and muscle strengthening (PT), and fall recovery techniques (PT). ***Control:*** Usual care.
Graff, M. J., Vernooij-Dassen, M. J., Thijssen, M., Dekker, J., Hoefnagels, W. H., & Rikkert, M. G. (2006)	1	8	3	***Intervention:*** 10 1-hour in-home OT sessions aimed at identifying and implementing compensatory strategies and environmental approaches to address issues in participation in daily occupations in which patients and caregivers identified and prioritized the daily occupation issues. ***Control:*** Usual care.
Niva, B., & Skar, L. (2006)	1	18	3	***Intervention:*** Participants' homes were assessed by an OT, and appropriate modifications to improve accessibility and usability were completed.
Campbell, A. J., Robertson M. C., La Grow, S. J., Kerse, N. M., Sanderson, G. F., Jacobs, R. J., et al. (2005)	1	24, 25	3	***Intervention:*** Home safety program (led by OT), Otago exercise program and vitamin D supplementation (led by PT), social visits (done by research staff).
Fange, A., & Iwarsson, S. (2005)	5	18	3	***Intervention:*** Home modification to remove physical barriers and increase usability of home.
Gitlin, L. N., Hauck, W. W., Dennis, M. P., & Winter, L. (2005)	4	8	3	***Intervention:*** An OT environmental skill-building program (5 home contacts and 1 telephone contact by OTs, who provided education, problem-solving training, and adaptive equipment) for caregivers of people with dementia. ***Control:*** Usual care.
Hendriks, M. R. C., van Haastregt, J. C. M., Diederiks, J. P. M., Evers, S. M. A. A., Crebolder, H. F. J. M., & van Eijk J. T. M. (2005)	1	24	3	***Intervention:*** Medical and OT assessment resulting in recommendations. Medical assessment identified and addressed risk factors for falling. OT assessment identified possible risk factors for falling in the home environment (recommendations made regarding adaptations to the home environment, assistive devices, home care, and behavioral change). ***Control:*** Usual care.

continued

Table 7-2 (continued)

Occupational Therapy Interventions Promoting Environmental Outcomes

Author (Date)	Pop	DX	Setting	Intervention
Chiu, C. W. Y., & Man, D. W. K. (2004)	4	3	3	***Intervention:*** A home-based training by OT in the use of assistive devices.
Clemson, L., Cumming, R. G., Kendig, H., Swann, M., Heard, R., & Taylor, K. (2004)	1	24	3	***Intervention:*** Aims to improve fall self-efficacy, encourage behavioral change, and reduce falls. Cognitive-behavioral approach used to improve lower-limb balance and strength, home and community environmental and behavioral safety, and to encourage regular visual screening, make adaptations to low vision, and promote medication review. 2-hour sessions were conducted weekly for 7 weeks, with a follow-up OT home visit. ***Control:*** Control group received up to 2 social visits.
Dooley, N. R., & Hinojosa, J. (2004)	1	8	3	***Intervention:*** Using the results of the baseline assessment, an OT visited the homes of participants and worked with the patient and caregiver to come up with a list of recommendations to maximize quality of life. A 30-minute follow-up visit was also scheduled, and the list of written recommendations was left with the caregiver. ***Control:*** Participants received usual care and no treatment related to the study.
Haines, T., Bennell, K., Osborne, R., & Hill, K. (2004)	4	24	4	***Intervention:*** Falls risk alert card, recommended by nurses. Exercise program led by PT. Educational program led by OT. Hip protectors implemented by nurses, PT, OT, and medical staff. ***Control:*** Regular care without falls prevention program.
Stark, S. (2004)	4	24	3	***Intervention:*** OT assessment of home and intervention plan provided to modify home and eliminate environmental barriers by strictly using compensatory strategies such as provision of adaptive equipment, architectural modifications, and bathroom and major home renovations.
Weatherall, M. (2004)	1	3, 16, 17, 18, 24	4	***Intervention:*** Received recommendations from the results of a fall risk assessment instrument such as provision of hip protectors, a card placed above the subject's bed stating that he or she was at risk of falls (as well as brochure to family), 3 extra 45 minutes of PT a week, and 2 extra 30-minute OT sessions a week. ***Control:*** Did not receive these recommendations but received usual care.
Gitlin, L. N., Winter, L., Corcoran, M., Dennis, M. P., Schinfeld, S., & Hauck, W. W. (2003)	4	8	3	***Intervention:*** An OT environmental skill-building program (5 home contacts and 1 telephone contact by OTs, who provided education, problem-solving training, and adaptive equipment) for caregivers of people with dementia. ***Control:*** Usual care.
McGruder, J., Cors, D., Tiernan, A. M., & Tomlin, G. (2003)	5	3, 7, 18	3,4	***Intervention:*** OT intervention that alternated conditions between treatment (application of weighted fabric wrist cuff) and control (identical cuff with weights removed) during mealtime to determine whether tremors were reduced and functional feeding increased.
Tolley, L. & Atwal, A. (2003)	4	24	4	***Intervention:*** Multifaceted falls prevention program (9 of 14 sessions with OT) where OT educated subjects about the causes of falls and home modifications as well as advising on ADL. PT conducted and provided information regarding exercise, and a podiatrist advised on footwear and the management of the foot.

continued

Table 7-2 (continued)

Occupational Therapy Interventions Promoting Environmental Outcomes

Author (Date)	Pop	DX	Setting	Intervention
Gosman-Hedstrom, G., Claesson, L., & Blomstrand, C. (2002)	1	3	4	**Intervention:** This group was in a stroke unit, which worked according to same medical treatment, rehabilitation (OT, PT, and stroke nurse), and active participation of family. **Control:** Subjects randomized to conventional treatment were on general wards at acute hospitals. They had medical treatment, but rehabilitation (OT and PT) only when especially referred by doctor. Subjects were involved in treatments for 3 and 12 months.
VanLeit, B., & Crowe, T. (2002)	2	18	4	**Intervention:** 8-week psychosocial OT intervention program for mothers of children with disabilities. An initial 60-minute individual intervention session preceded and proceeded 6 group problem-solving and support sessions. Individual and group sessions revolved around discussion of occupational routines and concerns. **Control:** Usual care.
Corcoran, M. A., & Gitlin, L. N. (2001)	5	8	3	**Intervention:** 5 90-minute OT sessions with caregivers to determine caregiving issues and generate environment-based solutions. Model of the environment used to understand the range of strategies. Tailored to enhance skills for caregivers in using physical and social environment to address troublesome behavior for family members with dementia.
Gitlin, L. N., Corcoran, M., Winter, L., Boyce, A., & Hauck, W. W. (2001)	4	8	3	**Intervention:** 5 90-minute home visits by an OT involving education and modifications. **Control:** Participants received printed educational materials.
Koppenhaver, D., Erickson, K., Harris, B., McLellan, J., Skotko, G., & Newton, R. (2001)	2	18	3	**Intervention:** Mothers and their daughters attended 5 individual, monthly, 2-hour assessment and informational sessions that consisted of explanation of plans, introduction of equipment, and explanation of procedures related to storybook reading. **Session 1:** Baseline of how mothers read to daughters. **Session 2:** Investigate effects of resting splint on non-dominant hand—OT delivered. **Session 3:** Impact of variety of assistive technologies. **Session 4:** Parent training on nature of interaction and communication.
Close, J., Ellis, M., Hooper, R., Glucksman, E., Jackson, S., & Swift, C. (1999)	1	24	3,4	**Intervention:** Medical assessment (focused on visual acuity, balance, cognition, affect, and prescribing practice) and referral to other disciplines (if appropriate). OT assessment to assess function, environmental hazards. Advice, education, and devices were supplied if appropriate. **Control:** Usual care.
Cumming, R. G., Thomas, M., Szonyi, G., Salkeld, G., O'Neill, E., Westbury, C., et al. (1999)	1	24	3	**Intervention:** Received home visit by OT who assessed the home for environmental hazards and facilitated any necessary home modifications. **Control:** Received usual care that did not include a home visit by OT.
Gitlin, L. N., Miller, K. S., & Boyce, A. (1999)	1	3, 10, 17, 18, 19, 24	3	**Intervention:** OT was involved in providing bathroom modifications for female elders who are non-homeowners.

continued

Table 7-2 (continued)
OCCUPATIONAL THERAPY INTERVENTIONS PROMOTING ENVIRONMENTAL OUTCOMES

Author (Date)	Pop	DX	Setting	Intervention
Mann, W. C., Ottenbacher, K. J, Fraas, L., Tomita, M., & Granger, C. V. (1999)	1	24	3	**Intervention:** Treatment group received comprehensive functional assessment by OT, which included an evaluation of home environment. Treatment provided were environmental interventions and assistive technology designed to maintain function. **Control:** Usual care.
Buri, H. (1997)	1	24	4	**Intervention:** Assessment of ADL, provision of adaptive equipment and temporary orthoses, and discharge planning. The interventions group received a group education program and a booklet regarding falls prevention. **Control:** Received the booklet about falls prevention only.
Yang, J. J., Mann, W. C., Nochajski, S., & Tomita, M. R. (1997)	1	3, 8, 19, 25, 26	3	**Intervention:** Previous OT instruction and prescription of assistive devices.
Liddle, J., March, L., Carfrae, B., Finnegan, T., Druce, J., Schwarz, J., et al. (1996)	1	24	3	**Intervention:** OT assessed participants in their homes and recommended community services, home modifications, or equipment. Participants in the intervention group received the recommendations or equipment provided. **Control:** Control group did not have recommendations carried out.
Finlayson, M., & Havixbeck, K. (1992)	4	3, 17, 18, 22	4	**Intervention:** OT prescribed assistive devices and educated clients on how they are used.
McClain, L., & Todd, C. (1990)	N/A	21	3	**Intervention:** OT assessed 8 accessibility areas relevant to grocery shopping at 20 institutions and provided constructive feedback to the store managers regarding areas that were not accessible (2 to 4 weeks later).
Chamberlain, M. A., Thornley, G., Stow, J., & Wright, V. (1981)	4	3, 7, 18, 19	3	**Intervention:** Treatment group received bath aids immediately on discharge and were instructed in their use at home by an OT. **Control:** Control group received aids through "the usual channels."

Population: 1=geriatric (65+); 2=adult (25 to 64); 3=young adult (18 to 24); 4=adult and geriatric; 5=young adult, adult, and geriatric; N/A=not applicable.

Diagnosis: 3=stroke; 5=multiple sclerosis; 7=acquired brain injury; 8=dementia or Alzheimer's disease; 10=limb amputation; 16=upper extremity injury; 17=lower extremity injury; 18=other; 19=arthritis; 21=no diagnosis; 22=joint injury; 24=frail elderly, at-risk elderly or acute geriatric inpatient; 25=sensory impairment; 26=cardiac condition.

Setting: 1=long-term care; 2=acute care; 3=home care; 4=rehabilitation; 5=primary care.

Table 7-3

EVIDENCE OF EFFECTIVENESS OF OCCUPATIONAL THERAPY ON ENVIRONMENTAL OUTCOMES

Author (Date)	Major Results	Study Design	Sample Size	Conclusion and Limitations
Positive Effects—Randomized Controlled Trial				
Gitlin, L. N., Winter, L., Dennis, M. P., Corcoran, M., Schinfeld, S., & Hauck, W. W. (2006)	At 6 months, intervention participants had less difficulty with ADL (p=0.03, 95% CI -0.21 to 0.02) and IADL (p=0.04, 95% CI -0.26 to 0.03) than controls. Intervention participants had less fear of falling at 6 months (p=0.001) and 12 months (p=0.008, 95% CI 0.15 to 0.97). Intervention participants had increased overall functional efficacy at 6 months (p=0.02, 95% CI -0.06 to 0.23). Intervention participants had fewer home hazards at 6 months (p=0.05, 95% CI -3.17 to 0.41). Intervention participants used more control-oriented strategies at 6 months (p=0.009) and 12 months (p=0.01, 95% CI 0.03 to 0.24). Intervention group had 1% mortality rate as compared to a rate of 10% for control participants (p=0.003, 95% CI 2.4 to 15.04%).	RCT	319	***Conclusions:*** This multicomponent intervention focused on modifiable environmental and behavioral factors and was associated with quality of life improvements, which were retained, for the most part, over a year. ***Limitations:*** Intervention was not described in detail and was difficult to reproduce, study participation was voluntary.
Graff, M. J., Vernooij-Dassen, M. J., Thijssen, M., Dekker, J., Hoefnagels, W. H., & Rikkert, M. G. (2006)	At 12 weeks: Statistically significant (p<0.0001) improvement for members of treatment group on all 3 outcome measures.	RCT	105	***Conclusions:*** In-home OT is effective at both improving care-recipient ADL performance and care-provider confidence. ***Limitations:*** Method of data collection not described.
Campbell, A. J., Robertson M. C., La Grow, S. J., Kerse, N. M., Sanderson, G. F., Jacobs, R. J., et al. (2005)	41% fewer falls in the participants of the home safety program compared with those who did not receive the program (incidence rate ratio 0.59, 95% CI 0.42 to 0.83). No significant difference in the reduction of falls at home compared with those away from the home environment (ratio of incidence rate ratios 0.60, 0.31 to 1.17). 15% more falls during the trial for participants randomized to the exercise program compared with those who did not receive this program (incidence rate ratio 1.15, 0.82 to 1.61).	RCT	361	***Conclusions:*** The home safety program reduced falls and injury, whereas the exercise program did not. The reason may be due to low levels of adherence. ***Limitations:*** Possible selection bias, co-intervention, outcome measures validity and reliability not reported, sample size too small to elicit difference in exercise program group.

continued

Table 7-3 (continued)

EVIDENCE OF EFFECTIVENESS OF OCCUPATIONAL THERAPY ON ENVIRONMENTAL OUTCOMES

Author (Date)	Major Results	Study Design	Sample Size	Conclusions and Limitations
Positive Effects—Randomized Controlled Trial				
Gitlin, L. N., Hauck, W. W., Dennis, M. P., & Winter, L. (2005)	This paper reports results at 12 months. Caregiver affect improved (p<0.05).	RCT	130	**Conclusions:** More frequent professional contact and ongoing skills training may be necessary to maintain the initial positive outcomes of treatment. **Limitations:** Participants were self-selected, high attrition rate.
Chiu, C. W. Y., & Man, D. W. K. (2004)	Significant pre-test/post-test differences in intervention groups as compared to control for following outcomes: Total FIM scores (motor ability) QUEST scores—satisfaction with assistive device Higher rate of device use (96% vs. 56%) and bathing independence in intervention group than in controls.	RCT	53	**Conclusions:** The intervention group improved significantly in functioning and satisfaction. In addition, the use of bathing devices was higher in the intervention group. **Limitations:** Generalizability of results limited by short follow-up period, subjects were recruited from one site, intervention costly, so may not always be feasible.
Clemson, L., Cumming, R. G., Kendig, H., Swann, M., Heard, R., & Taylor, K. (2004)	The intervention group experienced a 31% reduction in falls (RR=0.69, 95% CI=0.50 to 0.96; p=0.025). Secondary analysis of subgroups showed that it was particularly effective for men (n=80; RR=0.32, 95% CI=0.17 to 0.59).	RCT	310	**Conclusions:** The clinically meaningful results demonstrated that the Stepping On program was effective for reducing falls in community-residing elderly people. **Limitations:** Contact time varied between groups, methods to prevent co-intervention were not discussed.
Dooley, N. R., & Hinojosa, J. (2004)	Caregivers in the treatment group had a high level of adherence to the recommendations, employing on average 65% of the 5 most important recommended strategies. A significant improvement in caregiver burden, positive affect, activity frequency, and self-care status (p<0.001) was observed in the treatment group compared to control.	RCT	40	**Conclusions:** The results of this study support the value of OT in progressive conditions like Alzheimer's disease and demonstrate its effectiveness in preventing unnecessary decline and improving quality of life in patients and caregivers.
Haines, T., Bennell, K., Osborne, R., & Hill, K. (2004)	Intervention group experienced 30% fewer falls that participants in control group, and this was statistically significant (p=0.045). Intervention group experienced a trend in a reduction of the proportion of participants who fell (RR=0.78, 95% CI 0.56 to 1.06). Intervention group experienced 28% fewer falls, which resulted in injury, but this was not statistically significant.	RCT	626	**Conclusions:** The number and/or severity of falls decreased among intervention participants. **Limitations:** Dropouts were not reported, nor the reason for them, sample was recruited from one site, outcome measures lacked psychometric properties, difficulty in blinding all staff and participants.

continued

Table 7-3 (continued)
EVIDENCE OF EFFECTIVENESS OF OCCUPATIONAL THERAPY ON ENVIRONMENTAL OUTCOMES

Author (Date)	Major Results	Study Design	Sample Size	Conclusions and Limitations
Positive Effects—Randomized Controlled Trial				
Weatherall, M. (2004)	Research indicated fewer falls in intervention group although the difference in hazard function was not apparent until 45 days post-admission (intervention group decreased and usual care group increased falls). A targeted falls prevention program plus usual care significantly reduced the rate of falls by 30% compared with usual care alone (p=0.004). Fall-related injuries were reduced by 28% (p=0.20).	RCT	98	***Conclusions:*** A combination of targeted falls prevention plus usual care during hospital stay can reduce falls in older adults. ***Limitations:*** No psychometric properties for outcome measures.
Gitlin, L. N., Winter, L., Corcoran, M., Dennis, M. P., Schinfeld, S., & Hauck, W. W. (2003)	Caregivers in the experimental group reported less upset with memory-related behaviors, less need for assistance from others, and better affect (p<0.05).	RCT	190	***Conclusions:*** The intervention reduces caregiving burden and stress and has added benefit for women and spouses. ***Limitations:*** Participants were self-selected, high attrition rate.
Gosman-Hedstrom, G., Claesson, L., & Blomstrand, C. (2002)	Subjects in stroke unit/general ward, 82/77% had at least one assistive device prescribed at 12 months (p>0.20). A total of 41% of stroke unit group and 40% of general ward group were independent or modified independent after 12 months. There was no significant difference between the groups regarding the impact of assistive devices. However, the prescription of assistive devices increased the ability to perform daily activities for both groups.	RCT	173	***Conclusions:*** Although there was no significant difference between groups with respect to the impact of assistive devices, the prescription of assistive devices increased the ability for participants in both groups to perform daily activities. ***Limitations:*** Most outcome measures lack psychometric properties and are not standardized.
Corcoran, M. A., & Gitlin, L. N. (2001)	Of the 9 problem areas that formed the focus of intervention, the most problematic for caregivers were caregiver-centered concerns, catastrophic reactions, wandering, and incontinence. Caregivers tried 1068 strategies, which were part of the intervention. 869 of 1068 (81%) of the strategies were used independently by caregivers (including modifying the task, social environment, and physical environment).	RCT	100	***Conclusions:*** Caregivers were receptive to and use environmental strategies offered by OT. ***Limitations:*** No standardized assessments and measures did not have psychometric properties, OTs providing treatment were not blinded, unable to find inter-rater consistency between the 10 OTs in terms of coding procedures.

continued

Table 7-3 (continued)

EVIDENCE OF EFFECTIVENESS OF OCCUPATIONAL THERAPY ON ENVIRONMENTAL OUTCOMES

Author (Date)	Major Results	Study Design	Sample Size	Conclusions and Limitations
Positive Effects—Randomized Controlled Trial				
Gitlin, L. N., Corcoran, M., Winter, L., Boyce, A., & Hauck, W. W. (2001)	Intervention caregivers reported fewer declines in patients' IADL (p=0.03) and fewer behavior problems. Intervention caregivers reported less upset (p=0.049).	RCT	171	**Conclusions:** The environmental program appears to have a modest effect on dementia patients' IADL dependence. Among certain sub-groups of caregivers, the program improves self-efficacy and reduces upset in specific areas of caregiving. **Limitations:** High attrition rate, used only modified versions of standardized assessments.
Close, J., Ellis, M., Hooper, R., Glucksman, E., Jackson, S., & Swift, C. (1999)	Risk of falling in 12-month follow-up was lower in the intervention group than in the control group after adjustment for differences in ADL scores at baseline and number of falls in the 12 months before the index fall (odds ratio 0.39 [95% CI 0.23 to 0.6]). Lower risk of recurrent falling in the intervention group than in the control group after adjustment for the same baseline variables (0.33 [CI 0.16 to 0.68]). Odds of at least 1 hospital admission were lower in the intervention group than in the control group (0.61 [CI 0.35 to 1.05]). Difference between the groups (p=0.017) and change in scores over time (p<0.0001) for ADL scores.	RCT	397	**Conclusions:** The intervention showed promising results in terms of a reduced number of falls. Proven falls and injury prevention strategies should be incorporated into clinical service. **Limitations:** Dropouts were reported after randomization, and the reason for dropout was not provided by the subject in 19 cases; possible population bias. Sample size too small (352 would have the appropriate power). Regarding the referral to other disciplines, the other professions were not listed.
Cumming, R. G., Thomas, M., Szonyi, G., Salkeld, G., O'Neill, E., Westbury, C., et al. (1999)	Intervention appeared to reduce the risk of falling by 19% (p=0.050). For people with a history of falls, the OT intervention reduced the proportion of people falling during follow-up by 36% (p=0.001). This also indicated that about 36% of intervention population had at least 1 fall during follow-up, compared with 45% of controls (p=0.050).	RCT	530	**Conclusions:** Among all study subjects, there was some suggestion that OT intervention might have reduced risk of falling. **Limitations:** Possible that intervention group underreported falls due to attention effect from home visits, usual care for controls not specified.

continued

Table 7-3 (continued)

EVIDENCE OF EFFECTIVENESS OF OCCUPATIONAL THERAPY ON ENVIRONMENTAL OUTCOMES

Author (Date)	Major Results	Study Design	Sample Size	Conclusions and Limitations
Positive Effects—Randomized Controlled Trial				
Mann, W. C., Ottenbacher, K. J., Fraas, L., Tomita, M., & Granger, C. V. (1999)	Statistically significant outcome: Greater decline in motor and total scores on FIM for control group (p<0.001). Pain increased significantly for control group (p<0.05). Costs for environmental interventions and assistive technology were significantly greater for treatment group. Costs for institutional care significantly greater for control group. Costs for in-home care similar between groups; nursing care, case manager visit costs greater for control group.	RCT	104	**Conclusions:** Although the health status of the frail elderly participants did decline during the intervention period, the provision of assistive technology and environmental interventions slowed the decline. In addition, certain costs to participants were reduced. **Limitations:** Reasons for dropouts were not reported.
Chamberlain, M. A., Thornley, G., Stow, J., & Wright, V. (1981)	100% of treatment group were bathing at follow-up, compared to 82% of controls. 90% of treatment group bathed from seated position, compared to 50% of controls. 74% of treatment group received their bath aids within 2 weeks of discharge, compared to 39% of controls.	RCT	100	**Conclusions:** Participants in the intervention group showed a greater improvement in bathing ability in general as well as bathing from a seated position than did the control group. **Limitations:** Statistical analyses of the significance of results were not performed.
Positive Effects—Non-Randomized Controlled Trial				
Gentry, T. (2008)	All participants demonstrated complete independence in operating PDA 1 week after final training. At 8-week follow-up, 19 participants showed independence in the majority of functions, 3 participants required verbal cues to use the calendar and alarm clock features, and 1 participant required demonstrations to perform basic PDA functions. Improvement in scores for COPM performance and satisfaction with performance improved considerably during the treatment period with a large effect size (M=4.008, SE=3.90, p<0.001, r=0.79). Performance dropped slightly during post-treatment period but remained significantly higher than the initial assessment. Similar significant improvements were observed in subjects' CHART-R scores; however, the RBMT-E showed no significant change.	Non-RCT	20	**Conclusions:** All subjects showed continued ability in use of the PDA for a period of 8 weeks after training, and home-based OT was sufficient in providing instruction in the use of the PDA as an assistive device. Use of the PDA significantly improved participants' functional ability in everyday tasks and their satisfaction with daily function. **Limitations:** This study was non-controlled and was composed of a very small and select sample of MS patients whose hearing, vision, and dexterity were intact. The results of the study may not be applicable to other portions of the MS patient population.

continued

Table 7-3 (continued)

EVIDENCE OF EFFECTIVENESS OF OCCUPATIONAL THERAPY ON ENVIRONMENTAL OUTCOMES

Author (Date)	Major Results	Study Design	Sample Size	Conclusions and Limitations
Positive Effects—Non-Randomized Controlled Trial				
Petersson, I., Lilja, M., Hammel, J., & Kottorp, A. (2008)	Statistically significant improvements (p<0.05) were found between baseline and follow-up in perceived difficulty in 6 tasks: Getting in and out of home, bathing/showering, grooming, transferring to toilet, walking a block, and moving in and out of bed. There were also statistically significant improvements (p<0.05) in perceived safety between baseline and follow-up in 10 tasks related to self-care, transfers, instrumental activities, and leisure. Overall, participants indicated they had less difficulty and felt safer in performing everyday activities after the home modification.	Non-RCT	105	**Conclusions:** Removing physical environmental barriers in the home can reduce perceived difficulties of tasks and increase feelings of safety. Subject's perceptions regarding completion of everyday tasks showed significant positive change after home modifications were completed. This shows that home modification services may play an important part in reducing problems related to ability in everyday life. However, home modifications did not have any significant impact on self-rated functional independence. **Limitations:** Results of this study may suffer from bias due to the fact that subjects were not randomized but rather the control group was made up of people on a waiting list for home modification. Also, the majority of participants in this study were already at a high level of functional independence at baseline so the outcome measures may not have been sensitive enough to detect changes in this area.
Niva, B., & Skar, L. (2006)	Subject ratings of accessibility inside the house increased substantially from baseline to 10-week follow-up (4.4 average points to 6.7). Accessibility outside the home also increased from an average of 3.9 points at baseline to 5.8 at 10 weeks of follow-up. The results of OQ also showed that participants rated their ability to perform ADL and participate in leisure activities higher at the 10-week follow-up than at baseline. Furthermore, participants reported participating in a wider variety of leisure activities and spending less time resting during the day.	Non-RCT	5	**Conclusions:** Home modifications increased both accessibility and usability in study subjects' homes. This improvement in accessibility led to an increased ability to perform daily tasks and leisure activities, an increased variety of leisure activities, and a better balance of time use throughout the day. Activities performed were also perceived to be of greater importance after housing modifications were completed and the effects of the home modifications lasted up to 10 weeks. **Limitations:** The study sample was very limited and subject to a large amount of bias.

continued

Table 7-3 (continued)

EVIDENCE OF EFFECTIVENESS OF OCCUPATIONAL THERAPY ON ENVIRONMENTAL OUTCOMES

Author (Date)	Major Results	Study Design	Sample Size	Conclusions and Limitations
Positive Effects—Non-Randomized Controlled Trial				
Fange, A., & Iwarsson, S. (2005)	Results were considered significant at p<0.05. Significant improvement in housing accessibility was found between baseline and 2- to 3-month follow-up. Significant decreases in the sum of environmental barriers was found between baseline and 2 to 3 months of follow-up, 2 to 3 months of follow-up and 8 to 9 months of follow-up, and baseline and 8 to 9 months of follow-up. Client's perception of usability improved only between baseline and 2 to 3 months of follow-up and no other time period.	Non-RCT	104	**Conclusions:** Improvements in accessibility and decreases in functional limitations and dependence on mobility devices accompanied housing modifications. Clients' perceptions of usability also improved. **Limitations:** The housing enabler is unable to detect small changes in accessibility. Little improvement was detected in clients' perception of accessibility after 2 to 3 months of follow-up due to a "ceiling effect" in measurement.
Stark, S. (2004)	60% of modifications (45/75 identified barriers) were completed for all subjects. Overall, self-perception of satisfaction (pre-test=2.25, post-test=7.69) and performance (pre-test=3.19, post-test=7.81) of occupational performance issues indicated an improvement.	Non-RCT	16	**Conclusions:** The removal of environmental barriers from the homes of older adults with functional limitations can significantly improve occupational performance. **Limitations:** Small sample size, limited follow-up (only pre- and post-), sample not random of population (difficult to generalize), almost half of intervention incomplete (40%), outcome measures were limited to self-perception and not on functional abilities.
McGruder, J., Cors, D., Tiernan, A. M., & Tomlin, G. (2003)	All subjects demonstrated improvements during treatment in 1 or more dependent variables. But use of weighted wrist cuff was effective in significantly decreasing either the tremor or some effect of the tremor for 3 of 5 participants.	Non-RCT	5	**Conclusions:** Weights used to reduce tremors are effective for biomechanical reasons and because of the increased proprioceptive input. **Limitations:** Limited statistical analysis in results, small sample size, improvements were limited due to the length of elapsed time between injury and research intervention.

continued

Table 7-3 (continued)

EVIDENCE OF EFFECTIVENESS OF OCCUPATIONAL THERAPY ON ENVIRONMENTAL OUTCOMES

Author (Date)	Major Results	Study Design	Sample Size	Conclusions and Limitations
Positive Effects—Non-Randomized Controlled Trial				
Tolley, L., & Atwal, A. (2003)	45% of subjects completed both pre- and post-intervention questionnaire. 17% of participants made changes to the way they performed laundry by following OT advice. Also, bathing aids were successful in enhancing functional ability (21%). Post-program, some subjects perceived that their ability to perform ADL had been enhanced by attending program. Post-program, there was a decrease in the number of people who experienced anxiety after a fall (pre-program=50% and post-program=40% with anxiety).	Non-RCT	78	**Conclusions:** The inclusion of OT in a falls prevention program can reduce the impact of falls and thus increase quality of life by enhancing ability and confidence in performing ADL. **Limitations:** High attrition rate (possible volunteer bias), descriptive statistics used, outcome measures not standardized and lack psychometric properties, no follow-up assessment completed.
Koppenhaver, D., Erickson, K., Harris, B., McLellan, J., Skotko, G., & Newton, R. (2001)	Group and individual data indicated that all 6 girls became more active and successful participants in the interactions during storybook reading. Hand splints enabled some of the girls to choose to label by pointing, but only when picture symbols were made available. The girls increased their range of communication modes and increased their frequency of labeling.	Non-RCT	6	**Conclusions:** The use of storybook reading may enhance early participation and communication. **Limitations:** Small sample size.
Gitlin, L. N., Miller, K. S., & Boyce, A. (1999)	Participants receiving OT assessment demonstrated a statistically significant improvement in bathing (p<0.01), ADL performance (p<0.01), and transferring (p<0.000).	Non-RCT	34	**Conclusions:** Findings are considered clinically significant and point to the importance of OT assessment in home modifications and the need for follow-up to ensure safe and continued use of equipment. **Limitations:** Dropouts not reported but evident, no comparison group, non-standardized assessment used, and no psychometric properties given.
Finlayson, M., & Havixbeck, K. (1992)	A total of 83 assistive devices were distributed. At follow-up, all but 1 subject felt satisfied with the instruction they received (97% satisfaction). Of the total percentage of equipment distributed, 75% was in use at follow-up. Subjects with home visit were 2 times more likely to use all their prescribed equipment than those who did not receive home visit.	Non-RCT	29	**Conclusions:** Although further research is needed, participants in this study were satisfied with the assistive device education they received and showed a high rate of equipment utilization. **Limitations:** Length of treatment varied among subjects, no psychometric properties for outcomes measures, small sample size.

continued

Table 7-3 (continued)

EVIDENCE OF EFFECTIVENESS OF OCCUPATIONAL THERAPY ON ENVIRONMENTAL OUTCOMES

Author (Date)	Major Results	Study Design	Sample Size	Conclusions and Limitations
Positive Effects—Non-Randomized Controlled Trial				
McClain, L., & Todd, C. (1990)	5 of 20 managers made changes to deficient areas: 3 of 5 improved parking, 1 of 5 improved parking and restrooms and provided lap baskets, and 1 of 5 improved the restrooms only. None of the institutions made improvements to ramps, curbs, entrances, aisles, or telephones.	Non-RCT	20	***Conclusions:*** OTs can be effective advocates for accessibility and therefore provide a vital link to productive living for people in wheelchairs. ***Limitations:*** Small sample size, outcome measures lacked psychometric properties, and minimal statistical analysis.
No Effect				
De Craen, A., Gussekloo, J., Blauw, G. J., Willems, C. G., & Westendorp, R. (2006)	Progressive increases in disability were observed in both intervention (mean annual increase, 2 points; SE=0.2, p<0.001) and control (mean annual increase, 2.1 points; SE=0.2, p<0.001). However, the difference between groups was not significant (0.08 points; 95% CI=-1.1 to 1.2, p=0.75), and no significant differences were seen in secondary outcome measures.	RCT	297	***Conclusions:*** Unsolicited OT provided to community-living elders did not prevent or reduce a decline in functional ability. ***Limitations:*** Data were analyzed on an intention-to-treat basis; however, 55 subjects in the control group declined to complete the intervention. The presence of their results may have diluted any beneficial effect of the treatment.
Hendriks, M. R. C., van Haastregt, J. C. M., Diederiks, J. P. M., Evers, S. M. A. A., Crebolder, H. F. J. M., & van Eijk, J. T. M. (2005)	This study was a description of a previously done study design, no economic evaluation figures or effectiveness were reported.	RCT	333	***Conclusions:*** Study not complete at time of publication, and, therefore, results not available. ***Limitations:*** Researchers placed no restrictions on co-interventions, outcome measures lacked psychometric properties, intervention was described vaguely and thus would be difficult to reproduce.
VanLeit, B., & Crowe, T. (2002)	No significant differences were found between the groups on time use perceptions, but both groups improved significantly for satisfaction of time use. No significant differences were found between the 2 groups on the performance subscale; however, the treatment group demonstrated significantly greater score increases (p<0.05) on their perception of satisfaction.	RCT	38	***Conclusions:*** Attending to the time and occupational concerns of mothers of children with disabilities can have a positive impact on their satisfaction with occupational performance. ***Limitations:*** Small sample size, possible volunteer bias for sample selection, some outcome measures lacked psychometric properties.

continued

Table 7-3 (continued)

EVIDENCE OF EFFECTIVENESS OF OCCUPATIONAL THERAPY ON ENVIRONMENTAL OUTCOMES

Author (Date)	Major Results	Study Design	Sample Size	Conclusions and Limitations
No Effect				
Buri, H. (1997)	Knowledge scores between the 2 groups before intervention did not display significant differences (X2=0.43, df=1, ns). Immediately post-intervention, there was no significant difference (X2=2.01, df=1, ns). After 24 hours, there was a significant difference (X2=9.75, p<0.01). For change of attitude, there was very little change between groups before and 1-month post-intervention.	Non-RCT	37	**Conclusions:** Participants receiving the booklet and education program were most likely to show a very high knowledge score in terms of falls prevention strategies but very little changed between groups in regard to their attitudes/behavior toward risk taking 1 month after discharge. **Limitations:** Outcome measures designed for study, small sample, difficult to generalize, convenience sample, and non-random allocation to groups.
Yang, J. J., Mann, W. C., Nochanjski, S., & Tomita, M. R. (1997)	Functional status was decreased from a score of 70.6 to 45.6, and IADL performance mean moved lower from 5 to 3.4. Cognitive status decreased from 17 to 10. In regard to use of assistive devices, after 1 to 2 years of follow-up, the number of owned devices went down from 10 (8.8) to 8.6 (2.8), and the mean number of devices used went from 8.5 (7.7) to 6.3 (2.8). 75% of caregivers felt OT intervention was helpful.	Non-RCT	7	**Conclusions:** Although participants had degenerative changes in health and abilities, OT interventions appeared to be helpful for this small study sample. **Limitations:** Descriptive statistics, small sample size, significance testing impractical, follow-up time inconsistent for all subjects.
Liddle, J., March, L., Carfrae, B., Finnegan, T., Druce, J., Schwarz, J., et al. (1996)	No significant difference (p<0.01) between intervention and control groups at baseline or after 6 months. Both groups demonstrated some significant changes from baseline within groups.	RCT	105	**Conclusions:** It does not appear that, in the short term, acting on OT recommendations improves outcomes in this population. **Limitations:** Possible volunteer bias for sample selection.

CHART-R=Craig Handicap Assessment and Rating Technique–Revised, COPM=Canadian Occupational Performance Measure, FIM=Functional Independence Measure, OQ=Occupational Questionnaire, QUEST=Quebec User Evaluation of Satisfaction, RBMT-E=Rivermead Behavioural Memory Test–Extended.

Table 7-4

OUTCOME MEASURES USED TO CAPTURE ENVIRONMENTAL OUTCOMES

Author (Date)	Outcome(s) Investigated	Outcome Measure(s)	Method of Administration
Gentry, T. (2008)	Ability to use and frequency of use of PDA Functional performance and satisfaction with performance in everyday activities Change in behavioral/working memory	PDA usage checklist COPM CHART-R RBMT-E	PDA usage checklist was administered during the final training session and at 8-week post-training follow-up. COPM and CHART-R were administered at baseline 8 weeks prior to training, the first training session, the last training session, and at 8-week post-training follow-up. RBMT-E was administered at baseline 8 weeks prior to training and at post-training 8-week follow-up.
Petersson, I., Lilja, M., Hammel, J., & Kottorp, A. (2008)	Self-rated ability in everyday life	C-CAP Part I	Assessment was conducted as a structured interview with OT and client participating. Interviews were conducted at baseline and at 2-month follow-up.
De Craen, A., Gussekloo, J., Blauw, G. J., Willems, C. G., & Westendorp, R. (2006)	Primary: Changes in restrictions in ability to perform ADL Secondary: Subjects' self-perceived well-being and loneliness	GARS Cantril's Ladder de Jong-Gierveld Questionnaire	All assessments were provided by a research nurse at baseline, 6, 12, 18, and 24 months of follow-up. Administered by therapists blind to study's purpose.
Gitlin, L. N., Winter, L., Dennis, M. P., Corcoran, M., Schinfeld, S., & Hauck, W. W. (2006)	Mobility/transfer function ADL function IADL function Fear of falling Self-efficacy in tasks Adaptive strategy use Observed home hazards Mortality	Mobility/transfer index ADL index IADL index Falls efficacy scale Three items from Activities-Specific Balance Confidence Scale Functional self-efficacy index Mortality Rate	Self-report post-program (6 months) and follow-up (at 12 months). Home visit by independent research OT 3 to 6 months after discharge.
Graff, M. J., Vernooij-Dassen, M. J., Thijssen, M., Dekker, J., Hoefnagels, W. H., & Rikkert, M. G. (2006)	Care-recipient ADL performance Caregiver sense of competence/burden	Care recipients: AMPS IDDD Caregivers: SCQ Not reported	
Niva, B., & Skar, L. (2006)	Patients' perceived accessibility of home environment Effect of housing adaptations of activity patterns	Accessibility in My Home questionnaire Occupational Questionnaire	Assessments were mailed to participants and were completed by them at baseline (pre-modification) and at 5-day and 10-week follow-up.

continued

Table 7-4 (continued)

OUTCOME MEASURES USED TO CAPTURE ENVIRONMENTAL OUTCOMES

Author (Date)	Outcome(s) Investigated	Outcome Measure(s)	Method of Administration
Campbell, A. J., Robertson, M. C., La Grow, S. J., Kerse, N. M., Sanderson, G. F., Jacobs, R. J., et al. (2005)	Number of falls Injuries resulting from falls Cost of implementing the home safety program	Monthly postcard calendars recording falls Reviewing trial records Interview of participants Financial records of the research group and other equipment funders	Self-report during program. Researcher reported post-program.
Fange, A., & Iwarsson, S. (2005)	Change in accessibility and environmental barriers Client's perception of usability of physical environment Sum of physical barriers Changes in functional ability (ADL)/dependence on mobility devices	UIHM ADLS-R	Housing enabler delivered by OTs at baseline, 2 to 3 months after modification, and 8 to 9 months after modification. Self-administered UIHM completed at baseline, 2 to 3 months after modification, and 8 to 9 months after modification. ADLS-R provided by interviewer as combination of interview and observation.
Gitlin, L. N., Hauck, W. W., Dennis, M. P., & Winter, L. (2005)	Caregiver well-being Care recipient functioning (also looked at whether effects varied by caregiver gender, race, and relationship)	Self-report measures of caregiver objective and subjective burden, caregiver well-being Revised MBPC A modification of the FIM	Trained interviewers met with caregivers in their homes, obtained signed informed consent, and conducted the baseline interview and follow-up interview at 6, 12, and 18 months post-baseline.
Hendriks, M. R. C., van Haastregt, J. C. M., Diederiks, J. P. M., Evers, S. M. A. A., Crebolder, H. F. J. M., & van Eijk J. T. M. (2005)	Percentage of elderly people sustaining a fall during the 1-year follow-up Recurrent falls during follow-up Injurious falls during follow-up Daily functioning Perceived health ADL and IADL disability Mental health Quality of life	Falls calendar measures number of falls and if medical care was necessary after a fall FAI First 2 items of the SF-36 GARS HADS EuroQol Instrument	Self-administered questionnaires at baseline, 4, and 12 months.
Chiu, C. W. Y., & Man, D. W. K. (2004)	Self-care: Locomotion, sphincter control, transfers, communication, and social cognition Satisfaction with assistive technology devices Use of assistive devices Bathing independence	FIM QUEST Authors' own questionnaire on assistive device use and bathing independence	Administered by therapists blind to study's purpose.

continued

Table 7-4 (continued)
Outcome Measures Used to Capture Environmental Outcomes

Author (Date)	Outcome(s) Investigated	Outcome Measure(s)	Method of Administration
Clemson, L., Cumming, R. G., Kendig, H., Swann, M., Heard, R., & Taylor, K. (2004)	Fall history Functional mobility and balance Confidence in avoiding falls Perception of physical and mental health	Demographic and fall history questionnaire Get Up and Go Test Rhomberg test of balance SF-36 MES MFES	Self-administered questionnaires given at baseline and 14 months post-randomization assessment.
Dooley, N. R., & Hinojosa, J. (2004)	Ability to perform common ADL Caregiver burden Quality of life Self-care ability	AIF ZBI AAL-AD PSMS	Assessments were completed at baseline and 1-month follow-up.
Haines, T., Bennell, K., Osborne, R., & Hill, K. (2004)	Falls prevention	PJC-FRAT Standardized incident reports measured the severity of falls and fall-related injuries, for participants who fell	Reported by nurses, OTs, PTs, and medical staff at both baseline and post-program. Reported by hospital medical staff upon examination of fallen patient.
Stark, S. (2004)	Occupational performance (self-perception of performance and satisfaction)	FIM COPM Enviro-FIM Follow-up assessment used: COPM	Interview evaluation at baseline (home assessment) and again 3 to 6 months post-assessment (after medications were completed).
Weatherall, M. (2004)	Falls and injuries during hospital admission	Data were collected from hospital records	N/A.
Gitlin, L. N., Winter, L., Corcoran, M., Dennis, M. P., Schinfeld, S., & Hauck, W. W. (2003)	Caregiver well-being Care recipient functioning (also looked at whether effects varied by caregiver gender, race, and relationship)	Self-report measures of caregiver objective and subjective burden, caregiver well-being Revised MBPC A modification of the FIM	Trained interviewers met with caregivers in their homes, obtained signed informed consent, and conducted the baseline interview and follow-up interview at 6, 12, and 18 months post-baseline.
McGruder, J., Cors, D., Tiernan, A. M., & Tomlin, G. (2003)	Accuracy of feeding Feeding efficiency Amount of food consumed Food spills and compensation Self-perception of the use of the wrist-cuff Investigator tremor ratings	Stopwatch used to measure time Number of times participants spilled or dropped food was recorded Self-rating scale (0 to 10) for tremors	Videotaping throughout 8 meal sessions. Videotapes reviewed by co-investigators to rate tremors.
Tolley, L., & Atwal, A. (2003)	Implementation of falls prevention advice by OT Evaluating ability to participate in performing ADL Anxiety attributed to falls	Program-based questionnaire	Self-administered questionnaire completed pre-intervention (week 1 of intervention) and post-intervention (week 14 of intervention).

continued

Table 7-4 (continued)

Outcome Measures Used to Capture Environmental Outcomes

Author (Date)	Outcome(s) Investigated	Outcome Measure(s)	Method of Administration
Gosman-Hedstrom, G., Claesson, L., & Blomstrand, C. (2002)	Ability to perform daily activities Living and social conditions Utilization of health and social care including assistive devices (and use of the devices)	FIM Structured questionnaire	Blinded OTs evaluated subjects in their home environment 4 times within 1 year.
VanLeit, B., & Crowe, T. (2002)	Satisfaction with time use Perceptions of occupational performance Occupational satisfaction	TPI TUA COPM	Assessments delivered pre-test and post-test (2 weeks post-intervention).
Corcoran, M. A., & Gitlin, L. N. (2001)	Care recipient daily functioning and behaviors (problem areas, strategies recommended by OT, and strategies used)	OT structured interview with caregivers	OT interview.
Gitlin, L. N., Corcoran, M., Winter, L., Boyce, A., & Hauck, W. W. (2001)	Self-efficacy and upset in caregivers Daily function of dementia patients	MBPC Modification of the FIM 5-point Likert scale (self-efficacy of caregivers)	Participants were interviewed in their homes by a trained interviewer at baseline and 3 months post-intervention.
Koppenhaver, D., Erickson, K., Harris, B., McLellan, J., Skotko, G., & Newton, R. (2001)	Interactions between mother and daughter during storybook reading: Communication mode (vocalizations; pointing with eyes, fingers, or objects; facial expressions; actions on books; and activation of voice-output message device) Communication act (labeling pictures by any mode)	Interactions between mothers and daughters reading familiar or unfamiliar books were videotaped, coded, and analyzed	Videotapes were made, coded, and analyzed throughout treatment sessions.
Close, J., Ellis, M., Hooper, R., Glucksman, E., Jackson, S., & Swift, C. (1999)	Falls prevention Function Psychological consequences of fall	Postal questionnaire every 4 months for 1 year to measure the number of falls BI FHI	Self-reported on follow-up; by the therapist at baseline and follow-up every 4 months for 1 year (BI and FHI).
Cumming, R. G., Thomas, M., Szonyi, G., Salkeld, G., O'Neill, E., Westbury, C., et al. (1999)	Fall history and frequency over a 12-month period Demographics ADL	Interview-administered questionnaire Falls calendar SKI Smith's Modification of the RBHS	Baseline interview from blinded research assistant (pre-randomization). Follow-up calendars mailed to researchers monthly.
Gitlin, L. N., Miller, K. S., & Boyce, A. (1999)	Improvements in self-care Difficulties using equipment Continued use of equipment	An ADL and IADL rating scale developed by the researchers, based on the Katz ADL Scale	Participants were assessed by the OT. After recommendations for equipment were made and the equipment installed, the participants were re-assessed by same OT.

continued

Table 7-4 (continued)

OUTCOME MEASURES USED TO CAPTURE ENVIRONMENTAL OUTCOMES

Author (Date)	Outcome(s) Investigated	Outcome Measure(s)	Method of Administration
Mann, W. C., Ottenbacher, K. J, Fraas, L., Tomita, M., & Granger, C. V. (1999)	ADL/IADL function Participation Pain Health care costs	FIM CHART-R Functional Status Instrument Health care costs	18-month intervention period. Visits were made to home at baseline and every 6 months to administer the measures. Phone calls were made to participant once per month to discuss any issues they were having.
Buri, H. (1997)	Knowledge of falls prevention strategies Attitudes and behavior toward risk taking	2 questionnaires were designed for the study measures: Current knowledge Changes in attitudes and behavior	Questionnaires were administered pre-intervention. Current knowledge was tested immediately post-intervention and 24 hours later. Attitudes and behaviors were tested 1 month after discharge.
Yang, J. J., Mann, W. C., Nochanjski, S. & Tomita, M. R. (1997)	Physical health status Functional physical and cognitive status Perceptions of family care Current use of assistive devices	OARS FIM MMSE ZCBS UAD	Interviews were conducted in residences of participants 1 to 2 years post intervention.
Liddle, J., March, L., Carfrae, B., Finnegan, T., Druce, J., Schwarz, J., et al. (1996)	Quality of life Ability to perform daily activities	SIP PGCMS LSI Linear rating scale for "happiness in the last month" and "quality of life in the last 6 months"	Assessed at baseline and at 6 months follow-up.
Finlayson, M., & Havixbeck, K. (1992)	Specific aids prescribed Description of device use/disuse Satisfaction with the assistive device(s) Subject's participation	SIS Home Visit Questionnaire Telephone interview questionnaire (All developed by therapists at hospital)	Baseline information collected from SIS and follow-up interviews were conducted using the remaining measures.
McClain, L., & Todd, C. (1990)	Accessibility areas for grocery shopping store such as parking, ramps, curbs, entrances, aisles, telephones, baskets, and rest rooms	On-site survey designed based on specifications provided in relevant sections of the architectural and transportation barriers compliance board (1982) guidelines and requirements	On-site assessment and assessment of site 6 months post-recommendations provided.

continued

Table 7-4 (continued)

OUTCOME MEASURES USED TO CAPTURE ENVIRONMENTAL OUTCOMES

Author (Date)	Outcome(s) Investigated	Outcome Measure(s)	Method of Administration
Chamberlain, M. A., Thornley, G., Stow, J., & Wright, V. (1981)	Number of patients bathing Ability to bathe Use of bath aids Number of patients supplied with all their prescribed bath aids within 2 weeks of discharge	Client interviews developed by researchers	Home visit by independent research OT 3 to 6 months after discharge.

AAL-AD=Affect and Activity Limitation–Alzheimer's Disease Assessment, ADLS-R=ADL Staircase Revised, AIF=Assessment of Instrument Function, AMPS=Assessment of Motor and Process Skills, BI=Barthel Index, C-CAP=Client-Clinician Assessment Protocol, CHART-R=Craig Handicap Assessment and Rating Technique–Revised, COPM=Canadian Occupational Performance Measure, Enviro-FIM=Environmental Functional Independence Measure, EuroQol=European Quality of Life Instrument, FAI=Frenchay Activity Index, FHI=Falls Handicap Inventory, FIM=Functional Independence Measure, GARS=Groningen Activity Restriction Scale, HADS=Hospital Anxiety and Depression Scale, IDDD=Interpretation of Deterioration in Doing Activities in Dementia, LSI=Life Satisfaction Index, MBPC=Memory and Behavior Problems Checklist, MES=Mobility Efficacy Scale, MFES=Modified Falls-Efficacy Scale, MMSE=Mini Mental Status Examination, OARS=Older American Research and Service Centre Instrument, PGCMS=Philadelphia Geriatric Center Morale Scale, PJC-FRAT=Peter James Centre Falls Risk Assessment Tool, PSMS=Physical Self-Maintenance Scale, QUEST=Quebec User Evaluation of Satisfaction, RBHS=Rosow-Breslau Health Scale, RBMT-E=Rivermead Behavioural Memory Test–Extended, SCQ=Sense of Competence Questionnaire, SF-36=Short Form Health Survey, SIP=Sickness Impact Profile, SIS=Survey Information Sheet, SKI=Spectator-Katz Index, TPI=Time Perception Inventory, TUA=Time Use Analyzer, UAD=Use of Assistive Devices, UIHM=Usability in My Home, ZBI=Zarit Burden Interview, ZCBS=Zarit Caregiver Burden Scale.

and injuries for older adults having various medical diagnoses who are at risk for falls. The diagnostic groups in these studies include older adults at risk for falls and people with low vision, stroke, lower extremity injuries/fractures, arthritis, amputation, dementia, and other diagnoses that put a person at risk for lower ADL function and increased falls.

Two studies evaluated the outcomes of occupational therapy interventions that focused on educating and training clients on the use of assistive/technological aids (DeCraen, Gussekloo, Blauw, Willems, & Westendorp, 2006; Gentry, 2008). In a randomized controlled trial by DeCraen and colleagues (2006), two groups of geriatric clients who were characterized as "frail elderly" were compared, with one group receiving additional occupational therapy in the community to educate and train clients on the use of assistive devices. Although the results indicated no significant differences in the changes in restrictions of ADL, the high attrition rate within the control group may have influenced the results.

A second study evaluated the use of a technology device (personal digital assistant) as a cognitive aid after training by a home care occupational therapist for a population of adults with multiple sclerosis (Gentry, 2008). In this before-and-after study design, the results indicated significant improvements in the clients' functional abilities within their everyday tasks.

Several studies examined the effects of providing education to prevent falls as well as home modifications (Campbell et al., 2005; Close, Ellis, Hooper, Glucksman, Jackson, & Swift, 1999; Gitlin et al., 2006; Haines et al., 2004; Tolley & Atwal, 2003; Weatherall, 2004). Results indicated that the combined program of falls education and home modifications leads to physical environmental changes and associated decrease in falls. The provision of home modifications and education for caregivers of people with dementia led to increased use of environmental solutions, changes to the physical and social environment, and improved self-efficacy for caregivers (Corcoran & Gitlin, 2001).

The research also provides information about the level of intervention dose/number of visits required to lead to positive outcomes. Studies that used only one to two therapy visits (Gosman-Hedstrom, Claesson, & Blomstrand, 2002; Liddle et al., 1996) did not demonstrate significant effects after intervention. Studies that focused on specific modifications to a few areas of the home such as a bathroom (Gitlin et al., 1999) demonstrated significant differences after two to three visits. A couple of studies (Close et al., 1999; Stark, 2004) demonstrated significant improvements after two to three visits. Effective programs that were more extensive in providing modifications for the entire home and education to client and/or caregiver typically provided four to eight visits (Clemson, Cumming, Kendig, Swann, Heard, & Taylor, 2004; Corcoran & Gitlin, 2001; Gitlin & Chee, 2006; Gitlin et al., 2001, 2003, 2005; Haines et al., 2004; Koppenhaver, Erickson, Harris, McLellan, Skotko, & Newton, 2001; Mann et al., 1999; Weatherall, 2004).

Three studies exclusively examined the impact of home modifications by home care occupational therapy on physical barriers and usability of the home environment (Petersson, Lilja, Hammel, & Kottorp, 2008; Fange & Iwarsson, 2005; Niva & Skar, 2006). In two studies using before-and-after designs, geriatric clients demonstrated an increase in accessibility within the home and functional abilities (or usability) and a decrease in environmental barriers (Fange & Iwarsson, 2005; Niva & Skar, 2006). The study by Petersson and colleagues (2008) used a non-randomized two-group design (control group selected from a waitlist) to evaluate the impact of home modification on self-rated ability in everyday life. The results reported significant positive changes in completing everyday tasks after home modifications were completed.

Only two studies have investigated the effects of changing physical environmental outcomes on costs (Campbell et al., 2005; Mann et al., 1999). Campbell et al. (2005) demonstrated that a home safety program for older adults with low vision was more cost effective than an exercise program. Mann and colleagues (1999), in a randomized controlled trial comparing provision of environmental interventions and assistive technology for older adults living at home, found that these interventions led to physical environmental changes and associated reduced institutional and nurse/case manager costs.

Social Environment

Empirical Studies

In the previous section on changing the physical environment, several studies demonstrated the effectiveness of caregiver education and training (Corcoran & Gitlin, 2001; Gitlin & Chee, 2006; Gitlin et al., 1999, 2001, 2003, 2005, 2006). These interventions focused on training caregivers to improve their skills in using the physical and social environment to maintain client functioning and to address troublesome behavior for family members with dementia. The results indicate that these interventions decrease caregiver stress and increase their feelings of self-efficacy within the caregiving situation as well as lead to better maintenance of clients' ADL and IADL (instrumental activities of daily living) functioning.

Two studies have examined the effects of occupational therapy intervention to provide training and support to caregivers of children and youth with disabilities (Koppenhaver et al., 2001; VanLeit & Crowe, 2002). VanLeit and Crowe (2002) evaluated an 8-week support group intervention for mothers of children with disabilities as compared to a no-treatment control group. Results indicated no significant differences for time use, and the treatment group improved significantly on a measure of satisfaction with their occupational performance. Koppenhaver and colleagues (2001) conducted a small before-and-after study that found that training and provision of equipment to parents and their child through a story-telling intervention led to improved participation and interactions for these children. Dooley and Hinojosa (2004) used a pre-test/post-test control group design to examine the extent to which adherence to occupational therapy recommendations would increase the quality of life of community-dwelling people with Alzheimer's disease and their caregivers. Individualized occupational therapy interventions based on the Person-Environment Fit Model were effective in improving outcomes for both caregivers and patients. Further research for these types of interventions is warranted.

Measures Used to Capture Environmental Outcomes

When examining outcomes that are sensitive to occupational therapy intervention to change environmental factors, it is useful to distinguish between intermediate and long-term outcomes. When environmental changes are introduced, an intermediate outcome would center on an assessment of actual changes within the environment. This assessment determines if the intervention was successful in changing the targeted environmental factor. For example, if home modifications are completed to improve the safety of the home environment, a home safety assessment can be completed. Similarly, assessment of a client's or caregiver's knowledge will indicate the intermediate outcome after training is provided. Long-term outcomes center on the impact of the intervention on client and caregiver functioning.

Based on the scoping reviews completed for this chapter, there is evidence to support the impact of occupational therapy environmental intervention on the following intermediate outcomes:

▲ Safety knowledge
▲ Use of adaptive equipment
▲ Safety hazards present in the home
▲ Client satisfaction with environmental modification and equipment/devices

Table 7-5

OUTCOME MEASURES TO ASSESS ENVIRONMENTAL INTERVENTIONS

Measure	Population	Content Domains	Reliability and Validity
Craig Hospital Inventory of Environmental Factors (CHIEF)	Adults	A 25-item measure (or 12-item short form) based on WHO's ICIDH-2 that examines frequency of the following 5 types of environmental barriers that impact daily activities: accessibility, accommodation, resource availability, social support, equality.	Studies demonstrate test-retest and inter-rater reliability, and content and construct validity.
Environmental Functional Independence Measure (Enviro-FIM)	Adults	Measures behavior-in-environment situations using activities from the FIM.	Studies demonstrate test-retest and inter-rater reliability, and content and construct validity.
Home Falls and Accidents Screening Tool (HOME FAST)	Older adults	25-item screening instrument in which therapist assesses hazards inside and outside the client's residence that may contribute to falls.	Studies demonstrate internal consistency and observer reliability, and content validity.
Safety Assessment of Function and the Environment for Rehabilitation (SAFER Tool)	Older adults	An OT screening tool for assessing the ability of elderly people to function safely in the home. Items address the following areas: Living situation, mobility, kitchen, fire hazards, eating, wandering, memory aids, household, dressing, grooming, bathroom, medication, communication, general.	Studies demonstrate content validity, test-retest and inter-rater reliability.

Caregiver outcomes:

▲ Skills in adapting home environment to support client functioning
▲ Self-efficacy
▲ Stress/upset
▲ Perceived burden of caregiving
▲ Need for extra assistance in the home
▲ Mood/affect

Outcome measures used in occupational therapy to assess intermediate outcomes of environmental intervention, such as preventing falls/injury, increasing access, and improving safety include the following (Table 7-5):

▲ Craig Hospital Inventory of Environmental Factors (CHIEF)
▲ Environmental Functional Independence Measure (Enviro-FIM)
▲ Home Falls and Accidents Screening Tool (HOME FAST)
▲ Safety Assessment of Function and the Environment for Rehabilitation (SAFER Tool)

Outcomes can assess the goal to increase support for daily functioning. When the intervention is aimed at improving caregiver skills and caregiving, outcome measures include the following (Table 7-6):

▲ Canadian Occupational Performance Measure (COPM)
▲ Life Satisfaction Index (LSI)
▲ Sickness Impact Profile (SIP)
▲ Time Perception Inventory (TPI)
▲ Time Use Analyzer (TUA)
▲ Zarit Caregiver Burden Scale (ZCBS)

Conclusions and Recommendations for Future Research

Occupational therapy intervention to change environmental outcomes has focused more on products and technology, natural environment and human-made changes, and support and relationships. To date, there are few studies examining interventions focused on changing societal attitudes or services, systems, and policies. Interventions to clients across several diagnostic categories that combine home mod-

Table 7-6

OUTCOME MEASURES TO ASSESS ENVIRONMENTAL INTERVENTIONS FOR CAREGIVERS

Measure	Population	Content Domains	Reliability and Validity
Canadian Occupational Performance Measure (COPM)	All populations	Individualized assessment; client identifies occupational performance issues during interview with therapist; 5 most important issues are rated by client for performance and satisfaction.	Studies demonstrate test-retest reliability, construct validity, and responsiveness.
Life Satisfaction Index (LSI)	Older adults	20-item questionnaire that measures 5 aspects of well-being: Zest, resolution and fortitude, congruence between desired and achieved goal, positive self-concept, mood tone.	Studies demonstrate inter-rater and internal consistency reliability, and content and construct validity.
Sickness Impact Profile (SIP)	All populations	A health status questionnaire that measures the impact of illness on everyday behavior and activity.	Studies demonstrate test-retest reliability and content, construct, and criterion validity.
Time Perception Inventory (TPI)	Adults	A 56-item questionnaire that examines people's attitudes about time across 5 factors: Past-negative, present hedonistic, future, past-positive, present fatalistic.	Studies demonstrate acceptable internal and test-retest reliability and convergent, divergent, discriminant, and predictive validity.
Time Use Analyzer (TUA)	Adults	Assesses how people feel about how they use their time (satisfaction/dissatisfaction): At work, asleep, on personal hygiene, taking care of personal/family business, in community and church activities, with family or home members, in education and development, and on recreational hobbies.	Little/no evidence regarding this measure's reliability or validity.
Zarit Caregiver Burden Scale (ZCBS)	Adults	A 22-item questionnaire dealing with caregiving issues across a 5-point scale from "never" to "nearly always." Total scores indicate either little or no burden, mild to moderate burden, moderate to severe burden, or severe burden.	Studies demonstrate high test-retest reliability, internal consistency reliability, and good overall validity.

ifications with caregiver support and education have demonstrated significant changes in the home safety, reduced hazards, and improved caregiver outcomes.

References

Buri, H. (1997). A group programme to prevent falls in elderly hospital patients. *British Journal of Therapy and Rehabilitation, 4,* 550-556.

Campbell, A. J., Robertson, M. C., La Grow, S. J., Kerse, N. M., Sanderson, G. F., Jacobs, R. J., et al. (2005). Randomised controlled trial of prevention of falls in people aged 75 with severe visual impairment: The VIP trial. *British Medical Journal, 331,* 817-823.

Chamberlain, M. A., Thornley, G., Stow, J., & Wright, V. (1981). Evaluation of aids and equipment for the bath: II. A possible solution to the problem. *Rheumatology and Rehabilitation, 20,* 38-43.

Chang, J. T., Morton, S. C., Rubenstein, L. Z., Mojica, W. A., Maglione, M., Suttorp, M. J., et al. (2004). Interventions for the prevention of falls in older adults: Systematic review and meta-analysis of randomised clinical trials. *British Medical Journal, 328*(7441), 680-683.

Chiu, C. W. Y., & Man, D. W. K. (2004). The effect of training older adults with stroke to use home-based assistive devices. *OTJR: Occupation, Participation, and Health, 24,* 113-120.

Clemson, L., Cumming, R. G., Kendig, H., Swann, M., Heard, R., & Taylor, K. (2004). The effectiveness of a community-based program for reducing the incidence of falls in the elderly: A randomized trial. *Journal of the American Geriatrics Society, 52*(9), 1487-1494.

Close, J., Ellis, M., Hooper, R., Glucksman, E., Jackson, S., & Swift, C. (1999). Prevention of falls in the elderly trial (PROFET): A randomised controlled trial. *Lancet, 353,* 93-97.

Corcoran, M. A., & Gitlin, L. N. (2001). Family caregiver acceptance and use of environmental strategies provided in an occupational therapy intervention. *Physical and Occupational Therapy in Geriatrics, 19,* 1-20.

Cumming, R. G., Thomas, M., Szonyi, G., Salkeld, G., O'Neill, E., & Westbury, C., et al. (1999). Home visits by an occupational therapist for assessment and modification of environmental hazards: A randomized trial of falls prevention. *Journal of the American Geriatrics Society, 47*(12), 1397-1402.

DeCraen, A., Gussekloo, J., Blauw, G. J., Willems, C. G., & Westendorp, R. (2006). Randomised controlled trial of unsolicited occupational therapy in community-dwelling elderly people: The LOTIS trial. *PLoS Clinical Trials, 1*(1), e2.

Dooley, N. R., & Hinojosa, J. (2004). Improving quality of life for persons with Alzheimer's disease and their family caregivers: Brief occupational therapy intervention. *American Journal of Occupational Therapy, 58*(5), 561-569.

Erikson, A., Karlsson, G., Soderstrom, M., & Tham, K. (2004). A training apartment with electronic aids to daily living: Lived experiences of persons with brain damage. *American Journal of Occupational Therapy, 58*(3), 261-271.

Fange, A., & Iwarsson, S. (2005). Changes in accessibility and usability in housing: An exploration of the housing adaptation process. *Occupational Therapy International, 12*(1), 44-59.

Finlayson, M., & Havixbeck, K. (1992). A post-discharge study on the use of assistive devices. *Canadian Journal of Occupational Therapy, 59,* 201-207.

Friedland, J., & McColl, M. A. (1989). Social support for stroke survivors: Development and evaluation of an intervention program. *Physical and Occupational Therapy in Geriatrics, 7,* 55-69.

Gentry, T. (2008). PDAs as cognitive aids for people with multiple sclerosis. *American Journal of Occupational Therapy, 62*(1), 18-27.

Gillespie, L. D., Gillespie, W. J., Robertson, M. C., Lamb, S. E., Cumming, R. G., & Rowe, B. H. (2003). Interventions for preventing falls in elderly people. *Cochrane Database of Systematic Reviews*, Issue 3. Art. No.: CD000340. DOI: 10.1002/14651858.CD000340.

Gitlin, L. N., & Chee, Y. K. (2006). Use of adaptive equipment in caring for persons with dementia at home. *Alzheimer's Care Quarterly, 7,* 32-40.

Gitlin, L. N., Corcoran, M., Winter, L., Boyce, A., & Hauck, W. W. (2001). A randomized, controlled trial of a home environmental intervention: Effect on efficacy and upset in caregivers and on daily function of persons with dementia. *Gerontologist, 41*(1), 4-14.

Gitlin, L. N., Hauck, W. W., Dennis, M. P., & Winter, L. (2005). Maintenance of effects of the home environmental skill-building program for family caregivers and individuals with Alzheimer's disease and related disorders. *Journals of Gerontology. Series A: Biological Sciences and Medical Sciences, 60*(3), 368-374.

Gitlin, L. N., Miller, K. S., & Boyce, A. (1999). Bathroom modifications for frail elderly renters: Outcomes of a community-based program. *Technology and Disability, 10*(3), 141-149.

Gitlin, L. N., Winter, L., Corcoran, M., Dennis, M. P., Schinfeld, S., & Hauck, W. W. (2003). Effects of the home environmental skill-building program on the caregiver-care recipient dyad: 6-month outcomes from the Philadelphia REACH initiative. *Gerontologist, 43*(4), 532-546.

Gitlin, L. N., Winter, L., Dennis, M. P., Corcoran, M., Schinfeld, S., & Hauck, W. W. (2006). A randomized trial of a multi-component home intervention to reduce functional difficulties in older adults. *Journal of the American Geriatrics Society, 54,* 809-816.

Gosman-Hedstrom, G., Claesson, L., & Blomstrand, C. (2002). Assistive devices in elderly people after stroke: A longitudinal, randomized study—the Goteborg 70+ Stroke Study. *Scandinavian Journal of Occupational Therapy, 9,* 109-118.

Graff, M. J., Vernooij-Dassen, M. J., Thijssen, M., Dekker, J., Hoefnagels, W. H., & Rikkert, M. G. (2006). Community-based occupational therapy for patients with dementia and their care givers: Randomised controlled trial. *British Medical Journal, 333*(7580), 1196.

Greenhalgh, T. (2006). *How to read a paper: The basics of evidence-based medicine* (3rd ed.). London, England: Blackwell Publishing Ltd.

Haines, T., Bennell, K., Osborne, R., & Hill, K. (2004). Effectiveness of targeted falls prevention in sub-acute hospital setting: Randomised controlled trial. *British Medical Journal, 328,* 676-679.

Hendriks, M. R. C., van Haastregt, J. C. M., Diederiks, J. P. M., Evers, S. M. A. A., Crebolder, H. F. J. M., & van Eijk, J. T. M. (2005). Effectiveness and cost-effectiveness of a multidisciplinary intervention programme to prevent new falls and functional decline among elderly persons at risk: Design of a replicated randomised controlled trial. *BMC Public Health, 5,* 6.

Jongbloed, L., & Crichton, A. (1990). A new definition of disability: Implications for rehabilitation practice and social policy. *Canadian Journal of Occupational Therapy, 57,* 32-37.

Koppenhaver, D., Erickson, K., Harris, B., McLellan, J., Skotko, G., & Newton, R. (2001). Storybook-based communication intervention for girls with Rett syndrome and their mothers. *Disability and Rehabilitation, 23,* 149-159.

Law, M. (1991). 1991 Muriel Driver lecture. The environment: A focus for occupational therapy. *Canadian Journal of Occupational Therapy, 58,* 171-180.

Liddle, J., March, L., Carfrae, B., Finnegan, T., Druce, J., Schwarz, J., et al. (1996). Can occupational therapy intervention play a part in maintaining independence and quality of life in older people? A randomized controlled trial. *Australian and New Zealand Journal of Public Health, 20,* 574-578.

Lyons, R. A., John, A., Brophy, S., Jones, S. J., Johansen, A., Kemp, A., Lannon, S., Patterson, J., Rolfe, B., Sander, L. V., & Weightman, A. (2006). Modification of the home environment for the reduction of injuries. *Cochrane Database of Systematic Reviews*, Issue 3. Art. No.: CD003600. DOI: 10.1002/14651858.CD003600.pub2.

Mann, W. C., Ottenbacher, K. J., Fraas, L., Tomita, M., & Granger, C. V. (1999). Effectiveness of assistive technology and environmental interventions in maintaining independence and reducing home care costs for the frail elderly. A randomized controlled trial. *Archives of Family Medicine, 8*(3), 210-217.

McClain, L., & Todd, C. (1990). Food store accessibility. *American Journal of Occupational Therapy, 44,* 487-491.

McGruder, J., Cors, D., Tiernan, A. M., & Tomlin, G. (2003). Weighted wrist cuffs for tremor reduction during eating in adults with static brain lesions. *American Journal of Occupational Therapy, 57*(5), 507-516.

Niva, B., & Skar, L. (2006). A pilot study of the activity patterns of five elderly persons after a housing adaptation. *Occupational Therapy International, 13*(1), 21-34.

O'Brien, P., Dyck, I., Caron, S., & Mortenson, P. (2002). Environmental analysis: Insights from sociological and geographical perspectives. *Canadian Journal of Occupational Therapy, 69,* 229-238.

Petersson, I., Lilja, M., Hammel, J., & Kottorp, A. (2008). Impact of home modification services on ability in everyday life for people ageing with disabilities. *Journal of Rehabilitation Medicine, 40*(4), 253-260.

Shaw, F. E., Bond, J., Richardson, D. A., Dawson, P., Steen, I. N., McKeith, I. G., et al. (2003). Multifactorial intervention after a fall in older people with cognitive impairment and dementia presenting to the accident and emergency department: Randomised controlled trial. *British Medical Journal, 326,* 73-75.

Stark, S. (2004). Removing environmental barriers in the homes of older adults with disabilities improves occupational performance. *OTJR: Occupation, Participation, and Health, 24*(1), 32-39.

Steultjens, E., Dekker, J., Bouter, L., Jellema, S., Bakker, E., & van den Ende, C. (2004). Occupational therapy for community dwelling elderly people: A systematic review. *Age and Ageing, 33,* 453-460.

Tolley, L., & Atwal, A. (2003). Determining the effectiveness of a falls prevention programme to enhance quality of life: An occupational therapy perspective. *British Journal of Occupational Therapy, 66*(6), 269-276.

Tse, T. (2005). The environment and falls prevention: Do environmental modifications make a difference? *Australian Occupational Therapy Journal, 52*(4), 271-281.

VanLeit, B., & Crowe, T. (2002). Outcomes of an occupational therapy program for mothers of children with disabilities: Impact on satisfaction with time use and occupational performance. *American Journal of Occupational Therapy, 56,* 402-410.

Weatherall, M. (2004). A targeted falls prevention programme plus usual care significantly reduces falls in elderly people during hospital stays. *Evidence-Based Healthcare and Public Health, 8*(5), 273-275.

World Health Organization. (2001). *International classification of functioning, disability, and health.* Geneva, Switzerland: Author.

World Health Organization. (2007). International classification of functioning, disability and health children and youth version (ICF-CY). Retrieved from www.who.int/classifications/icf/site/onlinebrowser/icf.cfm on October 17, 2007.

Yang, J. J., Mann, W. C., Nochajski, S., & Tomita, M. R. (1997). Use of assistive devices among elders with cognitive impairment: A follow-up study. *Topics in Geriatric Rehabilitation, 13,* 13-31.

PHYSICAL DETERMINANTS OF OCCUPATION

Mary Ann McColl, PhD, MTS and Wendy Pentland, PhD, OT Reg. (Ont.)

The physical determinants of occupation refer to the musculoskeletal structures and functions that affect an individual's ability to undertake the occupations of his or her choice (McColl, Law, Stewart, Doubt, Pollock, & Krupa, 2002). The structures involved are primarily muscles, bones, and joints, and the functions include strength, endurance, and range of motion. Occupational therapy for the physical determinants of occupation focuses at the level of impairment. From a biomechanical frame of reference, therapy focuses on remediating the impairment, whereas from a rehabilitative framework, therapy focuses on adaptation and compensation for physical deficits (James, 2003; Seidel, 2003).

A physical impairment is highly influential for occupational performance. For most occupations, there is a requirement of some degree of physical participation, from simply positioning oneself to exerting muscular strength. Many occupational therapists, particularly those working within a rehabilitative tradition, seek to remediate physical abilities underlying daily occupations (Seidel, 2003). Their assumption is that if the physical organism is working to its optimal level, it will rely on existing patterns or problem solve new ones in order to restore occupation. This chapter reviews the evidence for the effectiveness of occupational therapy in promoting real and meaningful changes in musculoskeletal structures and functions.

Conceptual Background

The conceptual background supporting therapists seeking to change the physical components of occupation come directly from the basic sciences of anatomy, physiology, kinesiology, and biomechanics. To be effective in enhancing physical functioning, an occupational therapist needs a firm grounding in the composition and operation of the musculoskeletal system. It is important to know not only how tissues are structured and function under normal circumstances, but also how they are injured and how they repair.

There is often a question of how occupational and physical therapists relate to one another in this area of practice. In ideal circumstances, they communicate and collaborate to make the best uses of the skills and aptitudes of each. There is sometimes a belief that occupational therapists work on the top half of the body—the arms, hands, and head—while

M. Law & M. A. McColl (Eds.)
Interventions, Effects, and Outcomes in Occupational Therapy:
Adults and Older Adults (pp. 183-246)
© 2010 SLACK Incorporated

physical therapists work on the bottom half—trunk and legs. We suggest that this formulation is far too simplistic to make the best use of the skills of either profession; however, there is a considerable emphasis in this chapter on upper extremity outcomes, particularly hand function. It is an area of specialization that occupational therapists have cultivated.

Historically, occupational therapy began in the area of mental health near the beginning of the 20th century, but with the return of injured and disabled soldiers from World War I, occupational therapists began to turn their skills and methods to assisting injured and traumatized veterans to return to civilian life. Through the use of habits and activities in the hospital, the emerging profession of occupational therapy helped to add meaning to the lives of these individuals. Often called "reconstruction aides," they incorporated a focus on vocational as well as self-care and leisure activities (Baldwin, 1919; Billings, 1918).

After World War II, the physical specialty within the profession took another leap forward, as severely disabled individuals who would not previously have survived their wounds sought to be restored to citizenship in the countries for which they had fought. The moral imperative associated with this situation led to the development of rehabilitation as a medical specialty. The focus at that time was to restore function through training and skill development, orthotics and prosthetics, and vocational rehabilitation.

In the later part of the 20th century, the physical rehabilitative approach began to wane in popularity, coincident with the rise of the independent living movement. The biomedical view of disability gave way to the social model of disability, wherein disability is defined not as a property of the individual, but rather as a function of an environment that is inadequately supportive or even hostile toward people with disabilities (McColl & Bickenbach, 1998). Some commentators agree that a swing back to a more moderate position is currently underway, incorporating both the physical reality of disability and the sociopolitical emphasis on environmental accommodation and change.

Search Strategy

In this chapter, the focus is on several physical outcomes in particular that appear in the literature. As already mentioned, there is a significant focus on hand function. There is also considerable literature on fatigue, endurance, pain, and general mobility. There are also small bodies of evidence on joint protection, seating, and falls. The most common diagnoses addressed with occupational therapy for physical outcomes are orthopedic conditions, arthritis, amputations, trauma, and peripheral nerve injuries.

The scoping review focused on physical functioning as an outcome in occupational therapy. The search strategy sought intervention studies aimed at improving physical functioning and was guided by the keywords listed in Table 8-1. A systematic search of health care and occupational therapy databases, as well as hand-searched relevant references, yielded 97 papers that addressed physical outcomes associated with occupational therapy articles. These studies featured occupational therapy interventions aimed at improving physical functioning and offered empirical evidence for the effectiveness of those interventions on physical outcomes.

Tables 8-2 through 8-4 provide detailed information on the interventions used, the conclusions drawn about the effectiveness of occupational therapy for enhancing physical function, and the outcome measures applied.

Interventions Used to Improve Physical Outcomes

This review uncovered articles that described programs aimed at promoting physical outcomes in occupation therapy. They range across six categories of intervention and focus on different age groups depending on the approach. For example, training approaches are more likely to be addressed to younger individuals, while adaptive and preventive approaches, such as joint protection and energy conservation, are more likely to be directed to older adults. Some interventions are more likely to occur in the hospital, such as those requiring equipment for training or splint manufacturing. Educational interventions, on the other hand, are just as likely to occur in the community. These interventions are seldom used in isolation, but rather tend to be combined into a program of care, often multidisciplinary in nature. For example, a program for people with arthritis might include splinting, joint protection, environmental modifications, adapted tools and techniques, pain management, and support.

Physical Training

The scoping review contained 34 articles that took a training approach to intervention. In these articles, the nature of what was included as "occupational therapy intervention" varied, ranging from joint protection, energy conservation, activities of daily living (ADL) training, education, assistive devices, games, and activities to prescribing and monitoring exercise programs and/or administering therapeutic modalities. Many focused on the arm and/or hand, and eight focused on general physical functioning. Four used physical modalities, such as functional electrical

Table 8-1

SEARCH TERMS FOR OCCUPATIONAL THERAPY INTERVENTIONS TO IMPROVE PHYSICAL OUTCOMES

Occupation, occupational therapy (therapist), OR multidisciplinary team AND…

Primary terms: arm injury/injuries, artificial limbs, client education, conservative treatment, energy conservation, fatigue, finger injury, hand injuries, joint diseases, joint protection, limb prosthesis, orthotic devices, outcomes of education, patient education, preoperative education, prostheses and implants, prosthesis(es), prosthetics, psychoeducation, seating, splinting.

Secondary terms: casts, dynamic splint, education, fibromyalgia, foot orthoses, hand, hand therapy, health education, health promotion, joint(s), medical education, methods, muscle fatigue, myoelectric prosthesis, orthopaedic procedure, orthoses, orthoses design, orthotics, patient positioning, position, prevention, prosthesis design, splints, surgical, teaching, teaching methods.

Additional terms used to focus the search included clinical effectiveness, community health services, health care delivery, health care services, health service, health services for the aged, home care, home care services, home health care, home occupational therapy, home rehabilitation, interdisciplinary education, interdisciplinary research, interdisciplinary treatment approach, intervention treatment approach, multidisciplinary care team, outcomes, outcomes assessment patient care, outcomes (health care), outcomes research, patient care team, rehabilitation, rehabilitation care, rehabilitation centre, rehabilitation outcomes, teamwork, treatment effectiveness evaluation, treatment outcomes.

stimulation, robotic assistance, or continuous passive movement, to enhance physical functioning. In each of these, biofeedback is an important component of the treatment.

Nineteen articles involved exercise-based programs, which varied from intensive inpatient daily exercise to home exercise programs supervised weekly or even less frequently by the therapist. Four articles looked specifically at occupationally embedded exercise compared to rotely performed exercise. Two meta-analyses have shown the effectiveness of activity-oriented exercise for enhancing motor performance and promoting movement (Lin, Wu, Tickle-Degnen, & Coster, 1997; Wu, Trombly, Lin, & Tickle-Degnen, 1998).

Environmental Modification

Another common intervention found in this scoping review pertaining to people seeking occupational therapy for physical impairment is environmental modification. The modifications reported primarily entailed environmental applications applied directly to the person (e.g., splints). A few articles addressed the more distal environment (e.g., modifying the bathroom set-up during immediate recovery post-total hip replacement or re-arranging the environment to reduce falls risks) (Luukinen, Lehtola, Jokelainene, Vaananen-Sainio, Lotvonen, & Koistinen, 2007). Of 24 articles identified, 17 pertained specifically to splinting, orthotics, or prosthetics; the bulk of these were

related to conditions of the wrist or hand. Five articles pertained to wheelchair mobility and seating. These articles tended to focus on clients with spinal cord injuries, strokes, or amputations.

Splints are defined as "any medical device added to a person's body to support, align, position, immobilize, prevent or correct deformity, assist weak muscles, or improve function" (Deshaies, 2002). Occupational therapists may design and fabricate splints from scratch using a variety of techniques and materials or they may prescribe, fit, and train with pre-fabricated orthotics. In addition, occupational therapists may be involved in the fitting and training associated with prosthetics. There are various therapeutic goals in hand splinting: Immobilization, pain relief, prevention of mal-alignment, prevention/reduction of soft tissue overstretch, counteracting hypertrophic scars, support of weak muscles, and improvement of function to functional improvement (Paternostro-Sluga & Stieger, 2004). Pathological conditions that frequently require splint treatment as a part of their rehabilitation management are rheumatoid arthritis, osteoarthritis, tendinopathies, neurological diseases, burn injuries, and aftercare of hand surgery (Paternostro-Sluga & Stieger, 2004).

The literature cited here covers a mixture of both custom-made and ready-made splints, often comparing the two. Based on the results of several review articles, there seems to be little consensus around

text continues on page 240

Table 8-2

OCCUPATIONAL THERAPY INTERVENTIONS PROMOTING PHYSICAL OUTCOMES

Author (Date)	Pop	Dx	Setting	Intervention
Training				
Paes Lourencao, M. I., Battistella, L. R., Moran de Brito, C. M., Tsukimoto, G. R., & Miyazaki, M. H. (2008)	5	3	4	**Intervention:** Consisted of 1-hour OT sessions twice a week that included functional electrical stimulation of elbow and wrist extensor muscles. Participants also received 1 hour of surface electromyography and biofeedback once a week. **Control:** Participants received 1-hour OT sessions twice a week that included functional electrical stimulation of the elbow and wrist extensor muscles.
Rosenstein, L., Ridgel, A., Thota, A., Samame, B., & Alberts, J. (2008)	2	3	3	**Intervention:** The patient completed 4 hours of therapy each day for 15 days, including 2 hours with the Hand Mentor and 2 hours of repetitive task practice. The Hand Mentor is a robotic device that provides biofeedback regarding muscle activation and is designed to inhibit flexion in the fingers and wrist, provide neuro-reeducation, and increase strength and range of motion in the fingers and wrist. During repetitive task practice, the patient completed tasks of her choosing, focusing on the complete task or specific components and performing them repetitively for 15 to 30 minutes. The difficulty of the tasks was gradually increased over time. The patient completed 12 of 15 rehabilitation days, missing 3 due to illness.
Luukinen, H., Lehtola, S., Jokelainen, J., Vaananen-Sainio, R., Lotvonen, S., & Koistinen, P. (2007)	1	24	3	**Intervention:** Each subject was visited in their home by an OT and PT who evaluated environmental and medical risk factors for falls and then created an individualized exercise program including home and group exercise and self-care training. The program was evaluated and cleared by each subject's physician before he or she began. **Control:** Subjects continued with usual routine care including visits to their physician.
Li, L. C., Davis, A. M., Lineker, S. C., Coyte, P. C., & Bombardier, C. (2006)	4	19	3, 4	**Intervention:** Intervention time was 6 weeks, and visits depended on client needs. Experimental group had OT or PT who provided treatments: Education, physical modalities, exercise, prescriptions or assistive devices, splints and orthoses, psychosocial support, and advocacy. **Control:** Seen by a PT or OT and then referred to other professions as needed. Intervention provided as needed.
Pang, M., Harris, J., & Eng, J. (2006)	1, 2	3	3, 4	**Intervention:** Subjects took part in a 19-week upper arm exercise program that took place 3 times a week in 1-hour sessions facilitated by a PT, OT, and exercise instructor. Participants rotated through 3 activity stations during each session and completed brief warm-ups and cool-downs (5 minutes each) that included stretching and range of motion exercises. The exercise program was designed to prevent learned non-use and to improve function in the paretic UE through self-directed exercises. **Control:** Participants completed a similar exercise program that focused solely on the LEs and did not include any UE training.
Popovic, M. R., Thrasher, T. A., Adams, M. E., Takes, V., Zivanovic, V., & Tonack, M. I. (2006)	5	6	4	**Intervention:** Functional electrical stimulation for hand therapy. **Control:** Conventional OT for hand therapy.

continued

Table 8-2 (continued)
Occupational Therapy Interventions Promoting Physical Outcomes

Author (Date)	Pop	DX	Setting	Intervention
Training				
Aldehag, A. S., Jonsson, H., & Ansved, T. (2005)	1, 2	18	3	**Intervention:** Participants completed hand training exercises at home 3 times a week for 12 weeks and received guided training from an OT once every 3 weeks. The training program consisted of stretching and resistance exercises that focused on flexion and extension of the wrist and fingers in isolated and mass movements. The resistance exercises were completed using silicone putty (Theraputty), and the number of repetitions was increased by one every fourth week.
Dohnke, B., Knauper, B., & Muller-Fahrnow, W. (2005)	1, 2	22	4	**Intervention:** Post-surgery for hip joint replacement, patients were admitted to an inpatient rehabilitation ward where they underwent a multidisciplinary program that included exercise therapy, OT, patient education programs, and PT.
Lynch, D., Ferraro, M., Krol, J., Trudell, C. M., Christos, P., & Volpe, B. T. (2005)	5	3	4	Participants were randomly assigned to 1 of 2 groups: **Group 1:** Receive daily continuous passive motion treatments or participate in self range of motion groups under the supervision of an OT. **Group 2:** Device-delivered continuous passive range of motion exercises for the upper limb by OT and/or PT.
Ring, H., & Rosenthal, N. (2005)	4	3	4	Participants were randomly assigned to usual outpatient treatment group or neuroprosthesis group. Both groups had functional treatment to improve ADL, neuromuscular re-education using Bobath techniques, PT, OT, communication, psychological intervention, and cognitive deficits. **Intervention:** Neuroprosthesis group has a non-invasive microprocessor controlled simulation through 5 electrodes on an orthotic to stimulate select muscle groups.
Studenski, S., Duncan, P., Perera, S., Reker, D., Lai, S., & Richards, L. (2005)	1, 2	3	3	**Intervention:** Participants received 36 individual sessions of home exercise led by an OT or PT over 12 weeks. The exercises were targeted to improve strength, balance, and endurance and encouraged use of the affected UE. Participants also received written guidelines to continue exercising on their own once the 12 weeks of the program were finished. **Control:** Participants received usual care prescribed to them by their primary physician, including monitoring of health status and health education. Approximately half received formal OT or PT.
Sandqvist, G., Akesson, A., & Eklund, M. (2004)	5	18	4	**Intervention:** Consisted of paraffin bath treatments to 1 hand once a day. This was followed by hand exercise program adapted to each individual's needs (UEs and LEs). **Control:** (Other hand) was only provided with exercise program. Treatment continued for 1 month.
Tsuji, T., Liu, M., Hase, K., Masakado, Y., Takahashi, H., Hara, Y., et al. (2004)	4	3	4	Stroke program for 80 minutes of PT and OT sessions and daily rehabilitation nursing for 5 days a week for hospital stay.
Case-Smith, J. (2003)	2	16	4	Splinting, therapeutic exercise, therapeutic activities, manual therapy, ADL, ultrasound, hot/cold packs, whirlpool, electrical stimulation, moist heat.
Desrosiers, J., Malouin, F., Richards, C., Bourbonnais, D., Rochette, A., & Bravo, G. (2003)	5	3	4	Active post-stroke rehabilitation by both OT and PT.

continued

Table 8-2 (continued)

OCCUPATIONAL THERAPY INTERVENTIONS PROMOTING PHYSICAL OUTCOMES

Author (Date)	Pop	DX	Setting	Intervention
Training				
Fischer, T., Nagy, L., & Buechler, U. (2003)	2	16	4	Extensor carpi radialis longus was transferred to the adductor pollicis tendon, and one slip of the abductor pollicis longus was transferred to the first dorsal interosseus tendon.
Sandin-Aldehag, A., & Jonsson, H. (2003)	5	18	4	Hand therapy program that provided therapist-guided weekly sessions and 2 homework sessions a week.
Donnelly, C. J., & Wilton, J. (2002)	5	18	4	*Intervention:* Received customized hand rehabilitation program in conjunction with self-scar massage for duration of 4 weeks. This group was instructed on how to self-massage (given an illustrated handout and received a 10-minute therapist scar massage at each session). *Control:* Only received customized hand rehabilitation excluding massage.
Christensen, O. M., Kunov, A., Hansen, F. F., Christiansen, T. C., & Krasheninnikoff, M. (2001)	4	16	4	*Group 1:* Received only exercise instructions in movements for shoulder, arm, and hands. *Group 2:* Received exercises and OT. Active joint exercises for wrist, elbow, and shoulder, edema prevention, coordination exercise, coarse and fine motor function exercise, strengthening exercise, sensation exercise, and ADL training.
Ozdemir, F., Birtane, M., Tabatabaei, R., Kokino, S., & Ekuklu, G. (2001)	4	3	3, 4	*Hospitalized intervention:* 5 days a week included therapeutic exercises, neuromuscular facilitation exercises, physical agents, OT (hand or wrist splints, ankle-foot orthoses, tripods, canes). *Home intervention:* 7 days a week included family training (convenient bed positioning and exercises), splints, PT orthoses, assistive devices, and physician visits.
Wahi Michener, S. K., Olson, A. L., Humphrey, B. A., Reed, J. E., Stepp, D. R., Sutton, A. M., et al. (2001)	5	16	4	Grip strengthening intervention following hand trauma, aimed at promoting hand function.
Griffiths, T., Burr, M., Campbell, I., Lewis-Jenkins, V., Mullins, J., Shiels, K., et al. (2000)	4	27	4	Multidisciplinary team (OT, PT, and dietetic staff) provided rehabilitation program for 3 half days/week for 6 weeks. Sessions were 2 hours long. Educational sessions were followed by individual training exercise programs (30 minutes; treadmill started at 80% of max in 10 minute shuttle-walk test, cycling, stair machine, circuit training). Program ends with a "psychological issues" session related to chronic disability (stress management and relaxation techniques). Individualization in program available.
Jarus, T., Shavit, S., & Ratzon, N. (2000)	4	16	4	Both treatment groups 3 times a week for 5 weeks. *Group 1:* Computer-aided treatment training program following wrist fracture. *Group 2:* Low-technology brush-making machine exercise.
Bailey, A., Starr, L., Alderson, M., & Moreland, J. (1999)	5	18	4	Fibro-Fit intervention involves a 12-week exercise and education treatment program provided by an interdisciplinary team of a PT, OT, and social work. Pharmacist, dietitian, and kinesiologist supported program.
Baskett, J. J., Broad, J. B., Reekie, G., Hocking, C., & Green, G. (1999)	4	3	3, 4	*Intervention:* Weekly visits by an OT and/or PT who prescribed a program of exercises and activities for the following week. *Control:* Received outpatient or day hospital therapy.

continued

Table 8-2 (continued)
OCCUPATIONAL THERAPY INTERVENTIONS PROMOTING PHYSICAL OUTCOMES

Author (Date)	Pop	DX	Setting	Intervention
Training				
Hoppes, S. (1997)	1	3, 4 17, 18	1	Timed trials at elevated standing table, alternating between taking part in a game they liked (cards, dominos) or taking part in a non-playful activity (reading, chatting). Timing started when participants had independent balance and ended once they sat down. Trial took place on different days.
Hsieh, C. L., Nelson, D. L., Smith, D. A., & Peterson, C. Q. (1996)	4	3,18	4	Participants completed the same basic exercise (throwing) consecutively across 3 different conditions: *Intervention 1:* Added-materials occupation. *Intervention 2:* Imagery-based occupation. *Control:* Rote exercise.
Kohlmeyer, K. M., Hill, J. P., Yarkony, G. M., & Jaeger, R. J. (1996)	2	6	4	Participants were randomized to 4 treatment groups for 5 to 6 weeks: Conventional treatment. Electrical stimulation. Biofeedback. Combined electrical stimulation and biofeedback.
Nelson, D. L., Konosky, K., Fleharty, K., Webb, R., Newer, K., Hazboun, V. P., et al. (1996)	4	3	4	*Intervention:* Occupationally embedded exercise involving a simple dice game. *Control:* Rote exercise.
Thomes, L. J. & Thomes, B. J. (1995)	5	16	4	Participants took part in a 6-week treatment for early mobilization of surgically repaired extensor tendons in zone III.
King, T. I. (1993)	5	16	4	Participants at hand therapy clinic were randomly assigned to 1 of 2 treatment groups: *Group 1:* Completed a purposeful activity before the non-purposeful activity. The purposeful activity was a video game, and the non-purposeful was a grip or pinch activity. *Group 2:* Completed the non-purposeful activity before the purposeful one.
Sietsema, J. M., Nelson, D. L., Mulder, R. M., Mervau-Scheidel, D., & White, B. E. (1993)	2	7	4	*Intervention:* Occupationally embedded intervention: Computer-controlled game. *Control:* Rote exercise.
Trombly, C. A., Thayer-Nason, L., Bliss, G., Girard, C. A., Lyrist, L. A., & Brexa-Hooson, A. (1986)	2	3	4	*Intervention:* Participated in 3 hand exercises (requiring maximal loading of the extensor digitorum). *Control:* Were allowed to engage in any activity that did not involve the affected hand.
Greenberg, S., & Fowler, R. S., Jr. (1980)	4	3	4	*Intervention:* Audiovisual kinesthetic biofeedback (relaying information about actual movement of a body part to the client). *Control:* Conventional OT.

continued

Table 8-2 (continued)
OCCUPATIONAL THERAPY INTERVENTIONS PROMOTING PHYSICAL OUTCOMES

Author (Date)	Pop	DX	Setting	Intervention
Education				
Spadaro, A., De Luca, T., Massimiani, M., Ceccarelli, F., Riccieri, V., & Valesini, G. (2008)	2	18	3	***Intervention:*** Patients with ankylosing spondylitis were treated with anti-TNFα drugs for 12 weeks prior to entering the study and continued treatment while receiving additional OT. The program took a total of 6 hours to complete: 3 2-hour individual sessions held approximately every 6 weeks. Patients received individualized interventions developed by an OT based on their specific needs and priorities. Interventions used included information about ankylosing spondylitis and its treatment and management, relevant ADL training, joint protection, energy conservation, posture and positioning advice, advice on leisure or work, and a home exercise program to increase range of movement in the spine. ***Control:*** Patients received anti-TNFα drug treatment and routine care but no OT.
Matuska, K., Mathiowetz, V., & Finlayson, M. (2007)	2	5	3	***Intervention:*** Participants attended a 6-week energy conservation course that consisted of structured 2-hour group classes held weekly and facilitated by a certified OT. A variety of educational techniques were used including lectures, discussions, long- and short-term goal setting, activity stations, and take-home work. The program addressed a variety of topics including the importance of rest throughout the day, positive and effective communication, proper body mechanics, ergonomic principles, environment modification, activity analysis and modification, priority setting, and achieving a balanced lifestyle.
Gitlin, L., Hauck, W., Winter, L., Dennis, M., & Schulz, R. (2006)	1	24	3	***Intervention:*** OT and PT educated participants on environmental modifications, behavioral strategies, and cognitive strategies. ***Control:*** Had no contact but received educational material on home safety and performance techniques.
Finlayson, M. (2005)	2	5	3	A modified energy conservation program "managing fatigue" delivered through teleconference. Program developed and instructed by OT.
Lamb, A. L., Finlayson, M., Mathiowetz, V., & Chen, H. Y. (2005)	5	5	3	***Intervention:*** Patients attended the "managing fatigue" program, a 6-week patient education program designed to increase use of energy conservation skills and increase patient's confidence in managing fatigue. The program is community based and is delivered as group sessions facilitated by an OT. ***Control:*** Patients who missed any of the group sessions for medical or other reasons received a self-study module to complete at home that contained all of the information given in the group session.
Li, L. C., Davis, A. M., Lineker, S., Coyte, P., & Bombardier, C. (2005)	5	19	3	***Intervention:*** OT or PT was assigned as primary therapist, provided individual therapy based on client's needs (e.g., education, pain management, energy conservation, joint protection, splinting, exercise, assistive devices, and referral to community programs) in addition to medical care by a rheumatologist. Therapy lasted approximately 6 weeks long. ***Control:*** Received usual medical care.
Mathiowetz, V. G., Finlayson, M. L., Matuska, K. M., Chen, H. Y., & Luo, P. (2005)	5	5	3	6-session, 2 hours a week energy conservation course for groups of 8 to 10 participants.

continued

Table 8-2 (continued)
OCCUPATIONAL THERAPY INTERVENTIONS PROMOTING PHYSICAL OUTCOMES

Author (Date)	Pop	DX	Setting	Intervention
Education				
Hammond, A., & Freeman, K. (2004)	2	19	4	Educational and behavioral joint protection program for standard arthritis and control group.
Hammond, A., Young, A., & Kidao, R. (2004)	5	19	5	**Intervention:** Participants received usual rheumatology care in conjunction with an additional program of OT. The program was delivered by experienced rheumatology OTs and consisted of 4 1-hour individual sessions usually delivered weekly and 1 2-hour group arthritis education session. Patients were interviewed before treatment regarding their medical/social history and disease status, and an individual treatment plan was devised between the therapist and patient using this information. **Control:** Patients received usual rheumatology care, which normally did not include OT or PT unless specially requested.
Ward, C. D., Turpin, G., Dewey, M. E., Fleming, S., Hurwitz, B., Ratib, S., et al. (2004)	5	4, 5, 18	3	**Intervention:** Education group. Education and information and a 12-month health action plan. **Control:** Standardized printed information.
Hammond, A., Jeffreson, P., Jones, N., Gallagher, J., & Jones, T. (2002)	2	19	4	"Looking After Your Joints" program, an educational-behavioral program includes information about rheumatoid arthritis and disease management, joint protection, and energy conservation.
Hammond, A., & Freeman, K. (2001)	2	19	4	Educational and behavioral joint protection program for standard arthritis and control group.
Mathiowetz, V., Matuska, K. M., & Murphy, M. E. (2001)	5	5	3	6-session, 2 hours a week energy conservation course for groups of 8 to 10 participants.
Thomas, J. J. (1996)	5	26	2	**Intervention:** Collaborative education (OT and patients). **Control:** Traditional patient education.
Spalding, N. J. (1995)	4	22	4	Participants awaiting total hip replacement surgery were randomly assigned to 1 of 2 groups: **Intervention:** Received a preoperative education session. The training program consisted of 2 sessions taught by an OT, anesthesiologist, dietitian, senior nurse, and PT. **Control:** Did not attend the educational program.
Barry, M. A., Purser, J., Hazleman, R., McLean, A., & Hazleman, B. L. (1994)	4	19	4	1 OT treatment session (1 hour) consisting of instruction in energy conservation and joint protection techniques.
Hammond, A. (1994)	4	19	4	Participants took part in 2 joint protection education sessions, part of a 6-week (12 hour) arthritis program. Joint protection principles that were evaluated were either demonstrated, discussed, illustrated, or practiced during these sessions.
Furst, G. P., Gerber, L. H., Smith, C. C., & Fisher, S. (1987)	4	19	4	Energy conservation program.

continued

Table 8-2 (continued)
OCCUPATIONAL THERAPY INTERVENTIONS PROMOTING PHYSICAL OUTCOMES

Author (Date)	Pop	DX	Setting	Intervention
Education				
Gerber, L., Furst, G., Shulman, B., Smith, C., Thornton, B., Liang, M., et al. (1987)	-	19	3	**Intervention:** Workbook group. Group sessions for 6 weeks. The framework suggested that intervention must "foster and reinforce" behavioral change. **Control:** Received typical OT treatment, average of 2 sessions learning about joint protection and energy conservation and provided with splints/adaptive equipment, as necessary.
Skill Development				
van Houten, P., Achterberg, W., & Ribbe, M. (2007)	1	18	1	**Intervention:** Subjects received training in mobility and/or toileting skills on an individual basis from an OT or PT. Specific tasks were practiced for 30 minutes 3 times a week for a minimum of 1 week or a maximum of 8. Therapists could end the program when the patient could complete all tasks in the targeted time. **Control:** Subjects received care as usual in the long-term care facility.
Ip, W. M., Woo, J., Yue, S. Y., Kwan, M., Sum, S. M., Kwok, T., et al. (2006)	1, 2	21	4	**Intervention:** Participants were shown how to complete a set of daily tasks and completed them in the usual manner or by applying 1 of 3 conservation techniques. The energy conservation techniques used included use of labor-saving equipment, workspace set-up, and avoidance of reaching overhead. The tasks completed were carrying groceries using a basket/bag or a cart, hand washing clothing while standing or seated, and hanging clothes overhead or at waist height.
Storr, L. K., Sorensen, P. S., & Ravnborg, M. (2006)	5	5	4	**Intervention:** Subjects were admitted to a multiple sclerosis rehabilitation hospital for 3 to 5 weeks to complete a multidisciplinary rehabilitation program that included PTs, OTs, psychologists, social workers, nurses, and neurologists. The team consulted with each patient to devise an individual treatment plan suited to their needs and desires. **Control:** Subjects received their usual treatment and no additional therapy similar to that used in the study.
Mendelsohn, M. E., Overend, T. J., & Petrella, R. J. (2004)	1	17	4	Intervention is approximately 4 weeks carried out by OT and PT. Range of motion, flexibility, strengthening exercises, balance, gait, stair retraining, ADL training (assistive device use, coordination, dressing, grooming, eating/drinking, getting in and out of bed, rising from chair, going up and down stairs).
Maeshima, S., Ueyoshi, A., Osawa, A., Ishida, K., Kunimoto, K., Shimamoto, Y., et al. (2003)	4	3	4	**Intervention:** Received same PT as control group plus family-run therapy including orientation, assistance in gait rehabilitation, and stand-up exercises. Families were trained and conducted therapy after supervision. **Control:** Received PT, OT (functional ergotherapy, 5 hand movements, delicate motions, changing hand dominance, ADL exercises).
Rodgers, H., Mackintosh, J., Price, C., Wood, R., McNamee, P., Fearon, T., et al. (2003)	4	3	4	**Intervention:** Had usual stroke care plus enhanced upper limb rehabilitation by PT and OT. **Control:** Usual stroke care involved joint therapy sessions with PT (Bobath based) and OT (practicing normal movements with meaningful tasks).
Neistadt, M. E. (1994)	5	7	1, 4	**Group 1:** Parquetry block assembly group. **Group 2:** A meal preparation group. Treatment sessions were 30 minutes long, and each participant received 3 sessions per week for 6 weeks.

continued

Table 8-2 (continued)
OCCUPATIONAL THERAPY INTERVENTIONS PROMOTING PHYSICAL OUTCOMES

Author (Date)	Pop	DX	Setting	Intervention
Environmental Modification				
Lannin, N., Cusick, A., McCluskey, A., & Herbert, R. (2007)	1, 2	3	4	**Intervention:** Participants received usual post-stroke care and wore custom-made, static, palmar splints for up to 12 hours nightly for 4 weeks. Patients were divided further into 2 groups: One wore a hand splint that positioned the wrist in a neutral position (0 to 10 degrees of extension), while the other wore a splint that positioned the wrist in an end-of-range position (>45 degrees) and extended the fingers. **Control:** Patients received usual post-stroke rehabilitative care and did not wear any splints during the program.
van der Giesen, F. J., Nelissen, R., Rozing, P., Arendzen, J., de Jong, Z., Wolterbeek, R., et al. (2007)	5	18	2	**Intervention:** Patients were referred to a specialized hand clinic staffed by an orthopedic surgeon, rehabilitation specialist, rheumatologist, OT, and PT. At their first visit, patients were assessed by the PT, rheumatologist, and OT. At the second visit, the entire team along with the patient reviewed the findings of the assessment and devised a treatment plan. If any interventions were instituted, a 3-month follow-up visit was scheduled.
Pagnotta, A., Korner-Bitensky, N., Mazer, B., Baron, M., & Wood-Dauphinee, S. (2005)	5	19	4	Commercially available pre-fabricated circumferential wrist working splints (e.g., Futuro, Roylan).
Pizzi, A., Carlucci, G., Falsini, C., Verdesca, S., & Grippo, A. (2005)	5	19	4	Participants wore a custom-made immobilizing volar resting splint. Patients were asked to wear the splint for 3 months (at least 90 minutes a day). If participants did not meet this criterion, they were not admitted to follow-up.
Haskett, S., Backman, C., Porter, B., Goyert, J., & Palejko, G. (2004)	2	19	4	Over 4-week period using each of the 3 wrist splints in turn (custom leather splint, Rolyan, and Anatech).
Zijlstra, T. R., Heijnsdijk-Rouwenhorst, L., & Rasker, J. J. (2004)	5	19	4	Orthoses custom fabricates silver ring finger orthoses prescribed and fitted by an OT and a PT. (Rheumatologist involved in DAS28 and erythrocyte assessments.)
Lannin, N. A., Horsley, S. A., Herbert, R., McCluskey, A., & Cusick, A. (2003)	4	7	4	**Intervention:** Wore a static, palmar resting mitt splint on a daily basis, for a maximum of 12 hours each night, for the duration of a 4-week intervention period. **Control:** Routine therapy for individual motor training and upper limb stretches (5 weeks in total).
Akalin, E., El, O., Peker, O., Senocak, O., Tamci, S., Gulbahar, S. et al. (2002)	2	16	4	Participants in both groups received a custom-made neutral volar wrist splint. **Group 1:** Only wore splint all night and during the day as much as possible for 4 weeks. **Group 2:** Wore splint and also were instructed to perform nerve and tendon gliding exercises done for 4 weeks.
Shechtman, O., Hanson, C. S., Garrett, D., & Dunn, P. (2001)	5	3, 6, 10, 18	4	Use of 6 different pressure-relieving wheelchair cushions.
Bolin, I., Bodin, P., & Kreuter, M. (2000)	2	6	4	Interventions to improve the fit of the wheelchair to the individual, with an emphasis on reduction of kyphotic posture and pelvic obliquity.

continued

Table 8-2 (continued)
Occupational Therapy Interventions Promoting Physical Outcomes

Author (Date)	Pop	DX	Setting	Intervention
Environmental Modification				
Bishop, S. A., Bulla, N., DiLellio, E., Dy, M., Koski, J. H., Linnemeyer, C. B., et al. (1999)	1	21	1	Participants were asked to sit in 4 positions on 4 different wheelchair cushions that were placed on a standard wheelchair. They were instructed to hold each body position for a specified time frame while pressure ratings were taken.
Li, S., Liu, L., Miyazaki, M., & Warren, S. (1999)	5	16	4	OT provided the following treatment to all subjects: Education on carpal tunnel syndrome; fabricated a modified ulnar gutter wrist splint for each subject; and explained splint purpose, wearing times, care instructions, and precautions.
Pellow, T. R. (1999)	5	6	4	Tilt and recline positioning and 3 different wheelchair cushions.
Pagnotta, A., Baron, M., & Korner-Bitensky, N. (1998)	5	19	4	**Intervention:** Each patient was fitted with a Futuro wrist orthosis to wear during functional evaluation. **Control:** Incorporated repeating the evaluation without the splint.
Tijhuis, G. J., Vliet Vlieland, T. P., Zwinderman, A. H., & Hazes, J. M. (1998)	5	19	4	Orthoses fabricated custom wrist splint (other professionals). Participants were asked to wear as frequently as possible in cross-over design. **Group 1:** Custom-made wrist orthoses. **Group 2:** Commercially available wrist orthoses.
Callinan, N. J., & Mathiowetz, V. (1996)	5	19	4	Participants each took part in 3 experimental treatment periods. The order of treatment periods was randomized. OT provided wear and care instructions for each splint and instructed participants to wear the splint at night. **Group 1:** Treatment with a soft splint. **Group 2:** Treatment with a hard splint. **Control:** Unsplinted.
Stern, E. B., Ytterberg, S. R., Krug, H. E., & Mahowald, M. L. (1996)	5	19	4	Cross-over design: Each patient was randomly fitted with 1 of 3 commercially available wrist orthosis (Futuro, AliMed, Roylan) and was instructed to wear it on the dominant hand for a minimum of 4 hours daily for 5/7 days.
Stern, E. B., Ytterberg, S. R., Krug, H. E., Mullin, G. T., & Mahowald, M. L. (1996)	5	19	4	Each patient was randomly fitted with 1 of 3 commercially available wrist orthoses (Futuro, AliMed, Roylan) and was instructed to wear it on the dominant hand for a minimum of 4 hours daily for 5/7 days.
Conine, T. A., Hershler, C., Daechsel, D., Peel, C., & Pearson, A. (1994)	1	18	1	Participants were randomly assigned to receive either a foam wheelchair cushion (foam group) or a Jay wheelchair cushion (Jay group). Both groups were followed for 3 months. The OT adjusted wheelchairs and cushions and completed a weekly follow-up, as needed. Participants received the same medical, nursing, rehabilitation, and dietary care within their extended care facility.
Yuen, H. K., Nelson, D. L., Peterson, C. Q., & Dickinson, A. (1994)	2	19	3	**Intervention:** Prosthesis control training provided with object related visual input. Training consisted for 2 1.5-hour sessions. **Control:** Were instructed how to lift and lower the prosthesis by flexing and extending the right shoulder; 5 successful trials were allowed.
Cron, L., & Sprigle, S. (1993)	5	3, 10	1, 4	Use of the hemi wheelchair cushion for people self-propelling with 1 lower limb.

continued

Table 8-2 (continued)
OCCUPATIONAL THERAPY INTERVENTIONS PROMOTING PHYSICAL OUTCOMES

Author (Date)	Pop	DX	Setting	Intervention
Environmental Modification				
Fletchall, S., & Hickerson, W. L. (1991)	5	9, 16	2	Multidisciplinary group including a medical director, OT, prosthetist, and surgeon assessed burn patients prior to surgery to amputate limbs. OT role was to assess factors such as muscle function of both UEs and possible muscle sites for myoelectric prosthetic use, range of motion, both early problems, and anticipated problems after healing. OT received from admission to post-surgery for prosthetic training.
Poole, J. L., Whitney, S. L., Hangeland, N., & Baker, C. (1990)	2	3	4	**Intervention:** Inflatable pressure splints (applied 20 minutes a day) applied to counteract contracture in affected UE. **Control:** Received no treatment and engaged in regular weightbearing activity.
Mathiowetz, V., Bolding, D. J., & Trombly, C. A. (1983)	5	3, 18	4	The EMG activity of 4 participants with hemiplegia and 8 without hemiplegia were measured during 4 conditions: Wearing no positioning device. Wearing a volar resting splint. A finger spreader. A firm cone.
Occupational Development				
Lannin, N., Clemson, L., McCluskey, A., Lin, C-W., Cameron, I., & Barras, S. (2007)	1	18	2, 3	**Intervention:** 1 home-based OT visit prior to discharge from a rehabilitation center delivered by an OT. The visit included evaluation of the home environment, assessment of the subject's discharge risks, assessment of functional abilities, and a review of prescribed assistive equipment. **Control:** 1 hospital session with an OT that included assessment of functional abilities and home and community accessibility. An interview regarding duties at home and social and leisure activities as well as education regarding safe use of equipment and existing community services.
Masiero, S., Boniolo, A., Wassermann, L., Machiedo, H., Volante, D., & Punzi, L. (2007)	1, 2	19	5	**Intervention:** Participants continued their usual drug treatment and routine care and received additional joint protection training. The training consisted of 3-hour group sessions every 3 weeks, and patients were encouraged to bring a partner or family member. The program was developed and delivered by a multidisciplinary team that included a rheumatologist, physiatrist, PT, and OT. The topics covered in the education program included pathophysiology of rheumatoid arthritis, pain and stress management techniques, home exercises, energy conservation techniques, and joint protection methods. **Control:** Patients received routine care and the same drug treatment as the intervention but did not receive PT, OT, or any other treatments.
Stenvall, M., Olofsson, B., Lundstrom, M., Englund, U., Borssen, B., Svensson, O., et al. (2007)	1	17	2	**Intervention:** Patients were admitted to a geriatric ward that specialized in orthopedic patients. Nurses, 2 full-time PTs, 2 full-time OTs, geriatricians, and a part-time dietitian who all received special training in rehabilitation and teamwork staffed the ward. The staff coordinated closely to create individualized rehabilitation programs for each patient and provide comprehensive and active detection and prevention of postoperative complications and falls. **Control:** Patients were admitted to a regular orthopedic ward and received routine postoperative care.

continued

Table 8-2 (continued)
OCCUPATIONAL THERAPY INTERVENTIONS PROMOTING PHYSICAL OUTCOMES

Author (Date)	Pop	DX	Setting	Intervention
Occupational Development				
von Renteln-Kruse, W., & Krause, T. (2007)	1	24	2	***Intervention:*** A multidisciplinary team with experience in geriatrics consisting of a physician, 2 nurses, a PT, an OT, and a quality manager devised a series of preventative measures to reduce falls in a geriatric hospital. The program included a staff education and training program, written materials for patients and caregivers, fall-risk assessment upon admission, and individual patient and caregiver training.
Kaapa, E. H., Frantsi, K., Sarna, S., & Malmivaara, A. (2006)	5	20	4	***Intervention:*** 8 weeks of intervention involving cognitive-behavioral stress management and applied relaxation, back school education (based on principles by physician, PT, and OT). Team consisted of PTs, 2 OTs, a psychologist, and specialized rehabilitation medicine physician (low back pain). ***Control:*** PT based on individual assessment and treatment sessions for 6 to 8 weeks.
Wennemer, H. K., Borg-Stein, J., Gomba, L., Delaney, B., Rothmund, A., Barlow, D., et al. (2006)	5	18	3	***Intervention:*** Subjects received 3 2-hour training sessions per week for 8 weeks. The multidisciplinary training program was designed to be progressive and target physical functioning, not pain. Physical therapists delivered flexibility training, low-impact aerobics, and strength and balance training while OTs trained patients with simulated functional tasks, ergonomic techniques, and relaxation methods. Each program was individualized to meet the needs of the patient.
Davison, J., Bond, J., Dawson, P., Steen, I. N., & Kenny, R. A. (2005)	1	18, 24	3	***Intervention:*** Multidisciplinary falls prevention program with comprehensive medical assessment and appropriate interventions provided by physician. PT performed gait and balance assessment along with review of footwear and assistive devices providing functional training programs and prescribing assistive devices when necessary. OT completed home hazard assessment with User Safety and Environmental Risk (USER) checklist and appropriate modifications according to published criteria. ***Control:*** Received usual care upon admission to hospital for fall, did not undergo OT/PT assessment or receive individualized program.
Malcus-Johnson, P., Carlqvist, C., Sturesson, A., & Eberhardt, K. (2005)	1, 2	19	3, 4	***Intervention:*** Patients had scheduled visits with an OT every 3 months in the first 2 years of the study and every 6 months in the years following. During the visit, they could discuss problems with the OT and receive any necessary interventions. Patients could also contact the OT between scheduled visits if they desired. The most common interventions were prescriptions of assistive devices and orthotics followed by hand training, hand exercises, and patient education.
WaiShan Louie, S. (2004)	4	27	4	6 practice sessions of guided imagery using relaxation music and an OT's instructions on how to construct a pleasant mental picture and incorporate abdominal breathing.
Walsh, D. A., Kelly, S. J., Johnson, P. S., Rajkumar, S., & Bennetts, K. (2004)	5	20	4	Program at back pain unit for 7 hours a day for 9 days during 5 weeks. Intervention includes education, communication skills, medication usage, relaxation and imagery, graded exercise, and pacing (low back pain). Groups of 7 to 13 participants in each group. Team included clinical psychologist, OT, PT, pain nurse specialist, pharmacist (when needed), rheumatologist, and dietitian.

continued

Table 8-2 (continued)
OCCUPATIONAL THERAPY INTERVENTIONS PROMOTING PHYSICAL OUTCOMES

Author (Date)	Pop	DX	Setting	Intervention
Occupational Development				
Sterner, Y., Lofgren, M., Nyberg, V., Karlsson, A. K., Bergstrom, M., & Gerdle, B. (2001)	5	20	4	Rehabilitation program included ergonomics, physical activity including hydrotherapy, body awareness therapy, relaxation, education in pain, pharmacology, stress, psychological consequences of pain, and meetings in the workplace. The program had cognitive and behavioral components and was based on problem-based learning. **Intervention:** Included examination and treatment from physician, PT, OT, and social worker/psychologist.
Richards, S. H., Coast, J., Gunnell, D. J., Peters, T. J., Pounsford, J., & Darlow, M. A. (1998)	4	3, 17, 18	3, 4	**Intervention:** Home intervention team with a nurse coordinator, RN, PT, OT, support worker, and OT technician. **Control:** Hospital care ward receiving usual hospital care.
Hildebrandt, J., Pfingsten, M., Saur, P., & Jansen, J. (1997)	5	20	4	Pre-program (education, stretching, and callisthenic exercises over 3 weeks). Then, intensive treatment period (physical exercises, back school education, cognitive behavioral group therapy, relaxation training, OT, socioeconomic, and vocational counseling) for 5 weeks. [low back pain]

Population: 1=geriatric (65+); 2=adult (25 to 64); 3=young adult (18 to 24); 4=adult and geriatric; 5=young adult, adult, and geriatric.

Diagnosis: 3=stroke; 4=Parkinson's disease; 5=multiple sclerosis; 6=spinal cord injury; 7=acquired brain injury; 9=burns; 10=amputations; 16=upper extremity injury; 17=lower extremity; 18=other; 19=arthritis; 20=chronic pain; 21=no diagnosis; 22=joint injury (includes fracture and arthroplasty of hip and knee); 24=frail elderly, at-risk older adults, older adult acute hospital intake, acute inpatient geriatric admission; 26=cardiac conditions; 27=chronic obstructive pulmonary disease.

Setting: 1=long-term care; 2=acute care; 3=home care; 4=rehabilitation; 5=primary care.

Table 8-3

EVIDENCE OF EFFECTIVENESS OF OCCUPATIONAL THERAPY ON PHYSICAL OUTCOMES

Author (Date)	Major Results	Study Design	Sample Size	Conclusions and Limitations
Positive Effects—Randomized Controlled Trial				
Paes Lourencao, M. I., Battistella, L., Moran de Brito, C. M., Tsukimoto, G. R., & Miyazaki, M. H. (2008)	Significant differences were found between the intervention and control groups in hand function (p=0.02), elbow and wrist movement (p=0.002 and p=0.02, respectively). Improvements were seen between baseline and 6 months (p<0.001 and p=0.002); baseline and 12 months (p<0.001); and 6 and 12 months (p<0.01 and p<0.001). There were no differences between groups on manual dexterity or elbow/wrist spasticity; however, significant improvements over time in these outcomes were observed in both groups.	RCT	59	**Conclusions:** After 6 and 12 months of treatment, OT accompanied by electrical stimulation and biofeedback improved range of motion and UE function in hemiparetic stroke patients significantly more than OT and electrical stimulation alone. Patients in the intervention group also showed a clinically significant reduction in spasticity. **Limitations:** Relatively small sample size could have left this study underpowered to detect small but significant changes caused by the treatment.
Spadaro, A., De Luca, T., Massimiani, M., Ceccarelli, F., Riccieri, V., & Valesini, G. (2008)	The intervention group demonstrated significantly more improvement in functional ability (p<0.05), disease status (p<0.02), health status (p<0.02), and pain (p<0.02) than the control did. Subjects in the intervention group also reported using more self-management techniques and had higher adherence to treatment in general than the controls.	RCT	27	**Conclusions:** The results of this study show that OT is beneficial for patients with ankylosing spondylitis, especially in the reduction of pain and disability and the improvement of function. **Limitations:** Results of this study are limited by the small sample size, short duration of the study, and lack of follow-up.
Lannin, N., Clemson, L., McCluskey, A., Lin, C., Cameron, I., & Barras, S. (2007)	Aside from the FIM, all other outcome measures showed improvement over 3 months. ADL scores in the intervention group were higher at 2 weeks (p=0.012) and at 2 months (p=0.003). At 2 weeks and 2 and 3 months, a greater proportion of study subjects reported being able to leave the house (from 30% at baseline to 57%); however, there were no significant differences between the 2 groups. Community support levels decreased similarly in both groups, only 1 participant was re-admitted to hospital during follow-up, and 3 participants (2 controls and 1 intervention) reported falls during the follow-up period.	RCT	10	**Conclusions:** Clinically significant differences were found between the intervention and control groups especially in ADL scores. The study also showed that a randomized controlled trial comparing home visits vs. in-hospital assessment is feasible and possible to complete with a high methodological quality. **Limitations:** The study sample size was very small and experienced high attrition rate (20%) so the authors had to interpret their results very conservatively.

continued

Table 8-3 (continued)

EVIDENCE OF EFFECTIVENESS OF OCCUPATIONAL THERAPY ON PHYSICAL OUTCOMES

Author (Date)	Major Results	Study Design	Sample Size	Conclusions and Limitations
Positive Effects—Randomized Controlled Trial				
Masiero, S., Boniolo, A., Wassermann, L., Machiedo, H., Volante, D., & Punzi, L. (2007)	Significant improvements in functional status (p=0.01) were observed in the intervention group at follow-up while the control group demonstrated mild non-significant deterioration. Arthritis Impact Scale showed that the intervention group experienced significant improvements in the symptoms, social interaction, and physical function domains (p=0.02; p=0.04; p=0.05), but there was no significant change in the work and psychological dimensions (p=0.31; p=0.19). The control group demonstrated a slight downward trend over all the subscales (p values ranged from 0.36 to 0.64). Patients in the intervention also had significantly lower pain scores than control. Within-group analysis of the intervention subjects showed that the amount of exercise completed at home did not have an impact on any outcomes.	RCT	70	**Conclusions:** This study showed that patients with mild to moderate rheumatoid arthritis benefited from attending an education-behavioral joint protection program. They exhibited less disability, reported lower pain levels, implemented more self-management strategies, and had an overall better health status than control. The effects of the program were also maintained over an 8-month follow-up period. **Limitations:** During this study, physiological data on disease status that could have given insight on increased pain and disability in patients were not included in the final analysis for either group. Also, there was no immediate post-intervention assessment so certain trends in the data may have been missed at the 8-month follow-up, and the study did not include objective measures of disability like dexterity level and variation in range of motion.
Stenvall, M., Olofsson, B., Lundstrom, M., Englund, U., Borssen, B., Svensson, O., et al. (2007)	Fall incidence was significantly lower in the intervention group (p=0.006) as was fall rate (p=0.008). The fall risk, expressed as the time to the first fall, was significantly lower in the intervention as well (p=0.012). There were 3 mild or moderate injuries caused by falls in the intervention group compared to 15 in the control. There were also fewer postoperative complications in the intervention group, and they had a shorter average hospital stay.	RCT	199	**Conclusions:** Results of this study show that the number of falls, fall risk, and risk of postoperative complications can be greatly reduced in elderly patients after femoral neck fracture by a multidisciplinary geriatric care program. **Limitations:** A number of falls may have been missed by staff on the wards and not reported and the collection of fall data could not be blinded according to allocation.
Gitlin, L., Hauck, W., Winter, L., Dennis, M., & Schulz, R. (2006)	There was significantly less mortality among vulnerable seniors in the experimental group (p=0.003). Experimental group was significantly more likely to make home and behavioral modifications (p=0.003).	RCT	390	**Conclusions:** There was significantly less mortality among frail elderly receiving in-home intervention. **Limitations:** Volunteer bias, possibility of contamination, no psychometric properties of outcome measures reported, difficult to determine when outcome measures were used in the study.

continued

Table 8-3 (continued)
EVIDENCE OF EFFECTIVENESS OF OCCUPATIONAL THERAPY ON PHYSICAL OUTCOMES

Author (Date)	Major Results	Study Design	Sample Size	Conclusions and Limitations
Positive Effects—Randomized Controlled Trial				
Pang, M., Harris, J., & Eng, J. (2006)	Significant improvements in motor function for intervention group (p=0.003 to 0.001) over time and when compared to control. There were no significant changes in grip strength or motor activity. Patients classified as mildly impaired at baseline had significant improvement in functional usage of the paretic arm but no change in grip strength. Moderately impaired patients had significant improvement in all outcomes. Severely impaired patients showed improvement in level of impairment and usage of the paretic arm only.	RCT	60	**Conclusions:** The results of this study show that a community-based exercise program is feasible and effective in improving functional ability and usage of paretic UEs in stroke patients. **Limitations:** Baseline differences between the intervention and control groups and an underpowered sample size weaken the results of the study.
Davsion, J., Bond, J., Dawson, P., Steen, I. N., & Kenny, R. A. (2005)	Number of falls in intervention group was reduced by 36% (p<0.05). Proportion of subjects who fell did not change significantly. Falls efficacy was significantly better in intervention group at 1 year (p<0.05). No difference in number of hospital admissions resulting from falls; however, duration of hospital stay was significantly shorter in intervention group (0.8 days vs. 4.5; p<0.05).	RCT	282	**Conclusions:** Multidisciplinary intervention in cognitively intact older adults who were recurrent fallers was successful in reducing the fall burden on individuals, but did not reduce the number who continued to fall. Intervention group also experienced a greater reduction in "fear of falling." **Limitations:** Lack of comparable data regarding fall risk factors for control group. The control group also experienced significant contamination as 21% of subjects received some kind of specialist falls assessment or intervention. Design of study prevents identification of effects of any single intervention on the outcomes.
Mathiowetz, V. G., Finlayson, M. L., Matuska, K. M., Chen, H. Y., & Luo, P. (2005)	Significant increase in some subscales of the SF-36 (p<0.01), significant decrease in fatigue impact (p<0.001), a significant increase in self-efficacy (p<0.001).	RCT	169	**Conclusions:** The results support the use of energy conservation courses as non-pharmacological approaches to managing fatigue in people with multiple sclerosis. **Limitations:** Attrition was high and reasons not provided.

continued

Table 8-3 (continued)

EVIDENCE OF EFFECTIVENESS OF OCCUPATIONAL THERAPY ON PHYSICAL OUTCOMES

Author (Date)	Major Results	Study Design	Sample Size	Conclusions and Limitations
Positive Effects—Randomized Controlled Trial				
Pagnotta, A., Korner-Bitensky, N., Mazer, B., Baron, M., & Wood-Dauphinee, S. (2005)	Pain was significantly decreased on 3 work performance tasks with splint (p<0.05). Work performance did not vary significantly for any task with or without splint use. 5 of 14 tasks were reported to be less difficult while wearing a splint.	RCT	30	***Conclusions:*** Commercially available working wrist splints subjectively decrease task difficulty and generally reduce pain without negatively affecting work performance. ***Limitations:*** Small sample size; length of time participant had previously worn splint was not recorded or analyzed (affects validity if a practice effect exists).
Studenski, S., Duncan, P., Perera, S., Reker, D., Lai, S. M., & Richards, L. (2005)	Intervention group experienced significantly greater improvement than control in all domains including some scales of the SF-36 and SIS. However, at 6 months of follow-up, the benefits of the intervention were no longer observed due to continued recovery in the control group.	RCT	80	***Conclusions:*** A structured exercise intervention administered to patients during the sub-acute phase of stroke recovery produced accelerated gains in functional ability and quality of life but the effects of the intervention had dissipated by 6 months. ***Limitations:*** Patients could not be blinded to treatment allocation, and the majority of outcome measures were self-reported so knowledge of treatment could have biased responders. Participants in the intervention group also had substantially more contact with the researchers and therapists.
Hammond, A., & Freeman, K. (2004)	Intervention group experienced statistically significant improvement in joint protection behavior (p=0.001) and early morning stiffness (p=0.001).	RCT	107	***Conclusions:*** Educational-behavioral training is more effective than standard training in improving joint protection adherence; and joint protection can help maintain functional ability in early rheumatoid arthritis. ***Limitations:*** Possible floor effect for primary outcome measure (AIMS-2); the design did not include a no-treatment control group; possible volunteer bias from the selected sample based on the willingness of participation.
WaiShan Louie, S. (2004)	There was a statistically significant (p<0.05) increase in partial percentage of oxygen saturation in the treatment group using guided imagery for COPD.	RCT	26	***Conclusions:*** Exploring psychological effects of guided imagery can be helpful. Personal traits and individualized coping styles should be considered when planning to use imagery relaxation as an intervention. ***Limitations:*** Convenience sample.

continued

Table 8-3 (continued)

EVIDENCE OF EFFECTIVENESS OF OCCUPATIONAL THERAPY ON PHYSICAL OUTCOMES

Author (Date)	Major Results	Study Design	Sample Size	Conclusions and Limitations
Positive Effects—Randomized Controlled Trial				
Hammond, A., Jefferson, P., Jones, N., Gallagher, J., & Jones, T. (2002)	Joint protection adherence increased after the intervention (p=0.001). At 6 months post-intervention, there was less adherence.	RCT	30	**Conclusions:** OTs providing "Looking After Your Joints" program can help clients improve use of joint protection techniques. **Limitations:** Small sample size; psychometric properties of assessments not stated.
Hammond, A., & Freeman, K. (2001)	The intervention group scores improved or were maintained, and control group maintained or worsened. Most statistically significant results for intervention group were decrease in hand pain (p=0.001) and decrease in morning stiffness (p=0.01).	RCT	107	**Conclusions:** The study provides support for the use of joint protection programs that follow an educational-behavioral approach. **Limitations:** Possible floor effect for primary outcome measure (AIMS-2).
Ozdemir, F., Birtane, M., Tabatabaei, R., Kokino, S., & Ekuklu, G. (2001)	Significantly less time for rehabilitation in hospitalized group vs. home treatment group. Significantly better results for hospitalized group with motor status, functional independence, and cognitive status (p<0.05), but no significant differences in spasticity.	RCT	60	**Conclusions:** Clients with strokes do better on initial rehabilitation as inpatients rather than outpatients. **Limitations:** Interventions were not well-described; dropout rates not accounted for; follow-up time not standard for all clients; heterogeneous population (significantly difference of ages between groups).
Griffiths, T., Burr, M., Campbell, I., Lewis-Jenkins, V., Mullins, J., Shiels, K., et al. (2000)	COPD patients spent significantly fewer days in the hospital in experimental group (p=0.02). Intervention group made more visits to primary care (p=0.003) and had fewer primary care home visits (p=0.037). Lower rates of inhaler use (p=0.004) and oral medication (p=0.045) by the intervention group. Intervention group had greater improvements in walking ability and in general and disease-specific health status.	RCT	180	**Conclusions:** Overall, there was some evidence that 1-year follow-up in outpatient rehab was effective, but this was limited. **Limitations:** Missing data excluded from results; all outcome measures were not used at same point in study.
Nelson, D. L., Konosky, K., Fleharty, K., Webb, R., Newer, K., Hazboun, V. P., et al. (1996)	The experimental group was able to complete significantly more handle rotations than the control group (p<0.05).	RCT	26	**Conclusions:** The occupationally embedded exercise is more effective in increasing supination in clients with hemiplegia. **Limitations:** Small sample size; possible confounding variables; outcome measure does not have psychometric properties and is not related to functional performance; method of recruiting participants not indicated.

continued

Table 8-3 (continued)

EVIDENCE OF EFFECTIVENESS OF OCCUPATIONAL THERAPY ON PHYSICAL OUTCOMES

Author (Date)	Major Results	Study Design	Sample Size	Conclusions and Limitations
Positive Effects—Randomized Controlled Trial				
Yuen, H. K., Nelson, D. L., Peterson, C. Q., & Dickinson, A. (1994)	The experimental group scored significantly better on object-oriented prosthesis control (p=0.02).	RCT	52	***Conclusions:*** Object-oriented motor training is more effective than non-object-oriented motor training. ***Limitations:*** Results may have demonstrated a practice effect in treatment group.
Positive Effects—Non-Randomized Controlled Trial				
Rosenstein, L., Ridgel, A., Thota, A., Samame, B., & Alberts, J. (2008)	The patient displayed slight improvement in 4 tasks of the WMFT including lifting the forearm to a table, extending elbows to the side, reaching and retrieving, and lifting a basket. There was no change in the remaining tasks. She also displayed a 3-point improvement on the FMA specifically positive improvements in dysmetria, tremor, and finger flexion. Mild improvements in elbow flexor tone and range of movement in the shoulder, arm, and wrist were observed.	Non-RCT	1	***Conclusions:*** A robotically enforced regimen of repetitive task practice improved this patient's UE motor function and functional performance in tasks of daily living. ***Limitations:*** Due to the fact that this study was a case report, it is impossible to determine the individual effects of the repetitive task training or use of the Hand Mentor.
Matuska, K., Mathiowetz, V., & Finlayson, M. (2007)	All of the energy conservation strategies listed on the survey (14 total) were identified by respondents as effective (range of 7.0 to 8.2 on a 10-point scale). The strategies most implemented after the course (used by 70% of respondents) related to changing body position, planning for rest periods, adjusted priorities, reduced frequency of or simplified work, and communicated need for assistance. Among those respondents who did not report using these techniques, the primary reason for not doing so was because they already used these methods. The energy conservation strategies used least (51% or fewer of participants) were changed time of day of activity and used adaptive equipment. The primary reason for not employing these techniques was because they were already being used but 13% of respondents said they didn't use adaptive equipment because there were unsure of what to use or could not use it.	Non-RCT	123	***Conclusions:*** This study shows that people with multiple sclerosis who attended a structured group-based energy conservation course were able to successfully implement the techniques they were taught and perceived them to be effective. ***Limitations:*** The survey used in this study was self-reported, and no additional data were used, so it is unknown if participants were accurate reporters of their behavior. Participants who did not complete the course did not complete the survey, thus the results of this study may only be applicable to more motivated individuals who are willing to learn and implement new strategies.

continued

Table 8-3 (continued)
EVIDENCE OF EFFECTIVENESS OF OCCUPATIONAL THERAPY ON PHYSICAL OUTCOMES

Author (Date)	Major Results	Study Design	Sample Size	Conclusions and Limitations
Positive Effects—Non-Randomized Controlled Trial				
van der Giesen, F. J., Nelissen, R., Rozing, P., Arendzen, J., de Jong, Z., Wolterbeek, R., et al. (2007)	Patients who completed the recommended treatments showed a trend toward improvement in all outcomes except for range of motion and hand pain/stiffness. Improvements in MHQ scores and grip strength reached statistical significance (p<0.005 and p=0.01, respectively). There were no significant differences in the outcome measures between groups that underwent surgical treatment, conservative treatment, or both.	Non-RCT	69	***Conclusions:*** Approximately two-thirds of the patients followed treatment recommendations, which resulted in significant improvement in the majority of patients. ***Limitations:*** The study involved a small number of people with a variety of rheumatic conditions and a wide range of impairments at baseline. Also, the comparisons among the patients who received different types of treatment were conducted with very small groups, making it difficult to draw reliable conclusions.
Von Renteln-Kruse, W., & Krause, T. (2007)	There was a significant reduction in falls after the program was introduced from 893 to 468 (IRR=0.82; 95% CI 0.73 to 0.92; p<0.001). The rate of falls per 1000 hospital days also decreased significantly from 10 to 8.2 (p<0.001); however, there was no significant reduction in the total number of falls that caused injuries. In general, patients who fell had lower BI scores on admission and more men than women experienced falls. The number of falls was lower in those with higher BI scores on admission but, regardless of baseline mobility, the proportion of fallers was lower after the intervention was introduced.	Non-RCT	7253	***Conclusions:*** The introduction of a structured fall-prevention program into a clinical setting that already specialized in multidisciplinary geriatric care was highly effective in reducing the number of falls and the relative risk of falling. There was also a slight non-significant decline in the number of fall-related injuries. ***Limitations:*** The use of a historical control means there may be some confounding factors that were unaccounted for and may have caused an overestimation effect.

continued

Table 8-3 (continued)

EVIDENCE OF EFFECTIVENESS OF OCCUPATIONAL THERAPY ON PHYSICAL OUTCOMES

Author (Date)	Major Results	Study Design	Sample Size	Conclusions and Limitations
Positive Effects—Non-Randomized Controlled Trial				
Ip, W. M., Woo, J., Yue, S. Y., Kwan, M., Sum, S. M., Kwok, T., et al. (2006)	A significant inverse correlation was found between age and energy expenditure on all tasks regardless of the implementation of energy conservation techniques. Similar relationships were found between body mass index and energy expenditure. Use of labor-saving equipment (carrying groceries in a cart vs. a bag) resulted in significantly less energy expenditure in younger subjects (<60) as well as lower heart rate and less feeling of fatigue but it took longer to complete the task. In comparison, elderly subjects (>60) also had a reduced heart rate and less increase in blood pressure and fatigue but there was no difference in overall energy expenditure or time to complete the task. The workstation set-up and avoidance of overhead reaching techniques resulted in slightly less fatigue and shorter time required to complete the task in young and old subjects but none of the changes were significant.	Non-RCT	108	***Conclusions:*** The use of labor-saving equipment was the only clinically effective energy conservation technique and showed the biggest improvement in young subjects. ***Limitations:*** The ergonomics and efficiency of movement of the subjects while completing the tasks were not investigated and could have had an impact on energy expenditure. Also, the activity background of the subjects was not examined and could have been a confounding factor.
Wennemer, H. K., Borg-Stein, J., Gomba, L., Delaney, B., Rothmund, A., Barlow, D., et al. (2006)	After participating in the rehabilitation program, patients demonstrated significant improvement in physical functioning (p=0.01) and a trend toward improvement in disease status (p=0.40) and general health (p=0.14) that did not reach significance. There were significant improvements in range of motion both in the back and lower body (values range from p<0.001 to p<0.05) and in the distance traveled during the 6MWT (p<0.001).	Non-RCT	20	***Conclusions:*** A functionally oriented exercise and education program for fibromyalgia patients was effective in significantly improving physical function, flexibility, and endurance and in slightly improving perceived impairment and disability. The program was also well-tolerated and well-received by patients. ***Limitations:*** The absence of a control group leaves the possibility of a placebo effect.

continued

Table 8-3 (continued)

EVIDENCE OF EFFECTIVENESS OF OCCUPATIONAL THERAPY ON PHYSICAL OUTCOMES

Author (Date)	Major Results	Study Design	Sample Size	Conclusions and Limitations
Positive Effects—Non-Randomized Controlled Trial				
Aldehag, A. S., Jonsson, H., & Ansved, T. (2005)	There was a significant increase in muscle force in the wrist and finger flexors and extensors with the exception of the finger extensors of the left hand. 2 of the 5 participants demonstrated an improvement in grip force and pinch force but no significant differences were found in the overall analysis. However, individual and group analysis showed improvement in both fine motor control and self-rated performance of occupational task. 4 of the 5 participants also reported higher satisfaction with performance of occupational tasks, but none of the patients changed their level of self-rated myotonia.	Non-RCT	5	**Conclusions:** The findings of the study show that a 3-month hand-training program is safe and effective in improving muscle strength and hand function for patients with myotonic dystrophy type I. **Limitations:** Results of this study need to be confirmed in a larger sample of myotonic dystrophy patients and the possible long-term benefits of the exercise program must be investigated as well.
Dohnke, B., Knauper, B., & Muller-Fahrnow, W. (2005)	Patients were admitted to the inpatient rehabilitation program on average 3 weeks after surgery and stayed for 22.6 days. Results show that, upon discharge, patients had significantly lower scores (p<0.001) in pain, disability, and depressive symptoms. Significant increases (p<0.001) in self-efficacy related to pain management and compensating for disability were also found at discharge. Further analysis showed that high self-efficacy and confidence in the ability to recover were significant predictors of less pain, disability, and depressive symptoms. Results at 6 months of follow-up showed a continued significant decrease in disability (p<0.01) and a significant increase (p<0.01) in depressive symptoms; however, pain levels remained consistent (p=0.10). Levels of all 3 remained lower than admission scores at the 6-month follow-up.	Non-RCT	769	**Conclusions:** The results of this study show that a multidisciplinary rehabilitation program not specifically targeted to improve self-efficacy was still effective in improving self-efficacy and improved self-efficacy led to better physical and emotional health in patients. **Limitations:** When the patients who dropped out of the study and those who remained were compared, it was shown that the patients who dropped out were generally younger and significantly more affected by their pain and emotional status. Also, the variables that may have explained the health-promoting benefits of increased self-efficacy were not examined.

continued

Table 8-3 (continued)

EVIDENCE OF EFFECTIVENESS OF OCCUPATIONAL THERAPY ON PHYSICAL OUTCOMES

Author (Date)	Major Results	Study Design	Sample Size	Conclusions and Limitations
Positive Effects—Non-Randomized Controlled Trial				
Malcus-Johnson, P., Carlqvist, C., Sturesson, A., & Eberhardt, K. (2005)	The majority of hand impairment as measured by SOFI had already occurred at the start of the study (mean disease duration 1 year); however, the deterioration in function over the course of the study (10 years) was significant ($p<0.001$). Grip strength increased significantly ($p<0.001$) during the first year of the study and remained stable throughout. At follow-up, 101 of the patients had developed hand deformities, and mean activity scores had increased significantly (0.2 units; $p<0.001$).	Non-RCT	168	**Conclusions:** OT is important and beneficial to patients with rheumatoid arthritis, and regular appointments with an OT at least once a year is a viable option for patients in all stages of the disease. **Limitations:** External validity of the results are limited because all of the subjects included in the study were at a very early stage of the disease when they started (1 year or less post-onset) and received close surveillance throughout the duration of the study.
Pizzi, A., Carlucci, G., Falsini, C., Verdesca, S., & Grippo, A. (2005)	Mean splint use was 110 minutes a day. Statistically significant gains in wrist passive range of motion ($p<0.001$). Statistically significant decrease in elbow MAS scores ($p<0.002$). Statistically significant decrease on PSFS scores ($p<0.01$). Statistically significant H-Reflex:M response ratio ($p<0.01$).	Non-RCT	40	**Conclusions:** A static resting splint produces statistically significant benefits for patients with hemiplegia secondary to CVA. **Limitations:** No control group; potentially non-compliant participants were excluded from follow-up; dropouts not included in statistical analysis; no procedure to minimize contamination or co-intervention.
Ring, H., & Rosenthal, N. (2005)	No statistical significance for improvement in active motion between groups for patients without voluntary motion at baseline. Patients with voluntary motion at baseline showed significant improvements in wrist flexion, and neuroprosthesis group showed greater improvements in shoulder flexion ($p=0.03$), wrist extension ($p=0.02$), and wrist flexion ($p=0.04$). Neuroprosthesis group has significantly greater improvement in all functional hand tests ($p<0.05$). All neuroprosthesis participants improved in pain and edema.	Non-RCT	22	**Conclusions:** Some positive results indicated that daily home neuroprosthetic activation may be beneficial for stroke clients with hemiplegia. **Limitations:** No follow-up assessment to determine if results are maintained; small sample sizes.

continued

Table 8-3 (continued)

EVIDENCE OF EFFECTIVENESS OF OCCUPATIONAL THERAPY ON PHYSICAL OUTCOMES

Author (Date)	Major Results	Study Design	Sample Size	Conclusions and Limitations
Positive Effects—Non-Randomized Controlled Trial				
Haskett, S., Backman, C., Porter, B., Goyert, J., & Palejko, G. (2004)	Pain significantly reduced (p=0.007) compared with baseline. All 3 splints improved perceived wrist pain but only the change in the leather splint was statistically significant. Grip strength, 2- and 3-point pinch strength, aggregate applied dexterity, and pouring water were significantly improved from baseline (p<0.02). Each of the 3 splints significantly improved these variables compared with baseline. The Rolyan resulted in significantly stronger grip than the Anatech splint (p=0.04).	Non-RCT	45	**Conclusions:** After 4 weeks' use, wrist splints reduce pain, improve strength, and do not compromise dexterity. The leather and Rolyan splint had similar improvements and were superior to the Anatech splint. **Limitations:** Contamination and co-intervention were accounted for in procedure; all subjects were from a specialized arthritis treatment center; psychometric properties for outcomes not reported.
Mendelsohn, M. E., Overend, T. J., & Petrella, R. J. (2004)	Significant difference in proprioception from admission to discharge in injured knee (p<0.042) and injured hip (p<0.001). At discharge, significant differences between injured and non-injured hip (p=0.003) and knee (p<0.001). Significant increase from admission to discharge for BBS, FIM, gait speed, and 30-second chair stand. A significant decrease TUG (p<0.05), absolute angular error decreased significantly from admission to discharge in hip flexion and knee extension on injured side (p<0.05).	Non-RCT	40	**Conclusions:** The findings of the study show that there is a statistically significant increase in hip and knee proprioception in the injured limb as a result of rehabilitation. **Limitations:** Poor description of control group, intervention not described in detail, no randomization, no psychometric properties of outcome measures reported, no follow-up measures.
Sandqvist, G., Akesson, A., & Eklund, M. (2004)	At the follow-up, finger flexion and extension (p<0.01), thumb abduction (p<0.05), volar flexion in the wrist (p<0.05), and perceived stiffness and skin elasticity (both p<0.001) had improved significantly in the paraffin-treated hand compared with the baseline values. Improved hand function was independent of skin score and disease duration. Function improvements were significantly greater in the hands treated with paraffin bath and exercise than hands undergoing exercise only concerning extension deficit, perceived stiffness, and skin elasticity.	Non-RCT	17	**Conclusions:** Improvements in function were significantly greater in the hand that was treated with paraffin bath and exercise than in the hand treated with exercise only concerning extension deficit, perceived stiffness, and skin elasticity. **Limitations:** Not effective controls based on hand dominance and possible bias, small sample, no procedure to monitor compliance of exercises bilaterally.

continued

Table 8-3 (continued)
Evidence of Effectiveness of Occupational Therapy on Physical Outcomes

Author (Date)	Major Results	Study Design	Sample Size	Conclusions and Limitations
Positive Effects—Non-Randomized Controlled Trial				
Tsuji, T., Liu, M., Hase, K., Masakado, Y., Takahashi, H., Hara, Y., et al. (2004)	Metabolic function showed no significant improvements. Significant improvements in paresis/ADL, muscular function, and cardiopulmonary function ($p<0.05$).	Non-RCT	107	**Conclusions:** The study found that fitness in this population can be categorized into ADL/paresis, muscular function, metabolic function, and cardiopulmonary function. Overall, the clinical message is that emphasis should be placed on fitness promotion. **Limitations:** Measurement at discharge time was variable before and after study; many outcome measures.
Walsh, D. A., Kelly, S. J., Johnson, P. S., Rajkumar, S., & Bennetts, K. (2004)	Significant improvements in all outcomes ($p<0.05$).	Non-RCT	101	**Conclusions:** The study found that all outcomes measured were statistically improved, and self-reported improvements in performance and satisfaction are associated with observed improvement in performance and increased self-efficacy. **Limitations:** Heterogeneous population; no procedure accounting for possible co-intervention.
Case-Smith, J. (2003)	Significant ($p<0.001$) improvements for COPM. Significant ($p<0.001$) improvements in ADL ability and pain reduction. Significant improvement in physical health ($p=0.003$), physical roles ($p<0.001$), pain ($p<0.001$), and social participation ($p<0.001$) according to SF-36, but not general health.	Non-RCT	33	**Conclusions:** Clients with UE injury or surgery made strong, positive gains in functional measures following client-centered OT services. The COPM was the most sensitive to change, then the DASH, and then the SF-36. **Limitations:** Small sample size, interventions were named but not described.
Fischer, T., Nagy, L., & Buechler, U. (2003)	Improvement of overall functional performance from preop to postop of an average of 4 points on VAS. All 9 patients returned to their previous occupations (1 could not work preoperatively). 6 adductor pollicis and 6 first dorsal interosseus transfers were strong and produced good function. Key pinch strength doubled following the transfers in 3 cases. Wrist extension had a mean torque that was 96% of the force of the opposite wrist.	Non-RCT	9	**Conclusions:** After tendon transfers for ulnar paralysis, there were improvements in overall function, return to work, and wrist extension strength. **Limitations:** Contamination and co-intervention procedures were not reported, all participants were recruited from the same location, psychometric properties of outcome measures were not reported.

continued

Table 8-3 (continued)
EVIDENCE OF EFFECTIVENESS OF OCCUPATIONAL THERAPY ON PHYSICAL OUTCOMES

Author (Date)	Major Results	Study Design	Sample Size	Conclusions and Limitations
Positive Effects—Non-Randomized Controlled Trial				
Sandin-Aldehag, A., & Jonsson, H. (2003)	Statistically significant improvement in muscle strength scores for left hands (p=0.01) only. Statistically significant gains for right pinch grip strength (p=0.04). Statistically significant difference for 4 subjects in MCP joint extension (p=0.04) of the right index finger and for 6 patients in PIP joint extension (p=0.02) of same finger. Statistically significant improvement on ADL scale (p=0.01). No significant change on the life satisfaction checklist.	Non-RCT	11	***Conclusions:*** Specific interventions may be beneficial in restoring hand function for people affected with neuromuscular diseases. ***Limitations:*** No procedural control for contamination or co-intervention; no control group; small sample size; standardized outcome measures were modified without validation; limited description of intervention.
Donnelly, C. J., & Wilton, J. (2002)	Significant increases in active range of motion for both control and treatment group (p=0.003). Massage group had significantly more active range of motion than control group (p=0.023). Significant improvement in skin glide for both control (p=0.011) and treatment (p=0.046) groups. No significant difference between the groups for skin glide. No observable linear relationship between duration of massage and improvement in active range of motion and skin mobility.	Non-RCT	22	***Conclusions:*** Massage in conjunction with hand therapy does improve active range of motion and not skin mobility. ***Limitations:*** Treatment was not uniform across participants within each group; small sample size; heterogeneous between group diagnoses and overall range of motion at baseline.
Mathiowetz, V., Matuska, K. M., & Murphy, M. E. (2001)	Impact of fatigue decreased after intervention and was maintained 6 weeks after (p<0.01), a medium increase in self-efficacy (p<0.01), significant improvement of SF-36 subscales: Vitality, social functioning, and mental health (p<0.01).	Non-RCT	54	***Conclusions:*** The results provide strong evidence for the efficacy the program. ***Limitations:*** Follow-up period post-intervention short (6 weeks) to measure longer term effects; participants were self-selected.
Shechtman, O., Hanson, C. S., Garrett, D., & Dunn, P. (2001)	The ROHO high and low cushions were the most effective at relieving pressure for both the high and average body mass index participants (p<0.05). The ROHO high and low cushions were scored as the most comfortable (p=0.002).	Non-RCT	40	***Conclusions:*** The air-filled ROHO cushions were the most effective for reducing pressure, a clinically significant finding. ***Limitations:*** Sample selection not randomized; seating did not take into account individualized needs of participant; researchers not blinded to cushion type.

continued

Table 8-3 (continued)

EVIDENCE OF EFFECTIVENESS OF OCCUPATIONAL THERAPY ON PHYSICAL OUTCOMES

Author (Date)	Major Results	Study Design	Sample Size	Conclusions and Limitations
Positive Effects—Non-Randomized Controlled Trial				
Sterner, Y., Lofgren, M., Nyberg, V., Karlsson, A. K., Bergstrom, M., & Gerdle, B. (2001)	Pain intensity in neck and upper back were significantly decreased at follow-up (p=0.018; p=0.011). Indication of satisfaction with program through questionnaire and interview. Increased ability to cope and control pain (p=0.039 for distraction behavioral response on MPI). No significant change in other outcomes measured.	Non-RCT	90	*Conclusions:* Some positive effects for the program were seen retrospectively, although these results do not differ greatly from the prospective data of the same programs. *Limitations:* No control group, intervention not described in detail, programs conducted in various centers and varied in amount of time.
Jarus, T., Shavit, S., & Ratzon, N. (2000)	Range of motion indicated a significant linear main effect for time. Participants improved range of motion from before treatment to 5 weeks post-treatment. Grip strength indicated a significant linear main effect for time. Participants improved from before treatment to 5 weeks post-treatment. Edema indicated a significant linear main effect for time. Decrease in the edema for all participants from one initial to follow-up. Significant difference between the 2 treatment groups (low tech and high tech).	Non-RCT	47	*Conclusions:* The computer-aided group showed significantly more interest in treatment than did the brush machine group. The potential for more interesting motor treatment and rehabilitation of the wrist through the use of computer games is there. *Limitations:* Dropouts were not reported; brief duration of therapy may explain the lack of differences between the 2 treatment groups; psychometric properties of outcome measures not reported; intervention details were not adequate to reproduce it; sample size small to detect differences in the 2 treatment groups.
Bailey, A., Starr, L., Alderson, M., & Moreland, J. (1999)	Clinically significant improvements in all disability measures (largest with COPM). Statistically significant improvement in aerobic fitness, upper body strength, flexibility, abdominal strength, pain, self-efficacy, and disability (by FIQ, COPM, F-COPES) (p<0.001 for all). No significant difference in grip strength.	Non-RCT	149	*Conclusions:* Results showed significant changes in almost all outcomes investigated and stated that improvement in overall disability was clinically significant. *Limitations:* Intervention not described well enough to be reproduced; profession-specific intervention not described.

continued

Table 8-3 (continued)

EVIDENCE OF EFFECTIVENESS OF OCCUPATIONAL THERAPY ON PHYSICAL OUTCOMES

Author (Date)	Major Results	Study Design	Sample Size	Conclusions and Limitations
Positive Effects—Non-Randomized Controlled Trial				
Li, S., Liu, L., Miyazaki, M., & Warren, S. (1999)	Out of 22 subjects (29 hands), 77% had reduced symptom severity, 73% showed improvement in functional status. 23% and 27% of hands did not show improvement in symptoms and function, respectively. Statistically significant decrease in symptom severity after splinting (F=19.03, p<0.001) and in overall functional status improvement post-splinting (F=7.02, p<0.001). 3 months post-splinting: 68% showed significant decrease in symptom severity and 36% showed significant improvement in functional status.	Non-RCT	22	***Conclusions:*** Splinting for 3 months was effective in relieving carpal tunnel syndrome symptoms and improved functional status for subjects in the study. ***Limitations:*** No control group; convenient sample from 1 hospital; long-term follow-up was set up due to time constraints only; small sample size; outcomes were evaluated based on self-reported questionnaire.
Hildebrandt, J., Pfingsten, M., Saur, P., & Jansen, J. (1997)	Significant improvement in flexibility, strength, lifting capacity, and endurance measurements (p<0.001) by the end of treatment for experimental group. Pain, disability, depression, and psycho-vegetative reports reduced in experimental group (p<0.001); experimental group reported significant increase in activity levels at home; self-evaluation for predicting a return to work, length of absence from work, application for pension, decrease in disability after treatment (p<0.05).	Non-RCT	90	***Conclusions:*** There is evidence that this program is effective for the low back pain population. ***Limitations:*** Psychometric properties of outcomes measures not reported; poor description of outcome measures; no control group.
Hoppes, S. (1997)	The effect of treatment was analyzed using a Wilcoxon signed-ranks test. "From the standard normal probability table, we find that the probability of an observation Sn being this large is than 1%. Therefore, we can safely reject the null hypothesis, and conclude that tolerance with play is significantly greater than tolerance without play. The analysis indicated that game-playing increases standing tolerance significantly" (significance level 0.01).	Non-RCT	10	***Conclusions:*** Game-playing was shown to increase standing tolerance for participants in the study. ***Limitations:*** Small, non-randomized sample. In future studies, standardized procedures with a control group and blinded pre- and post-evaluation after treatments based on game playing during standing tolerance is needed.

continued

Table 8-3 (continued)

EVIDENCE OF EFFECTIVENESS OF OCCUPATIONAL THERAPY ON PHYSICAL OUTCOMES

Author (Date)	Major Results	Study Design	Sample Size	Conclusions and Limitations
Positive Effects—Non-Randomized Controlled Trial				
Callinan, N. J., & Mathiowetz, V. (1996)	Arthritis pain was considerably less during both splinted periods when compared with the pre-test (p<0.001). Subjects identified fewer joints as being painful during the soft splint condition than during the unsplinted condition (p<0.05). There were no significant differences among conditions on hand function measures (p<0.001). However, participants were significantly more satisfied with their hand function after splinting (splint preference was 57% for the soft splint, 33% for the hard splint, and 10% for no splint).	Non-RCT	39	***Conclusions:*** Findings indicate that "resting hand splints are effective for pain relief and that persons with rheumatoid arthritis are more likely to prefer and comply with soft splint use for this purpose." ***Limitations:*** Outcomes measures may not be sensitive enough to detect small changes in hand function; short treatment periods may have been too short to see improvements in hand function; no washout periods between treatment conditions, possible carryover effect.
Hsieh, C. L., Nelson, D. L., Smith, D. A., & Peterson, C. Q. (1996)	No significant order effects were found. A significant difference between the 3 conditions was shown (F [2,40]=16.8, p<0.001) with participants performing more repetitions using the added-materials and imagery-based conditions compared to the rote exercise condition.	Non-RCT	21	***Conclusions:*** Difference in exercise performance was not significantly different between the added-materials and imagery-based conditions. ***Limitations:*** Difficult to control variables between participants (e.g., differences in imagining the ball and the difference in level of challenge in hitting the target)
Spalding, N. J. (1995)	The mean and standard deviation were lower for the experimental group as compared to the control group for number of days it took to achieve frame independence (5 ± 2 vs. 7 ± 4) and number of days it took to be discharged from hospital (12 ± 3 vs. 16 ± 5). Participants in the experimental group received fewer OT home visits than the control group.	Non-RCT	41	***Conclusions:*** The length of hospitalization was reduced for people who took part in the education session leading authors to suggest that pre-operative educational programs may have cost-saving benefits. ***Limitations:*** The method was quasi-experimental, a risk to reliability.
Thomas, L. J., & Thomas, B. J. (1995)	All patients had MP joint active range of motion within normal limits for their repaired hands as compared with their unaffected hands. No patient experienced tendon rupture, re-repair, or secondary tendon surgery.	Non-RCT	27	***Conclusions:*** The technique helped to reduce pain and re-establish early hand use. ***Limitations:*** Not a comparative study to a control group.

continued

Table 8-3 (continued)

EVIDENCE OF EFFECTIVENESS OF OCCUPATIONAL THERAPY ON PHYSICAL OUTCOMES

Author (Date)	Major Results	Study Design	Sample Size	Conclusions and Limitations
Positive Effects—Non-Randomized Controlled Trial				
Barry, M. A., Purser, J., Hazleman, R., McLean, A., & Hazleman, B. L. (1994)	Statistically significant improvement of questionnaire scores both 1 and 6 months post-treatment (p<0.001). Scores not influenced by age, gender, or disease duration.	Non-RCT	47	**Conclusions:** OT intervention is effective in improving client knowledge and performance, and this is sustained for at least 6 months. **Limitations:** Reasons for dropouts not reported; outcome measure does not have psychometric properties; intervention was not described in detail, difficult to be reproduced; no justification for the sample size.
Neistadt, M. E. (1994)	Participants in the functional meal preparation group showed significantly greater improvement in dominant hand dexterity for picking up small objects than participants in the tabletop puzzle activity group (F=5.23, p=0.027). Other coordination test results were comparable for the 2 treatment groups.	Non-RCT	45	**Conclusions:** The findings showed that "functional activities may be better than tabletop activities for fine motor coordination with this population." **Limitations:** Co-intervention evident and no procedures to eliminate effects.
King, T. I. (1993)	Dependent t-tests indicated that the mean number of repetitions for the purposeful activity was significantly greater than for the non-purposeful activity for both the grippers (p<0.001) and the pinchers (p<0.05).	Non-RCT	146	**Conclusions:** The use of computer games may be valuable for treatment-related activities like dexterity and range of motion. **Limitations:** Purposeful activity was not chosen by the participant.
Sietsema, J. M., Nelson, D. L., Mulder, R. M., Mervau-Scheidel, D., & White, B. E. (1993)	Range of motion from hip to wrist during active reach of affected arm was significantly higher during the occupationally embedded exercise (p<0.001).	Non-RCT	20	**Conclusions:** Results are clinically significant, and they support the incorporation of occupationally embedded exercise in neurodevelopmental therapy. **Limitations:** Small sample size.
No Effect				
Lannin, N., Cusick, A., McCluskey, A., & Herbert, R. (2007)	Overall, there was high adherence to the splinting program with patients assigned to neutral splints showing slightly higher compliance. On average, all participants experienced a moderate loss of range of motion over the course of the study with splinting having little to no effect. The effects of splinting on all other outcomes were also clinically and statistically insignificant.	RCT	62	**Conclusions:** This study found that an intensive 4-week splinting program did not increase extensibility of the wrist and finger flexor muscles in adult stroke patients and had no impact on arm function and disability as a whole. **Limitations:** Participants were not blinded to allocation, so the possibility of responder bias in some of the subjective measures exists.

continued

Table 8-3 (continued)
EVIDENCE OF EFFECTIVENESS OF OCCUPATIONAL THERAPY ON PHYSICAL OUTCOMES

Author (Date)	Major Results	Study Design	Sample Size	Conclusions and Limitations
No Effect				
Luukinen, H., Lehtola, S., Jokelainen, J., Vaananen-Sainio, R., Lotvonen, S., & Koistinen, P. (2007)	No significant difference was found between intervention and control regarding the number of total falls or the proportion of subjects in each group who fell. Among subjects who were able to move outdoors, the hazard ratios of the first 4 falls were slightly lower in the intervention group, but the difference did not reach significant levels. There were no significant differences between the groups on any of the other outcomes except for a significant improvement in balance that was observed in the intervention group (p<0.05). Use of public health services was roughly equal in both groups, and private health service use was slightly lower in the intervention group.	RCT	358	***Conclusions:*** The implementation of pragmatic home-based exercise was not effective in reducing falls in elderly home-dwelling people but did significantly delay impairment of balance. ***Limitations:*** The positive effects on fall rates demonstrated in the study were determined through secondary outcomes, limiting the validity of the results. There was also a large space of time between the baseline assessments and beginning of the intervention, and the number of falls reported in the intervention group during this period was higher than control.
van Houten, P., Achterberg, W., & Ribbe, M. (2007)	Though it did not reach statistical significance, the intervention resulted in 8% to 35% less urine loss in intervention subjects compared to control. 3 women in the intervention group showed a reduction in urine loss of more than 90%. 6 women were able to move from dependent toileting to independent toileting compared to 2 in the control. The intervention group also showed significant positive improvement on the daytime sum score for the toilet training test under stabilized circumstances while improvement on the night time scores approached but did not reach significance. No significant effect on BI or Prafab scores was observed in either group.	RCT	53	***Conclusions:*** The results show that the intervention was effective in causing a slight positive improvement in the time needed to perform toilet tasks and allowed some participants to achieved independence. However, it was not able to significantly reduce incontinence as a whole. ***Limitations:*** The toilet facilities in many of the nursing homes were very poor and lacked privacy, which may have had a negative influence on the motivation to use the toilet and improve toileting skills.
Kaapa, E. H., Frantsi, K., Sarna, S., & Malmivaara, A. (2006)	No statistically significant differences between control and experimental groups in main outcomes after intervention or at 6, 12, or 24 months follow-up. General well-being statistically better in experimental group just after rehabilitation (p=0.02). Both experimental and control group improved and maintained improvements at 2 years follow-up—trend toward decreased health care consumption in experimental group.	RCT	120	***Conclusions:*** Overall, the study found that there is no benefit for semi-light multidisciplinary rehabilitation for women with chronic low back pain in an outpatient setting compared to PT. ***Limitations:*** Psychometric properties of outcome measures not included and limited description of outcome measures; potential for contamination due to volunteer bias.

continued

Table 8-3 (continued)
EVIDENCE OF EFFECTIVENESS OF OCCUPATIONAL THERAPY ON PHYSICAL OUTCOMES

Author (Date)	Major Results	Study Design	Sample Size	Conclusions and Limitations
No Effect				
Li, L. C., Davis, A. M., Lineker, S. C., Coyte, P. C., & Bombardier, C. (2006)	Intervention group statistically higher disease knowledge from baseline to discharge and 6 months follow-up compared to control group (p<0.01). No statistically significant differences in physical functions or pain between groups. Intervention group had a decline in coping efficacy at 6-month follow-up compared to improvement in control group (p=0.03). No statistically significant differences in self-efficacy or activities between groups. Both interventions showed statistically significant improvements for clients over time.	RCT	78	***Conclusions:*** There is some evidence to show that the primary therapist model is beneficial for people with rheumatoid arthritis, although the study had a high attrition rate. ***Limitations:*** High attrition rate; comparison of 2 completely different services (not controlling for therapist or setting); unequal number of visits between groups; no procedure addressing contamination and co-intervention; low treatment adherence by populations.
Popovic, M. R., Thrasher, T. A., Adams, M. E., Takes, V., Zivanovic, V., & Tonack, M. I. (2006)	No statistically significant differences found between control and experimental groups. The participants in experimental group had positive views about the treatment. The authors conclude that functional electrical therapy administered by OTs in clinical settings has the potential to be effective in increasing grasping function in people with quadriplegia.	RCT	21	***Conclusions:*** Though the results are not statistically significant, the authors conclude that functional electrical therapy is a practical and efficient OT modality and that further studies with larger sample sizes are needed to demonstrate its effectiveness. ***Limitations:*** Small sample size; limited statistical significance; dropouts not reported.
Storr, L. K., Sorensen, P. S., & Ravnborg, M. (2006)	None of the outcome measures reached a level of significant change either in the intervention or control group. There were some positive trends in the intervention group regarding upper limb function and physical impairment and slight improvement in the control group in pain level.	RCT	90	***Conclusions:*** The results of this study failed to show any benefit in multidisciplinary rehabilitation for multiple sclerosis patients. ***Limitations:*** The study was underpowered due to a limited time period and low recruitment rate (small sample size).
Finlayson, M. (2005)	Non-statistically significant improvements in severity of fatigue, the impact of fatigue, and the quality of life (SF-36 subscales of Bodily Pain and General Health). Greatest percent change from use of strategies occurred in following areas: Resting, planning, changing work heights, using gadgets, and adapted devices. Results considered clinically important.	Non-RCT	29	***Conclusions:*** Results were not statistically significant, but the researchers concluded that the results support the need for more rigorous studies on this topic. ***Limitations:*** Sample size small.

continued

Table 8-3 (continued)

EVIDENCE OF EFFECTIVENESS OF OCCUPATIONAL THERAPY ON PHYSICAL OUTCOMES

Author (Date)	Major Results	Study Design	Sample Size	Conclusions and Limitations
No Effect				
Lamb, A., Finlayson, M., Mathiowetz, V., & Chen, H. Y. (2005)	Changes in mean scores on all the assessments except for the emotional and mental health subscales of the SF-36 were similar in both groups. However, statistical analysis showed only a weak difference between groups on the mental health subscale of the SF-36. All other outcomes were non-significant.	Non-RCT	92	**Conclusions:** Participants who used the self-study modules because of missed group sessions received the same benefits as patients who attended all the group sessions in the program. **Limitations:** The groups in this study were naturally occurring and not randomized, so unknown potential biases may not have been accounted for.
Li, L., Davis, A., Lineker, S., Coyte, P., & Bombardier, C. (2005)	Decreased pain for experimental group (54.4% improvement). Larger increase in health perceptions by experimental group (50% improvement compared to 9% for control). Trend toward improvement for all clinical measures from experimental group. Control group had increased pain at 6 weeks and deterioration of disease knowledge at 6 months.	RCT	22	**Conclusions:** There is a trend toward improvement through use of a primary therapist model for adults with rheumatoid arthritis. **Limitations:** Weak statistical analysis; small sample size; intervention not well described (difficult to reproduce); sample size did not meet power calculation of study; only 10 clients completed all of the core measurements; control was incomplete for baseline characteristics.
Lynch, D., Ferraro, M., Krol, J., Trudell, C. M., Christos, P., & Volpe, B. T. (2005)	Results indicate greater improvement in stability in experimental group; however, not statistically significant.	RCT	35	**Conclusions:** Authors conclude that results support the use of continuous passive motion devices to reduce adverse symptoms associated with shoulder instability. **Limitations:** Limited sample size, no power calculations.

continued

Table 8-3 (continued)

EVIDENCE OF EFFECTIVENESS OF OCCUPATIONAL THERAPY ON PHYSICAL OUTCOMES

Author (Date)	Major Results	Study Design	Sample Size	Conclusions and Limitations
No Effect				
Hammond, A., Young, A., & Kidao, R. (2004)	There were no significant differences and no trends approaching significance found between intervention and control groups on any of the outcome measures used. Within-group comparisons found that both groups had significant improvement on the physical function scores (intervention: p=0.002; control: p=0.001) in the AISM-2 and total self-efficacy scores (p=0.001 for both). However, pain scores on the VAS changed little (p=0.31; p=0.78). Further analysis based on disease status at baseline (American College of Rheumatology classes I, II, and III) revealed this did not have a significant impact on primary outcomes.	RCT	261	***Conclusions:*** The OT program designed for this study was effective in improving adherence to and use of self-management programs in rheumatoid arthritis patients, but over a 2-year follow-up did not have any greater effect on health status than usual care. ***Limitations:*** A majority of the patients in the sample were classified with "mild" OT and did not have functional deficits, thus a longer-term follow-up (5 to 10 years) would be more beneficial in determining if the program had a positive effect on health status. Also, some of the measurement instruments used may not have been sensitive enough to detect changes over the short time period (a "floor" effect).
Ward, C. D., Turpin, G., Dewey, M. E., Fleming, S., Hurwitz, B., Ratib, S., et al. (2004)	Experimental group sustained more falls (p=0.036) and had more skin sores (p=0.039) than the control group at follow-up and at 12 months post-intervention. The experimental group showed a significant rise in Nottingham Extended ADL scores (p=0.002).	RCT	114	***Conclusions:*** The experimental group had more negative effects (falls, skin sores) than the control group, prompting the authors to caution against the assumption that all educational interventions are beneficial for these populations. ***Limitations:*** Follow-up period might not have been long enough to produce positive effects.
Zijlstra, T. R., Heijnsdijk-Rouwenhorst, L., & Rasker, J. J. (2004)	There was a statistically significant change in DAS28 (−0.5; p=0.019); however, no other statistically significant changes were observed.	Non-RCT	17	***Conclusions:*** The authors conclude that silver ring splints can be an effective treatment method for certain individuals after a careful screening process. ***Limitations:*** Lack of control group; limited attempt to control for co-intervention or contamination; lack of description of intervention (e.g., wearing instructions/duration).

continued

Table 8-3 (continued)

EVIDENCE OF EFFECTIVENESS OF OCCUPATIONAL THERAPY ON PHYSICAL OUTCOMES

Author (Date)	Major Results	Study Design	Sample Size	Conclusions and Limitations
No Effect				
Desrosiers, J., Malouin, F., Richards, C., Bourbonnais, D., Rochette, A., & Bravo, G. (2003)	After rehabilitation discharge, the rate of motor recovery was maintained in the UE, though dropped in the LE. There was a faster rate of functional improvement in the LE during active rehabilitation ($p < 0.05$ for all results).	Non-RCT	132	*Conclusions:* The study suggests that the level of motor improvement of the UE and LE is similar during active rehabilitation, but the UE has higher rate of motor recovery after discharge. *Limitations:* High attrition rate; sample size not justified and no power calculation conducted; psychometric properties of outcome measures not reported.
Lannin, N. A., Horsley, S. A., Herbert, R., McCluskey, A., & Cusick, A. (2003)	Splinting increased wrist extension by a mean of 1 degree after the intervention, and it reduced wrist extension by a mean of 2 degrees at follow-up (within 95% CI). Splinting decreased upper limb function, performance of hand movements, advanced hand activities, and upper limb function after intervention and at follow-up (within 95% CI). No evidence of clinically significant effects. Splinting increased the reported intensity of upper limb pain after the intervention and reduced the reported pain intensity at follow-up (95% CI).	RCT	28	*Conclusions:* Use of overnight splints with the affected hand in the functional position did not produce clinically beneficial effects in adults with acquired brain impairment. *Limitations:* N/A.
Maeshima, S., Ueyoshi, A., Osawa, A., Ishida, K., Kunimoto, K., Shimamoto, Y., et al. (2003)	No significant difference between groups for non-paretic lower limb strength at end of intervention; significant difference in the torque value between exercise types in family participation group only ($p < 0.05$). No significant difference between groups for mobility scores. No statistically significant difference in average number of days of inpatient treatment for each group.	Non-RCT	60	*Conclusions:* There were no significant results at first evaluation but, with further statistical testing, patients' strength and mobility improved with family participation. *Limitations:* Control and experimental groups vary in size; short experimental time and no follow-up measures; not randomized; no procedures reported to account for co-intervention, non-homogeneous population.
Rodgers, H., Mackintosh, J., Price, C., Wood, R., McNamee, P., Fearon, T., et al. (2003)	No significant differences on any outcomes at 3 and 6 months after stroke.	RCT	96	*Conclusions:* The increased intensity program was not effective. *Limitations:* Intervention time differed between groups; high dropout rates; intervention descriptions not clear; no procedure accounting for possible contamination.

continued

Table 8-3 (continued)

EVIDENCE OF EFFECTIVENESS OF OCCUPATIONAL THERAPY ON PHYSICAL OUTCOMES

Author (Date)	Major Results	Study Design	Sample Size	Conclusions and Limitations
No Effect				
Akalin, E., El, O., Peker, O., Senocak, O., Tamci, S., Gulbahar, S., et al. (2002)	After 8 weeks of the treatment, there was a statistically significant improvement in all parameters in both groups, except for the 2-point discrimination in group 1. The improvement in group 2 was slightly greater than group 1, but this difference was not statistically significant, except for pinch strength.	RCT	28	**Conclusions:** There were no significant differences between the splint and exercise group compared with the splint-only group. **Limitations:** Dropouts not reported; small sample size.
Christensen, O. M., Kunov, A., Hansen, F. F., Christiansen, T. C., & Krasheninnikoff, M. (2001)	There was no difference between the 2 groups.	RCT	30	**Conclusions:** There are no significant differences between the 2 groups at the specified time periods indicating that for non-surgically treated patients with a distal radius fracture, only instructions are necessary. **Limitations:** Dropouts were not reported; contamination and co-intervention were not discussed; psychometric properties for outcome measure not reported.
Wahi Michener, S. K., Olson, A. L., Humphrey, B. A., Reed, J. E., Stepp, D. R., Sutton, A. M., et al. (2001)	Moderate correlation between grip strength and hand function score at discharge (r=0.59). No correlation was observed between VAS scores and MHQ or VAS and grip strength scores.	Non-RCT	15	**Conclusions:** No differences were observed between scores of participants who underwent surgery and those who did not. **Limitations:** Small sample size; compliance may not have been accurately measured with outcomes measure used; variability in evaluators may have contributed to variance in measurements; no description of OT intervention (difficult to reproduce).
Bolin, I., Bodin, P., & Kreuter, M. (2000)	Statistical significance was not considered.	Non-RCT	4	**Conclusions:** Authors conclude that the interventions improved sitting position and reduced or solved specific problems. However, tables indicating clients' subjective views of the intervention demonstrate that not all interventions led to improvement. **Limitations:** Small sample size; psychometric properties of outcome not reported.

continued

Table 8-3 (continued)
EVIDENCE OF EFFECTIVENESS OF OCCUPATIONAL THERAPY ON PHYSICAL OUTCOMES

Author (Date)	Major Results	Study Design	Sample Size	Conclusions and Limitations
No Effect				
Baskett, J. J., Broad, J. B., Reekie, G., Hocking, C., & Green, G. (1999)	No statistical differences in changes in neurological, physical, and ADL function between the control and experimental (p<0.05). Caregivers in the experimental group thought there had been an improvement (not statistically significant).	RCT	100	***Conclusions:*** Having the OT or PT visit clients in their homes is just as effective as having clients attend an outpatient stroke rehabilitation clinic. ***Limitations:*** Psychometric properties of assessments not described; small sample size.
Bishop, S. A., Bulla, N., DiLellio, E., Dy, M., Koski, J. H., Linnemeyer, C. B., et al. (1999)	No significant differences in dynamic pressure ratings were found between the 4 different low-cost wheelchair pads. Some descriptive trends between body type and wheelchair cushion type were seen. Individuals categorized as possessing a normal body type, gel cushion, and foam layers may facilitate a favorable pressure distribution.	Non-RCT	32	***Conclusions:*** For thin individuals, the cushion of gel and foam layers may be favorable. For obese individuals, a cushion of gel/foam mixture may be favorable. ***Limitations:*** Small sample size; recording device did not record pressure ratings above 200 mm Hg, so some pressure ratings may have been higher; unequal distribution of participants in each body type category.
Pellow, T. R. (1999)	The High Profile Roho cushion caused the least amount of pressure on the ischial tuberosities. Forty-five degrees of tilt provided the best pressure relief on the ischial tuberosities. No statistical analysis.	Non-RCT	2	***Conclusions:*** Roho cushion and tilt position can offer best pressure relief, but seating must be tailored to the individual. ***Limitations:*** Small sample size; no statistical analysis.
Pagnotta, A., Baron, M., & Korner-Bitensky, N. (1998)	Work performance while wearing splint was significantly inferior (p<0.001) to performance without a splint for the screwdriver task. No significant differences observed between work performance levels on the shears task. Dexterity was significantly negatively affected by splint use (p=0.0086). Pain was reported to be higher while subjects performed tasks without a splint. No correlation between pain and work performance.	RCT	40	***Conclusions:*** While splints decrease pain, they also decrease hand output. ***Limitations:*** Evaluators not blinded to intervention.

continued

Table 8-3 (continued)
EVIDENCE OF EFFECTIVENESS OF OCCUPATIONAL THERAPY ON PHYSICAL OUTCOMES

Author (Date)	Major Results	Study Design	Sample Size	Conclusions and Limitations
No Effect				
Richards, S. H., Coast, J., Gunnell, D. J., Peters, T. J., Pounsford, J., & Darlow, M. A. (1998)	Length of hospital care was significantly longer for home patients (p<0.001). No significant differences between group mortality rates. No significant differences between groups for functional ability with ADL. No significant differences in reported quality of life. There was significantly higher satisfaction of care for home group in some questions (p<0.05).	RCT	207	**Conclusions:** The results of the study indicate that in-hospital care reduces the amount of treatment time. **Limitations:** Study not blind for interviewers; interventions not described; dropouts not described in detail; control treatment not described.
Tijhuis, G. J., Vliet Vlieland, T. P., Zwinderman, A. H., & Hazes, J. M. (1998)	No statistically significant differences between the 2 interventions for any outcome measure.	RCT	10	**Conclusions:** The increased cost of a custom-made orthoses is not justified by the results of the study. **Limitations:** Small sample size; short duration of intervention; short time between cross-over may confound treatment results; not all assessors were blind to treatment.
Kohlmeyer, K. M., Hill, J. P., Yarkony, G. M., & Jaeger, R. J. (1996)	All treatment groups improved. Addition of biofeedback and electrical stimulation both alone and in concert did not prove to be more effective than standard therapy for wrist extensor recovery during the acute phase of rehabilitation.	Non-RCT	45	**Conclusions:** Electrical stimulation and biofeedback were no more effective than conventional treatment. **Limitations:** Procedures to prevent co-intervention were not reported; psychometric properties of outcome measures were not reported.
Stern, E. B., Ytterberg, S. R., Krug, H. E., & Mahowald, M. L. (1996)	No significant differences between the 3 splints on either outcome measure. A significant and equally negative effect was observed on both outcome measures when comparing performance with all 3 splints vs. free hand activity (p=0.01).	RCT	42	**Conclusions:** The study concludes that none of the orthoses are more effective than any of the others at improving hand function or dexterity and that wrist orthoses negatively affect hand function and dexterity. **Limitations:** Evaluators not blind to treatment; no procedure to minimize contamination or co-intervention.
Stern, E. B., Ytterberg, S. R., Krug, H. E., Mullin, G. T., & Mahowald, M. L. (1996)	Grip strength was equally and significantly reduced (F=13.07; p=0.001) after participants first donned a splint. Only one splint (Roylan) was associated with significantly improved grip strength (while wearing splint) 1 week later (F=7.49; p=0.01). No splints significantly improved non-splinted grip strength after 1 week. No statistical differences among splints' effects on daily tasks questionnaire.	RCT	36	**Conclusions:** 1 orthoses may be slightly more effective than the 2 others. **Limitations:** Evaluators not blind to treatment; no psychometric data were provided for questionnaire; no procedure to minimize contamination or co-intervention.

continued

Table 8-3 (continued)

EVIDENCE OF EFFECTIVENESS OF OCCUPATIONAL THERAPY ON PHYSICAL OUTCOMES

Author (Date)	Major Results	Study Design	Sample Size	Conclusions and Limitations
No Effect				
Thomas, J. J. (1996)	No significant difference between experimental and control groups on post-test knowledge scores. Authors noticed an improvement in scores if a pretest had been taken (not statistically significant).	RCT	96	***Conclusions:*** The results show no difference between the 2 approaches; however, more research should be conducted on this subject and on the effects of pretesting in patient education. ***Limitations:*** None identified.
Conine, T. A., Hershler, C., Daechsel, D., Peel, C., & Pearson, A. (1994)	A lower proportion of the patients in the Jay group (25%) experienced pressure ulcer formation during the 3 months of observation as compared to the foam group (41%). No statistically significant differences were found between groups on the location, severity, or healing duration of the pressure ulcers. Most lesions (65%) were limited to persistent erythema of intact skin and healed in 3 to 4 weeks. Higher proportions of patients in the Jay groups (7%) rejected their cushion because of discomfort as compared to foam (1%).	Non-RCT	141	***Conclusions:*** The Jay foam group experienced less pressure ulcer formation during the observation period compared to the foam group but no differences were found on the location, severity, or healing duration of the ulcers. ***Limitations:*** A larger sample needed to control type II error.
Hammond, A. (1994)	No significant differences between pre- and post-assessment scores on the HJC, HAQ, and VAS. Education did not appear to significantly improve scores, as only 4 patients had increased JPBA scores at 6 weeks. Hand pain, as assessed by VAS, was significantly associated with JPBA scores both before ($p<0.02$) and after ($p<0.05$). No participant achieved a clinically significant change in scores, as based on pre-determined calculation.	Non-RCT	11	***Conclusions:*** The joint protection education did not lead to significant change in behavior, in terms of the activities that were assessed. ***Limitations:*** Small sample size; limited timeframe for patient follow-up.
Cron, L., & Sprigle, S. (1993)	No significant difference between the cushions.	Non-RCT	11	***Conclusions:*** The hemi wheelchair cushion is economical and appropriate for people propelling with use of one leg. ***Limitations:*** Confounding variables not examined; small sample size.

continued

Table 8-3 (continued)

EVIDENCE OF EFFECTIVENESS OF OCCUPATIONAL THERAPY ON PHYSICAL OUTCOMES

Author (Date)	Major Results	Study Design	Sample Size	Conclusions and Limitations
No Effect				
Fletchall, S., & Hickerson, W. L. (1991)	All patients exhibited a decrease in stump edema once fitted with the prosthesis. By the completion of the prosthetic program, all patients were wearing their prostheses for at least 8 hours a day, 7 days a week. 4 participants reached independence using their prosthesis for basic self-care activities within 1 week, and the other 3 within 3 weeks of being fitted. After the final fitting of the prosthesis, clients returned to their pre-amputation activities within 1.5 to 5 months, and all returned to work/school within 2 to 9 months. All patients remained free of skin breakdown on the fitted extremity.	Non-RCT	7	***Conclusions:*** Early-prosthetic fit is beneficial for patients requiring amputation. ***Limitations:*** Small sample size, no statistical analyses performed with outcome measures.
Poole, J. L., Whitney, S. L., Hangeland, N., & Baker, C. (1990)	No statistical differences between control and experimental groups on FMA.	RCT	18	***Conclusions:*** No statistical differences between control and experimental groups on FMA. ***Limitations:*** No procedures to control for contamination or co-intervention in control group; assessor was not blind to treatment method; small sample size; limited description of intervention.
Furst, G. P., Gerber, L. H., Smith, C. C., & Fisher, S. (1987)	Results show improvement for experimental group; however, no results were statistically significant.	RCT	28	***Conclusions:*** The study provides some support for energy conservation programs. ***Limitations:*** Small sample size; dropouts not reported.
Gerber, L., Furst, G., Shulman, B., Smith, C., Thornton, B., Liang, M., et al. (1987)	In terms of disease activity, RAI, timed walk, and grip strength, there were no differences between the treatment and control groups at baseline or 3 months after intervention. No significant differences between groups on the HAQ or VAS of pain, either before treatment or after. For PAIS subscales, no statistically significant differences between the control group and intervention groups. 50% of the treatment group and 11% of controls spent more time in physical activity over the 3 months.	RCT	28	***Conclusions:*** The significant differences between groups, in terms of activity level and rest periods may suggest that a "systematic" approach to education is successful in changing behavior. ***Limitations:*** Outcome measures used may not have been sensitive to slow level of change in disability; small sample size.

continued

Table 8-3 (continued)

EVIDENCE OF EFFECTIVENESS OF OCCUPATIONAL THERAPY ON PHYSICAL OUTCOMES

Author (Date)	Major Results	Study Design	Sample Size	Conclusions and Limitations
No Effect				
Trombly, C. A., Thayer-Nason, L., Bliss, G., Girard, C. A., Lyrist, L. A., & Brexa-Hooson, A. (1986)	No statistical differences between control and experimental groups on any outcome measure.	RCT	20	***Conclusions:*** No statistical differences were observed between treatment and control. ***Limitations:*** No procedure to control for contamination or co-intervention in control group; assessor was not blind to treatment method; small sample size.
Mathiowetz, V., Bolding, D. J., & Trombly, C. A. (1983)	Results showed significantly greater EMG activity for the finger spreader compared to no device in the flexor carpi radialis of non-hemiplegic subjects during the grasping period (significant at the 0.05 level). Hemiplegic subjects did not show significantly less EMG activity when using positioning devices compared to no device. In fact, the volar splint appeared to increase the EMG activity while the subjects were grasping.	Non-RCT	12	***Conclusions:*** There were no significant positive effects found between use of any of the positioning devices vs. using no device for the hemiplegic patients, and, in fact, use of the volar resting splint appeared to increase spasticity for hemiplegic patients in this study. ***Limitations:*** Small sample size; variability of their outcomes measures based on positioning devices and grasping.
Greenberg, S. & Fowler, R. S., Jr. (1980)	The increase in elbow extension in the experimental group was similar to that in the control group. However, the results are not statistically significant.	RCT	20	***Conclusions:*** The authors conclude that kinesthetic biofeedback might more effective if used in conjunction with other forms of therapy. ***Limitations:*** Small sample size; potentially confounding variables; functional outcome measures not used.

6MWT=6-Minute Walk Test, AIMS-2=Arthritis Impact Measurement Scales 2, BBS=Berg Balance Scale, BI=Barthel Index, COPM=Canadian Occupational Performance Measure, DAS28=Disease Activity Score, DASH=Disabilities of the Arm, Shoulder, and Hand Outcome Measure, F-COPES= Family Crisis Oriented Personal Evaluation Scales, FIM=Functional Independence Measure, FIQ=Fibromyalgia Impact Questionnaire, FMA=Fugl-Meyer Assessment, HAQ=Health Assessment Questionnaire, HJC=Hand Joint Count, JPBA=Joint Protection Behaviour Assessment, MAS=Motor Assessment Scale, MHQ=Michigan Hand Questionnaire, PAIS=Psychosocial Adjustment to Illness Scale, Prafab=Dutch subjective measure of incontinence, PSFS=Penn Spasm Frequency Score, RAI=Rheumatology Attitudes Index, SF-36=Short Form Health Survey, SOFI=Signals of Functional Impairment, TUG=Timed Up and Go Test, VAS=Visual Analog Scale, WMFT=Wolf Motor Function Test.

Table 8-4
OUTCOME MEASURES USED TO CAPTURE PHYSICAL OUTCOMES

Author (Date)	Outcome(s) Investigated	Outcome Measure(s)	Method of Administration
Hand and Upper Extremity			
Paes Lourencao, M. I., Battistella, L. R., Moran de Brito, C. M., Tsukimoto, G. R.,& Miyazaki, M. H. (2008)	Hand function Manual dexterity Elbow/wrist movement Elbow/wrist spasticity	Hand function test Minnesota manual dexterity test Joint range of motion scale Modified Ashworth Scale	Patients were evaluated at baseline, 6, and 12 months.
Rosenstein, L., Ridgel, A., Thota, A., Samame, B., & Alberts, J. (2008)	Functional ability Motor function (affected UE) Spasticity	WMFT FMA Modified Ashworth Scale	Assessments were completed by independent OTs before and after the intervention.
Lannin, N., Cusick, A., McCluskey, A., & Herbert, R. (2007)	Extension in wrist and fingers Upper limb spasticity Self-reported disability	Wrist extension range (with fingers extended) MAS Tardieu scale DASH	Assessments were completed at baseline, 4, and 6 weeks by an independent blinded assessor.
van der Giesen, F. J., Nelissen, R., Rozing, P., Arendzen, J., de Jong, Z., Wolterbeek, R., et al. (2007)	Joint swelling/deformity Assistive devices Hand function Range of motion Grip strength Pain	ICF impairment categories Goniometry Jamar dynamometer VAS SODA AIMS-2 MHQ	Clinical assessment by rheumatologist, PT, and 5 OTs, all specially trained for the study. Training and calibration sessions repeated every 3 months.
Pang, M., Harris, J., & Eng, J. (2006)	UE function Motor impairment in paretic UE Grip strength Use of paretic UE in daily activities	WMFT FMA Jamar dynamometer MAL	Outcomes were measured by independent assessors at baseline and after completion of the exercise program.
Popovic, M. R., Thrasher, T. A., Adams, M. E., Takes, V., Zivanovic, V., & Tonack, M. I. (2006)	Grasping function in people with quadriplegia Consumer perception of the intervention	FIM SCIM RELHFT Consumer perceptions of intervention	Administered before and after the intervention by the researchers.
Aldehag, A.S., Jonsson, H., & Ansved, T. (2005)	Hand function Occupational performance Degree of myotonia	Hand-held myometer Grippit (instrument for grip force) Purdue Pegboard COPM Self-rated myotonia (VAS)	Hand function measurements were performed on the first and last weeks of training—a total of 9 times each week (3 times daily for 3 days). Measurements for occupational performance and myotonia were completed once before and once after training.
Lynch, D., Ferraro, M., Krol, J., Trudell, C. M., Christos, P., & Volpe, B. T. (2005)	Shoulder joint instability Pain Tone Impairment Disability	FMA MSS MRCMP Observed gleno-humeral stability, pain, and tone FIM	An OT blinded to groups administered at admission and discharge.

continued

Table 8-4 (continued)
OUTCOME MEASURES USED TO CAPTURE PHYSICAL OUTCOMES

Author (Date)	Outcome(s) Investigated	Outcome Measure(s)	Method of Administration
Hand and Upper Extremity			
Malcus-Johnson, P., Carlqvist, C., Sturesson, A., & Eberhardt, K. (2005)	Hand impairment Grip strength Hand deformity Activity level	SOFI Stanford Health Assessment Questionnaire Disability Index	Assessments were completed upon inclusion in the study and during scheduled visits with the OT (every 3 months in the first 2 years and every 6 months in the following years).
Pizzi, A., Carlucci, G., Falsini, C., Verdesca, S., & Grippo, A. (2005)	Spasticity Passive range of motion Pain Spasms	VAS MAS Goniometry PSES	Observed/semi-structured interview.
Ring, H., & Rosenthal, N. (2005)	Range of motion for flexion and abduction of shoulder Flexion and extension of elbow and wrist Flexion and extension of fingers Thumb opposition Muscle tone at shoulder elbow, wrist, finger, and thumb Functional use of hand Presence of pain or edema	Goniometry 7-point scale for thumb opposition AS Blocks and box test JHFT	Therapist administered; baseline, 6 weeks.
Hammond, A., & Freeman, K. (2004)	Adherence to joint protection Functional ability Hand impairment Disease status	JPBA AIMS-2 ASES VAS for hand pain EULAR 28 Tender and swollen joint count Jamar dynamometer	Independent assessors blinded to groups conducted assessments in participants' homes at 0 and 4 years; questionnaires also completed by participants.
Hammond, A., Young, A., & Kidao, R. (2004)	Functional ability Disease status Hand function Psychosocial status	HAQ AIMS-2 Tender/swollen joint count (0 to 3 scale rating) American College of Rheumatology functional grade Duration of early morning stiffness (in minutes) Pain level in past week (VAS) Jamar dynamometer JHFT ASES RAI	Assessments were completed at baseline, 6, 12, and 24 months by the same assessor who was blinded to group allocation.
Haskett, S., Backman, C., Porter, B., Goyert, J., & Palejko, G. (2004)	Wrist pain Hand function Patient perception of UE function Disease activity measures	VAS AHFT MACTAR	Taken by therapist at baseline and end of 4-week splint phase, and at the end of the 1-week washout period between splints.

continued

Table 8-4 (continued)

OUTCOME MEASURES USED TO CAPTURE PHYSICAL OUTCOMES

Author (Date)	Outcome(s) Investigated	Outcome Measure(s)	Method of Administration
Hand and Upper Extremity			
Sandqvist, G., Akesson, A., & Eklund, M. (2004)	Range of motion Mobility of fingers and wrist Grip force Perceived pain Stiffness/elasticity of skin Thickness of skin	Goniometry HAMIS Grippit VAS (for pain and stiffness) RSS—modified	Both hands (control and intervention) measured at baseline and 1-month post-treatment.
Zijlstra, T. R., Heijnsdijk Rouwenhorst, L., & Rasker, J. J. (2004)	Dexterity Self-reported hand function Hand pain Grip and pinch strength Patient satisfaction	SODA Pressure balloon with mercury manometer AIMS-2 DAS28 Erythrocyte sedimentation rate	Observed, self-report.
Case-Smith, J. (2003)	UE functional performance	COPM DASH SF-36 CIQ	Self-report with therapist at baseline and just before discharge for all except CIQ. CIQ also measured at follow-up.
Desrosiers, J., Malouin, F., Richards, C., Bourbonnais, D., Rochette, A., & Bravo, G. (2003)	UE and LE impairments UE and LE disabilities	FMA Finger-to-nose test TEMPA-French Walking balance	OT/research assistant assessed participants.
Fischer, T., Nagy, L., & Buechler, U. (2003)	Strength Power grip Thumb adduction Index finger abduction Various thumb to index pinch grips and wrist extension. Functional performance	Jamar dynamometer PPGD BTE VAS	Hand therapist (mean of 3 times) administered tests preoperatively and postoperatively. Self-report measures were also completed preoperatively and postoperatively.
Lannin, N. A., Horsley, S. A., Herbert, R., McCluskey, A., & Cusick, A. (2003)	Length of wrist and finger flexor muscles Hand and arm function Pain levels	Torque-controlled measure of wrist and finger extension Modified Ashworth Scale VAS	Measured by therapist at baseline, post-program, and 1-week follow-up (after program completed).
Rodgers, H., Mackintosh, J., Price, C., Wood, R., McNamee, P., Fearon, T., et al. (2003)	Upper limb impairment Upper limb pain Ability to do ADL Costs to health and social services	ARAT MI FAT Upper limb pain BI Nottingham Extended ADL Scale Costs to health and social services	Therapist administered; baseline, 3, and 6 months after stroke.
Sandin-Aldehag, A., & Jonsson, H. (2003)	Hand function Basic and instrumental ADL Life satisfaction	Manual muscle testing Grippit Goniometry ADL-T LSC	Observation, self-report, and structured interview.

continued

Table 8-4 (continued)
OUTCOME MEASURES USED TO CAPTURE PHYSICAL OUTCOMES

Author (Date)	Outcome(s) Investigated	Outcome Measure(s)	Method of Administration
Hand and Upper Extremity			
Akalin, E., El, O., Peker, O., Senocak, O., Tamci, S., Gulbahar, S., et al. (2002)	Grip strength Pinch strength Subjective carpal tunnel syndrome symptoms Symptom status Functional status	MV Tinel's sign/Phalen's sign SSS FSS	Measured by therapist pre- and post-treatment.
Donnelly, C. J., & Wilton, J. (2002)	Active range of motion Skin mobility	Goniometry Rating scale modified from skin slide grade scale	Therapist assessment; baseline and 4 weeks (both at beginning of therapy session).
Hammond, A., Jeffreson, P., Jones, N., Gallagher, J., & Jones, T. (2002)	Ability to increase clients' use of joint protection strategies Continued use of joint protection techniques	JPBA PKQ ASES VAS HAQ Jamar dynamometer RAI	Conducted by an independent assessor, blinded to group allocation, at 3-month intervals.
Christensen, O. M., Kunov, A., Hansen, F. F., Christiansen, T. C., & Krasheninnikoff, M. (2001)	Functional performance	SMGW	At cast removal by 5 weeks, and after 3 and 9 months.
Hammond, A., & Freeman, K. (2001)	Adherence Functional ability Hand impairment Disease status	AIMS-2 ASES JPBA VAS EULAR 28 Jamar dynamometer	Independent assessors blinded to groups conducted assessments in participant homes at baseline, 6, and 12 months.
Wahi Michener, S. K., Olson, A. L., Humphrey, B. A., Reed, J. E., Stepp, D. R., Sutton, A. M., et al. (2001)	Hand function Grip strength Program compliance	MHQ Jamar dynamometer VAS	Observation.
Jarus, T., Shavit, S., & Ratzon, N. (2000)	Range of motion Grip strength Edema Level of interest	Goniometry Jamar dynamometer Volumeter VAS	Evaluated by therapist at baseline and every week for 5-week program.
Li, S., Liu, L., Miyazaki, M., & Warren, S. (1999)	Carpal tunnel syndrome severity Functional status	SSS FSS	Self-administered questionnaires (both scales) were completed twice before splinting (1 to 2 weeks prior and immediately before splinting) and twice post-splinting (2 weeks and 10 to 12 weeks post-splinting).
Pagnotta, A., Baron, M., & Korner-Bitensky, N. (1998)	Work performance Dexterity Pain during activity	BTE JHFT VAS	Observed/semi-structured interview.

continued

Table 8-4 (continued)
OUTCOME MEASURES USED TO CAPTURE PHYSICAL OUTCOMES

Author (Date)	Outcome(s) Investigated	Outcome Measure(s)	Method of Administration
Hand and Upper Extremity			
Tijhuis, G. J., Vliet Vlieland, T. P., Zwinderman, A. H., & Hazes, J. M. (1998)	Tender joint count Swelling of the MCP, PIP, IP, and wrist Wrist range of motion Grip strength with/without orthoses	RS MV	Observed.
Callinan, N. J., & Mathiowetz, V. (1996)	Pain Hand function Splint preference	AIMS-2 Pain Localization Diagram Jamar dynamometer Daily diary of splint and morning stiffness Subjective splint rating form	The AIMS-2, pain localization diagram, and Jamar dynamometer testing were completed before and after each experimental and control condition (4 measurement times in total). The AIMS-2 is a self-administered questionnaire. All testing was taken at the same time of day for each patient. The daily diary and the subjective splint rating were self-administered at completion of each experimental condition.
Kohlmeyer, K. M., Hill, J. P., Yarkony, G. M., & Jaeger, R. J. (1996)	Tenodesis grasp Manual muscle grade and function	Manual muscle testing Function score	Assessed by evaluator at baseline and post-program.
Nelson, D. L., Konosky, K., Fleharty, K., Webb, R., Newer, K., Hazboun, V. P., et al. (1996)	Changes in supination	Degrees of handle rotation of an apparatus used in the hand therapy (non-standardized)	Measured by OT before and after each treatment session for 4 weeks.
Stern, E. B., Ytterberg, S. R., Krug, H. E., & Mahowald, M. L. (1996)	Finger dexterity Hand function	JHFT PT	Observed.
Stern, E. B., Ytterberg, S. R., Krug, H. E., Mullin, G. T., & Mahowald, M. L. (1996)	Maximum grip strength (splinted and non-splinted) Effect of orthosis on daily tasks	Jamar dynamometer ADL questionnaire	Observed/semi-structured interview.
Thomas, L. J., & Thomas, B. J. (1995)	Success of treatment method (joint action)	JTAM (computation joint range of motion using the Strickland and Glogovac method)	Not specified.
Barry, M. A., Purser, J., Hazleman, R., McLean, A., & Hazleman, B. L. (1994)	Patient knowledge and performance of joint protection maneuvers, and whether these outcomes were sustained over a 6-month period	Photographic questionnaire	Prior to treatment, 1 month, and 6 months after treatment, by independent assessor.
Hammond, A. (1994)	Joint protection behaviors Classification of disease Hand joint count of pain and deformity Functional ability Pain measurement Activity during ADL	JPBA American College of Rheumatology HJC HAQ VAS	Clinical data were collected at first and last assessments. Pre-test evaluation occurred at 1 week and post-test occurred at 2 and 6 weeks. Assessments were conducted in an OT kitchen.

continued

Table 8-4 (continued)

Outcome Measures Used to Capture Physical Outcomes

Author (Date)	Outcome(s) Investigated	Outcome Measure(s)	Method of Administration
Hand and Upper Extremity			
Neistadt, M. E. (1994)	Fine motor performance/coordination skills	Line Bisection Test JHFT WAIS-R PBT RKE-R	Measures were administered by trained independent evaluators (13 in total). Evaluators were blind to treatment group with the exception of 1 evaluator. Patients were evaluated by the same evaluator. All measures administered at the pre-test. All measures but the Line Bisection Test were administered post-test.
Yuen, H. K., Nelson, D. L., Peterson, C. Q., & Dickinson, A. (1994)	UE prosthesis control	Speed and accuracy of tracing a path on a maze-line. Time required to complete the maze.	Observed.
King, T. I. (1993)	Assess number of times the patient gripped or pinched the device	A grip and pinch strengthening device hooked up to a computer (with appropriate software)	The participants were instructed on how to use the grip or pinch strengthening device.
Sietsema, J. M., Nelson, D. L., Mulder, R. M., MervauScheidel, D., & White, B. E. (1993)	Range of motion	Measurement of range of motion using motion analysis equipment	Subjects' range of motion recorded during both intervention and control and analyzed afterwards.
Fletchall, S., & Hickerson, W. L. (1991)	Type of injury Type of amputation needed Length of hospital stay Length of time until independent with prosthesis on self-care activities Length of time until return to work/school	Patient data form to collect needed information	Not specified.
Poole, J. L., Whitney, S. L., Hangeland, N., & Baker, C. (1990)	UE motor function in adults with hemiparesis secondary to CVA	FMA	Observation.
Trombly, C. A., Thayer-Nason, L., Bliss, G., Girard, C. A., Lyrist, L. A., & Brexa-Hooson, A. (1986)	Hand function	Goniometry HFOT Pegboard test	Observation.
Mathiowetz, V., Bolding, D. J., & Trombly, C. A. (1983)	Flexor muscle activity of the forearm	EMG activity	The EMG activity was measured 4 times during the intervention—1 minute each time for each condition.
Greenberg, S., & Fowler, R. S., Jr. (1980)	Active elbow extension	Goniometry	Trained evaluator.

continued

Table 8-4 (continued)

OUTCOME MEASURES USED TO CAPTURE PHYSICAL OUTCOMES

Author (Date)	Outcome(s) Investigated	Outcome Measure(s)	Method of Administration
Pain			
Masiero, S., Boniolo, A., Wassermann, L., Machiedo, H., Volante, D., & Punzi, L. (2007)	Pain intensity Functional status Disability and health status	VAS HAQ AIMS-2	Assessments were completed at baseline and completion of the study (approximately 8 months later).
Kaapa, E. H., Frantsi, K., Sarna, S., & Malmivaara, A. (2006)	Changes in back pain Sciatic pain intensity Disability Sick leave(s) Health care consumption Symptoms of depression Beliefs of working ability	VAS Subjective working capacity ODI Sick leave due to back pain Health care consumption due to back pain DEPS General well-being after back rehabilitation	Self-report at baseline, after rehabilitation, 6-, 12-, and 24-month follow-up.
Li, L. C., Davis, A. M., Lineker, S. C., Coyte, P. C., & Bombardier, C. (2006)	Changes in physical function Pain Disease knowledge Changes in self-efficacy Activities Coping management	HAQ VAS RAKQ SSES Rheumatoid arthritis disease activity index CES	Self-report at baseline, discharge, and 6 months after baseline.
Dohnke, B., Knauper, B., & Muller-Fahrnow, W. (2005)	Perceived self-efficacy Physical health (pain and disability) Depressive symptoms	ASES VAS Activity questionnaire CES-D	Assessments were performed at admission (baseline), discharge, and 6-month follow-up.
Li, L., Davis, A., Lineker, S., Coyte, P., & Bombardier, C. (2005)	Changes in pain Functional ability Disease-specific knowledge Patient's health perception Health resource use	VAS HAQ RAKQ EuorQOL HRU	Self-report in booklet format. Completed at baseline (immediately prior to randomization), discharge or 6 weeks, and 6 months. HRU was completed every month.
Pagnotta, A., Korner-Bitensky, N., Mazer, B., Baron, M., & Wood-Dauphinee, S. (2005)	Pain Work performance Endurance Perceived task difficulty (with/without splint)	BTE VAS	Observed.
Walsh, D. A., Kelly, S. J., Johnson, P. S., Rajkumar, S., & Bennetts, K. (2004)	Occupational concerns of patient disability specific to lower back pain Confidence in activities Walking performance	COPM RMDQ PSEQ 5-minute walk test	Self-report and therapist administered; baseline, after therapy, 9 months follow-up.

continued

Table 8-4 (continued)

OUTCOME MEASURES USED TO CAPTURE PHYSICAL OUTCOMES

Author (Date)	Outcome(s) Investigated	Outcome Measure(s)	Method of Administration
Pain			
Sterner, Y., Lofgren, M., Nyberg, V., Karlsson, A. K., Bergstrom, M., & Gerdle, B. (2001)	Pain, disability, and life quality Comparison to pre-morbid stage Satisfaction with rehabilitation program Pain intensity of 4 anatomical regions Life satisfaction Depression Coping ability Amount of sick leave	Questionnaire on pain, disability, life quality, function Semi-structured interview on satisfaction with program Medical record audit VAS LSQ BDI MPI CRI	Self-report for questionnaire; retrospective data immediately after program and at 6 months follow-up; prospective data before, after, and 6 months follow-up (for pain intensity, life satisfaction questionnaire, depression, coping, and sick leave).
Hildebrandt, J., Pfingsten, M., Saur, P., & Jansen, J. (1997)	Return to work Pain reduction Treatment rating Factors affecting return to work Factors affecting satisfaction with program	Medical examination for impairment Subjective description of worksite variables VAS PDI Deficiencies in daily activities Depression scale Pain-related coping behavior Physical assessment (strength, endurance, range of motion)	Self-report and therapist assessed; baseline, discharge, 6-month follow-up, 12-month follow-up.
Spalding, N. J. (1995)	Length of stay in hospital Level of preparation for discharge	Number of days postoperatively walked with frame or cane Patient-controlled analgesia usage in the first 24 hours after surgery Number of postoperative home visits by the OT	Chart audit.
Fatigue/Endurance			
Matuska, K., Mathiowetz, V., & Finlayson, M. (2007)	Usage of energy conservation strategies Perceived effectiveness of energy conservation strategies	ECSS	The assessment was completed by participants 6 weeks after completion of the energy conservation course.
Ip, W. M., Woo, J., Yue, S. Y., Kwan, M., Sum, S. M. W., Kwok, T., et al. (2006)	Energy expenditure Fatigue	Portable indirect calorimetry system Heart rate monitor Blood pressure cuff VAS Borg Scale	Energy expenditure was measured throughout the completion of the tasks via the calorimetry system and the heart rate monitor, and a resting heart rate was recorded prior to completing the tasks. Blood pressure and fatigue were measured before and after completing the tasks.

continued

Table 8-4 (continued)
Outcome Measures Used to Capture Physical Outcomes

Author (Date)	Outcome(s) Investigated	Outcome Measure(s)	Method of Administration
Fatigue/Endurance			
Finlayson, M. (2005)	Fatigue severity Fatigue impact Self-efficacy for fatigue management Quality of life Self-reported use of energy conservation strategies	FSS SEPEC SF-36 Energy conservation strategies survey	Administered by a research assistant 1 to 2 weeks before the intervention and within 10 days after intervention.
Lamb, A., Finlayson, M., Mathiowetz, V., & Yun Chen, H. (2005)	Fatigue Health status Self-efficacy in energy conservation	FIS SF-36 SEPEC	All assessments were completed at baseline and once the training program was completed.
Mathiowetz, V. G., Finlayson, M. L., Matuska, K. M., Chen, H. Y., & Luo, P. (2005)	Fatigue impact Quality of life Self-efficacy	FIS SF-36 SEPEC	Research assistants administered the 3 outcome measures before and after intervention.
WaiShan Louie, S. (2004)	Physiological symptoms	Partial percentage of oxygen saturation Heart rate Upper thoracic surface electromyography Skin conductance Peripheral skin temperature Modified Borg Scale for Breathlessness	Following the 6 intervention sessions, the Pro-comp biofeedback measured upper thoracic surface electromyography, skin conductance, and peripheral skin temperature; Pulsox 3i (oxygen saturation monitor) measured partial percentage of oxygen saturation and heart rate.
Mathiowetz, V., Matuska, K. M., & Murphy, M. E. (2001)	Fatigue impact Self-efficacy Quality of life	FIS SEG SF-36	Participants given the assessments to complete individually (at weeks 1, 7, 13, 19). Note that control group preceded intervention (weeks 1 to 6), and no intervention followed experimental group (weeks 13 to 19).
Hsieh, C. L., Nelson, D. L., Smith, D. A., & Peterson, C. Q. (1996)	Frequency and duration of exercise repetitions Frequency of discontinuities lasting 5 seconds or more	Stopwatch and frequency counts	A stopwatch and 2 counters (silent and out the participant's sight) were used to determine frequency and duration of the exercise.
Furst, G. P., Gerber, L. H., Smith, C. C., & Fisher, S. (1987)	ADL status Psychosocial adjustment to illness Knowledge of disease activity Pain Fatigue	SHAQ PAIS RCAI VAS Activity record	Subjects tested by OTs before treatment, and at 3 months and 9 months after treatment.

continued

Table 8-4 (continued)

OUTCOME MEASURES USED TO CAPTURE PHYSICAL OUTCOMES

Author (Date)	Outcome(s) Investigated	Outcome Measure(s)	Method of Administration
Fatigue/Endurance			
Gerber, L., Furst, G., Shulman, B., Smith, C., Thornton, B., Liang, M., et al. (1987)	Participation in physical activities Pain Fatigue Grip strength Timed walking Joint swelling ADL function Psychological adjustment to illness	PAIS HAQ RAI	Patients were assessed before the intervention and at 3 months after the intervention. A physician conducted the assessments involving grip strength, the RAI, and the timed walking test.
Mobility			
Spadaro, A., De Luca, T., Massimiani, M., Ceccarelli, F., Riccieri, V., & Valesini, G. (2008)	Functional ability Disease status Spinal/hip mobility Health status Pain	BASFI BASDAI BASMI SF-36 VAS	Assessments were completed at baseline and 16 weeks later.
Storr, L. K., Sorensen, P. S., & Ravnborg, M. (2006)	Quality of Life Disability Upper limb function/ambulation Physical impairment	Life Appreciation and Satisfaction Questionnaire Functional Assessment in Multiple Sclerosis Guy's Neurological Disability Scale 9HPT Timed 10-meter walking test MSIS EDSS	Assessments were completed twice over the span of 10 weeks (once before and once after intervention) In patients' homes by the same blinded assessor.
Wennemer, H. K., Borg-Stein, J., Gomba, L., Delaney, B., Rothmund, A., Barlow, D., et al. (2006)	Range of motion Physical function Disease status General health status	Straight leg-raise 6MWT FIQ FHAQ SF-36	Participants completed the questionnaires and assessment before and after entry to the program.
Mendelsohn, M. E., Overend, T. J., & Petrella, R. J. (2004)	Range of motion in knees Proprioception of hip and knees Difference active vs. passive range of motion	Electro-goniometry Proprioception assessment TUG BBS FIM Gait speed 30-second chair stand	Therapist administered at baseline and 48 hours prior to discharge.
Maeshima, S., Ueyoshi, A., Osawa, A., Ishida, K., Kunimoto, K., Shimamoto, Y., et al. (2003)	Changes in nonparetic lower limb strength Mobility	Isokinetic machine Rivermead Mobility Index	Therapist administered at baseline, 1 week after baseline, 2 weeks after baseline.

continued

Table 8-4 (continued)

OUTCOME MEASURES USED TO CAPTURE PHYSICAL OUTCOMES

Author (Date)	Outcome(s) Investigated	Outcome Measure(s)	Method of Administration
Mobility			
Ozdemir, F., Birtane, M., Tabatabaei, R., Kokino, S., & Ekuklu, G. (2001)	Spasticity Motor status Functional status Cognitive status	AS Brunnstrom's stages for motor development FIM MMSE	Therapist administered; history was taken at baseline and mean follow-up of 60 days.
Bolin, I., Bodin, P., & Kreuter, M. (2000)	Balancer Transfers Wheelchair skills Physical strain during wheelchair propulsion Spasticity Respiration	FRT FIM MAS Other measures designed by researchers	Researchers assessed 3 to 6 weeks before intervention and 6 to 8 weeks after intervention.
Griffiths, T., Burr, M., Campbell, I., Lewis-Jenkins, V., Mullins, J., Shiels, K., et al. (2000)	Days spent in hospital Respiratory medication use Walking capacity Health status Anxiety Depression	Chart audit ICD-9 codes Respiratory medication use 10-meter shuttle-walk test SF-36 SGRQ HADS	Self-report and therapist assessed; walking capacity and health status at baseline, 6 weeks, and 1 year; hospital stay information at end of year.
Hoppes, S. (1997)	Standing tolerance	Stop watch	Investigator timed.
Seating			
Shechtman, O., Hanson, C. S., Garrett, D., & Dunn, P. (2001)	Perceived comfort Sitting pressure	Perceived comfort VAS XPMS	Participants were positioned on a wheelchair with no cushion, and pressure was measured after 5 minutes. Participants sat on one of the cushions for 5 minutes, and pressure was again measured. Repeated for 6 cushions.
Bishop, S.A., Bulla, N., DiLellio, E., Dy, M., Koski, J.H., Linnemeyer, C.B., et al. (1999)	Dynamic sitting pressure while using 4 different low-cost wheelchair cushions Body type and relationship with this to peak sitting pressure	Simko body type (height, weight, age) XPMS	Researchers were in charge of the Xsensor device, which consists of a pressure mapping pad, a power supply, a computer interface cable, and computer software. The computer shows pressure images in 2- and 3-dimensional map grid and gives pressure readings in mm Hg.
Pellow, T. R. (1999)	Pressure on the ischial tuberosities and the sacrum	T2PM	Pressure readings taken by the student OT in the neutral position and after every change in position and cushion.
Conine, T. A., Hershler, C., Daechsel, D., Peel, C., & Pearson, A. (1994)	Severity of the pressure ulcer/tissue lesion Interface pressure while seated in wheelchair with cushion	NS ESS SE	Measures were completed on admission and weekly thereafter.

continued

Table 8-4 (continued)
OUTCOME MEASURES USED TO CAPTURE PHYSICAL OUTCOMES

Author (Date)	Outcome(s) Investigated	Outcome Measure(s)	Method of Administration
Seating			
Cron, L., & Sprigle, S. (1993)	Seat interface pressure Sitting balance Wheelchair mobility	Pressure monitor Wheelchair propulsion scale Sitting posture scale	Measured by OTs first on regular cushion, then again 4 days after the use of the hemi cushion.
Falls			
Lannin, N. A., Clemson, L., McCluskey, A., Lin, C., Cameron, I. D., & Barras, S. (2007)	Re-integration to community living Mobility Functional status Fear of falling Quality of life Number of falls Hours and type of community support Number of hospital readmissions	RNLI Tinnetti Performance-Oriented Mobility Assessment FIM Nottingham Extended ADL Scale FES-I EQ-5D Instrument	All assessments and outcome measures were completed at baseline (pre-intervention) and at 2 week, 1, 2, and 3 month follow-up (post-discharge).
Luukinen, H., Lehtola, S., Jokelainen, J., Vaananen-Sainio, R., Lotvonen, S., & Koistinen, P. (2007)	Falls and fall-related injuries Health status Physical ability Use of health services	Interview and questionnaire developed by researchers	Number of falls and fall-related injury data were collected every 2 weeks by a research nurse via a telephone interview and medical records check. All other outcomes measures were recorded at baseline and 2-year follow-up.
Stenvall, M., Olofsson, B., Lundstrom, M., Englund, U., Borssen, B., Svensson, O., et al. (2007)	Falls Complications/injuries from fall Depressive symptoms Pre-injury ADL performance	Medical records OBS GDS-15 Staircase of Activities of Daily Living	Assessments were completed upon admission and discharge from the hospital by an independent researcher blinded to allocation.
von Renteln-Kruse, W., & Krause, T. (2007)	Falls Functional ability	Questionnaire developed by researchers BI	Falls and all related data were collected continuously during patients' stay, and functional ability was assessed at admission and discharge.
Davison, J., Bond, J., Dawson, P., Steen, I. N., & Kenny, R. A. (2005)	Number of falls and number of subjects that fell during 1-year follow-up Injury rates, fall-related hospitalization, mortality, and changes in fall efficacy	Fall diaries ABC Hospital and emergency visits	Fall diaries collected weekly (self-reported). Interviews conducted at 3, 6, and 12 months. ABC administered at baseline and 1 year. Hospital visits recorded prospectively prompted by fall diary. Retrospective audit hospital records at 1 year.

continued

Table 8-4 (continued)

Outcome Measures Used to Capture Physical Outcomes

Author (Date)	Outcome(s) Investigated	Outcome Measure(s)	Method of Administration
Falls			
Ward, C. D., Turpin, G., Dewey, M. E., Fleming, S., Hurwitz, B., Ratib, S., et al. (2004)	Number of falls Skin sores	BBS Self-reported service utilization Nottingham Extended ADL Scale GHQ	An assessor administered in home at baseline and 12 months post-intervention.
Other, Including General Health			
van Houten, P., Achterberg, W., & Ribbe, M. (2007)	Incontinence Toilet usage	Pad test Toilet Timing Test	Assessments were completed at baseline and at the end of the 8-week intervention period.
Gitlin, L., Hauck, W., Winter, L., Dennis, M., & Schulz, R. (2006)	Health and physical function changes Mortality Control-oriented strategy use	5-point scale (1=no difficulty, 5=unable to do due to health problems) Mortality was reported by family 4-point scale (1=not at all true, 4=very much true)	Self-report. Health and physical function measured at baseline. Mortality measured over 14 months.
Studenski, S., Duncan, P., Perera, S., Reker, D., Lai, S. M., & Richards, L. (2005)	Daily functioning Quality of life	FIM BI Lawton and Brody IADL SIS SF-36	Assessments were completed at baseline and 3 and 6 months.
Tsuji, T., Liu, M., Hase, K., Masakado, Y., Takahashi, H., Hara, Y., et al. (2004)	Primary pathology and impairment Disability Muscular function Metabolic function Cardiopulmonary function	SIAS FIM Grip strength Knee extensor torque Body mass index and fat accumulation Heart rate oxygen coefficient 12-minute propulsion distance	Therapist assessed, baseline and discharge (variable).
Bailey, A., Starr, L., Alderson, M., & Moreland, J. (1999)	Changes in self-efficacy, aerobic fitness, strength, flexibility, and disability	Fibro-Fit Questionnaire CST FIQ COPM F-COPES	Therapist administered and self-report. At baseline (day 1 and week 2 for fitness evaluation), and post.
Baskett, J. J., Broad, J. B., Reekie, G., Hocking, C., & Green, G. (1999)	Characteristics of both groups Gait speed Limb function ADL Time with therapists Mood of both subjects and caregivers Anticipation of outcome at entry compared with perceived outcome at exit	MAS BI 9HPT FAT Jamar dynamometer HADS GHQ-28	Assessments conducted by 2 independent research officers.

continued

Table 8-4 (continued)
Outcome Measures Used to Capture Physical Outcomes

Author (Date)	Outcome(s) Investigated	Outcome Measure(s)	Method of Administration
Other, Including General Health			
Richards, S. H., Coast, J., Gunnell, D. J., Peters, T. J., Pounsford, J., & Darlow, M. A. (1998)	Cognitive ability ADL capabilities Quality of life Mortality Post-randomization length of stay ADL functional ability Satisfaction with care services	MMSE BI EuroQol COOP-WONCA Mortality rate and length of stay in care Patient satisfaction with care	Combination of self-report and therapist-administered assessments; baseline, 4 weeks, and 3 months after randomization.
Thomas, J. J. (1996)	Knowledge of cardiac rehabilitation principles Anxiety Self-efficacy	Cardiac Knowledge Questionnaire	During initial interview with OT and 24 hours before hospital discharge.

6MWT=6-Minute Walk Test, 9HPT=Nine-Hole Peg Test, ABC=Activities-Specific Balance Confidence, ADL-T=ADL-Taxonomy, AHFT=Arthritis Hand Function Test, AIMS-2=Arthritis Impact Measurement Scales 2, ARAT=Action Research Arm Test, AS=Ashworth Scale for Spasticity, ASES=Arthritis Self-Efficacy Scale, BASDAI=Bath Ankylosing Spondylitis Disease Activity Index, BASFI=Bath Ankylosing Spondylitis Functional Index, BASMI=Bath Ankylosing Spondylitis Metrology Index, BBS=Berg Balance Scale, BDI=Beck Depression Inventory, BI=Barthel Index, BTE=Baltimore Therapeutic Equipment Company, CES=Coping Efficacy Scale, CES-D=Centre for Epidemiologic Studies Depression Scale, CIQ=Community Integration Questionnaire, COOP-WONCA=Name of a generic quality of life measure, COPM=Canadian Occupational Performance Measure, CRI=Coping Resources Inventory, DAS28=Disease Activity Score, DASH=Disability of Arm, Shoulder, and Hand, DEPS=Assessment to measure symptoms of depression, ECSS=Energy Conservation Strategies Survey, EDSS=Expanded Disability Status Scale, EQ-5D=EuroQol 5D, ESS=Exton-Smith Scale, EULAR 28=Assessing Disease Activity in Rheumatoid Arthritis (name of a handbook of standard methods), EuroQol=European Quality of Life Scale, FAT=Frenchay Arm Test, F-COPES=Family Crisis Oriented Personal Evaluation Scales, FES-I=Falls Efficacy Scale International Scale, FHAQ=Fibromyalgia Health Assessment Questionnaire, FIM=Functional Independence Measure, FIQ=Fibromyalgia Impact Questionnaire, FIS=Fatigue Impact Scale, FMA=Fugl-Meyer Assessment, FRT=Functional Reach Test, FSS=Functional Status Scale, GDS-15=Geriatric Depression Scale, GHQ=General Health Questionnaire, HADS=Hospital Anxiety and Depression Scale, HAMIS=Hand Mobility in Scleroderma, HAQ=Health Assessment Questionnaire, HFOT=Halstead Finger Oscillation Test, HJC=Hand Joint Count, HRU=Health Resource Utilization, JHFT=Jebsen Hand Function Test, JPBA=Joint Protection Behaviour Assessment, LSC=Life Satisfaction Checklist, LSQ=Life Satisfaction Questionnaire, MACTAR=McMaster-Toronto Arthritis Patient Function Performance, MAL=Motor Activity Log, MAS=Motor Assessment Scale, MHQ=Michigan Hand Questionnaire, MI=Motoricity Index, MMSE=Mini Mental Status Examination, MPI=Multidimensional Pain Inventory, MRCMP=Medical Research Council Motor Power, MSIS=Multiple Sclerosis Impairment Scale, MSS=Motor Status Scale, MV=Martin Vigorimeter, NS=Norton Scale, OBS=Organic Brain Syndrome Scale, ODI=Oswestry Disability Index, PAIS=Psychosocial Adjustment to Illness Scale, PBT=Parquetry Block Test, PDI=Pain Disability Index, PKQ=Patient Knowledge Questionnaire, PPGD=Preston Pinch Gauge Device, PSEQ=Pain Self-Efficacy Questionnaire, PSES=Patient Self-Efficacy Scale, PT=Purdue Test, RAI=Rheumatology Attitudes Index, RAKQ=Rheumatoid Arthritis Knowledge Questionnaire, RCAI=Richey-Camp Articular Index, RELHFT=Rehabilitation Engineering Laboratory, RKE-R=Rabideau Kitchen Evaluation-Revised, RMDQ=Rolland and Morris Disability Questionnaire, RNLI=Reintegration to Normal Living Index, RS=Ritchie Scale, RSS=Rodnan Skin Score, SCIM=Spinal Cord Independence Measure, SE=Synergy electromyography, SEG=Self-Efficacy Gauge, SEPEC=Self-Efficacy for Performing Energy Conservation Strategies, SF-36=Short Form Health Survey, SGRQ=St. George Respiratory Questionnaire, SHAQ=Stanford Health Assessment Questionnaire, SIAS=Stroke Impairment Assessment Set, SIS=Stroke Impact Scale, SODA=Sequential Occupational Dexterity Assessment, SOFI=Signals of Functional Impairment Index, SMGW=Solgaard Modified Gartland and Werley, SSES=Stanford Self-Efficacy Scale, SSS=Symptom Severity Scale, T2PM=Talley II Pressure Monitor, TEMPA=Test evaluating upper extremity function in aging persons, TUG=Timed Up and Go Test, VAS=Visual Analog Scale, WAIS-R=Weschler Adult Intelligence Scale, WMFT=Wolf Motor Function Test, XPMS=Xsensor pressure mapping system.

the use of splints (Adams, 1996; Egan & Brousseau, 2007; Egan et al., 2001), with the exception of resting splints for conditions like carpal tunnel syndrome (Gelberman, Szabo, & Mortenson, 1984; O'Connor, Marshall, & Massy-Westropp, 2006).

Educational Approach

The educational approach is also popular in occupational therapy for physical impairment. Of 19 articles cited in this literature review, 15 pertained to energy conservation and joint protection. There was also a cardiac rehabilitation program featured and a pre-surgical education program for older patients awaiting joint replacement surgery. Intervention environments examined included inpatient, outpatient, and community (home and nursing homes).

These interventions tended to focus on individuals with neuromuscular diseases, such as multiple sclerosis, or with arthritic conditions. These approaches tend to combine a number of basic occupational therapy principles, such as avoiding placing stress on joints, adapting tools and environments to enhance proper joint use, balancing rest and activity, and supporting proximal joints to allow distal joints to work. The educational methods used ranged from highly individualized approaches where the occupational therapist met one-on-one with the client either in the hospital or in the client's home to therapists teaching pre-designed multisession patient education programs to groups of clients (Hammond, Young, & Kidao, 2004; Lamb, Finlayson, Mathiowetz, & Chen, 2005; Melvin, 1989).

Occupational Development

Thirteen studies were identified that considered occupational development in a broader sense. These tended to be multidisciplinary, multifocused interventions aimed at promoting occupation more generally. These included programs aimed at falls prevention, low back pain, and chronic lung disease. They tended to include education, training, and support elements in intensive programming. Some were individually tailored, and some were offered in a group context. Several included pain management and relaxation exercises.

Skill Development

Seven articles focused on the development of specific skills, particularly ADL and IADL (instrumental activities of daily living) skills. These programs tended to be of shorter duration and more specifically focused on a particular skill or set of skills such as toileting, eating, rising from a chair, and climbing stairs (Mendelsohn, Overend, & Petrella, 2004; van

Houten, Achterberg, & Ribbe, 2007), rather than on occupational performance overall.

Effects of Occupational Therapy in Promoting Physical Outcomes

Table 8-2 summarizes the evidence for effectiveness of occupational therapy interventions addressing the physical determinants of occupation. There is evidence from 19 randomized clinical trials for positive effects of occupational therapy. The vast majority of these have been published in the past 5 years, suggesting a growing trend in generating randomized controlled trial-based evidence for occupational therapy interventions. There are five studies that provide positive evidence for joint protection programs, especially those using the educational-behavioral approach (Hammond & Freeman, 2001, 2004; Hammond, Jeffreson, Jones, Gallagher, & Jones, 2002; Masiero, Boniolo, Wassermann, Machiedo, Volante, & Punzi, 2007; Spadaro, De Luca, Massimiani, Ceccarelli, Riccieri, & Valesini, 2008). Other programs that appear to be successful include energy conservation (Mathiowetz, Finlayson, Matuska, Chen, & Luo, 2005), falls prevention (Davison, Bond, Dawson, Steen, & Kenny, 2005; Stenvall et al., 2007), home safety (Gitlin, Hauck, Winter, Dennis, & Schulz, 2006), and guided relaxation (WaiShan Louie, 2004). These appear to be multidimensional programs with some degree of educational focus.

With regard to training and exercise programs, it appears that early intervention is useful for stroke recovery, but that gains may not be sustained (Studenski, Duncan, Perera, Reker, Min Lai, & Richards, 2005). Two studies supported occupationally embedded exercise (Nelson et al., 1996; Yuen, Nelson, Peterson, & Dickinson, 1994), and one supported the importance of biofeedback during exercise (Paes Lourencao, Battistella, Moran de Brito, Tsukimoto, & Miyazaki, 2008). There is support for both inpatient (Ozdemir, Birtane, Tabatabaei, Kokino, & Ekuklu, 2001) and community-based rehabilitation programs (Griffiths et al., 2000; Pang, Harris, & Eng, 2006), as well as for a pre-discharge home visit for assessing physical demands of the home environment (Lannin, Clemson, McCluskey, Lin, Cameron, & Barras, 2007). Finally, only one randomized trial supports the effectiveness of a commercially available working wrist splint (Pagnotta, Korner-Bitensky, Mazer, Baron, & Wood-Dauphinee, 2005).

There were 36 non-randomized controlled trial studies in the set that also produced positive results, furnishing more evidence of effectiveness of occupational therapy interventions. For example, six additional studies were found that concluded that occupationally embedded exercise was more effective than rote exercise for improving physical functioning (Hoppes, 1997; Hsieh, Nelson, Smith, & Peterson, 1996; Jarus, Shavit, & Ratzon, 2000; King, 1993; Neistadt, 1994; Sietsema, Nelson, Mulder, Mervau-Scheidel, & White, 1993). Hand and upper extremity function were responsive to occupational therapy interventions addressing factors such as strength, pain, and functional activity performance (Aldehag, Jonsson, & Ansved, 2005; Case-Smith, 2003; Fischer, Nagy, & Buechler, 2003). Energy conservation programs and hand function programs were also afforded some support by non-randomized controlled trial studies.

In the category of no effect, 43 studies were found, both randomized controlled trials and non-randomized controlled trials. Several findings stand out as being of interest for further research. Investigators were unable to show significant results, but did observe trends suggesting the need for further investigation of educational interventions including joint protection and energy conservation.

On the other hand, there were also some interventions that could not be supported with empirical evidence. For example, there was no clear direction on seating. The selection and use of wheelchair cushions and seating systems seems sufficiently individually unique to each client as to preclude standardized approaches for effectiveness.

Furthermore, the evidence for splinting is not strong. With the exception of reducing pain, such as resting splints for carpal tunnel syndrome, the evidence was weak for the effectiveness of splinting in general and explicitly negative on splinting for people post-stroke and acquired brain injury (Lannin, Cusick, McCluskey, & Herbert, 2007; Matheiowetz, Bolding, & Trombly, 1983). One group of researchers suggests that custom splinting cannot be justified, given the ambivalence of their results comparing custom with pre-fabricated splints (Tijhuis, Vliet Vlieland, Zwinderman, & Hazes, 1998).

Measures Used to Capture Physical Outcomes

Outcome measures for the physical determinants of occupation fall broadly into seven categories: Measures of arm and hand function (e.g., strength, range of motion, morning stiffness), pain, fatigue, mobility, seating, falls, and general health. In the area of arm and hand function, we are not surprised to see manual muscle testing, goniometry, and dyna-mometry as staples in the measurement of physical performance components. These basic, low-technology measures are standard clinical and research tools in rehabilitation and are recognized for their validity and reliability when administered by trained clinicians. Several other common assessments are the Fugl-Meyer Assessment (FMA) of Sensorimotor Recovery, the Motor Assessment Scale (MAS), the Jebsen Hand Function Test (JHFT), and the Arthritis Impact Measurement Scale (AIMS-2). As their names suggest, these measures are designed for specific populations in some instances, such as arthritis and stroke. Another interesting measure that does not specifically address hand function, but that does pertain to arthritis, is the Arthritis Self-Efficacy Scale (ASES).

In the area of pain, the most common measure by far was the visual analog scale (VAS). It has become virtually an industry standard to invite patients to rate their pain on a 10-cm line, from least to most severe. There are of course other measures of pain, such as the Multidimensional Pain Inventory (MPI) or the McGill Pain Questionnaire (MPQ), but none was as prevalent as the VAS in this review.

With regard to fatigue, in addition to more qualitative diary-type questionnaires, the most common measure used in these studies was the Fatigue Impact Scale (FIS). Measures of mobility tended to be timed tests, like the Timed Up and Go Test (TUG), or other tests of distance, strength, and speed. Mobility tests tended to be disease-specific, such as those mentioned in Table 8-4 for ankylosing spondylitis or fibromyalgia. Seating measures tended to involve pressure monitoring. Measures associated with falls included the Berg Balance Scale (BBS) and the Falls Efficacy Scale (FES).

Finally, a number of measures were often included in these studies that assessed overall functioning, health, and well-being. Functional measures, such as the Functional Independence Measure (FIM) and the Barthel Index (BI), assessed ADL independence as an indication of physical functioning and overall recovery. Other more distal measures included the Return to Normal Living Index (RNLI), the Sickness Impact Profile (SIP), the Health Assessment Questionnaire (HAQ), and the SF-36 and SF-12 of the Medical Outcomes Study Health Survey. These measures are readily recognized by researchers in other fields and, thus, have the advantage of transferability and credibility. However, there is a danger that measures like this will not be sufficiently sensitive to the physical changes achieved and, therefore, will not show significant change over a period of therapy. When interpreting lack of significance in results that use these global measures, consideration needs to be given to the fact that they may simply be measuring too broad a concept to detect changes in outcomes at a specific physical function level.

Conclusions and Recommendations for Future Research

In summary, this chapter has identified five types of interventions used by occupational therapists to promote improvements in physical functioning: Physical training, education, environmental modifications, skills development, and occupational development.

Of particular interest is the support for occupationally embedded activities for therapeutic purposes in the physical area. There was sound evidence from both randomized controlled trial and non-randomized controlled trial studies that occupationally embedded activities enhanced engagement in therapy and promoted positive outcomes. This finding was true across a number of different diagnoses and clinical conditions, and upholds one of the basic tenets of occupational therapy.

Educational interventions also appear to be very effective. Occupational therapists use educational approaches to promote joint protection, energy conservation, home safety, falls prevention, and pain management (Palmer & Simons, 1991). The most successful techniques were those that combined cognitive and behavioral aspects, furnishing patients with new knowledge while also affording them opportunities to try on new behaviors.

A potentially controversial finding of this review is the lack of strong evidence supporting the splinting approaches studied (Pratt, 2004). With the exception of carpal tunnel syndrome, the literature reviewed was equivocal about splints (Gelberman et al., 1984). In a systematic review of conservative techniques to treat carpal tunnel syndrome, evidence supports a short-term positive effect of resting hand splints on symptoms (O'Connor et al., 2006).

For the most part, the effectiveness of splinting is not well documented (Paternostro-Sluga & Stieger, 2004). There seems to be little consensus on the effect of splints in preventing deformity and increasing hand function for both acute and chronic rheumatoid hands (Adams, 1996). One systematic review looked at the impact of splints on people with rheumatoid arthritis and found weak evidence for the effectiveness of working splints, resting splints, and shoe inserts on pain relief at any joint, with the exception of joints of the neck or back (Egan et al., 2006).

Hand splinting is also used to prevent contractures for clients after strokes, but evidence from a systematic review by Lannin and Herbert (2003) indicates limited research and poor methodology. Alternatively, serial casting may be used to prevent contractures and has been shown to be effective in improving range of motion and clinical measures of spasticity in individuals with spastic limbs, but more research is required (Preissner, 2001).

Another controversial topic is the use of physical training and modalities in occupational therapy. There may be international and geographic variations in occupational therapy practices in this regard. In the treatment of upper extremity injuries, physical modalities are sometimes used as an adjunct to engagement in occupation (American Occupational Therapy Association, 1997). A survey by Cornish-Painter, Peterson, and Lindstrom-Hazel (1997) indicated that many occupational therapists use at least one of the following modalities in their practice: Hot/cold packs, paraffin, contrast baths, functional electrical stimulation (FES), neuromuscular electrical stimulation (NES), fluidotherapy, ultrasound, whirlpool, and transcutaneous electrical stimulation (TENS). In a meta-analysis, electrotherapeutic agents were shown to have a potentially positive effect on shoulder function for clients with stroke, facilitating grasp patterns in the affected upper extremity (Handy, Salinas, Blanchard, & Aitken, 2003).

The literature offers a number of systematic reviews of occupational therapy with specific physical conditions. A few examples of the findings of these reviews follow. For osteoarthritis, occupational therapy intervention typically includes splinting, technical aids, and joint protection. A systematic review of occupational therapy practice for people with osteoarthritis indicates some evidence supporting the benefits of these occupational therapy interventions (Towheed, 2005). In a systematic review of occupational therapy for people with Huntington's disease, programs involved re-education and provision of adaptive aids to assist in ADL (Bilney, Morris, & Perry, 2003). In a meta-analysis of treatment for clients with multiple sclerosis, occupational therapy was effective with interventions such as exercise, fatigue management, cooling, and TENS application. A smaller effect was seen for occupational therapy treatment of emotional and cognitive outcomes, such as stress management, skills training in socialization, and attention training (Baker & Tickle-Degnen, 2001).

With regard to outcome measures used in occupational therapy research on the physical components of occupation, there is a broad array indeed and a dizzying list of acronyms. Greater specificity in measurement in this area, as in other areas of occupational therapy research, seems to be associated with a greater likelihood of positive findings. This area of research would benefit greatly from some consensus about the best measures to demonstrate the effects of occupational therapy. Based on this scoping review, it would appear that some promising candidates might be the MAS, the Physical subscale of the SF-36, the VAS, and other proximal measures of physical performance, such as muscle strength and joint range. The nature of biomedical, quantitative, evidence-based research such as that focusing on physical determinants mandates that the researchers pre-identify the outcomes to be measured. This can create a paradoxical challenge for occupational therapy. It is a profession concerned with enabling clients to participate in those occupations that they find meaningful and satisfying. The challenge then for occupational therapy researchers on physical determinants is to also be able to demonstrate the link between occupational therapy interventions at the physical level and outcomes in occupational well-being.

In conclusion, this review offers clear guidance to occupational therapists with regard to occupationally embedded activity. Although we stated at the outset that it was overly simplistic to draw the distinction between occupational and physical therapy at the patient's waist, there does appear to be a concentration in the research on upper extremity and hand function. However, the more important distinction perhaps is the focus on occupationally embedded activity versus straight exercise. It appears that, for the most part, occupational therapy for physical impairment occurs in the context of a multidisciplinary team. Perhaps the most important contribution that future research can make is to further distinguish the contribution of occupational therapy through its association with real and meaningful activities in patients' lives.

References

Adams, J. (1996). Splinting the rheumatoid wrist and hand: Evidence for its effectiveness. *British Journal of Therapy and Rehabilitation, 3*(11), 621-624.

Akalin, E., El, O., Peker, O., Senocak, O., Tamci, S., Gulbahar, S., et al. (2002). Treatment of carpal tunnel syndrome with nerve and tendon gliding exercises. *American Journal of Physical Medicine and Rehabilitation, 81*, 108-113.

Aldehag, A. S., Jonsson, H., & Ansved, T. (2005). Effects of a hand training programme in five patients with myotonic dystrophy type 1. *Occupational Therapy International, 12*(1), 14-27.

American Occupational Therapy Association. (1997). Physical agent modalities: A position paper. *American Journal of Occupational Therapy, 51*, 870-871.

Bailey, A., Starr, L., Alderson, M., & Moreland, J. (1999). A comparative evaluation of a (No Suggestions) rehabilitation program. *Arthritis Care and Research, 12*(5), 336-340.

Baker, N. A., & Tickle-Degnen, L. (2001). The effectiveness of physical, sychological and functional interventions in treating clients with multiple sclerosis: A meta-analysis. *American Journal of Occupational Therapy, 55*, 324-331.

Baldwin, B. T. (1919). Helping the wounded soldier to "come back." *The Modern Hospital, 10*, 370-374.

Barry, M. A., Purser, J., Hazleman, R., McLean, A., & Hazleman, B. L. (1994). Effect of energy conservation and joint protection education in rheumatoid arthritis. *British Journal of Rheumatology, 33*(12), 1171-1174.

Baskett, J. J., Broad, J. B., Reekie, G., Hocking, C., & Green, G. (1999). Shared responsibility for ongoing rehabilitation: A new approach to home-based therapy after stroke. *Clinical Rehabilitation, 13*(1), 23-33.

Billings, F. (1918). Reconstruction and rehabilitation of disabled workers. *Journal of the American Medical Association, 70*, 1924-1931.

Bilney, B., Morris, M., & Perry, A. (2003). Effectiveness of physiotherapy, occupational therapy, and speech pathology for people with Huntington's disease: A systematic review. *Neurorehabilitation and Neural Repair, 17*, 12-24.

Bishop, S. A., Bulla, N., DiLellio, E., Dy, M., Koski, J. H., Linnemeyer, C. B., et al. (1999). The effects of low-cost wheelchair cushions and body-type on dynamic sitting pressure in nursing home residents. *Physical and Occupational Therapy in Geriatrics, 17*(1), 29-41.

Bolin, I., Bodin, P., & Kreuter, M. (2000). Sitting position—posture and performance in C5-C6 tetraplegia. *Spinal Cord, 38*(7), 425-434.

Callinan, N. J., & Mathiowetz, V. (1996). Soft versus hard resting hand splints in rheumatoid arthritis: Pain relief, preference, and compliance. *American Journal of Occupational Therapy, 50*(5), 347-353.

Case-Smith, J. (2003). Outcomes in hand rehabilitation using occupational therapy services. *American Journal of Occupational Therapy, 57*, 499-506.

Christensen, O. M., Kunov, A., Hansen, F. F., Christiansen, T. C., & Krasheninnikoff, M. (2001). Occupational therapy and Colles' fractures. *International Orthopaedics, 25*, 43-45.

Conine, T. A., Hershler, C., Daechsel, D., Peel, C., & Pearson, A. (1994). Pressure ulcer prophylaxis in elderly patients using polyurethane foam of Jay wheelchair cushions. *International Journal of Rehabilitation Research, 17*, 123-137.

Cornish-Painter, C., Peterson, C. Q., & Lindstrom-Hazel, D. K. (1997). Skill acquisition and competency testing for physical agent modality use. *American Journal of Occupational Therapy, 51*, 681-685.

Cron, L., & Sprigle, S. (1993). Clinical evaluation of the hemi wheelchair cushion. *American Journal of Occupational Therapy, 47*(2), 141-144.

Davison, J., Bond, J., Dawson, P., Steen, I. N., & Kenny, R. A. (2005). Patients with recurrent falls attending accident and emergency benefit from multifactorial intervention—a randomised controlled trial. *Age and Ageing, 34*(2), 162-168.

Deshaies, L. D. (2002). Upper extremity orthoses. In: C. A. Trombly & M. V. Radomski (Eds.), *Occupational therapy for physical dysfunction* (5th ed., pp. 313-349). Baltimore, MD: Lippincott Williams & Wilkins.

Desrosiers, J., Malouin, F., Richards, C., Bourbonnais, D., Rochette, A., & Bravo, G. (2003). Comparison of changes in upper and lower extremity impairments and disabilities after stroke. *International Journal of Rehabilitation Research, 26*(2), 109-116.

Dohnke, B., Knauper, B., & Muller-Fahrnow, W. (2005). Perceived self-efficacy gained from, and health effects of, a rehabilitation program after hip joint replacement. *Arthritis and Rheumatism, 53*(4), 585-592.

Donnelly, C. J., & Wilton, J. (2002). The effect of massage to scars on active range of motion and skin mobility. *British Journal of Hand Therapy, 7*(1), 5-11.

Egan, M., & Brousseau, L. (2007). Splinting for osteoarthritis of the carpometacarpal joint: A review of the evidence. *American Journal of Occupational Therapy, 61*(1), 70-78.

Egan, M., Brosseau, L., Farmer, M., Ouimet, M., Rees, S., Tugwell, P., & Wells, G. (2001). Splints and orthosis for treating rheumatoid arthritis (review). *The Cochrane Collaboration*, Vol. 4.

Finlayson, M. (2005). Pilot study of an energy conservation education program delivered by telephone conference call to people with multiple sclerosis. *Neurorehabilitation, 20*(4), 267-277.

Fischer, T., Nagy, L., & Buechler, U. (2003). Restoration of pinch grip in ulnar nerve paralysis: Extensor carpi radialis longus to adductor pollicis and abductor pollicis longus to first dorsal interosseus tendon transfers. *Journal of Hand Surgery (British Volume), 28B*, 28-32.

Fletchall, S., & Hickerson, W. L. (1991). Early upper-extremity prosthetic fit in patients with burns. *Journal of Burn Care and Rehabilitation, 12*(3), 234-236.

Furst, G. P., Gerber, L. H., Smith, C. C., & Fisher, S. (1987). A program for improving energy conservation behaviors in adults with rheumatoid arthritis. *American Journal of Occupational Therapy, 41*(2), 102-111.

Gelberman, R. H., Szabo, R. M., & Mortenson, M. M. (1984). Carpal tunnel pressures and wrist position in patients with Colles fractures. *Journal of Trauma, Injury, Infection and Critical Care, 24*, 747-749.

Gerber, L., Furst, G., Shulman, B., Smith, C., Thornton, B., Liang, M., et al. (1987). Patient education program to teach energy conservation behaviors to patients with rheumatoid arthritis: A pilot study. *Archives of Physical Medicine and Rehabilitation, 68*, 442-445.

Gitlin, L., Hauck, W., Winter, L., Dennis, M., & Schulz, R. (2006). Effect of an in-home occupational and physical therapy intervention on reducing mortality in functionally vulnerable older people: Preliminary findings. *Journal of the American Geriatrics Society, 54*(6), 950-955.

Greenberg, S., & Fowler, R. S., Jr. (1980). Kinesthetic biofeedback: A treatment modality for elbow range of motion in hemiplegia. *American Journal of Occupational Therapy, 34*(11), 738-743.

Griffiths, T., Burr, M., Campbell, I., Lewis-Jenkins, V., Mullins, J., Shiels, K., et al. (2000). Results at 1 year of outpatient multidisciplinary pulmonary rehabilitation: A randomized controlled trial. *Lancet, 355*(9201), 362-368.

Hammond, A. (1994). Joint protection behavior in patients with rheumatoid arthritis following an education program: A pilot study. *Arthritis Care and Research, 7*, 5-9.

Hammond, A., & Freeman, K. (2001). One-year outcomes of a randomized controlled trial of an educational-behavioural joint protection programme for people with rheumatoid arthritis. *Rheumatology (Oxford, England), 40*(9), 1044-1051.

Hammond, A., & Freeman, K. (2004). The long-term outcomes from a randomized controlled trial of an educational behavioural joint protection programme for people with rheumatoid arthritis. *Clinical Rehabilitation, 18*(5), 520-528.

Hammond, A., Jefferson, P., Jones, N., Gallagher, J., & Jones, T. (2002). Clinical applicability of an educational-behavioural joint protection programme for people with rheumatoid arthritis. *British Journal of Occupational Therapy, 65*(9), 405-412.

Hammond, A., Young, A., & Kidao, R. (2004). A randomised controlled trial of occupational therapy for people with early rheumatoid arthritis. *Annals of the Rheumatic Diseases, 63*(1), 23-30.

Handy, J., Salinas, S., Blanchard, S., & Aitken, M. (2003). Meta-analysis examining the effectiveness of electrical stimulation in improving functional use of the upper limb in stroke patients. *Physical and Occupational Therapy, 21*(4), 67-78.

Haskett, S., Backman, C., Porter, B., Goyert, J., & Palejko, G. (2004). A crossover trial of custom-made and commercially available wrist splints in adults with inflammatory arthritis. *Arthritis and Rheumatism, 51*, 792-799.

Hildebrandt, J., Pfingsten, M., Saur, P., & Jansen, J. (1997). Prediction of success from a multidisciplinary treatment program for chronic low back pain. *Spine, 22*(9), 990-1001.

Hoppes, S. (1997). Can play increase standing tolerance? A pilot-study. *Physical and Occupational Therapy in Geriatrics, 15*(1), 65-73.

Hsieh, C. L., Nelson, D. L., Smith, D. A., & Peterson, C. Q. (1996). A comparison of performance in added-purpose occupations and rote exercise for dynamic standing balance in persons with hemiplegia. *American Journal of Occupational Therapy, 50*(1), 10-16.

Ip, W. M., Woo, J., Yue, S. Y., Kwan, M., Sum, S. M., Kwok, T., et al. (2006). Evaluation of the effect of energy conservation techniques in the performance of activity of daily living tasks. *Clinical Rehabilitation, 20*(3), 254-261.

James, A. B. (2003). Biomechanical frame of reference. In E. B. Crepeau, E. S. Cohen, & B. A. B. Schell (Eds.), *Willard & Spackman's occupational therapy* (pp. 240-242). Philadelphia, PA: Lippincott Williams & Wilkins.

Jarus, T., Shavit, S., & Ratzon, N. (2000). From hand twister to mind twister: Computer-aided treatment in traumatic wrist fracture. *American Journal of Occupational Therapy, 54*, 176-182.

Kaapa, E. H., Frantsi, K., Sarna, S., & Malmivaara, A. (2006). Multidisciplinary group rehabilitation versus individual physio-

therapy for chronic nonspecific low back pain: A randomized trial. *Spine, 31*(4), 371-376.

King, T. I. (1993). Hand strengthening with a computer for purposeful activity. *American Journal of Occupational Therapy, 47*(7), 635-637.

Kohlmeyer, K. M., Hill, J. P., Yarkony, G. M., & Jaeger, R. J. (1996). Electrical stimulation and biofeedback effect on recovery of tenodesis grasp: A controlled study. *Archives of Physical Medicine and Rehabilitation, 77*, 702-706.

Lamb, A. L., Finlayson, M., Mathiowetz, V., & Chen, H. Y. (2005). The outcomes of using self-study modules in energy conservation education for people with multiple sclerosis. *Clinical Rehabilitation, 19*(5), 475-481.

Lannin., N., Clemson, L., McCluskey, A., Lin, C-W., Cameron, I., & Barras, S. (2007). Feasibility and results of a randomized pilot-study of pre-discharge occupational therapy home visits. *BMC Health Services Research, 7*, 42-49.

Lannin, N., Cusick, A., McCluskey, A., & Herbert, R. (2007). Effects of splinting on wrist contracture after stroke: A randomized controlled trial. *Stroke, 38*, 111-116.

Lannin, N. A., & Herbert, R. D. (2003). Is hand splinting effective for adults following stroke? A systematic review and methodological critique of published research. *Clinical Rehabilitation, 17*(8), 807-816.

Lannin, N. A., Horsley, S. A., Herbert, R., McCluskey, A., & Cusick, A. (2003). Splinting the hand in the functional position after brain impairment: A randomized, controlled trial. *Archives of Physical Medicine and Rehabilitation, 84*, 297-302.

Li, L. C., Davis, A. M., Lineker, S., Coyte, P. C., & Bombardier, C. (2005). Outcomes of home-based rehabilitation provided by primary therapists for patients with rheumatoid arthritis: Pilot study. *Physiotherapy Canada, 57*(4), 255-264.

Li, L. C., Davis, A. M., Lineker, S. C., Coyte, P. C., & Bombardier, C. (2006). Effectiveness of the primary therapist model for rheumatoid arthritis rehabilitation: A randomized controlled trial. *Arthritis and Rheumatism, 55*(1), 42-52.

Li, S., Liu, L., Miyazaki, M., & Warren, S. (1999). Effectiveness of splinting for work-related carpal tunnel syndrome: A three-month follow-up study. *Technology and Disability, 11*, 51-64.

Lin, K-C., Wu, C-Y., Tickle-Degnen, L., & Coster, W. (1997). Enhancing occupational performance through occupationally embedded exercise: A meta-analytic review. *Occupational Therapy Journal of Research, 17*(1), 25-47.

Luukinen, H., Lehtola, S., Jokelainene, J., Vaananen-Sainio, R., Lotvonen, S., & Koistinen, P. (2007). Pragmatic exercise-oriented prevention of falls among the elderly: A population-based, randomized controlled trial. *Preventative Medicine, 44*, 256-271.

Lynch, D., Ferraro, M., Krol, J., Trudell, C. M., Christos, P., & Volpe, B. T. (2005). Continuous passive motion improves shoulder joint integrity following stroke. *Clinical Rehabilitation, 19*(6), 594-599.

Maeshima, S., Ueyoshi, A., Osawa, A., Ishida, K., Kunimoto, K., Shimamoto, Y., et al. (2003). Mobility and muscle strength contralateral to hemiplegia from stroke: Benefit from self-training with family support. *American Journal of Physical Medicine and Rehabilitation, 82*(6), 456-462.

Malcus-Johnson, P., Carlqvist, C., Sturesson, A. L., & Eberhardt, K. (2005). Occupational therapy during the first 10 years of rheumatoid arthritis. *Scandinavian Journal of Occupational Therapy, 12*(3), 128-135.

Masiero, S., Boniolo, A., Wassermann, L., Machiedo, H., Volante, D., & Punzi, L. (2007). Effects of an educational–behavioural joint protection program on people with moderate to severe rheumatoid arthritis: A randomized controlled trial. *Clinical Rheumatology, 26*(12), 2043-2050.

Mathiowetz, V., Bolding, D. J., & Trombly, C. A. (1983). Immediate effects of positioning devices on the normal and spastic hand measured by electromyography. *American Journal of Occupational Therapy, 37*(4), 247-254.

Mathiowetz, V. G., Finlayson, M. L., Matuska, K. M., Chen, H. Y., & Luo, P. (2005). Randomized controlled trial of an energy conservation course for persons with multiple sclerosis. *Multiple Sclerosis, 11*(5), 592-601.

Mathiowetz, V., Matuska, K. M., & Murphy, M. E. (2001). Efficacy of an energy conservation course for persons with multiple sclerosis. *Archives of Physical Medicine and Rehabilitation, 82*(4), 449-456.

Matuska, K., Mathiowetz, V., & Finlayson, M. (2007). Use and perceived effectiveness of energy conservation strategies for managing multiple sclerosis fatigue. *American Journal of Occupational Therapy, 61*(1), 62-69.

McColl, M. A., & Bickenbach, J. (1998). *Introduction to disability.* London, England: W. B. Saunders Ltd.

McColl, M. A., Law, M., Stewart, D., Doubt, L., Pollock, N., & Krupa, T. (2002). *Theoretical basis of occupational therapy* (2nd ed.). Thorofare, NJ: SLACK Incorporated.

Melvin, J. L. (1989). *Rheumatic disease in the adult and child* (3rd ed.). Philadelphia, PA: F. A. Davis.

Mendelsohn, M. E., Overend, T. J., & Petrella, R. J. (2004). Effect of rehabilitation on hip and knee proprioception in older adults after hip fracture: A pilot study. *American Journal of Physical Medicine and Rehabilitation, 83*(8), 624-632.

Neistadt, M. E. (1994). The effects of different treatment activities on functional fine motor coordination in adults with brain injury. *American Journal of Occupational Therapy, 48*(10), 877-882.

Nelson, D. L., Konosky, K., Fleharty, K., Webb, R., Newer, K., Hazboun, V. P., et al. (1996). The effects of an occupationally embedded exercise on bilaterally assisted supination in persons with hemiplegia. *American Journal of Occupational Therapy, 50*(8), 639-646.

O'Connor, D., Marshall, S., & Massy-Westropp, N. (2006). Non-surgical treatment (other than steroid injection) for carpal tunnel syndrome. *Cochrane Database of Systematic Reviews,* Issue 4.

Ozdemir, F., Birtane, M., Tabatabaei, R., Kokino, S., & Ekuklu, G. (2001). Comparing stroke rehabilitation outcomes between acute inpatient and nonintense home settings. *Archives of Physical Medicine and Rehabilitation, 82*(10), 1375-1379.

Paes Lourencao, M. I., Battistella, L. R., Moran de Brito, C. M., Tsukimoto, G. R., & Miyazaki, M. H. (2008). Effect of biofeedback accompanying occupational therapy and functional electrical stimulation in hemiplegic patients. *International Journal of Rehabilitation Research, 31*(1), 33-41.

Pagnotta, A., Baron, M., & Korner-Bitensky, N. (1998). The effect of a static wrist orthosis on hand function in individuals with rheumatoid arthritis. *Journal of Rheumatology, 25*(5), 879-885.

Pagnotta, A., Korner-Bitensky, N., Mazer, B., Baron, M., & Wood-Dauphinee, S. (2005). Static wrist splint use in the performance of daily activities by individuals with rheumatoid arthritis. *Journal of Rheumatology, 32*(11), 2136-2143.

Palmer, P., & Simons, J. (1991). Joint protection: A critical review. *British Journal of Occupational Therapy, 54,* 453-458.

Pang, M., Harris, J., & Eng, J. (2006). A community-based upper-extremity group exercise program improves motor function and performance of functional activities in chronic stroke: A randomized controlled trial. *Archives of Physical Medicine and Rehabilitation, 87*(1), 1-9.

Paternostro-Sluga, T., & Stieger, M. (2004). Hand splints in rehabilitation. *Critical Reviews in Physical and Rehabilitation Medicine, 16,* 233-256.

Pellow, T. R. (1999). A comparison of interface pressure readings to wheelchair cushions and positioning: A pilot study. *Canadian Journal of Occupational Therapy, 66*(3), 140-149.

Pizzi, A., Carlucci, G., Falsini, C., Verdesca, S., & Grippo, A. (2005). Application of a volar static splint in post stroke spasticity of the upper limb. *Archives of Physical Medicine and Rehabilitation, 86*(9), 1855-1859.

Poole, J. L., Whitney, S. L., Hangeland, N., & Baker, C. (1990). The effectiveness of inflatable pressure splints on motor function in stroke patients. *Occupational Therapy Journal of Research, 10*(6), 360-366.

Popovic, M. R., Thrasher, T. A., Adams, M. E., Takes, V., Zivanovic, V., & Tonack, M. I. (2006). Functional electrical therapy: Retraining grasping in spinal cord injury. *Spinal Cord, 44*(3), 143-151.

Pratt, A. L. (2004). Is eight weeks' immobilisation of the distal interphalangeal joint adequate treatment for acute closed mallet finger injuries of the hand? A critical review of the literature. *British Journal of Hand Therapy, 9,* 4-10.

Preissner, K. S. (2001). The effects of serial casting in spasticity: A literature review. *Occupational Therapy in Health Care, 14,* 99-106.

Richards, S. H., Coast, J., Gunnell, D. J., Peters, T. J., Pounsford, J., & Darlow, M. A. (1998). Randomized controlled trial comparing effectiveness and acceptability of an early discharge, hospital at home scheme with acute hospital care. *British Medical Journal, 316*(7147), 1796-1801.

Ring, H., & Rosenthal, N. (2005). Controlled study of neuroprosthetic functional electrical stimulation in sub-acute post-stroke rehabilitation. *Journal of Rehabilitation Medicine, 37*(1), 32-36.

Rodgers, H., Mackintosh, J., Price, C., Wood, R., McNamee, P., Fearon, T., et al. (2003). Does an early increased-intensity interdisciplinary upper limb therapy programme following acute stroke improve outcome? *Clinical Rehabilitation, 17*(6), 579-589.

Rosenstein, L., Ridgel, A., Thota, A., Samame, B., & Alberts, J. (2008). Effects of combined robotic therapy and repetitive-task practice on upper-extremity function in a patient with chronic stroke. *American Journal of Occupational Therapy, 62*(1), 28-35.

Sandin-Aldehag, A., & Jonsson, H. (2003). Evaluation of a hand-training programme for patients with welander distal myopathy. *Scandinavian Journal of Occupational Therapy, 10*(4), 188-192.

Sandqvist, G., Akesson, A., & Eklund, M. (2004). Evaluation of paraffin bath treatment in patients with systemic sclerosis. *Disability and Rehabilitation, 26*(16), 981-987.

Seidel, A. C. (2003). Rehabilitative frame of reference. In E. B. Crepeau, E. S. Cohen, & B. A. B. Schell (Eds.), *Willard & Spackman's occupational therapy* (pp. 238-239). Philadelphia, PA: Lippincott Williams & Wilkins.

Shechtman, O., Hanson, C. S., Garrett, D., & Dunn, P. (2001). Comparing wheelchair cushions for effectiveness of pressure relief: A pilot study. *Occupational Therapy Journal of Research, 21*(1), 29-48.

Sietsema, J. M., Nelson, D. L., Mulder, R. M., Mervau-Scheidel, D., & White, B. E. (1993). The use of a game to promote arm reach in persons with traumatic brain injury. *American Journal of Occupational Therapy, 47*(1), 19-24.

Spadaro, A., De Luca, T., Massimiani, M., Ceccarelli, F., Riccieri, V., & Valesini, G. (2008). Occupational therapy in ankylosing spondylitis: Short-term prospective study in patients treated with anti-TNF-alpha drugs. *Joint Bone Spine, 75,* 29-33.

Spalding, N. J. (1995). A comparative study of the effectiveness of a preoperative education programme for total hip replacement patients. *British Journal of Occupational Therapy, 58*(12), 526-531.

Stenvall, M., Olofsson, B., Lundstrom, M., Englund, U., Borssen, B., Svensson, O., et al. (2007). A multidisciplinary, multifactorial intervention program reduces postoperative falls and injuries after femoral neck fracture. *Osteoporosis International, 18*(2), 167-175

Stern, E. B., Ytterberg, S. R., Krug, H. E., & Mahowald, M. L. (1996). Finger dexterity and hand function: Effect of three commercial wrist extensor orthoses on patients with rheumatoid arthritis. *Arthritis Care and Research, 9*(3), 197-205.

Stern, E. B., Ytterberg, S. R., Krug, H. E., Mullin, G. T., & Mahowald, M. L. (1996). Immediate and short-term effects of three commercial wrist extensor orthoses on grip strength and function in patients with rheumatoid arthritis. *Arthritis Care and Research, 9*(1), 42-50.

Sterner, Y., Lofgren, M., Nyberg, V., Karlsson, A. K., Bergstrom, M., & Gerdle, B. (2001). Early interdisciplinary rehabilitation programme for whiplash associated disorders. *Disability and Rehabilitation, 23*(10), 422-429.

Storr, L. K., Sorensen, P. S., & Ravnborg, M. (2006). The efficacy of multidisciplinary rehabilitation in stable multiple sclerosis patients. *Multiple Sclerosis, 12*(2), 235-242.

Studenski, S., Duncan, P., Perera, S., Reker, D., Min Lai, S., & Richards, L. (2005). Daily functioning and quality of life in a randomized controlled trial of therapeutic exercise for subacute stroke survivors. *Stroke, 36,* 1764-1770.

Thomas, J. J. (1996). Comparison of patient education methods: Effects on knowledge of cardiac rehabilitation principles. *Occupational Therapy Journal of Research, 16*(3), 166-178.

Thomas, L. J., & Thomas, B. J. (1995). Early mobilization method for surgically repaired zone III extensor tendons. *Journal of Hand Therapy, 8,* 195-198.

Tijhuis, G. J., Vliet Vlieland, T. P., Zwinderman, A. H., & Hazes, J. M. (1998). A comparison of the futuro wrist orthosis with a synthetic thermo-Lyn orthosis: Utility and clinical effectiveness. *Arthritis Care and Research, 11*(3), 217-222.

Towheed, T. E. (2005). Systematic review of therapies for osteoarthritis of the hand. *Osteoarthritis and Cartilage, 13,* 455-462.

Trombly, C. A., Thayer-Nason, L., Bliss, G., Girard, C. A., Lyrist, L. A., & Brexa-Hooson, A. (1986). The effectiveness of therapy in improving finger extension in stroke patients. *American Journal of Occupational Therapy, 40*(9), 612-617.

Tsuji, T., Liu, M., Hase, K., Masakado, Y., Takahashi, H., Hara, Y., et al. (2004). Physical fitness in persons with hemiparetic stroke: Its structure and longitudinal changes during an inpatient rehabilitation programme. *Clinical Rehabilitation, 18*(4), 450-460.

van der Giesen, F. J., Nelissen, R., Rozing, P., Arendzen, J., de Jong, Z., Wolterbeek, R., et al. (2007). A multidisciplinary hand clinic for patients with rheumatic diseases: A pilot study. *Journal of Hand Therapy, 20*(3), 251-261.

van Houten, P., Achterberg, W., & Ribbe, M. (2007). Urinary incontinence in disabled elderly women: A randomized clinical trial on the effect of training mobility and toileting skills to achieve independent toileting. *Gerontology, 53*(4), 205-210.

von Renteln-Kruse, W., & Krause, T. (2007). Incidence of in-hospital falls in geriatric patients before and after the introduction of an interdisciplinary team-based fall-prevention intervention. *Journal of the American Geriatrics Society, 55*(12), 2068-2074.

Wahi Michener, S. K., Olson, A. L., Humphrey, B. A., Reed, J. E., Stepp, D. R., Sutton, A. M., et al. (2001). Relationship among grip strength, functional outcomes, and work performance following hand trauma. *Work, 16*(3), 209-217.

WaiShan Louie, S. (2004). The effects of guided imagery relaxation in people with COPD. *Occupational Therapy International, 11*(3), 145-159.

Walsh, D. A., Kelly, S. J., Johnson, P. S., Rajkumar, S., & Bennetts, K. (2004). Performance problems of patients with chronic low-back pain and the measurement of patient-centered outcome. *Spine, 29*(1), 87-93.

Ward, C. D., Turpin, G., Dewey, M. E., Fleming, S., Hurwitz, B., Ratib, S., et al. (2004). Education for people with progressive neurological conditions can have negative effects: Evidence from a randomized controlled trial. *Clinical Rehabilitation, 18*(7), 717-725.

Wennemer, H. K., Borg-Stein, J., Gomba, L., Delaney, B., Rothmund, A., Barlow, D., et al. (2006). Functionally oriented rehabilitation program for patients with fibromyalgia: Preliminary results. *American Journal of Physical Medicine and Rehabilitation, 85*(8), 659-666.

Wu, C-Y., Trombly, C. A., Lin, K-C., & Tickle-Degnen, L. (1998). Effects of object. Affordances on reaching performance in persons with and without cerebrovascular accident. *American Journal of Occupational Therapy, 52*(6), 447-456.

Yuen, H. K., Nelson, D. L., Peterson, C. Q., & Dickinson, A. (1994). Prosthesis training as a context for studying occupational forms and motoric adaptation. *American Journal of Occupational Therapy, 48*(1), 55-61.

Zijlstra, T. R., Heijnsdijk-Rouwenhorst, L., & Rasker, J. J. (2004). Silver ring splints improve dexterity in patients with rheumatoid arthritis. *Arthritis and Rheumatism, 51*(6), 947-951.

9

SOCIO-CULTURAL DETERMINANTS OF OCCUPATION

Mary Ann McColl, PhD, MTS

Occupational therapists understand that one of the major components of the person is the values, beliefs, and perspectives that he or she holds. A significant part of what makes people who they are is determined by the social and cultural groups in which they were brought up and in which they interact every day. To the extent that the beliefs, values, and expectations of those groups are taken on by people and become part of their identity, they influence the way people enact their occupation. These internalized values, attributions, and perceptions make up socio-cultural aspects of occupation.

The socio-cultural aspect of the individual, however, must be differentiated from the socio-cultural environment (discussed more fully in Chapter 7). The socio-cultural aspect of the person, featured in this chapter, refers to internalized values, beliefs, and expectations that affect occupation. The socio-cultural environment, on the other hand, exists outside of the person. It too affects occupation, but it does so by exerting external demands, expectations, and pressures on individuals. In addition, the socio-cultural environment, in the form of family, friends, social organizations, and groups, may also provide support and aid to individuals in fulfilling their occupations.

This distinction is illustrated in the following example. If a woman holds the role of a wife, she will have a set of beliefs about what it means to be a wife, what is expected of her in that role, what occupations she should fulfill, and what benefits she may expect. These beliefs, values, and expectations will have been learned over the course of her life, through her interactions with family, friends, and the broader culture. But these beliefs are a part of her identity and shape how she makes occupational choices and executes particular occupations. These are all socio-cultural aspects of the individual, and they have obvious effects on her occupation—how she spends her time, what activities she does, what satisfaction she derives from her pursuits. On the other hand, her socio-cultural environment will also have its own definitions of the role of a wife and what she should and should not be doing within that role. Her husband, family, in-laws, and friends will also have their own ideas about what wives should and should not do. They will make their values and beliefs known to her in a variety of ways—some subtle and some direct. As long as these two sets of expectations (from the socio-cultural

M. Law & M. A. McColl (Eds.)
Interventions, Effects, and Outcomes in Occupational Therapy:
Adults and Older Adults (pp. 247-259)
© 2010 SLACK Incorporated

environment and the socio-cultural aspect of the individual) are in harmony, then occupational problems within this area do not arise. However, when beliefs, values, and expectations differ, there is considerable scope for conflict, and the individual is vulnerable to potential distress.

Conceptual Background

The socio-cultural aspects of occupation were what initially interested psychiatrists and nurses at the beginning of the 20th century and led to the founding of the profession that we now call occupational therapy. The North American founder, Adolph Meyer, observed that the use of time and a healthy social milieu were essential determinants of mental health (Meyer, 1977). To the extent that patients thought healthy thoughts and participated in healthy habits, they stood a good chance of actually being healthy. He and his associates aimed to promote a healthy lifestyle as a means of enhancing mental health.

The socio-cultural components of occupational therapy emerged again as prominent concepts in occupational therapy in the 1980s and 1990s, with the popular acceptance of the Model of Human Occupation (Kielhofner, 1992, 1995). Based as it was in the socio-behavioral tradition, the Model of Human Occupation significantly raised the profile of a number of important socio-cultural concepts, such as values, interests, habits, temporal patterns, and roles. These concepts have received considerably more attention in recent years, both singly and in combination, for their possible effects on overall occupational performance and life satisfaction.

Socio-cultural concepts are derived from being a member of a society or a culture. They are constructed phenomena that reflect a particular social and cultural context. For example, time is a socio-cultural concept. Anyone who has traveled will be aware that different cultures view time differently, and, consequently, the occupational expectations associated with time will be different depending on the culture to which one adheres or in which one attempts to operate. Some other socio-cultural concepts include habits, values, meaning, spirituality, social groups, and roles, to name a few of the most prevalent and influential ones (McColl, 2002). The measurement, use, and evaluation of these concepts as they relate to occupation are at the heart of the socio-cultural aspect of occupational therapy.

Search Strategy

This literature review focuses on socio-cultural outcome in occupational therapy. The search strategy sought intervention studies aimed at enhancing or reconciling socio-cultural aspects of the person. The search for articles was guided by the keywords listed in Table 9-1. A systematic search of health care and occupational therapy databases, as well as hand-searched relevant references, yielded 26 papers that addressed socio-cultural outcomes associated with occupational therapy. Of these, 15 qualified for inclusion in the chapter because they featured occupational therapy interventions aimed at improving socio-cultural components and offered empirical evidence for the effectiveness of those outcomes.

Tables 9-2 through 9-4 provide detailed information on the interventions used, the conclusions drawn about the effectiveness of occupational therapy for enhancing leisure, and the outcome measures applied.

Interventions Used to Improve Socio-Cultural Outcomes

This review uncovered 15 articles that described programs aimed at promoting socio-cultural outcomes in occupation therapy. They were directed almost equally at all age groups from youth to seniors, although the focus differed between age groups. Those aimed at older adults tended to focus more on social skills, whereas those aimed at younger adults tended to focus on functional and vocational skills. These interventions were also more likely to occur in hospital—nine took place either in rehab or in long-term care, while six were situated in the community. Not surprisingly, no socio-cultural programming took place in acute care. In terms of diagnostic groups, these programs tended to focus on people with no particular diagnosis (e.g., mothers of disabled children) and on people with mental illness (schizophrenia, depression).

Skills Development

Six of the programs identified in the literature fell into the category of skills development. In all six, there was some element of activity programs, such as crafts, hobbies, and group activities. These programs feature occupational therapists using activities that have been a part of the profession's history from its origins and are still used to provide a vehicle or a medium through which skills can be learned and practiced. For example, patients with HIV living in a residential facility were offered a program of manual and dramatic arts as a means of social interaction and skill development (Parruti et al., 2007). Reeder and colleagues (Reeder, Newton, Frangou, & Wykes, 2004) offered an occupational therapy activity group as the control group for a cognitive remediation program, but the specific activities used were not specified.

Table 9-1

SEARCH TERMS FOR OCCUPATIONAL THERAPY INTERVENTIONS TO IMPROVE SOCIO-CULTURAL OUTCOMES

Occupation, occupational therapy (therapist), OR multidisciplinary team AND...

Primary terms: cultural, culture, family, group, habit, life skills, lifestyle, meaning, role, social, socialization, social skills, spirituality, temporal adaptation, time, values.

Secondary terms: family, group, habit, life skills, lifestyle, meaning, role, spirituality, temporal adaptation, time, values.

Additional terms used to focus the search included clinical effectiveness, interdisciplinary education, interdisciplinary research, interdisciplinary treatment approach, outcomes, outcomes assessment, outcomes (health care), outcomes research, patient care, patient care team, rehabilitation outcomes, treatment effectiveness evaluation, treatment outcomes.

Liberman and associates (1998) also used an artistic and recreational activity group as a comparison with social and life skills training.

Hayes and colleagues (1991) compared activity therapy with social skills training as a means of improving social engagement and decreasing symptoms. Activity training involved parallel social participation in a specific product-oriented task. DeCarlo and Mann (1985) compared communication skills training with activity therapy including games and crafts to promote social interaction.

Occupational Development

Five of the articles identified described programs aimed at developing, balancing, or promoting occupation. These included life skills programs (DeMars, 1992; Mairs & Bradshaw, 2004), lifestyle re-design (Clark et al., 2001; Horowitz & Chang, 2004), and occupational engagement programs (Holm, Santangelo, Fromuth, Brown, & Walter, 2000). They focused on a broad range of occupations and sought to optimize their performance and satisfaction. These programs tended to emphasize selecting and balancing occupations, as well as strictly performing. Two programs focused on cultural competence, seeking to take into account a particular cultural context for occupation (Clark et al., 2001; DeMars, 1992).

Educational Approach

The remaining four articles took an educational approach to enhancing socio-cultural components. Elinge and associates (2003) sought to increase social participation with a falls prevention and osteoporosis education program for seniors who had recently incurred a fracture. This 20-hour program was supplemented by a home program aimed at increasing physical training and activity. VanLeit and Crowe (2002) and McGuire and associates (2004) both report on a program aimed at mothers of disabled children. Their focus is on the health of the mother and on teaching strategies to balance occupational demands. Parush and Hahn-Markowitz (1997) also attempted to influence maternal role participation with an educational program aimed at teaching new mothers about child development and modeling handling techniques for enhancing development.

Support Provision and Enhancement

Many of the programs, and in particular the educational programs, included an element of support provision by the therapist, or support enhancement by peer and social network, as an adjunct to the main program focus. Occupational therapists realize how difficult it is to make lifestyle changes and address issues in the socio-cultural area, given how fundamental they are to identity. Accordingly, they accompany these interventions with an intentional enhancement of support.

Effects of Occupational Therapy in Promoting Socio-Cultural Outcomes

Only 13 of the 15 articles cited offered quantitative evaluation results of the programs described. These findings are summarized in Table 9-2, and they suggest that social outcomes are amenable to occupational

text continues on page 257

Table 9-2

OCCUPATIONAL THERAPY INTERVENTIONS PROMOTING SOCIO-CULTURAL OUTCOMES

Author (Date)	Pop	DX	Setting	Intervention
Skills Development				
Parruti, G., Manzoli, L., Giansante, A., Deramo, C., Re, V., Graziani, R. V., & D'Amico, G. (2007)	5	18	1	**Intervention:** Patients with advanced HIV living in a residential facility were invited to participate in a wide range of arts and crafts and theatre activities. Subjects also received psychological counseling and some pre-vocational counseling.
Reeder, C., Newton, E., Frangou, S., & Wykes, T. (2004)	2	14	4	**Intervention:** Individualized cognitive remediation sessions; 40 sessions, 1 hour each, 3 times per week. **Control:** Individualized OT activities program.
Liberman, R. P., Wallace, C. J., Blackwell, G., Kopelowicz, A., Vaccaro, J. V. , & Mintz, J. (1998)	5	14	4	**Intervention:** 3 2-hour OT sessions per week for 6 months; total 72 hours. **Group 1:** Psychosocial OT comprised of expressive, artistic, and recreational activities. **Group 2:** Life skills and social skills training from 1 OT and 3 paraprofessionals.
Hayes, R., Halford, W., & Varghese, F. (1991)	5	14	4	**Intervention Group 1:** Activity therapy: Task-oriented group activity aimed at producing tangible product or service (e.g., wood-working, sewing). **Intervention Group 2:** Social skills training: Highly structured behavioral approach aimed at increasing the social interaction.
Arnetz, B. (1985)	4	21	1	**Intervention:** Social activation program: 6-month program including arts, history, physical activity, outings. **Control:** No change to daily routines.
DeCarlo, J., & Mann, W. (1985)	2	12, 14	4	**Intervention Group 1:** Activity therapy including role play, problem solving, games, crafts. **Intervention Group 2:** Verbal therapy consisting of discussion of interpersonal communication; both groups received 1 hour a week for 8 weeks. **Control:** Consisted of normal milieu therapy.
Occupational Development				
Horowitz, B. P., & Chang, P. F. (2004)	1	18, 24	3	**Intervention:** A 16-week group program to maximize performance in self-identified occupations through lifestyle redesign OT program that consisted of a 1.5-hour group every week and optional home visits once per month. **Control:** Usual care.
Mairs, H., & Bradshaw, T. (2004)	5	14	3	Individualized life skill training by trained OT; 12 sessions over a 4-month period; OTs trained 25 hours and supervised by researcher bi-weekly.
Clark, F., Azen, S. P., Carlson, M., Mandel, D., LaBree, L., Hay, J., et al. (2001)	1	21	3	**Intervention:** Well elderly program; preventive OT including lifestyle design, health promotion, support, and education. Alternate intervention: Generalized social activity group. **Control:** Non-treatment control.
Holm, M. B., Santangelo, M. A., Fromuth, D. J., Brown, S. O., & Walter, H. (2000)	3	12, 13, 18	3	**Intervention:** Occupation-based intervention within Community Living Arrangement program, coupled with either behavior modification programming or positive reinforcement strategies. Participants were involved in 3 alternating conditions within a multiple baseline single-case design, with activities introduced at different times and environments.
DeMars, P. (1992)	3	21	5	**Intervention:** Multi-level community development program of culturally distinct life skills and pre-vocational programming for Native Canadian community.

continued

Table 9-2 (continued)

OCCUPATIONAL THERAPY INTERVENTIONS PROMOTING SOCIO-CULTURAL OUTCOMES

Author (Date)	Pop	DX	Setting	Intervention
Education/Support				
McGuire, B., Crowe, T. K., Law, M., & VanLeit, B. (2004)	2	21	3	**Intervention:** 2 individual and 6 group sessions of lifestyle management, including exploring personal interests, goals, needs, supports, problem solving, self-awareness.
Elinge, E., Lofgren, B., Gagerman, E., & Nyberg, L. (2003)	4	17	4	**Intervention:** Multidisciplinary group learning program focusing on osteoporosis education, falls prevention; home program focused on physical exercise training and weightbearing; 2 hours a week for 10 weeks plus home program. **Control:** No intervention.
VanLeit, B., & Crowe, T. (2002)	2	21	4	**Intervention:** 8-week program for mothers of children with disabilities. Initial 60-minute individual session followed by 6 group problem-solving and support sessions. Individual and group sessions revolved around discussion of occupational routines and concerns. **Control:** Usual care.
Parush, S., & Hahn-Markowitz, J. (1997)	2	21	4	**Intervention:** Early intervention program to enhance learned maternal role behavior among mothers of newborns; teaching of sensory, perceptual, and cognitive development and modeling of techniques for enhancing development; 30 minutes every 8 weeks during the first year of the child's life (3 hours total over 1 year). **Control:** No intervention.

Population: 1=geriatric (65+); 2=adult (25 to 64); 3=young adult (18 to 24); 4=adult and geriatric; 5=young adult, adult, and geriatric.

Diagnosis: 12=depression; 13=bipolar disorder; 14=schizophrenia; 17=lower extremity; 18=other; 21=no diagnosis; 24=frail elderly.

Setting: 1=long-term care; 2=acute care; 3=home care; 4=rehabilitation; 5=primary care.

Table 9-3

Evidence of Effectiveness of Occupational Therapy on Socio-Cultural Outcomes

Author (Date)	Major Results	Study Design	Sample Size	Conclusions and Limitations
Positive Effects—Randomized Controlled Trial				
Elinge, E., Lofgren, B., Gagerman, E., & Nyberg, L. (2003)	Intervention group significantly improved ability to participate in social activity. No change in ADL or performance of preferred activities for either group.	RCT	1218	Multidisciplinary educational program effective in promoting purposeful activity, group participation, empowerment, and self-reliance.
Clark, F., Azen, S. P., Carlson, M., Mandel, D., LaBree, L., Hay, J., et al. (2001)	Statistically significant improvement ($p<0.05$) in quality of interaction, physical functioning, role functioning, vitality, social functioning, role emotional, general mental health.	RCT	285	**Conclusions:** The study identified long-term health benefits related to preventative OT. **Limitations:** Reasons for dropouts not reported. No record of preventing contamination or co-intervention. No reports of evaluators or participants blinded to treatment.
Liberman, R. P., Wallace, C. J., Blackwell, G., Kopelowicz, A., Vaccaro, J. V., & Mintz, J. (1998)	Statistically significant change was found for both groups measuring frequency of social activity, general psychological function, and symptoms of schizophrenia. OT skills training group showed statistically significant improvement over psycho-social OT group on frequency of IADL and ADL, self-esteem, symptoms of mental illness, and ability to adapt to life.	RCT	70	**Conclusions:** The skills training group scored significantly better on all scales that indicated improvement in both groups and on some scales where the psycho-social group did not improve. **Limitations:** No record of preventing contamination or co-intervention.
DeCarlo, J., & Mann, W. (1985)	Significant increase in interpersonal communication skills for activity group.	RCT	766	**Conclusions:** Findings suggest that activity groups are more effective in improving interpersonal communication skills than are verbal groups during OT in a psychiatric day program. **Limitations:** Possible influence of pre-test evaluation on treatment outcomes and similar treatments for all subjects.
Positive Effects—Non-Randomized Controlled Trial				
Parruti, G., Manzoli, L., Giansante, A., Deramo, C., Re, V., Graziani, R. V., & D'Amico, G. (2007)	Social function scores showed significant improvement ($p<0.001$) between baseline and 1-year follow-up (42% increase after 1 year; 70% increase at 2 years). Social distress mean scores significantly lower ($p<0.001$) than baseline after 1 year (reduced by 11% at 1 year and 22% at 2 years).	Non-RCT	14	**Conclusions:** OT with psychological counseling and pharmacological treatments was effective in reducing social stress and increasing social function in advanced HIV patients with multiple disabilities. **Limitations:** Results difficult to generalize due to ideal conditions, all health and social costs covered. Small sample size and no comparison group.

continued

Table 9-3 (continued)

EVIDENCE OF EFFECTIVENESS OF OCCUPATIONAL THERAPY ON SOCIO-CULTURAL OUTCOMES

Author (Date)	Major Results	Study Design	Sample Size	Conclusions and Limitations
Positive Effects—Non-Randomized Controlled Trial				
Holm, M. B., Santangelo, M. A., Fromuth, D. J., Brown, S. O., & Walter, H. (2000)	Using multiple baseline study with 2 developmentally disabled adults, systematic implementation of occupational engagement with reinforcement in home and work routines reduced number of anti-social and dysfunctional behaviors.	Non-RCT	2	**Conclusions:** "The use of everyday occupations, paired with positive reinforcement, was effective in decreasing dysfunctional and increasing functional behaviors" (quote from p. 361 of article). **Limitations:** Small sample size, attention due to nature of Community Living Arrangement program may have an effect on outcomes, no record of blinding of the assessment of performance.
Parush, S., & Hahn-Markowitz, J. (1997)	Intervention group had significantly higher scores for knowledge, attitudes, and practices; also had increased commitment to provide positive environment for infants.	Non-RCT	55, 54	Maternal role knowledge, attitudes, and behaviors cannot only be taught, they can be sustained up to 2 years post-program.
Hayes, R., Halford, W., & Varghese, F. (1991)	Social skills training resulted in significant improvement in social skills (p<0.05). No effect for activity therapy. No evidence of transfer of skills to naturalistic setting.	Non-RCT	8	Multiple baseline design with replication. Social skills training can improve social skills, but not ensure their use in social situation, despite proximity of setting.
Arnetz, B. (1985)	Social activity level increased after 3 months, 6 months of the program. The program was successful in enhancing social participation.	Non-RCT	3030	**Conclusions:** Social activation therapy may play an important role in preventing social isolation in institutional living. Those with low social activity level increased their participation the most after the initiation of the program. **Limitations:** Possible sample selection bias, outcome measures lack psychometric properties.
No Effect				
Horowitz, B. P., & Chang, P. F. (2004)	No statistical differences between control and experimental groups on any outcome measure. No effect of lifestyle intervention group.	RCT	24	**Conclusions:** Small sample size contributed to inability to find statistically significant differences between the groups. **Limitations:** Small sample size, reasons for dropouts not reported.
Mairs, H., & Bradshaw, T. (2004)	Significant improvement in overall symptomatology (p=0.018). Changes in symptomatology positively correlated with number of intervention sessions completed (r=0.613, p=0.026). No significant change in social functioning.	Non-RCT	13	Guarded conclusions given the absence of control group. Support for further exploration of life skills training in schizophrenia, but no conclusions about social skills improvements.

continued

Table 9-3 (continued)

EVIDENCE OF EFFECTIVENESS OF OCCUPATIONAL THERAPY ON SOCIO-CULTURAL OUTCOMES

Author (Date)	Major Results	Study Design	Sample Size	Conclusions and Limitations
No Effect				
Reeder, C., Newton, E., Frangou, S., & Wykes, T. (2004)	Cognitive remediation training associated with significant improvement in verbal working memory, but no improvement in social behavior. No effect of OT activity group. Psychological symptoms most influential in social outcomes.	RCT	18, 14	No evidence for effect of individualized activity therapy or cognitive remediation on social behavioral outcomes.
VanLeit, B., & Crowe, T. (2002)	No significant differences were found between the groups on time use or time perceptions. No significant differences were found between the groups on COPM performance subscale, but treatment group had significantly greater satisfaction scores (p<0.05).	RCT	38	***Conclusions:*** Focus on time and occupational concerns of mothers of children with disabilities can have a positive impact on satisfaction with occupational performance. ***Limitations:*** Small sample size, possible volunteer bias for sample selection, some outcome measures lacked psychometric properties.

COPM=Canadian Occupational Performance Measure.

Table 9-4

OUTCOME MEASURES USED TO CAPTURE SOCIO-CULTURAL OUTCOMES

Author (Date)	Outcome(s) Investigated	Outcome Measure(s)	Method of Administration
Social Functioning			
Parruti, G., Manzoli, L., Giansante, A., Deramo, C., Re, V., Graziani, R. V., & D'Amico, G. (2007)	Social and occupational abilities Social stress	GAFS SDRS	Assessments were completed in interviews when participants entered the study and yearly for the 5 years of the study.
Horowitz, B. P., & Chang, P. F. (2004)	Health and well-being of frail older adults	SF-36 LSI-Z MMSE FSQ MOS	Self-report interview.
Mairs, H., & Bradshaw, T. (2004)	Social functioning Psychiatric symptoms	SFS PANSS	PANSS by independent observer, completed at pre-test; SFS is self-report, completed at post-test.
Reeder, C., Newton, E., Frangou, S., & Wykes, T. (2004)	Social functioning	SBS BPRS and other psychological and psychiatric symptom measures	Social information provided by key informant at conclusion of program.
Elinge, E., Lofgren, B., Gagerman, E., & Nyberg, L. (2003)	Participation in activities with family and friends Activity preferences ADL	Single-item Branholm activity profile BI	Pre-test at 3 months post-fracture. Post-test at 10 weeks. Follow-up at 1 year.
Clark, F., Azen, S. P., Carlson, M., Mandel, D., LaBree, L., Hay, J., et al. (2001)	Social functioning Psychosocial functioning Physical and psychological health	SF-36 FSQ LSI-Z CES-D MOS	Not reported.
Holm, M. B., Santangelo, M. A., Fromuth, D. J., Brown, S. O., & Walter, H. (2000)	Frequency of behavior (verbal disruptions, distracting others, and appropriate social interactions) Duration of behavior (time engaged in appropriate activities	Frequency counts of behavior within 15-minute time frame Timer used to record total time engaged in activity during each 15-minute observation	Each participant was observed separately by a researcher during 15-minute segments under the 3 conditions.
Liberman, R. P., Wallace, C. J., Blackwell, G., Kopelowicz, A., Vaccaro, J. V., & Mintz, J. (1998)	Retention of skills learned in outpatient therapy	ILSS SAS PAL GSA Expanded BPRS BSI RSE LQL	Not reported.

continued

Table 9-4 (continued)
Outcome Measures Used to Capture Socio-Cultural Outcomes

Author (Date)	Outcome(s) Investigated	Outcome Measure(s)	Method of Administration
Social Functioning			
Hayes, R., Halford, W., & Varghese, F. (1991)	Level of social engagement Social skills Psychiatric symptomatology	Counts of social interactions in 15-second intervals during coffee breaks BPRS GSA SANS SRAS SSIT	Trained observers monitor behavior in naturalistic setting. Baseline pre-test. At end of social skills training. Follow-up—3 months.
Arnetz, B. (1985)	Social factors Social activity levels	Based on interview question-naire developed for study	All measures were conducted pre-treatment and 3 and 6 months post-treatment.
DeCarlo, J., & Mann, W. (1985)	Communication social skills	ICI	Pre-group baseline and immediately post-group.
Time Use			
VanLeit, B., & Crowe, T. (2002)	Satisfaction with time use Perceptions of occupational performance Occupational satisfaction	TPI TUA COPM	Assessments delivered pre-test and post-test (2 weeks post intervention).
Roles			
Parush, S., & Hahn-Markowitz, J. (1997)	Maternal role development	Adapted KAPQ	1987—immediately post-program. 1997—1.5 to 2 years post-program.

BI=Barthel Index, BPRS=Brief Psychiatric Rating Scale, BSI=Brief Symptom Inventory, CES-D=Center for Epidemiologic Studies Depression Scale, COPM=Canadian Occupational Performance Measure, FSQ=Functional Status Questionnaire, GAFS=Global Assessment of Functioning Scale, GSA=Global Scale Assessment, ICI=Interpersonal Communication Inventory, ILSS=Independent Living Skills Survey, Adapted KAPQ=Knowledge, Attitude, and Practices Questionnaire, LQL=Lehman Quality of Life Scale, LSI-Z=Life Satisfaction Index-Z, MMSE=Mini Mental Status Examination, MOS=Medical Outcomes Study Health Perception Scale, PAL=Profile of Adaptation to Life, PANSS=Positive and Negative Syndrome Scale, RSE=Rosenberg Self-Esteem, SANS=Schedule for the Assessment of Negative Symptoms, SAS=Social Activities Scale, SBS=Social Behavioural Scale, SDRS=Social Dysfunction Rating Scale, SF-36=Short Form Health Survey, SFS=Social Functioning Scale, SRAS=Simple Rathus Assertiveness Schedule, SSIT=Simulated Social Interaction Test, TPI=Time Perception Inventory, TUA=Time Use Analyzer.

therapy. Nine of the 13 articles described evaluations producing positive results on socio-cultural outcomes, particularly social functioning—four randomized trials and five observational studies. These articles show that skill development programs incorporating traditional occupational therapy activity programs are notably successful in promoting social skills, social participation, and appropriate social behavior. Hayes and colleagues (1991) caution against the assumption that enhanced social skills will generalize to other social situations. The combination of social skills training with purposeful activity appears to promote confidence and lead to a belief in improved ability to participate in social situations.

Life skills and lifestyle programs do not appear to have spill-over effects on social skills or social activity (Horowitz & Chang, 2004; Mairs & Bradshaw, 2004); however, programs promoting social and occupational engagement do appear to be successful (Clark et al., 2001; Holm et al., 2000). The one study dealing with role development suggests that role functioning can be improved using an educational approach and, furthermore, that this learning is durable over time (Parush & Hahn-Markowitz, 1997).

Four articles were unable to show positive effects of occupational therapy on socio-cultural outcomes. Although two were randomized trials and two were not, small samples sizes and measurement deficiencies may have affected the power of these studies. For example, Reeder and colleagues (2004) used a proxy measure for social engagement, and Horowitz and Chang (2004) had no specific social functioning measure, while Mairs and Bradshaw (2004) lacked a control group. VanLeit and Crowe (2002) focused on time use and were unable to detect an effect.

Measures Used to Capture Socio-Cultural Outcomes

Of the 13 articles where quantitative evaluation was conducted, 11 measured social function or dysfunction as the outcome of choice from a socio-cultural perspective (see Table 9-4). Instruments such as the Social Functioning Scale (SFS), Social Dysfunction Rating Scale (SDRS), Social Behaviour Schedule (SBS), and Social Activities Scale (SAS) were all measures used in these evaluations. These tend to count socially appropriate or inappropriate interactions and to offer scores that represent frequencies of desirable or undesirable social behavior. They also tend be relatively well-developed and well-researched measures that have some degree of recognition.

Another important measure of success in occupational therapy in the socio-cultural area is social engagement. Hayes and colleagues (1991) used an ingenious method of standardized observation to determine if learned social behaviors could be translated into the naturalistic setting. Elinge and associates (2003) used a single item that asked participants in their study if they felt they were better able to participate in activities with family and friends (yes/no). This study also used activities of daily living (ADL) and instrumental activities of daily living (IADL) as a measure of social engagement.

Many of the studies reviewed also considered outcomes of psychiatric symptomatology as indications of the efficacy of occupational therapy programs. It is important to acknowledge that psychological or affective symptoms ought not to be considered a direct measure of socio-cultural attainment, but rather a by-product of improved socio-cultural component performance. This emphasis on psychiatric symptomatology may signal an overidentification with the medical model, or it may suggest an underdevelopment of the socio-cultural area in terms of conceptual development and measurement tools. It is particularly surprising, in view of the historical importance of the socio-cultural area, that occupational therapy theory and measurement in the socio-cultural area are not more prominent. And yet perhaps it is not so surprising when one considers the subtlety and abstractness of these concepts.

Role performance is another important socio-cultural concept. Only one study addressed roles in a systematic way, focusing particularly on the maternal role and using a paper-and-pencil test of knowledge, attitudes, and practices of child development (Parush & Hahn-Markowitz, 1997). This is an important aspect of the maternal role without a doubt; however, it falls far short of the complexity of assessing the satisfactory fulfillment of the maternal role. Burke and Lomba (2005) review measures of occupational role and note that there are seven measures that could be useful to occupational therapists in this area. Although all are at relatively early stages in their psychometric development, it would be gratifying to see research using these measures for outcomes of occupational therapy programs directed at enhancing role performance.

One study also considered time use as an outcome of interest. VanLeit and Crowe (2002) used two measures of time use to see if an education program on child development could enhance effectiveness and satisfaction with time use among mothers of disabled children. Although the Canadian Occupational Performance Measure (COPM) showed increased satisfaction with occupation, the time use measures did not detect significant effects. Backman (2005) explores time use as a means of examining occupational balance. She reviews three approaches to time use measurement and several instruments associated with each. She concludes that time use measures offer only a partial picture of the complex concept of occupational balance. Pentland and McColl (2008) also offer an interesting view of time use as occupational integrity, or the extent to which occupational choices regarding time allocation are made consistently with the individual's values.

Conclusions and Recommendations for Future Research

In summary, this chapter has identified four types of interventions typically used by occupational therapists in attempts to have a positive impact on the socio-cultural components of occupation: activity groups, life skills, educational programs, and support initiatives. Of interest is the extent to which traditional occupational therapy activity groups continue to appear in the literature, despite a perceived bias against them.

This review offers a very sparse representation of the enormous range of occupational therapy programming that is possible for this very influential area. We have found very little research that meets the selection criteria relating to roles, habits, time use, values, beliefs, or other possible socio-cultural determinants of occupation. There is clearly a need not only for more research, but also for more creativity in the development, application, and evaluation of occupational therapy interventions in this area of practice.

With regard to effectiveness, occupational therapy programs have been shown in this review to be effective in promoting social functioning outcomes. This finding is compatible with the results of an impressive meta-analysis on social skills training, showing that it can be effective, even in a challenging population like people with schizophrenia (Kurtz & Mueser, 2008). Those authors underscore the importance of measuring what they call "proximal" outcomes, meaning those directly addressed in the intervention programming. They found greater likelihood of effectiveness of social skills training for proximal outcomes than for more distal outcomes, such as symptomatology or affective states.

In conclusion, this review offers encouraging findings regarding the ability of occupational therapy programs to promote significant and sustained effects on social functioning. However, it underlines the need for more attention to the socio-cultural area more broadly. Observational studies provide considerable evidence of the importance of socio-cultural factors for occupational performance. For example, McIntyre and Howie (2002) have shown the importance of role performance for occupational adaptation in widowhood. Segal (2000), Nygard and Johansson (2001), and Bejerholm and Eklund (2004) have shown the utility of time management, even for patients with severe occupational dysfunction. Banks (2008), Spadone (1992), and Price (2005) have all discussed the importance of culture as a determinant of occupation. Promising results like these extend a challenge to occupational therapists to develop programming and intervention approaches that are evidence based and conceptually sound in this historically rich area of occupational therapy.

References

Arnetz, B. (1985). Gerontic occupational therapy—psychological and social predictors of participation and therapeutic benefits. *American Journal of Occupational Therapy, 39*(7), 460-465.

Backman, C. (2005). Occupational balance: Measuring time use and satisfaction across occupational performance areas. In M. Law, C. Baum, & W. Dunn (Eds.), *Measuring occupational performance: Supporting best practice in occupational therapy* (2nd ed., pp. 287-300). Thorofare, NJ: SLACK Incorporated.

Banks, M. (2008). Women with disabilities: Cultural competence in rehabilitation psychology. *Disability and Rehabilitation, 30*(3), 184-190.

Bejerholm, U., & Eklund, M. (2004). Time use and occupational performance among persons with schizophrenia. *Occupational Therapy in Mental Health, 20*, 27-47.

Burke, J. P., & Lomba, T. B. (2005). Measurement of occupational role. In M. Law, C. Baum, & W. Dunn (Eds.), *Measuring occupational performance: Supporting best practice in occupational therapy* (2nd ed., pp. 277-286). Thorofare, NJ: SLACK Incorporated.

Clark, F., Azen, S. P., Carlson, M., Mandel, D., LaBree, L., Hay, J., et al. (2001). Embedding health-promoting changes into the daily lives of independent-living older adults: Long-term follow-up of occupational therapy intervention. *Journals of Gerontology. Series B: Psychological Sciences and Social Sciences, 56B*(1), P60-P63.

DeCarlo, J., & Mann, W. (1985). The effectiveness of verbal versus activity groups in improving self-perceptions of interpersonal communication skills. *American Journal of Occupational Therapy, 39*(1), 20-26.

DeMars, P. A. (1992). An occupational therapy life skills curriculum model for a native American tribe: A health promotion program based on ethnographic field research. *American Journal of Occupational Therapy, 46*, 727-736.

Elinge, E., Lofgren, B., Gagerman, E., & Nyberg, L. (2003). A group learning programme for old people with hip fracture: A randomized study. *Scandinavian Journal of Occupational Therapy, 10*(1), 27-33.

Hayes, R., Halford, W., & Varghese, F. (1991). Generalization of the effects of activity therapy and social skills training on the social behavior of low functioning schizophrenic patients. *Occupational Therapy in Mental Health, 11*(4), 3-20.

Holm, M. B., Santangelo, M. A., Fromuth, D. J., Brown, S. O., & Walter, H. (2000). Effectiveness of everyday occupations for changing client behaviours in a community living arrangement. *American Journal of Occupational Therapy, 54*, 361-371.

Horowitz, B. P., & Chang, P. F. (2004). Promoting well-being and engagement in life through occupational therapy lifestyle redesign: A pilot study within adult day programs. *Topics in Geriatric Rehabilitation, 20*(1), 46-58.

Kielhofner, G. (1992). *A model of human occupation: Therapy and application*. Baltimore, MD: Williams & Wilkins.

Kielhofner, G. (1995). *A model of human occupation: Therapy and application* (2nd ed.). Baltimore, MD: Williams & Wilkins.

Kurtz, M., & Mueser, K. (2008). A meta-analysis of controlled research on social skills training for schizophrenia. *Journal of Consulting and Clinical Psychology, 76*(3), 491-504.

Liberman, R. P., Wallace, C. J., Blackwell, G., Kopelowicz, A., Vaccaro, J. V., & Mintz, J. (1998). Skills training versus psychosocial occupational therapy for persons with persistent schizophrenia. *American Journal of Psychiatry, 155*(8), 1087-1091.

Mairs, H., & Bradshaw, T. (2004). Life skills training in schizophrenia. *British Journal of Occupational Therapy, 67*(5), 217-224.

McColl, M. A. (2002). Introduction: A basis for theory in occupational therapy. In M. A. McColl, M. Law, D. Stewart, L. Doubt, N. Pollock, & T. Krupa (Eds.), *Theoretical basis of occupational therapy* (2nd ed., pp. 1-6). Thorofare, NJ: SLACK Incorporated.

McGuire, B., Crowe, T. K., Law, M., & VanLeit, B. (2004). Mothers of children with disabilities: Occupational concerns and solutions. *Occupational Therapy Journal of Research, 24,* 54-63.

McIntyre, G., & Howie, L. (2002). Adapting to widowhood through meaningful occupation: A case study. *Scandanavian Journal of Occupational Therapy, 9,* 54-62.

Meyer, A. (1977). The philosophy of occupational therapy. *American Journal of Occupational Therapy, 31,* 639-642.

Nygard, L., & Johansson, M. (2001). The experience and management of temporality in five cases of dementia. *Scandinavian Journal of Occupational Therapy, 8,* 85-95.

Parruti, G., Manzoli, L., Giansante, A., Deramo, C., Re, V., Graziani, R. V., & D'Amico, G. (2007). Occupational therapy for advanced HIV patients at a home care facility: A pilot study. *AIDS Care, 19*(4), 467-470.

Parush, S., & Hahn-Markowitz, J. (1997). The efficacy of an early prevention program facilitated by occupational therapists: A follow-up study. *American Journal of Occupational Therapy, 51*(4), 247-251.

Pentland, W., & McColl, M. A. (2008). Occupational integrity: Another perspective on "life balance." *Canadian Journal of Occupational Therapy, 75,* 135-138.

Price, P. (2005). Measuring occupational performance within a socio-cultural context. In M. Law, C. Baum, & W. Dunn (Eds.), *Measuring occupational performance: Supporting best practice in occupational therapy* (2nd ed., pp. 347-366). Thorofare, NJ: SLACK Incorporated.

Reeder, C., Newton, E., Frangou, S., & Wykes, T. (2004). Which executive skills should we target to affect social functioning and symptom change? A study of a cognitive remediation therapy program. *Schizophrenia Bulletin, 30,* 87-100.

Segal, R. (2000). Adaptive strategies of mothers with children with attention deficit hyperactivity disorder: Enfolding and unfolding occupations. *American Journal of Occupational Therapy, 54,* 300-306.

Spadone, R. (1992). Internal-external control and temporal orientation among Southeast Asians and white Americans. *American Journal of Occupational Therapy, 46*(8), 713-719.

VanLeit, B., & Crowe, T. (2002). Outcomes of an occupational therapy program for mothers of children with disabilities: Impact on satisfaction with time use and occupational performance. *American Journal of Occupational Therapy, 56,* 402-410.

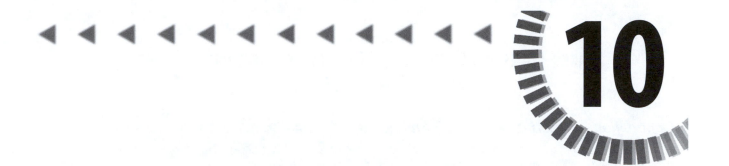

PSYCHO-EMOTIONAL OUTCOMES

Mary Law, PhD, FCAOT and Rebecca Gewurtz, MSc (OT), OT Reg. (Ont.)

In this chapter, we explore occupational therapy-sensitive outcomes that are psychological or emotional in nature. Psycho-emotional outcomes, according to the taxonomy developed by McColl and colleagues (2002), refer to both the thoughts and feelings that are intrinsic and learned responses of individuals to internal and external stimuli. Outcomes for people participating in daily occupations can be based on psychological and emotional responses toward these experiences.

Within this chapter, we include only research that focuses on these psychological and/or emotional outcomes. Interventions that focus on the use of cognitive and cognitive-behavioral strategies are reported in Chapter 11.

Conceptual Background

From the earliest days of our profession, the value of occupational engagement for individuals with psycho-emotional impairments has been promoted. Our theoretical literature and the foundational assumptions of our profession embrace a belief in the potential of occupation to improve mental health and well-being (Rebeiro, 1998). We believe that through occu-

pation, individuals can find meaning in life, organize their behaviors, and improve their performance and satisfaction (Canadian Association of Occupational Therapists [CAOT], 1997).

However, Rebeiro (1998) noted that there is a discrepancy between what the profession theoretically advances about the potential of psycho-emotional occupational therapy and the existing empirical evidence. Although, in recent years, some occupational therapists have conducted research on occupation-based interventions, our evidence base in this area is still developing. In the many years since the inception of our profession, the relationship between occupational therapy interventions and psycho-emotional outcomes has been largely grounded in our assumptions and beliefs about occupation and health rather than evidence from well-conducted research (Rebeiro, 1998).

Occupational therapists provide intervention individually or as a part of a multidisciplinary team with a goal to improve psycho-emotional outcomes. Such outcomes include feelings such as pain, motivation, mood, and anxiety and social communication and

M. Law & M. A. McColl (Eds.)
Interventions, Effects, and Outcomes in Occupational Therapy:
Adults and Older Adults (pp. 261-283)
© 2010 SLACK Incorporated

Table 10-1

SEARCH TERMS FOR OCCUPATIONAL THERAPY INTERVENTIONS TO IMPROVE PSYCHO-EMOTIONAL OUTCOMES

Occupation, occupational therapy (therapist), OR multidisciplinary team AND...

Primary terms: affective disorders, agoraphobia, anxiety, behavior therapy, bipolar disorder, cognitive-behavioral therapy, community mental health services, depression, depressive disorders, mental health, mood disorder, pain management, panic, personality disorder, post-traumatic stress disorder, psychosis, psychotic disorders, schizophrenia, stress management, substance-related disorders, suicide.

Secondary terms: alcoholism, anxiety disorder, backache, chronic pain, chronic pain control, community mental health, emotional disorder, interdisciplinary team, interdisciplinary treatment approaches, learning, low back pain, mental disease, mental disorders, mental health care, mental health service, mental patient, multidisciplinary care team, multidisciplinary team, muscle pain, myofascial pain, occupational therapist, occupational therapists, occupational therapy, occupational therapy techniques, pain, pain clinics, pain control, pain control behavior, pain: disruptive effects, pain (intractable), pain level, patient care team, psychosocial rehabilitation therapy, reflex sympathetic dystrophy, substance abuse, substance dependence, stress disorders, suicide attempted, teamwork, therapy effect, treatment effect, treatment outcome(s).

Additional terms used to focus the search included clinical effectiveness, community health services, health care delivery, health care services, health service, health services for the aged, home care, home care services, home health care, home occupational therapy, home rehabilitation, interdisciplinary education, interdisciplinary research, interdisciplinary treatment approach, intervention treatment approach, multidisciplinary care team, outcomes, outcomes assessment patient care, outcomes (health care), outcomes research, patient care team, psychotherapeutic outcomes, rehabilitation, rehabilitation care, rehabilitation centre, rehabilitation outcomes, teamwork, treatment effectiveness evaluation, treatment outcomes.

interpersonal interactions. Occupational therapists in this area provide various types of interventions including comprehensive occupation-based programs (sometimes carried out in collaboration with other disciplines) and cognitive-behavioral therapy (CBT) in combination with self-management or relaxation. Occupational therapists are also essential to various comprehensive community mental health treatment approaches such as assertive community treatment (ACT) teams and intensive case management teams (Krupa, Radloff-Gabriel, Whippey, & Kirsh, 2002). Although these models of practice have been well studied and are often considered best-practice approaches, it is often hard to isolate the contribution of occupational therapists.

Findings from the review have been organized according to area of intervention indicated in the literature appraised for this project. Further research regarding these interventions and outcomes is needed before firm conclusions can be drawn about occupational therapy-sensitive outcomes in those areas.

Search Strategy

The methodology to search the literature, identify studies, and select them based on specific inclusion criteria was discussed in Chapter 2. A systematic search of health care and occupational therapy databases, as well as hand-searched relevant references, yielded both review and empirical (qualitative and quantitative) papers that addressed the occupational therapy outcomes when providing psycho-emotional interventions. Selected studies met specific inclusion criteria, which consisted of the study being published between 1980 and 2008, an adult population, an intervention involving occupational therapist independently or on a multidisciplinary team, and being categorized as level of evidence 1 to 4 based on criteria by Greenhalgh (2006). For this chapter, the search terms used to capture occupational therapy-sensitive outcomes are listed in Table 10-1. A total of 22 empirical articles met the inclusion criteria and are reviewed in this chapter in more detail in Tables 10-2 through 10-4.

Interventions Used to Improve Psycho-Emotional Outcomes

In this section, we examine the occupational therapy interventions whose purpose is to impact a client's psycho-emotional outcomes. After that, the studies are

text continues on page 277

Table 10-2

OCCUPATIONAL THERAPY INTERVENTIONS PROMOTING PSYCHO-EMOTIONAL OUTCOMES

Author (Date)	Pop	DX	Setting	Intervention
Graff, M., Adang, E., Vernooij-Dassen, M., Dekker, J., Jonsson, L., Thijssen, M., et al. (2008)	1	8	3	**Intervention:** Subjects received 10 1-hour sessions of OT over 5 weeks. Therapy focused on both patients and their caregivers and began with clients identifying problems for them to work on and developing strategies to deal with them in conjunction with the OT. **Control:** Subjects received usual care that did not include any OT.
Hooten, W. M., Townsend, C., Sletten, C., Bruce, B., & Rome, J. D. (2007)	5	18	4	**Intervention:** Patients participated in the program 8 hours a day for 15 consecutive days. The treatment program consisted of CBT, PT, OT, and withdrawal of analgesic pain medications led by a physician.
Lambert, R. A., Harvey, I., & Poland, F. (2007)	2, 3	11	5	**Intervention:** Subjects received treatment in 4 stages: A lifestyle review, education to increase patient awareness of the negative effect of lifestyle behaviors, specific lifestyle changes negotiated between the therapist and patient, and monitoring and review of the subsequent lifestyle changes. **Control:** Subjects received routine care through their general practitioner.
Rosenberg, N. K., & Hougaard, E. (2005)	5	11	4	**Intervention:** 14 weekly group CBT interventions; OT treatment consisted of exposure to agoraphobic situations; PT treatment for breathing exercises and relaxation. **Control:** Waitlist.
Gutman, S. A., Diamond, H., Holness-Parchment, S. E., Brandofino, D. N., Pacheco, D. G., Jolly-Edouard, M., et al. (2004)	2	1, 7, 15, 18	3	Revised version of a program described by Gutman and Swarbrick (1998) to educate about safety, safe sex, assertiveness and advocacy, anger management, stress management, vocational/educational skills, money management, boundary establishment, housing application, hygiene, medication routine, nutrition, and leisure.
Nobili, A., Riva, E., Tettamanti, M., Lucca, U., Liscio, M., Petrucci, B., et al. (2004)	1	8	3	**Intervention:** Received a home visit by both a psychologist (to assess and give advice on relationships within family) and an OT (to suggest strategies for control of reactive behaviors and modification to home barriers). **Control:** Provided access to a free helpline, information about rights of patients and families, addresses of community services and specialized clinical centers.
Buchain, P. C., Vizzotto, A. D., Henna Neto, J., & Elkis, H. (2003)	2	14	4	**Intervention:** OT (free choice activities [individual and group activities]) in addition to the use of Clozapine. **Control:** Clozapine on its own.
Pfeiffer, A., Thompson, J. M., Nelson, A., Tucker, S., Luedtke, C., Finnie., S., et al. (2003)	4	18	4	The fibromyalgia treatment program includes education about fibromyalgia syndrome, self-management techniques using a cognitive-behavioral approach adapted from traditional chronic pain rehabilitation programs conducted by registered nurses. After this introduction, OT and PT take place. OT focused on energy conservation, techniques for moderation, and ergonomics (intervention over 1.5 days).
Sood, J. R., Cisek, E., Zimmerman, J., Zaleski, E. H., & Fillmore, H. H. (2003)	1	12	4	Geriatric wellness program: Treatment of depression through CBT and pleasant events. This included relaxation and imagery for anxiety reduction, mood ratings, positive reinforcement for functional gains, pleasurable events to reduce depressive symptoms.

continued

Table 10-2 (continued)

Occupational Therapy Interventions Promoting Psycho-Emotional Outcomes

Author (Date)	Pop	DX	Setting	Intervention
Lippert-Gruner, M., Wedekind, C., & Klug, N. (2002)	4	7	2	1 year of continuous rehabilitation following severe brain injury. Clients received: Early multimodal sensory stimulation, PT, OT, CBT, and speech-language pathology. After discharge had subacute rehabilitation with individual complex rehabilitation (OT, PT, speech, and behavioral therapy) for 4 hours a day for 12 weeks. Ambulatory rehabilitation focused on social and occupational reintegration.
Wu, C-Y. (2001)	5	14, 18	4	OTs randomly assigned to an experimental or control group. Intervention was 12 weeks, for 1 hour, 2 times a week. Therapy sessions for both groups were conducted on an individual, as opposed to group, basis. Experimental group received sessions based on the motivational frame of reference. Control group received standard OT (based on treatment protocol of the therapists).
Vines, S. W., Ng, A. K., Breggia, A., & Mahoney, R. (2000)	2	20	4	Multimodal rehabilitation program including nursing, physiatry, psychology, social work, PT, OT, and vocational rehabilitation. Participants attended classes for 4 weeks learning effective communication, problem solving, conflict resolution, stress management, relaxation for pain control, stretching and strengthening exercises, proper body mechanics, pool therapy, and nutritional classes.
Eklund, M. (1999)	2	14	3	*Intervention:* 4 to 30 months of weekly supervision, individual and group sessions for 20 hours a week over 4 days. Group-based OT program involved: Group meeting, group activities (art, clay, modeling, gardening, cooking, and body awareness), individual verbal sessions, and a group meeting at the end of the day.
Raweh, D. V., & Katz, N. (1999)	5	14	3	*Intervention:* Treatment according to Allen's Cognitive Disability Model using tasks from the Allen Diagnostic Module (1993): 24 treatment hours 3 times a week (for approximately 2 months). *Control:* Worked at community activity center.
Sellwood, W., Thomas, C. S., Tarrier, N., Jones, S., Clewes, J., James, A., et al. (1999)	2	14	3	Hospital outpatient rehab: Follow-up every 2 to 3 months—psychiatrist or trainee. As required: Community psychiatric nursing, day hospital and outpatient OT, outpatient psychology. Home-based rehab: Standard outpatient treatment plus individualized home-based treatments designed by OT and clinical psychologist with patient, informal carers, and agencies.
Turk, D. C., Okifuji, A., Sinclair, J. D., & Starz, T. W. (1998)	2	18	4	Interdisciplinary outpatient treatment: 6.5-day sessions in 4-week period, groups of 4 to 7. Medical sessions=led by physician (pain specialty). PT=Didactic sessions and exercise sessions. OT=Educational sessions regarding body mechanics, energy conservation, pacing, homework provided/reviewed. Psychology=Group sessions based on CBT.
DeWilliams, C. A. C., Nicholas, M. K., Richardson, P. H., Pither, C. E., Justins, D. M., Chamberlain, J. H., et al. (1993)	5	20	4	4-week inpatient program. All staff (psychologists, anesthetist, PT, OT, nurse) used behavioral methods to encourage client to reduce behaviors associated with pain, such as grimacing, limping, etc. Cognitive principles taught to enable patients to estimate their abilities and limitations realistically. Exercise, stretch, and relaxation routines taught. Advice given on improving sleep. Pain medication withdrawal encouraged.

continued

Table 10-2 (continued)
OCCUPATIONAL THERAPY INTERVENTIONS PROMOTING PSYCHO-EMOTIONAL OUTCOMES

Author (Date)	Pop	DX	Setting	Intervention
Roberts, A. H., Sternbach, R. A., & Polich, J. (1993)	5	18, 20	4	OT, PT, and behavioral psychologists. Each patient had 5 to 6 weeks of PT and OT as well as biofeedback. OT and PT treatment was individualized for each participant. Behavioral psychology also involved relevant family members. Biofeedback sessions involved muscle relaxation and stress management training. Patients returned home and continued their exercise.
Boswell, S. (1989)	5	12, 13, 14	4	The support group program consisted of 1-hour sessions a week for 9 weeks. OT and social worker were group leaders and taught a series of lessons and exercises to help participants develop supportive relationships, to relieve feelings of depression, to improve feelings of self-esteem, and to improve communication skills.
Strong, J., Cramond, T., & Maas, F. (1989)	4	20	4	Tape-recorded relaxation training and EMG biofeedback.
Cole, M. B., & Greene, L. R. (1988)	5	18	4	Subjects participated in either unstructured psychotherapy group or structured task-focused OT group (6 to 7 participants in each group).
Lushbough, R. S., Priddy, J. M., Sewell, H. H., Lovett, S. B., & Jones, T. C. (1988)	4	18	1	**Intervention:** OT and psycho-social groups for treatment included a 4-month intervention consisting of stress management from the staff psychologist, arts and crafts with OT, sports by all staff, "creative pen" writing assignments, and a goals group with one-on-one opportunities if needed. **Control:** Also had one-on-one opportunities and groups such as outdoor walks, music, and socials.

Population: 1=geriatric (65+); 2=adult (25 to 64); 3=young adult (18 to 24); 4=adult and geriatric; 5=young adult, adult, and geriatric.

Diagnosis: 1=developmental delay; 7=acquired brain injury; 8=dementia or Alzheimer's disease; 11=anxiety; 12=depression; 13=bipolar; 14=schizophrenia; 15=addiction/substance abuse; 18=other; 20=chronic pain.

Setting: 1=long-term care; 2=acute care; 3=home care; 4=rehabilitation; 5=primary care.

Table 10-3

EVIDENCE OF EFFECTIVENESS OF OCCUPATIONAL THERAPY ON PSYCHO-EMOTIONAL OUTCOMES

Author (Date)	Major Results	Study Design	Sample Size	Conclusions and Limitations
Positive Effects—Randomized Controlled Trial				
Graff, M., Adang, E., Vernooij-Dassen, M., Dekker, J., Jonsson, L., Thijssen, M., et al. (2008)	At 3-month follow-up, statistically significant differences were found between both groups. Successful treatment (clinically and statistically relevant improvement in all measures of functional ability and caregiver competence) was found in 26 patients and their caregivers, 25 of whom were in the control group.	RCT	132	**Conclusions:** The use of home-based OT was effective in improving patients' functional ability and caregivers' sense of competence. The treatment was also highly cost-effective. **Limitations:** Reasons for dropouts were not reported. Data analysis was completed on an intention-to-treat basis, which may have diluted the results.
Lambert, R. A., Harvey, I., & Poland, F. (2007)	At 20-week follow-up, fewer than 20% of patients in the intervention group experienced moderate to severe anxiety. BAI scores were significantly lower for the intervention group at 20 weeks ($p<0.001$, mean difference -9.8, 95% CI -15 to -4.6), and they remained most improved at 10-month follow-up though the difference between groups was no longer significant. At 20-week follow-up, 63.6% of patients in the intervention had been panic free for the previous month compared to 40% in the control. Results were similar at 10 months though the differences between the 2 groups never reached significance. Other secondary outcome measures showed significant or near significant results at 20 weeks, and only the general health item on the SF-36 showed significance at 10 months.	RCT	67	**Conclusions:** There is evidence that an OT-based lifestyle approach to the treatment of panic disorders may be as clinically effective as routine general practitioner care and may be more effective over the short term. **Limitations:** A small starting sample size and high dropout rate left the study very underpowered.
Buchain, P. C., Vizzotto, A. D., Henna Neto, J., & Elkis, H. (2003)	OT sessions combined with psychopharmacological treatment were more effective than psychopharmacological treatment on its own ($p=0.033$).	RCT	26	**Conclusions:** The combination of OT and Clozapine was shown to be more effective than Clozapine on its own. **Limitations:** Intervention not described, small sample size with significant dropouts.

continued

Table 10-3 (continued)

EVIDENCE OF EFFECTIVENESS OF OCCUPATIONAL THERAPY ON PSYCHO-EMOTIONAL OUTCOMES

Author (Date)	Major Results	Study Design	Sample Size	Conclusions and Limitations
Positive Effects—Randomized Controlled Trial				
Wu, C-Y. (2001)	Effects of change on intrinsic motivation, the effects of treatment group, and motivation type were not significant. Significant differences between control and experimental groups for the autonomy-oriented participants (p=0.041) and for the combined control-oriented and impersonal group (p=0.026). Positive change in intrinsic motivation among participants with control-oriented, autonomy-oriented and impersonal-oriented styles.	RCT	99	**Conclusions:** Results suggested that OT intervention was effective in facilitating intrinsic motivation in individuals with various motivational styles, such as those with autonomy-oriented, control-oriented, and impersonal types. **Limitations:** Psychometric properties of the assessments had limitations, sample sizes were small due to a high dropout rate.
Strong, J., Cramond, T., & Maas, F. (1989)	Participants receiving only relaxation showed a significant reduction in pain intensity at discharge (p<0.01) while the group receiving relaxation and biofeedback showed no significant changes in pain intensity over time. Both groups showed significantly lower pain rating index scores at discharge (p<0.01 and p<0.05). Participants receiving both treatments showed a significant difference in pain rating at follow-up (p<0.01).	RCT	40	**Conclusions:** The addition of EMG biofeedback to applied relaxation training has a long-term benefit. **Limitations:** Co-intervention not controlled for.
Positive Effects—Non-Randomized Controlled Trial				
Hooten, W. M., Townsend, C., Sletten, C., Bruce, B., & Rome, J. D. (2007)	MPI scores showed significant reductions (p<0.001) in pain severity, life interference, and psychological distress between admission and dismissal. Patients also reported significant improvements (p<0.001) in life control, social activity, and physical activity. Scores from all 4 subscales of the SF-36 also showed significant increases in physical and emotional health attributes. Significantly lower levels of pain catastrophizing and depressive symptoms were also observed between admission and dismissal. A significant number of patients also reported a decrease in the use of pain medications and muscle relaxants after completing the rehabilitation program.	Non-RCT	142	**Conclusions:** The interdisciplinary pain rehabilitation program in conjunction with the withdrawal of pain medications and muscle relaxants caused significant improvements in psycho-social functioning, health attributes, negative pain-related emotions, and depressive symptoms. **Limitations:** The lack of a control or comparison group makes it difficult to determine if the reduction in use of pain medication was a result of symptomatic improvement or medical direction during the rehabilitation program. Patients were also specially referred to the program, and all had the motivation and resources to complete the outpatient program.

continued

Table 10-3 (continued)

EVIDENCE OF EFFECTIVENESS OF OCCUPATIONAL THERAPY ON PSYCHO-EMOTIONAL OUTCOMES

Author (Date)	Major Results	Study Design	Sample Size	Conclusions and Limitations
Positive Effects—Non-Randomized Controlled Trial				
Rosenberg, N. K., & Hougaard, E. (2005)	Investigation group achieved better outcomes on most analyses with 47.2% found to be panic free after treatment compared to 12.5% in control group (p=0.001).	Non-RCT	93	***Conclusions:*** A naturalistic comparison between a group receiving this cognitive-behavioral intervention and a waiting list control group found that significantly more members of the intervention group were panic free after the study than members of the waiting list control group. ***Limitations:*** No random assignment to groups, contamination and co-intervention were not accounted for.
Gutman, S. A., Diamond, H., Holness-Parchment, S. E., Brandofino, D. N., Pacheco, D. G., Jolly-Edouard, M., et al. (2004)	All participants achieved their expected outcome or greater. Self-reported results indicate that 81% of participants achieved their most favorable outcome and 19% their expected outcome.	Non-RCT	26	***Conclusions:*** Self-reported results indicate that 81% of participants achieved their most favorable outcome and 19% their expected outcome. ***Limitations:*** The participants were a convenience sample, and there was no control group.
Pfeiffer, A., Thompson, J. M., Nelson, A., Tucker, S., Luedtke, C., Finnie, S., et al. (2003)	Significant overall improvement on FIQ (p<0.002). On entry into program, 44/78 subjects (56%) were depressed, and scores improved from 23 to 20.7, but this was not statistically significant. No significant improvements in CES-D, the physical impairment and depression subscales of the FIQ, CES-D, or LFSS. In the short term, treatment can have positive effects, but unlikely to impact depression.	Non-RCT	78	***Conclusions:*** Statistically significant improvements were identified in the FIQ (impact of illness scale). ***Limitations:*** Contamination and co-intervention possible given the length of follow-up.
Lippert-Gruner, M., Wedekind, C., & Klug, N. (2002)	83% of patients independent of care, 2% totally dependent, 4% dependent on help, 8% restrictedly independent. Only 35% able to work after 1 year. 10% able to work but unemployed or retired. 15% able to perform selected activities. 4% integrated in workshop for disabled people.	Non-RCT	79	***Conclusions:*** The majority of clients reached high levels of independence in their ADL, but many continued to have behavioral and speech deficits that impacted reintegration into school and work life. ***Limitations:*** Interventions not sufficiently detailed for replication, assessors not blinded.

continued

Table 10-3 (continued)

EVIDENCE OF EFFECTIVENESS OF OCCUPATIONAL THERAPY ON PSYCHO-EMOTIONAL OUTCOMES

Author (Date)	Major Results	Study Design	Sample Size	Conclusions and Limitations
Positive Effects—Non-Randomized Controlled Trial				
Eklund, M. (1999)	The participants showed statistically significant improvement in psychiatric symptoms ($p<.001$), global mental health ($p<.000$), and the 3 aspects of occupational functioning: Volition ($p<0.001$), habituation ($p<0.001$), and communication and interpersonal skills ($p<0.005$), but no improvement in quality of life.	Non-RCT	25	***Conclusions:*** This OT program within a psychiatric day care was shown to be beneficial for improvement for some psychiatric patients on a variety of outcome variables covering occupational performance, global mental health, and psychiatric symptoms. ***Limitations:*** Small sample size, participants not randomly allocated to groups.
Raweh, D. V., & Katz, N. (1999)	The intervention showed significant improvement over control group for cognitive functional ability; no significant difference on RTI scores.	Non-RCT	19	***Conclusions:*** The study group had improved significantly in cognitive functional ability (ACL-90 level) in comparison to the control. The study group also showed greater improvement in ability to perform routine tasks (RTI-2 level). ***Limitations:*** Small sample size, low participation of control group.
Turk, D. C., Okifuji, A., Sinclair, J. D., & Starz, T. W. (1998)	t-tests indicate significant changes, at $p<0.001$, over time between pre- and post-treatment on MPI variables, CES-D, and FIQ variables. Clinically significant treatment effects examined through reliable change index: 41.8% of treatment responders reported significantly lower pain severity than non-responders. Significant results ($p<0.005$) for outcome maintenance at follow-up for MPI and FIQ variables.	Non-RCT	58	***Conclusions:*** Pre-treatment and post-treatment measures revealed significant improvements in pain severity, life interference, sense of control, affective distress, depression, perceived physical impairment, fatigue, and anxiety. A 6-month follow-up indicated continued treatment gains in pain, life interference, sense of control, affective distress, and depression. ***Limitations:*** Relationship between adherence and treatment response unclear, possible heterogeneity of study participants with FMS subgroups, no control group, outcome variables based on self-report with no observed or objective variables.

continued

Table 10-3 (continued)

EVIDENCE OF EFFECTIVENESS OF OCCUPATIONAL THERAPY ON PSYCHO-EMOTIONAL OUTCOMES

Author (Date)	Major Results	Study Design	Sample Size	Conclusions and Limitations
Positive Effects—Non-Randomized Controlled Trial				
DeWilliams, C. A. C., Nicholas, M. K., Richardson, P. H., Pither, C. E., Justins, D. M., Chamberlain, J. H., et al. (1993)	Assessment immediately after treatment revealed statistically significant (p<0.001) improvements on all measures. Improvements well-maintained at 6-month follow-up.	Non-RCT	212	***Conclusions:*** Improvements in patients' physical functioning and self-reported emotional functioning between pre-treatment and follow-up interviews indicate that the program was effective in reducing impact of pain on functioning. Patients also reduced their use of analgesic medications over this time period, and results stayed steady to 6 months of follow-up. ***Limitations:*** No control group.
Roberts, A. H., Sternbach, R. A., & Polich, J. (1993)	Results indicated that pain in a number of areas declined across the treatment period. For example, pain during sitting, sleeping, standing, family interaction, and playing all decreased across time (p<0.001). There were also decreases in pain interference related to work and home activities, over the course of treatment (p<0.001). At 24 months, some of the variables show a non-significant trend toward baseline. Results of reduced pain remained over the 2-year follow-up period.	Non-RCT	354	***Conclusions:*** Results indicated that patients experienced decreased pain in a number of domains, such as sitting, standing, walking, and playing, over the treatment period. There was also a decrease in terms of pain interference on work- and home-related activities. ***Limitations:*** Lack of a control group, limited discussion of outcomes measures, related methods may make replication difficult.
Boswell, S. (1989)	Statistically significant changes in the depression (p<0.01) and anxiety (p<0.05) levels, as measured by both assessment tools. Although there were no statistically significant changes in social behavior, there were positive trends.	Non-RCT	10	***Conclusions:*** Statistical improvements were seen for depression and anxiety scores over the course of the program. Participants also began to form supportive relationships. ***Limitations:*** No control group, small sample size.
Cole, M. B., & Greene, L. R. (1988)	Data revealed a significant main effect of kind of group on evaluative ratings. Specifically, task-oriented OT groups were more highly regarded than the psychotherapy groups by all subjects (p<0.05). OT groups tended to be seen as more potent and active and their leaders as more significantly valuable (p<0.05), potent (p<0.05), and active (p<0.05).	Non-RCT	20	***Conclusions:*** Results demonstrated preference for OT groups over psychotherapeutic groups by all subjects involved. ***Limitations:*** Small sample size, no randomization to treatment groups, unclear about treatment length, baseline data and follow-up data not collected, no indication of blinded assessment.

continued

Table 10-3 (continued)

EVIDENCE OF EFFECTIVENESS OF OCCUPATIONAL THERAPY ON PSYCHO-EMOTIONAL OUTCOMES

Author (Date)	Major Results	Study Design	Sample Size	Conclusions and Limitations
Positive Effects—Non-Randomized Controlled Trial				
Lushbough, R. S., Priddy, J. M., Sewell, H. H., Lovett, S. B., & Jones, T. C. (1988)	Improved ratings for interpersonal effectiveness for the treatment group on COTE compared to controls. No other measures demonstrated significant treatment effects. Clinical improvements in voluntary group attendance, patient-to-patient interactions in group, and sustained task-oriented behaviors.	Non-RCT	12	***Conclusions:*** The OT and psycho-social groups resulted in clinical improvements evident in improved COTE scores, voluntary group attendance, peer interaction, and engagement in tasks. No significant changes were observed in the NOSIE and BPRS. ***Limitations:*** Evaluations not blinded, small sample size.
No Effect				
Nobili, A., Riva, E., Tettamanti, M., Lucca, U., Liscio, M., Petrucci, B., et al. (2004)	No differences between control and intervention groups in terms of patients' cognitive and functional changes, or time spent caregiving and caregivers' RSS scores. SBI-C score was significantly lower in intervention than in control group.	RCT	69	***Conclusions:*** The effect of a structured intervention on caregiver stress was examined, and results indicated that this intervention lowered problem behaviors in clients but did not reduce caregiver stress directly. ***Limitations:*** Small sample size, relatively short duration of study may have limited effect.
Sood, J. R., Cisek, E., Zimmerman, J., Zaleski, E. H., & Fillmore, H. H. (2003)	No significant group differences were found in physical or mental health; however, 75% of the control group members compared with 33% of the treatment group members were depressed at the end of the study. There was no significant difference in ADL functioning between groups.	Non-RCT	14	***Conclusions:*** While differences between the control group receiving standard occupational therapy and the treatment group receiving the general wellness program are not statistically significant, there was a difference in depressive symptoms between both groups, which is encouraging. ***Limitations:*** Small sample size, education level different between groups.
Vines, S. W., Ng, A. K., Breggia, A., & Mahoney, R. (2000)	Group mean changes over time for immune response were not statistically significant; statistically significant reductions in depression scores from baseline to end of program (p=0.001); no significant changes in pain intensity or health behaviors over 4 weeks.	Non-RCT	23	***Conclusions:*** Immune function, depression, and health behaviors were measured before and after a multimodal pain program. Blood test results fail to support a relationship between multimodal pain rehabilitation and improved immune response, although a decrease in depression scores was noted. ***Limitations:*** No control group, co-intervention was not avoided (due to ethical reasons), small sample size, convenience sample from clinic's patients.

continued

Table 10-3 (continued)

EVIDENCE OF EFFECTIVENESS OF OCCUPATIONAL THERAPY ON PSYCHO-EMOTIONAL OUTCOMES

Author (Date)	Major Results	Study Design	Sample Size	Conclusions and Limitations
No Effects				
Sellwood, W., Thomas, C. S., Tarrier, N., Jones, S., Clewes, J., James, A., et al. (1999)	No significant differences were found between the 2 groups at 9-month follow-up. Home group: Significant reduction in socially embarrassing behaviors p=0.03, significant improvements in interpersonal functioning and recreational activities p=0.019, significant reduction in suspiciousness p=0.016. Home group had a decreased amount of days spent in hospital: Home group 233 days and outpatient treatment group 467 days.	RCT	65	***Conclusions:*** Significant differences between the 2 groups at 9-month follow-up were not found. ***Limitations:*** Possible volunteer bias from sample selection, intervention not described well in order to reproduce, small sample size, no record of preventing contamination or co-intervention.

ACL-90=Allen Cognitive Level, BAI=Beck Anxiety Inventory, BPRS=Brief Psychiatric Rating Scale, CES-D=Center for Epidemiologic Studies Depression Scale, COTE=Comprehensive Occupational Therapy Evaluation, FIQ=Fibromyalgia Impact Questionnaire, LFSS=Life Fulfillment and Satisfaction Scales, MPI=Multidimensional Pain Inventory, NOSIE=Nurses Observation Scale for Inpatient Evaluation, RSS=Relative's Stress Scale, RTI-2=Routine Task Inventory, SBI-C=Spontaneous Behavior Inventory (Section C), SF-36=Short Form Health Survey.

Table 10-4

OUTCOME MEASURES USED TO CAPTURE PSYCHO-EMOTIONAL OUTCOMES

Author (Date)	Outcome(s) Investigated	Outcome Measure(s)	Method of Administration
Graff, M., Adang, E., Vernooij-Dassen, M., Dekker, J., Jonsson, L., Thijssen, M., et al. (2008)	Daily function Functional performance Caregiver competence	AMPS Interview of Deterioration in Daily Activities in Dementia Sense of Competence Questionnaire	OTs assessed the patients and caregivers at baseline, 6-week, and 3-month follow-up.
Hooten, W. M., Townsend, C., Sletten, C., Bruce, B., & Rome, J. D. (2007)	Pain severity and life interference Perceived life control Physical and emotional health status Pain catastrophizing	MPI SF-36 CES-D	The 4 questionnaires were administered at admission and dismissal.
Lambert, R. A., Harvey, I., & Poland, F. (2007)	Anxiety severity Panic attack frequency and severity Depression Phobic symptoms Quality of life	BAI ADIS-IV BDI-II Fear Questionnaire SF-36 EuroQol Health Questionnaire	Assessments were conducted at baseline and at follow-up 20 weeks and 10 months after randomization. Data were collected by research therapists who had not delivered the intervention.
Rosenberg, N. K., & Hougaard, E. (2005)	Symptoms of depression and anxiety Number of panic attacks in past 3 weeks	SCL-90R	SCL-90R completed by client; number of panic attacks self-reported by client; clients assessed immediately before treatment, at end of 4 months of treatment, and at follow-up 1.5 to 2 years after end of treatment.
Gutman, S. A., Diamond, H., Holness-Parchment, S. E., Brandofino, D. N., Pacheco, D. G., Jolly-Edouard, M., et al. (2004)	Addressing cognitive deficits to enhance life circumstances or quality of life	GAS	Self-report and pre-/post-tests (multiple choice and short answer).
Nobili, A., Riva, E., Tettamanti, M., Lucca, U., Liscio, M., Petrucci, B., et al. (2004)	Level of caregiver stress Cognitive and functional deficits Problem behaviors of clients	RSS SBI MMSE	SBI administered by OT over telephone upon entry to study and in initial in-person interview. RSS administered by OT during initial interview.
Buchain, P. C., Vizzotto, A. D., Henna Neto, J., & Elkis, H. (2003)	Performance of activity Reduction in psychotic symptoms Social interaction Self-care	EOITO	By OT at baseline and monthly for 6 months.
Pfeiffer, A., Thompson, J. M., Nelson, A., Tucker, S., Luedtke, C., Finnie, S., et al. (2003)	Fibromyalgia impact Life fulfillment Depression	FIQ LFSS CES-D	3 outcome measures were completed prior to the intervention. 1 month following the intervention program, the measures were mailed out to the subjects. Follow-up telephone calls were made to facilitate the completion and return of questionnaires.

continued

Table 10-4 (continued)
OUTCOME MEASURES USED TO CAPTURE PSYCHO-EMOTIONAL OUTCOMES

Author (Date)	Outcome(s) Investigated	Outcome Measure(s)	Method of Administration
Sood, J. R., Cisek, E., Zimmerman, J., Zaleski, E. H., & Fillmore, H. H. (2003)	Depression Physical and mental health Behavioral competence with ADL	GDS SF-12 MLAI	The SF-12 and MLAI were measured by self-report.
Lippert-Gruner, M., Wedekind, C., & Klug, N. (2002)	Changes in ADL or functional outcomes Occupational and social reintegration 1-year post brain injury	GCS CRS BI FIM DRS	1 year after trauma, patients were interviewed, and a standardized neurological exam was performed as well as a battery of tests to examine functional outcomes. Does not specify person who completes tests.
Wu, C-Y. (2001)	Intrinsic Motivation (and related behaviors)	CGOS COTE	The CGOS is a self-report measure and was filled out by the subjects before and after intervention. Pre- and post-evaluations were also conducted using the COTE. The COTE was administered by OTs uninvolved in the intervention.
Vines, S. W., Ng, A. K., Breggia, A., & Mahoney, R. (2000)	Level of depression Health behaviors Pain intensity Immunological response	BDI PLA MPQ-SF T-lymphocyte proliferation after stimulation with mitogens Concanavalin and Phytohemagglutinin measured immunological response	BDI, PLA, and MPQ-SF administered by client self-report; t-cell proliferation measured through blood tests. All measures taken at beginning and end of treatment period (4 weeks apart).
Eklund, M. (1999)	Changes in psychiatric symptoms, quality of life, and occupational performance.	SCL-90R HSRS SQoL AOF	Administered at admission and discharge: SCL-90R (self-report), HSRS (interview and observation), SQoL (self-report), AOF (semi-structured interview)
Raweh, D. V., & Katz, N. (1999)	Cognitive functional ability Ability to perform routine tasks and awareness	RTI-2 ACL-90 Awareness questionnaire	All measures were administered pre- and post-treatment.
Sellwood, W., Thomas, C. S., Tarrier, N., Jones, S., Clewes, J., James, A., et al. (1999)	Positive and negative symptoms of schizophrenia Cognitive impairment Social functioning Caregiver morbidity	BPRS MMSE SBS SFS LQL GHQ	Measures were administered pre-treatment and after 9 months of treatment. Individuals who administered tests received training and were not aware of treatment group.

continued

Table 10-4 (continued)

OUTCOME MEASURES USED TO CAPTURE PSYCHO-EMOTIONAL OUTCOMES

Author (Date)	Outcome(s) Investigated	Outcome Measure(s)	Method of Administration
Turk, D. C., Okifuji, A., Sinclair, J. D., & Starz, T. W. (1998)	Changes in clients' perceptions and interpretation of pain conditions Enhancing self-management skills Enhancing self-efficacy	MPI CES-D ODI LWMAS FIQ	3-hour pre-treatment assessment: Medical, physical, psychological, and self-report inventories. At end of last treatment session, completed questionnaires administered pre-treatment. 6-month mail follow-up.
DeWilliams, C. A. C., Nicholas, M. K., Richardson, P. H., Pither, C. E., Justins, D. M., Chamberlain, J. H., et al. (1993)	Impact of pain on patients' day-to-day functioning Average pain intensity Depression severity Confidence performing activities despite pain Walking speed and distance walked in 10 minutes Physical endurance Pain medication use	SIP 0-100 scale BDI PSEQ 20-meter indoor course used to measure walking speed Number of stairs climbed up or down in 2 minutes and number of sit-ups completed to tolerance measured physical endurance	Sickness impact profile given by interview; pain impression, confidence, and depression were self-reported by patients; physical aspects measured by observation; pain medication use measured by chart review. All measures completed at pre-treatment interview, 1 month, and 6 months after discharge.
Roberts, A. H., Sternbach, R. A., & Polich, J. (1993)	Self-reported pain Functional ability at work and home	Questionnaires included VAS Other questionnaire items assessed amount of time sitting, standing, walking, lying, and medication usage	Self-report questionnaires were given to participants before treatment then at 1, 6, 12, and 24 months after treatment began.
Boswell, S. (1989)	Level of depression Level of anxiety Frequency of positive behaviors How patient is feeling	BDI SSEQ Diary of daily activities	All measures were self-administered. BDI and SSEQ were given at the first and last program visit. The diary was given out on at session 8 to be completed over the week and returned at session 9 (final session).
Strong, J., Cramond, T., & Maas, F. (1989)	Chronic low back pain	McGill Pain Questionnaire Pain measurement instrument containing word descriptors of pain	Administered by self-report at baseline, discharge, and follow-up (3 to 15 months later).
Cole, M. B., & Greene, L. R. (1988)	Patients' reactions toward the groups, their leaders, and themselves	6-item semantic differential form Tapping Osgood, Suci, and Tannenbaum's (1957) basic factors of evaluation, potency, and activity	Not described.

continued

Table 10-4 (continued)
OUTCOME MEASURES USED TO CAPTURE PSYCHO-EMOTIONAL OUTCOMES

Author (Date)	Outcome(s) Investigated	Outcome Measure(s)	Method of Administration
Lushbough, R. S., Priddy, J. M., Sewell, H. H., Lovett, S. B., & Jones, T. C. (1988)	Functional ability, social interactions, and psychiatric symptoms	COTE NOSIE BPRS	Measures administered before interventions and after the 4-month program. COTE administered by OT, NOSIE administered by director of nurses, BPRS administered by staff psychiatrist.

ACL-90=Allen Cognitive Level, ADIS-IV=Anxiety Disorders Interview Schedule, AMPS=Assessment of Motor and Process Skills, AOF=Assessment of Occupational Functioning, BAI=Beck Anxiety Inventory, BDI=Beck Depression Inventory, BDI-II=Beck Depression Inventory II, BI=Barthel Index, BPRS=Brief Psychiatric Rating Scale, CES-D=Center for Epidemiologic Studies Depression Scale, CGOS=Chinese General Causality Orientations Scale, COTE=Comprehensive Occupational Therapy Evaluation, CRS=Coma Remission Scale, DRS=Disability Rating Scale, EOITO=Scale of Interactive Observation in Occupational Therapy, EuroQol=European Quality of Life Instrument, FIM=Functional Independence Measure, FIQ=Fibromyalgia Impact Questionnaire, GAS=Goal Attainment Scaling, GCS=Glasgow Coma Scale, GDS=Geriatric Depression Scale, GHQ=General Health Questionnaire, HSRS=Health Sickness Rating Scale, LFSS=Life Fulfillment and Satisfaction Scales, LQL=Lancashire Quality of Life, LWMAS=Locke-Wallace Marital Adjustment Scale, MLAI=Multi-Level Assessment Instrument, MMSE=Mini Mental Status Examination, MPI=Multidimensional Pain Inventory, MPQ-SF=McGill Pain Questionnaire-Short Form, NOSIE=Nurses Observation Scale for Inpatient Evaluation, ODI=Oswestry Disability Index, PLA=Personal Lifestyle Activities Questionnaire, PSEQ=Pain Self-Efficacy Questionnaire, RSS=Relative's Stress Scale, RTI-2=Routine Task Inventory, SBI=Spontaneous Behavior Inventory, SBS=Socially Embarrassing Behavior Scale, SCL-90R=Symptom Distress Checklist 90, SF-12=Short Form 12, SF-36=Short Form Health Survey, SFS=Social Functioning Scale, SIP=Sickness Impact Profile, SQoL=Subjective Estimation of Quality of Life, SSEQ=Speilberges Self-Evaluation Questionnaire, VAS=Visual Analog Scale.

reviewed and summarized, providing information on the strength of evidence linking occupational therapy interventions to these outcomes. The interventions are in three areas—comprehensive occupation-based programs, cognitive-behavioral interventions with a focus on self-management and pacing, and cognitive-behavioral programs with a focus on relaxation and guided imagery. The results of our empirical reviews are organized by these areas of intervention. The sections conclude with recommendations on how clinical treatment can proceed and/or where future research directions lie.

Occupation-Based Programs to Improve Psycho-Emotional Function

Occupational therapy programs for people with significant mental illness (addiction, anxiety disorder, bipolar disorder, depression, schizophrenia) often use occupation as the means to develop and/or achieve psycho-emotional outcomes. Such programs may include occupational therapy intervention by itself or may be part of a comprehensive multidisciplinary program. The goal of these programs is to facilitate clients' involvement in occupations as a means to achieve improvements in participation and improvements in psychological and emotional body functions. Occupational therapists are also involved in providing services directed at preventing health risks among older adults. Although such preventative occupational therapy services are generally directed at improving overall health outcomes among older adults, there is typically a large psychosocial focus.

Cognitive-Behavioral Training Interventions to Improve Psycho-Emotional Function

Several studies have evaluated the use of cognitive-behavioral strategies combined with self-management or relaxation interventions to change psychological and/or emotional symptoms. Typically, these programs are multidisciplinary in nature. In one type of intervention, occupational therapy focused on the use of CBT in conjunction with strategies to educate clients about energy conservation, pacing, and body mechanics. The second type of study focused on the use of CBT in combination with relaxation and guided imagery.

Occupational Therapy on a Mental Health Team

The program for ACT model is a continuous, comprehensive, and highly flexible community care program for people with mental illnesses who have a his-

tory of repeated psychiatric hospitalizations (Krupa et al., 2002). ACT teams include medical, psychosocial, and rehabilitation services that are available 7 days a week and 24 hours a day (Burns & Santos, 1995). Occupational therapy has been identified as one of the required disciplines required to fulfill the rehabilitative goals of the ACT model (Krupa et al., 2002).

Effects of Occupational Therapy in Promoting Psycho-Emotional Outcomes

Occupation-Based Programs to Improve Psycho-Emotional Function

Systematic Reviews

Two systematic reviews provide evidence that occupational therapy intervention improves psychosocial well-being (including depressive symptoms) (Ma & Trombly, 2002; Murphy & Tickle-Degnen, 2001). When the focus of occupational therapy intervention is on psychosocial areas, the outcomes of depression or psychological well-being improved significantly in the experimental groups providing occupation-based treatment versus its control group (Ma & Trombly, 2002).

A review of the research over the past 20 years regarding occupation-based work activities in sheltered settings for people with long-term schizophrenia concluded that these programs improve outcomes (Durham, 1997). Typically, these programs encompass work skills assessed, work adjustment, and job skill training through sheltered employment, transitional and supported employment, job finding, and job maintenance (Durham, 1997). This review found that while engaged in structured activity in occupational therapy, participants were less likely to exhibit negative symptoms such as lack of drive, social withdrawal, and emotional apathy (Durham, 1997). The review by Durham (1997) indicated that interventions involving occupational therapy and recreational therapy were more effective in delaying relapse of mental illness.

The findings reported by Durham (1997), however, must be interpreted with caution. Many of the studies included in the review were quite old (from the 1970s and 1980s) and, thus, were inconsistent with current trends in psychosocial occupational therapy, psychiatric rehabilitation, and recovery-oriented services. For example, in Canada, there are currently very few sheltered workshops for people with serious mental illnesses, and those that continue to exist have moved beyond their traditional philosophical roots to incorporate ideas around growth, recovery, and self-actualization (Kirsh,

Krupa, Cockburn, & Gewurtz, 2006). Occupational therapists have begun to focus on outcomes associated with work in integrated settings (Kirsh, Cockburn, & Gewurtz, 2005; Moll, Huff, & Detwiler, 2003) and promoting growth and career development among individuals with schizophrenia and other serious mental illnesses (Auerbach & Richardson, 2005; Gewurtz & Kirsh, 2007; Krupa, 2004).

Empirical Studies

Twelve empirical studies have examined the effect of occupation-based programs on psychological and emotional outcomes (Boswell, 1989; Buchain, Vizzotto, Henna Neto, & Elkins, 2003; Cole & Greene, 1988; Eklund, 1999; Graff et al., 2008; Gutman et al., 2004; Lambert, Harvey, & Poland, 2007; Lushbough, Priddy, Sewell, Lovett, & Jones, 1988; Nobili et al., 2004; Raweh & Katz, 1999; Sellwood et al., 1999; Wu, 2001). Eight of the interventions were occupational therapy alone (Boswell, 1989; Cole & Greene, 1988; Eklund, 1999; Graff et al., 2008; Gutman et al., 2004; Lambert et al., 2007; Raweh & Katz, 1999; Wu, 2001) while four were multidisciplinary in nature (Buchain et al., 2003; Lushbough et al., 1988; Nobili et al., 2004; Sellwood et al., 1999). The programs typically included involvement in individual and group activities whose purpose was to improve specific skills such as interpersonal relations and communication, decrease anxiety and stress, decrease depressive and other negative symptoms, and improve feelings of self-worth. Two studies used a social skills model. In this approach, complex social skills are broken down into simpler steps and taught by therapists modeling correct behavior and the clients learning by repeated exposure and practice (Lauriello, Bustillo, & Keith, 1999). Two of the studies in part directed intervention at decreasing caregiver stress or burden (Graff et al., 2008; Nobili et al., 2004).

The research in this intervention category included six randomized controlled trials (Buchain et al., 2003; Graff et al., 2008; Lambert et al., 2007; Nobili et al., 2004; Sellwood et al., 1999; Wu, 2001), two cohort studies (Eklund, 1999; Raweh & Katz, 1999), and four before-and-after studies (Boswell, 1989; Cole & Greene, 1988; Gutman et al., 2004; Lushbough et al., 1988). The sample sizes are not large, and each study has important limitations (see Table 10-3). Outcomes of two of the randomized controlled trials (Buchain et al., 2003; Sellwood et al., 1999) indicate that these interventions improved activity performance, decreased negative symptoms such as suspiciousness and socially embarrassing behaviors, and improved social interaction skills. Lambert and colleagues (2007) showed a short-term decrease in anxiety levels after occupational therapy-based intervention with people with panic disorders. In the randomized controlled trial by Wu

(2001), occupational therapy intervention was reported to be effective in facilitating intrinsic motivation with individuals having various motivation styles. The last two randomized controlled trials demonstrated the impact of occupational therapy in decreasing caregiver burden (Graff et al., 2008) and occupational therapy on a multidisciplinary team decreasing caregiver stress (Nobili et al., 2004).

Raweh's pilot study of the effect of Allen's cognitive disability treatment for people with schizophrenia found that the treatment group improved significantly in cognitive functioning but both groups improved in the performance of routine tasks. Eklund (1999) found that an occupation-based treatment approach improved communication skills and decreased psychiatric symptoms.

The four before-and-after studies (Boswell, 1989; Cole & Greene, 1988; Gutman et al., 2004; Lushbough et al., 1988) also found positive outcomes, but these studies did not include blinded measurement, and the sample sizes were small.

In addition, Rebeiro and her colleagues have conducted qualitative and mixed-method studies to explore the impact of occupation-based interventions on people with mental illnesses. One study explored experiences of engagement for eight female participants involved in an occupation-based mental health group (Rebeiro & Cook, 1999). This study found that occupation served as a means to enhance subjective well-being and perceived self-confidence and self-competence. The authors suggest that such interventions help individuals define and re-define their sense of self and serve as a means to sustain psychological well-being over time. In another study, Rebeiro and her consumer/survivor colleagues (Rebeiro, Day, Semeniuk, O'Brian, & Wilson, 2001) used a mixed-method approach to explore participating in a consumer-run, occupation-based, non-profit organization for individuals with mental illnesses. The qualitative findings highlight an increased sense of well-being and an increased sense of belonging among participants. These positive outcomes are further supported by the quantitative findings that point to reduced use of crisis services and hospitalizations and improved quality of life, socioeconomic status, and rates of paid employment among participants. However, the quantitative findings from this study are meant for descriptive purposes only and must be interpreted with caution due to the small sample size (n=10).

There is additional evidence from three studies exploring the impact of occupational therapy intervention among independently living older adults. These studies include one randomized controlled trial (Clark et al., 1997), one study examining the impact of the intervention from the randomized controlled trial at 6-month follow-up without any further treatment (Clark et al., 2001), and one before-and-after study (Matuska, Giles-Heinz, Flinn, Neighbor, & Bass-Haugen, 2003). The occupational therapy intervention in the studies typically included a program designed for adults over 65 years living independently.

The occupational therapy program used in both studies included a mixture of educational classes and direct experience focused on helping participants appreciate the importance of meaningful occupation to achieve a healthy and satisfying lifestyle, strategies to remove personal and environmental barriers that prevent or restrict participation, and exercises to help participants better understand the effect of occupation on their health, well-being, and daily lives. In the study by Matuska and colleagues (2003), the program involved 6 months of weekly 1.5-hour educational classes taught by occupational therapy faculty. The participants in the occupational therapy group of the study by Clark and colleagues (1997) received 2 hours per week of group occupational therapy and a total of 9 hours of individual occupational therapy during the 9-month treatment period.

The findings from both studies revealed that older adults who participated in the occupational therapy interventions showed significant improvements in various indicators of quality of life measures such as vitality, social functioning, and general mental health (Clark et al., 1997; Matuska et al., 2003). Clark and colleagues (2001) followed the participants who completed the trial for an additional 6 months without further intervention and then re-evaluated. The findings showed that approximately 90% of the therapeutic gains observed following occupational therapy intervention were retained at 6-month follow-up including improved physical functioning, role functioning, vitality, social functioning, role emotional, and general mental health.

In summary, there is evidence from eight studies with more rigorous designs that occupation-based interventions have a positive impact on psychological and emotional outcomes. The qualitative studies by Rebeiro enhance our understanding of how occupation-based interventions work to improve psycho-emotional outcomes and begin to unravel the power and potential of occupation-based intervention. However, further research with larger sample sizes is needed.

Cognitive-Behavioral Training Interventions to Improve Psycho-Emotional Outcomes

Empirical Studies

Two before-and-after studies have evaluated the effect of occupational therapy intervention using CBT

and self-management strategies focused on energy conservation, pacing, and proper body mechanics for people with fibromyalgia (Pfeiffer et al., 2003; Turk, Okifuji, Sinclair, & Starz, 1998). Results indicate that the programs led to decreased pain and stress. These studies are small and do not include a control group. In a larger (N=212) before-and-after study, DeWilliams and colleagues (1993) found significant improvements in self-reported emotional function of people with chronic pain after a 4-week inpatient multidisciplinary CBT program. A small (N=23) before-and-after study of CBT for chronic pain reported significant decreases in depression scores after a 4-week inpatient treatment (Vines, Ng, Breggia, & Mahoney, 2000). In another before-and-after study by Hooten and colleagues (2007), a multidisciplinary CBT program (including occupational therapy) to address pain in subjects with fibromyalgia showed improvements in psychosocial functioning, health attributes, negative pain-related emotions, and depressive symptoms.

Rosenberg and Hougaard (2005) compared a group CBT program for people with anxiety and agoraphobia to a waitlist control group. After 14 weekly sessions, the treatment group had 47% fewer panic attacks compared to 12.5% fewer in the control group (p<0.001). Three studies have evaluated the use of CBT along with relaxation and guided imagery. Results from a large before-and-after study by Roberts, Sternbach, and Polich (1993), a cohort study by Sood, Cisek, Zimmerman, Zaleski, and Fillmore (2003), and a randomized controlled trial by Strong, Cramond, and Maas (1989) found that CBT combined with relaxation and biofeedback or guided imagery led to significant decreases in depressive symptoms or pain for people with chronic pain.

Occupational Therapy on a Mental Health Team to Promote Psycho-Emotional Outcomes

Systematic Reviews

Marshall and Lockwood (1998) conducted a systematic review of ACT as an alternative to standard community care and traditional hospital-based rehabilitation on outcomes including remaining in contact with the psychiatric services, extent of psychiatric hospital admissions, clinical and social outcomes, and costs. They found that those receiving ACT services were more likely to remain in contact with services than those receiving standard community care but not hospital-based rehabilitation. Those receiving ACT services were also less likely to be admitted to the hospital and spent less time in the hospital than people receiving standard community care or hospital-based care. Compared to standard community care and hospital-based rehabilitation, individuals receiving ACT services were more likely to be living independently in stable accommodations and less likely to be unemployed. However, there were no differences in terms of mental state, social functioning, self-esteem, and quality of life.

Coldwell and Bender (2007) conducted a meta-analysis of the effectiveness of ACT with individuals who are homeless with severe mental illnesses. Of the 10 studies that met their inclusion criteria, six were randomized controlled trials and four were observational studies. Among all the studies, they found that ACT resulted in a greater reduction in homelessness and greater improvement in psychiatric symptoms such as anxiety, depression, and thought disturbances compared with standard case management treatment.

Although these studies suggest the clinical effectiveness of ACT provided services to individuals living with severe mental illnesses in the community who have high service needs, the contributions of occupational therapists are not always clear. Despite the explicit inclusion of occupational therapists on ACT teams in Ontario (Ministry of Health and Long-Term Care, 2004), there is often only one occupational therapist on each team, and it is sometimes unclear whether or not the teams evaluated in the studies reviewed included occupational therapists.

Measures Used to Capture Psycho-Emotional Outcomes

Because this chapter focuses on the impact of occupational therapy intervention on psychological and emotional outcomes, this section includes only those measures that assess these outcomes. Outcome measures for the outcomes of personal care and activity performance are included in other chapters.

Based on the scoping reviews completed for this chapter, there is evidence to support the impact of occupational therapy intervention on the following psychological and emotional outcomes:

▲ Body function
  △ Pain
  △ Depressive symptoms
  △ Anxiety
  △ Interpersonal interactions
  △ Motivation
▲ Activity
  △ Social communication
  △ Role functioning
  △ Social functioning

Outcome Measures

Drawing on reviews of measures already completed within occupational therapy (Law, Baum, & Dunn, 2005) and the measures used in studies reviewed for this project, we have compiled a table of measures most suitable for use in occupational therapy to assess outcomes of intervention focused on psycho-emotional components. These outcome measures are reviewed in Table 10-5.

Conclusions and Recommendations for Future Research

The scope and depth of the research in this area does not seem to be in tune with our theoretical beliefs about the potential and power of occupation embraced by our profession since its inception. Although we are firmly committed to the potential of occupation to improve and promote psycho-emotional outcomes, the research in this area is relatively weak and underdeveloped. This review reiterates the importance of Rebeiro's (1998) call to action and highlights the need for occupational therapists to conduct research to demonstrate the outcomes of their interventions in this area. We need to narrow the gap between what we believe in terms of the potential of our work to improve psycho-emotional functioning and the existing research evidence in the area.

Table 10-5

OUTCOME MEASURES TO ASSESS PSYCHO-EMOTIONAL INTERVENTIONS

Measure	Population	Content Domains	Reliability and Validity
Beck Anxiety Inventory (BAI)	Adults	A 21-item self-report questionnaire designed to distinguish anxiety from depression.	Studies demonstrate convergent and discriminant validity and internal consistency reliability.
Beck Depression Inventory (BDI)	Age 13 and over	Self-report questionnaire that produces an overall depression score. Participants answer questions about the behavioral, cognitive, and emotional symptoms recently experienced.	Studies demonstrate internal consistency and test-retest reliability and concurrent and construct validity.
Brief Psychiatric Rating Scale (BPRS)	Adults	Clinician interview of patient to assess the level psychiatric symptoms across 18 conditions such as hostility, suspiciousness, hallucination, and grandiosity.	Studies demonstrate internal consistency and inter-rater reliability and good overall validity.
Center for Epidemiologic Studies Depression Scale (CES-D)	Adults	20-item self-assessment measurement tool to identify patients at risk for depression.	Studies demonstrate internal consistency and test-retest reliability and construct validity.
Comprehensive Occupational Therapy Evaluation (COTE)	Adults	OTs rate patient behaviors in the following areas during structured and non-structured OT interactions or activities: General behaviors, interpersonal behaviors, and task behaviors.	Studies demonstrate inter-rater reliability and construct and criterion validity.
Disability Rating Scale (DRS)	Older teenagers and adults	Measures general changes in functional recovery after traumatic brain injury on a 5-point scale (level of functioning) from totally independent to totally dependent. Some sample items are eye opening, communication ability, toileting, feeding.	Studies demonstrate inter-rater and test-retest reliability and concurrent and predictive validity.
Health Sickness Rating Scale (HSRS)	Adults	A self-report measure of global mental health status with 7 key factors: Ability to function autonomously, symptom severity, degree of discomfort, effect on environment, quality of interpersonal relationships, utilization abilities, breadth and depth of interests.	Studies demonstrate inter-rater reliability and construct validity across different countries.
Mini Mental Status Examination (MMSE)	Adults and older adults	30-item questionnaire that assesses memory (retention and recall), concentration, and language.	Studies show test-retest, internal consistency, and inter-rater reliability and reliability and construct validity.
Multidimensional Pain Inventory (MPI)	Adults	A 61-item self-report measure of the impact of chronic pain that examines pain intensity, emotional distress, cognitive and functional adaptation, and social support.	Studies demonstrate inter-rater reliability and concurrent and predictive validity.

continued

Table 10-5 (continued)
Outcome Measures to Assess Psycho-Emotional Interventions

Measure	Population	Content Domains	Reliability and Validity
Multi-Level Assessment Instrument (MLAI)	Older adults	101 interview-administered questions that produces scores in 8 domains: Physical health, cognitive functioning, performance of ADL, personal adjustment, mobility, social support, meaningful time-use, and physical environment.	Studies demonstrate internal consistency and test-retest reliability.
Symptom Distress Checklist 90 (SCL-90R)	Age 13 and older	90-item self-report measure that assesses a range of psychological issues and symptoms: Somatization obsessive-compulsive, interpersonal sensitivity, depression, anxiety, hostility, phobic anxiety, paranoid ideation, psychoticism. It produces 3 global distress indices.	Studies demonstrate internal consistency and test-retest reliability, and concurrent, convergent, discriminant, and construct validity.
Volitional Questionnaire	Adults	A 14-item observation tool used by OTs to assess patient motives and gain information about how the environment affects volition.	Studies demonstrate criterion and construct validity and inter-rater reliability.

References

Auerbach, E., & Richardson, P. (2005). The long-term work experiences of persons with severe and persistent mental illness. *Psychiatric Rehabilitation Journal, 28*(3), 267-273.

Boswell, S. (1989). A social support group for depressed people. *Australian Occupational Therapy Journal, 36*(1), 34-41.

Buchain, P. C., Vizzotto, A. D., Henna Neto, J., & Elkis, H. (2003). Randomized controlled trial of occupational therapy in patients with treatment-resistant schizophrenia. *Revista Brasileira de Psiquiatria, 25*(1), 26-30.

Burns, B. J., & Santos, A. B. (1995). Assertive community treatment: An update of randomized trials. *Psychiatric Services, 46,* 669-675.

Canadian Association of Occupational Therapists. (1997). *Enabling occupation: An occupational therapy perspective.* Ottawa, Ontario, Canada: CAOT Publications.

Clark, F., Azen, S. P., Carlson, M., Mandel, D., LaBree, L., Hay, J., et al. (2001). Embedding health-promoting changes into the daily lives of independent-living older adults: Long-term follow-up of occupational therapy intervention. *Journal of Gerontology, 56B,* 60-63.

Clark, F., Azen, S. P., Zemke, R., Jackson, J., Carlson, M., Mandel, D., et al. (1997). Occupational therapy for independent-living older adults: A randomized controlled trial. *Journal of the American Medical Association, 278*(16), 1321-1326.

Coldwell, C. M., & Bender, W. S. (2007). The effectiveness of assertive community treatment for homeless populations with severe mental illness: A meta-analysis. *American Journal of Psychiatry, 164,* 293-299.

Cole, M. B., & Greene, L. R. (1988). A preference for activity: A comparative study of psychotherapy groups vs. occupational therapy groups for psychotic and borderline inpatients. *Occupational Therapy in Mental Health, 8*(3), 53-67.

DeWilliams, C. A. C., Nicholas, M. K., Richardson, P. H., Pither, C. E., Justins, D. M., Chamberlain, J. H., et al. (1993). Evaluation of a cognitive behavioural programme for rehabilitating patients with chronic pain. *British Journal of General Practice, 43*(377), 513-518.

Durham, T. (1997). Work-related activity for people with long-term schizophrenia: a review of the literature. *British Journal of Occupational Therapy, 60,* 248-252.

Eklund, M. (1999). Outcome of occupational therapy in a psychiatric day care unit for long-term mentally ill patients. *Occupational Therapy in Mental Health, 14*(4), 21-45.

Gewurtz, R., & Kirsh, B. (2007). How consumers of community mental health services come to understand their potential for work: Doing and becoming revisited. *Canadian Journal of Occupational Therapy, 74*(3), 173-185.

Graff, M., Adang, E., Vernooij-Dassen, M., Dekker, J., Jonsson, L., Thijssen, M., Hoefnagels, W., & Olde-Rikkert, M. (2008). Community occupational therapy for older patients with dementia and their care givers: Cost effectiveness study. *British Medical Journal, 336*(7636), 134-138.

Greenhalgh, T. (2006). *How to read a paper: The basics of evidence-based medicine* (3rd ed.). London, England: Blackwell Publishing Ltd.

Gutman, S. A., Diamond, H., Holness-Parchment, S. E., Brandofino, D. N., Pacheco, D. G., Jolly-Edouard, M., et al. (2004). Enhancing independence in women experiencing domestic violence and possible brain injury: An assessment of an occupational therapy intervention. *Occupational Therapy in Mental Health, 20*(1), 49-79.

Hooten, W. M., Townsend, C., Sletten, C., Bruce, B., & Rome, J. D. (2007). Treatment outcomes after multidisciplinary pain rehabilitation with analgesic medication withdrawal for patients with fibromyalgia. *Pain Med, 8*(1), 8-16.

Kirsh, B., Cockburn, L., & Gewurtz, R. (2005). Best practice in occupational therapy: Program characteristics that influence vocational outcomes for people with serious mental illnesses. *Canadian Journal of Occupational Therapy, 72,* 265-279.

Kirsh, B., Krupa, T., Cockburn, L., & Gewurtz, R. (2006). Work initiatives in Canada: A decade of development. *Canadian Journal of Community Mental Health, 25*(2), 173-191.

Krupa, T. (2004). Employment, recovery and schizophrenia: Integrating health and disorder at work. *Psychiatric Rehabilitation Journal, 28*(1), 8-15.

Krupa, T., Radloff-Gabriel, D., Whippey, E., & Kirsh, B. (2002). Occupational therapy and assertive community treatment. *Canadian Journal of Occupational Therapy, 69*(3), 153-157.

Lambert, R. A., Harvey, I., & Poland, F. (2007). A pragmatic, unblinded randomised controlled trial comparing an occupational therapy-led lifestyle approach and routine GP care for panic disorder treatment in primary care. *Journal of Affective Disorders, 99*(1-3), 63-71.

Lauriello, J., Bustillo, J., & Keith, S. (1999). A critical review of research on psychosocial treatment of schizophrenia. *Society of Biological Psychiatry, 46*, 1409-1417.

Law, M., Baum, C., & Dunn, W. (2005). *Measuring occupational performance: Supporting best practice in occupational therapy* (2nd ed.). Thorofare, NJ: SLACK Incorporated.

Lippert-Gruner, M., Wedekind, C., & Klug, N. (2002). Functional and psychosocial outcome one year after severe traumatic brain injury and early-onset rehabilitation therapy. *Journal of Rehabilitation Medicine, 34*(5), 211-214.

Lushbough, R. S., Priddy, J. M., Sewell, H. H., Lovett, S. B., & Jones, T. C. (1988). The effectiveness of an occupational therapy program in an inpatient geropsychiatric setting. *Physical and Occupational Therapy in Geriatrics, 6*(2), 63-73.

Ma, H. I., & Trombly, C. A. (2002). A synthesis of the effects of occupational therapy for persons with stroke, part II: Remediation of impairments. *American Journal of Occupational Therapy, 56*(3), 260-274.

Marshall, M., & Lockwood, A. (1998). Assertive community treatment for people with severe mental disorders. *Cochrane Database of Systematic Reviews*, Issue 2. Art. No.: CD001089. DOI: 10.1002/14651858.CD001089.

Matuska, K., Giles-Heinz, A., Flinn, N., Neighbor, M., & Bass-Haugen, J. (2003). Outcomes of a pilot occupational therapy wellness program for older adults. *American Journal of Occupational Therapy, 57*(2), 220-224.

McColl, M., Law, M., Stewart, D., Doubt, L., Pollock, N., & Krupa, T. (2002). *Theoretical basis of occupational therapy* (2nd ed.). Thorofare, NJ: SLACK Incorporated.

Ministry of Health and Long-Term Care. (2004). Ontario program standards for ACT teams (2nd ed.). Downloaded on December 27, 2007 from www.ontarioactassociation.com/on_standards.php.

Moll, S., Huff, J., & Detwiler, L. (2003). Supported employment: Evidence for a best practice model in psychosocial rehabilitation. *Canadian Journal of Occupational Therapy, 70*(5), 298-310.

Murphy, S., & Tickle-Degnen, L. (2001). The effectiveness of occupational therapy-related treatments for persons with Parkinson's disease: A meta-analytic review. *American Journal of Occupational Therapy, 55*(4), 385-392.

Nobili, A., Riva, E., Tettamanti, M., Lucca, U., Liscio, M., Petrucci, B., et al. (2004). The effect of a structured intervention on caregivers of patients with dementia and problem behaviors: A random-ized controlled pilot study. *Alzheimer's Disease and Associated Disorders, 18*(2), 75-82.

Pfeiffer, A., Thompson, J. M., Nelson, A., Tucker, S., Luedtke, C., Finnie, S., et al. (2003). Effects of a 1.5-day multidisciplinary outpatient treatment program for fibromyalgia: A pilot study. *American Journal of Physical Medicine and Rehabilitation, 82*(3), 186-191.

Raweh, D. V., & Katz, N. (1999). Treatment effectiveness of Allen's cognitive disabilities model with adult schizophrenic outpatients: A pilot study. *Occupational Therapy in Mental Health, 14*(4), 65-77.

Rebeiro, K. (1998). Occupation-as-means to mental health: A review of the literature, and a call for research. *Canadian Journal of Occupational Therapy, 65*(1), 12-19.

Rebeiro, K., & Cook, J. V. (1999). Opportunity, not prescription: An exploratory study of the experience of occupational engagement. *Canadian Journal of Occupational Therapy, 66*(4), 176-187.

Rebeiro, K., Day, D. G., Semeniuk, B., O'Brian, M. C., & Wilson, B. (2001). Northern Initiative for social action: An occupation-based mental health program. *American Journal of Occupational Therapy, 55*(5), 493-500.

Roberts, A. H., Sternbach, R. A., & Polich, J. (1993). Behavioral management of chronic pain and excess disability: Long-term follow-up of an outpatient program. *Clinical Journal of Pain, 9*, 41-48.

Rosenberg, N. K., & Hougaard, E. (2005). Cognitive-behavioural group treatment of panic disorder and agoraphobia in a psychiatric setting: A naturalistic study of effectiveness. *Nordic Journal of Psychiatry, 59*(3), 198-204.

Sellwood, W., Thomas, C. S., Tarrier, N., Jones, S., Clewes, J., James, A., et al. (1999). A randomised controlled trial of home-based rehabilitation versus outpatient-based rehabilitation for patients suffering from chronic schizophrenia. *Social Psychiatry and Psychiatric Epidemiology, 34*(5), 250-253.

Sood, J. R., Cisek, E., Zimmerman, J., Zaleski, E. H., & Fillmore, H. H. (2003). Treatment of depressive symptoms during short-term rehabilitation: An attempted replication of the DOUR project. *Rehabilitation Psychology, 48*(1), 44-49.

Strong, J., Cramond, T., & Maas, F. (1989). The effectiveness of relaxation techniques with patients who have chronic low back pain. *Occupational Therapy Journal of Research, 9*(3), 184-192.

Turk, D. C., Okifuji, A., Sinclair, J. D., & Starz, T. W. (1998). Interdisciplinary treatment for fibromyalgia syndrome: Clinical and statistical significance. *Arthritis Care and Research, 11*(3), 186-195.

Vines, S. W., Ng, A. K., Breggia, A., & Mahoney, R. (2000). Multimodal chronic pain rehabilitation program: Its effect on immune function, depression, and health behaviors. *Rehabilitation Nursing, 25*(5), 185-191.

Wu, C-Y. (2001). Facilitating intrinsic motivation in individuals with psychiatric illness: A study on the effectiveness of an occupational therapy intervention. *Occupational Therapy Journal of Research, 21*, 142-167.

INTERVENTIONS TO IMPROVE COGNITIVE-NEUROLOGICAL OUTCOMES

Briano Di Rezze, MSc (OT), OT Reg. (Ont.)

Impairments that affect a person's central nervous system (CNS) can have a great and sudden impact on his or her daily occupations. Occupational therapy-specific rehabilitation addressing the cognitive and neurological deficits that accompany an insult to the CNS aim to overcome such barriers and re-establish client participation in meaningful activities. The "cognitive-neurological determinants of occupation include the cognitive, sensory, perceptual, and neurological integration of input essential to one's ability to carry out daily activities with success and satisfaction" (McColl, 2002, p. 3).

This chapter examines the research evidence that has studied occupational therapy interventions focused on the cognitive-neurological deficits of the client. The evidence for these intervention outcomes, addressing these specific cognitive-neurological barriers, is divided into two areas: (1) interventions that aim to improve cognitive outcomes (i.e., cognitive and perceptual components) and (2) interventions that target neuro-sensorimotor outcomes (i.e., sensory and neuro-motor components). The chapter will begin by providing a conceptual background of these two areas of intervention and describe their relevance to both the client and occupational therapy. This is followed by a description of the search strategy that captured the relevant studies selected for this chapter. The nature of the selected intervention research is reviewed and summarized to provide information on linking the impact of occupational therapy-based cognitive-neurological interventions to client outcomes. The remaining section will address outcome measures sensitive to occupational therapy intervention, which are predominantly used in cognitive-neurological intervention. The chapter concludes with recommendations on how clinical treatment can proceed and/or direct future research.

Conceptual Background

This section defines the areas of cognitive and neuro-sensorimotor occupational therapy intervention that impact on client cognitive-neurological outcomes. These outcome areas will be described in the context of their benefit to client health and how occupational therapists address these outcomes.

M. Law & M. A. McColl (Eds.)
Interventions, Effects, and Outcomes in Occupational Therapy:
Adults and Older Adults (pp. 285-323)
© 2010 SLACK Incorporated

Interventions to Improve Cognitive Outcomes

Cognition is one of the major components that impacts on client occupational performance because most daily occupations require some cognitive and perceptual abilities (Uomoto, 1992). Cognitive processes in cognitive-neurological theory are distinct from theory related to psycho-emotional cognition because it aims to understand the inability to engage in particular cognitive process, whereas cognition in the latter deals with thoughts that are maladaptive (discussed in Chapter 10) (McColl, 2002, p. 14).

Interventions for both cognitive and perceptual deficits impacting on daily occupation are addressed in cognitive outcomes rehabilitation. Cognitive rehabilitation is an area of rehabilitation practice that is not exclusively conducted by occupational therapists, but when occupation-based treatments are often implemented, occupational therapists are primarily involved. Within occupational therapy practice, the components of cognitive deficits are made up of level of arousal, orientation, recognition, attention span, initiation of activity, termination of activity, memory, sequencing, categorization, concept formation, spatial operations, problem solving, learning, and generalization (Lamport, Coffey, & Hersch, 2001). Targeted components that are perceptual in nature can consist of stereognosis, kinesthesia, pain response, body scheme, right-left discrimination, form constancy, position in space, visual-closure, figure-ground, depth perception, spatial relations, and topographical orientation (Lamport et al., 2001).

Interventions to Improve Neuro-Sensorimotor Outcomes

Research evidence has reported that the CNS has a stronger capacity of brain plasticity in adults than the previous theories indicated (Sterr, Szameitat, Shen, & Freivogel, 2006). The sensory systems (i.e., olfactory, gustatory, visual, auditory, somatosensory, proprioceptive, and vestibular) and motor systems (i.e., somatic, cerebellum, basal ganglia network, and thalamic integration) exhibit principles that underlie all neuro-sensorimotor abilities, which influence occupational performance by controlling movement, modulating sensory input, and coordinating and integrating sensory information (Baum & Christiansen, 2005). Occupational therapy interventions can also aim to improve both neuro-motor and sensory components that cause impaired function. These neuro-sensorimotor determinants are distinct from impairments based on physical components based on the understanding that problems are associated with damage to the CNS rather than the peripheral nervous system, addressed in the physical interventions chapter in this book (McColl, 2002).

Clients experiencing cognitive-neurological issues can benefit from occupational therapy intervention based on principles to remediate their ability toward their previous ability and/or provide adaptive strategies to enable new methods to conduct their daily occupations. The evidence for interventions impacting on cognitive-neurological outcomes is gathered based on the search strategy conducted by this scoping review.

Search Strategy

The methodology to search the literature, identify studies, and select them based on specific inclusion criteria was discussed in Chapter 2. A systematic search of health care and occupational therapy databases, as well as hand-searched relevant references, yielded both review and empirical (qualitative and quantitative) papers that addressed the occupational therapy outcomes when providing cognitive-neurological interventions. Selected studies met specific inclusion criteria, which consisted of the study being published between 1980 and 2008, an adult population, an intervention involving occupational therapist independently or on a multidisciplinary team, and categorized as level of evidence 1 to 4 based on criteria by Greenhalgh (2006). For this chapter, the search terms used to capture occupational therapy-sensitive outcomes are listed in Table 11-1. A total of 42 empirical studies met the inclusion criteria and are reviewed in this chapter.

Interventions Used to Improve Cognitive-Neurological Outcomes

As previously described, interventions addressing cognitive-neurological outcomes can be examined as either challenges related to cognitive-perceptual or neuro-sensorimotor deficits. The approaches to these interventions used by occupational therapists have typically been grounded in strategies to remediate the client's ability to its pre-morbid form, to adapt the occupation to enable client participation with their new abilities, or to combine both approaches to facilitate success in their desired occupations (Lee, Powell, & Esdaile, 2001).

Cognitive-Perceptual Outcomes

The nature of occupational therapy interventions in areas addressing cognitive and perceptual

Table 11-1

SEARCH TERMS FOR OCCUPATIONAL THERAPY INTERVENTIONS TO IMPROVE COGNITIVE-NEUROLOGICAL OUTCOMES

Occupation, occupational therapy (therapist), OR multidisciplinary team AND...

Primary terms: attention, brain function, chronic pain, chronic pain control, cognition, cognition disorders, cognitive ability, cognitive defect, cognitive disorders, cognitive processes, cognitive rehabilitation, cognitive re-training, complex regional pain syndrome, decision making, executive function, memory, memory disorders, memory (impairment), memory short term, memory training, mental function, mental processes, metacognition, pain, pain clinics, pain control, pain: disruptive effects, pain (intractable), pain level, pain management, perception, problem solving, reflex sympathetic dystrophy, sequencing.

Secondary terms: acquired brain injury (ABI), brain damage (chronic), brain injury, brain lesions, brain stem injury, cerebral vascular accident (CVA), cerebrovascular accident, cerebrovascular disorders, cognitive therapy, craniocerebral trauma, head injury, motor learning, muscle spasticity, neuro-developmental therapy, sensory motor integration, spasticity, stroke, traumatic brain injury (TBI).

Additional terms used to focus the search included clinical effectiveness, community health services, health care delivery, health care services, health service, health services for the aged, home care, home care services, home health care, home occupational therapy, home rehabilitation, interdisciplinary education, interdisciplinary research, interdisciplinary treatment approach, intervention treatment approach, multidisciplinary care team, outcomes, outcomes assessment patient care, outcomes (health care), outcomes research, patient care team, rehabilitation, rehabilitation care, rehabilitation centre, rehabilitation outcomes, teamwork, treatment effectiveness evaluation, treatment outcomes.

deficits involves each of these approaches. Intervention involving remediation specifically targets restoring the cognitive and perceptual performance components underlying the impairment (Lee et al., 2001; Toglia, 2003). These components are treated by changing body functions to enable improvements in daily occupations (World Health Organization [WHO], 2001). An adaptive approach can involve various ways to minimize the impact of cognitive-perceptual deficits through adapting the task or environment, functional skill training, or using compensatory devices (Lee et al., 2001; Toglia, 2003). These areas of treatment address activity/participation domains of the International Classification of Functioning, Disability, and Health (ICF) intervention framework (WHO, 2001). Combining approaches of remediation and adaptation to improve cognitive and perceptual abilities is also a method enabling the occupational therapist to facilitate activity engagement by targeting changeable areas of function and compensating in areas where skills may be lost or slow to recover.

Neuro-Sensorimotor Outcomes

Neurological impairments can affect various motor and sensory abilities of the client. Motor control and motor learning theories provide occupational therapists with an understanding of the nature, cause, acquisition, and modification of movement supporting optimal occupational performance given the impairment (Giuffrida, 2003). Neuro-motor impairments treated by occupational therapists can initially provide adaptive approaches upon early onset (i.e., compensatory aids), but often aim to initially change body functions (WHO, 2001) that impact on a client's occupations. Sensory-based occupational therapy intervention seems to aid in supporting the person's motor system for more effective performance, which can also improve occupational performance capabilities. Sensory-focused intervention can include adaptive strategies to prepare the client for activity and/or remedial exercises that require client involvement in occupation-based activities (Dolhi, Leibold, & Schreiber, 2003).

This section has discussed the approaches to intervention used in cognitive-neurological interventions, including remediation, adaptation, or both. The evidence for the impact of these interventions on clients for cognitive-neurological outcomes will be described in the following section.

Effects of Occupational Therapy in Promoting Cognitive-Neurological Outcomes

Evidence for Cognitive Outcomes

The empirical evidence of various cognitive and perceptually focused interventions included 15 studies of clients receiving only occupational therapy treatment and seven studies involving occupational therapy in a multidisciplinary setting. Most of the studies (10) involved a comparison of adaptive and remediation approaches to intervention with occupational therapy providing treatment in one or both treatment arms in any given study. The full details of all cognitive-perceptual quantitative empirical evidence are seen in greater detail in Tables 11-2 through 11-4.

Remediation-Based Cognitive Occupational Therapy Interventions

Systematic Reviews

Overall, there were four systematic reviews that looked at cognitive rehabilitation outcomes—one for people with schizophrenia and the other three related to the stroke population.

Within a Cochrane Collaboration Review that analyzed the effects of cognitive rehabilitation for people with schizophrenia, three small studies were analyzed regarding various outcomes (including cognitive functioning) based on cognitive intervention (Hayes & McGrath, 2000). Only one of these studies involved occupational therapy within the intervention (Wykes, Reeder, Corner, Williams, & Everitt, 1999), which was also selected within our search and summarized in the pool of empirical evidence (see Table 11-2).

In the stroke literature, one review synthesizing the effects of occupational therapy was conducted for people who had a stroke. In a critical review by Ma and Trombly in 2002, 29 studies were analyzed regarding the effects of occupational therapy intervention to remediate psychosocial, cognitive-perceptual, and sensorimotor impairments. This systematic review demonstrated that use of activity- or occupation-based treatment leads to significant improvements in client capacities and abilities at the level of body function and structure. The results of the review reported that cognitive abilities and capacities improved using occupation-based tasks and activities and that visual perceptual abilities can improve more during task-specific practice (breaking a complex task into simpler steps).

The remaining two reviews were Cochrane Collaboration Publications evaluating cognitive remediation intervention in the stroke literature, which demonstrated results that were less convincing of its benefit. One review explored studies that involved programs to help retrain memory function or to help patients cope despite impairment post-stroke, and only one study met their stroke-specific inclusion criteria (Majid, Lincoln, & Weyman, 2000). This study by Doornhein and deHaan (1998) measured outcomes of memory impairment, as well as functional disability. It was unclear as to the intervention team or professionals conducting the study's intervention, and the review concluded that the evidence was insufficient to support or refute the effectiveness of cognitive-based rehabilitation for people with memory deficits (Majid et al., 2000). A second Cochrane Review examining 15 multidisciplinary studies for spatial neglect interventions post-stroke also reported inconclusive effects of cognitive rehabilitation at the level of the disability (Bowen, Lincoln, & Dewey, 2002). Overall, the results were inconclusive as to the effect of rehabilitation at the level of disability due to the variability of the impairment level assessments used (Bowen et al., 2002).

Empirical Studies

Occupational therapy interventions that exclusively remediate functional ability for cognitive or perceptual deficits have been documented in the literature, predominantly for a population of people with traumatic brain injuries (TBI) and schizophrenia and stroke survivors. A total of six empirical studies offer insight on remediation intervention for cognitive-perceptual intervention.

One study used a single-case experimental design to examine the incidence of frequently occurring memory lapses for people with a TBI (Campbell, Wilson, McCann, Kernahan, & Rogers, 2007). The intervention involved facilitating caregiver implementation of errorless learning with the participants with TBI, in order to remediate their memory to reduce the occurrence of specific everyday memory problems. Outcomes were statistically significant for this single case, but were only evaluated up to 3 months post-intervention. Longer term follow-up and a larger sample size would be necessary to strengthen this research.

For clients with schizophrenia, the literature has emphasized occupational therapy outcomes relevant to interventions to remediate cognitive components. One randomized controlled trial by Wykes and colleagues (1999) aimed to compare intensive occupational therapy (involving subjects in activities) to a group receiving both intensive occupational therapy

text continues on page 303

Table 11-2

OCCUPATIONAL THERAPY INTERVENTIONS PROMOTING COGNITIVE-PERCEPTUAL OUTCOMES

Author (Date)	Pop	DX	Setting	Intervention
Campbell, L., Wilson, F. C., McCann, J., Kernahan, G., & Rogers, R. G. (2007)	2	7	3	**Intervention:** The patient's caregiver received training in errorless learning from an OT. The OT also worked with patient and caregiver to develop a series of memory prompts to be used during the intervention. The intervention focused on 2 memory problems the patient and caregiver identified: Remembering to use a notebook as a memory aid and walking the dog each day. The intervention was applied over 2 separate periods (one to address each problem) with periods of no intervention in between where baseline data and outcome measures were collected.
Geusgens, C., van Heughten, C., Donkervoort, M., van den Ende, E., Jolles, J., & van den Heuvel, W. (2006)	5	3	4	**Intervention:** 8-week OT treatment implementing strategy training to increase independence by teaching participants strategies that are aimed at compensating for apraxia. **Control:** (Usual OT treatment) includes focus on motor, perceptual, and cognitive subcomponents for maximization of ability to complete ADL.
Ng, S., Lo, A., Lee, G., Lam, M., Yeong, E., Koo, M., et al. (2006)	1, 2	24	3	3-month duration. OT group session similar between facilities. Session themes: Education on memory and aging, memory games, problem solving, adaptive methods and usage of adaptive devices, schedule planning, relaxation, introduction to the community, resources and mutual help, visual and auditory attention training, mnemonics, reminiscence classes and games, outings, arts and crafts, money usage, and stress management.
Boman, I., Lindstedt, M., Hemmingsson, H., & Bartfai, A. (2004)	5	7	4	Individual cognitive training was provided 3 times per week for 3 weeks focusing on attention and memory. **Part 1:** Attention training: Used attention process training techniques. **Part 2:** Strategy generalization to everyday activities: Time teaching participants to use strategies independently and to incorporate them into daily activities. **Part 3:** Education: Compensatory strategies.
Cicerone, K. D., Mott, T., Azulay, J., & Friel, J. C. (2004)	2	7	4	**Intervention:** 16-week intensive cognitive rehabilitation, which consisted of group and individual cognitive therapy, as well as OT and PT as needed. **Control:** Standard neurorehabilitation consisted primarily of PT, OT, speech-language pathology and neuropsychologic therapies.
Gutman, S., Diamond, H., Holness-Parchment, S., Brandofino, D., Pacheco, D., Jolly-Edouard, M., et al. (2004)	5	12, 15, 18	3	Designed to enhance quality of life from revised version of a program by Gutman and Swarbrick (1998). Intervention was designed to address cognitive deficits that may prevent women experiencing domestic abuse from making positive life-altering changes. Activities were graded to skill level and used compensatory strategies. Practiced skills and adaptive devices were used to attain functional independence.
Wykes, T., Reeder, C., Williams, C., Corner, J., Rice, C., & Everitt, B. (2003)	5	14	4	In addition to day care programming, subjects received one of the following treatments for 3 months: **Intervention:** Cognitive remediation therapy group. **Control:** Intensive OT activities.
Hadas-Lidor, N., Katz, N., Tyano, S., & Weizman, A. (2001)	1, 5	14	4	**Intervention:** 2 to 3 weekly sessions (provided by OT) to increase participants' self-awareness of their abilities and to maximize cognitive performance and independence (treated by instrumental enrichment). **Control:** Received traditional OT both individually and in groups.

continued

Table 11-2 (continued)

OCCUPATIONAL THERAPY INTERVENTIONS PROMOTING COGNITIVE-PERCEPTUAL OUTCOMES

Author (Date)	Pop	DX	Setting	Intervention
Edmans, J. A., & Webster, J. (2000)	4	3	4	**Intervention:** 6-week OT intervention comparing the functional and transfer of training approaches. Functional approach—repetitive practice on specific tasks with the ultimate goal of increasing independence; does not expect transference. Transfer of training approach—practice of specific perceptual tasks aimed at remediating the perceptual problem; expectation that this will transfer over to functional tasks.
Dirette, D., & Hinojosa, J. (1999)	5	7	4	**Intervention:** OT sessions with strategy instruction. Strategies: Verbalization, chunking, and pacing. IQ builder program was used during instruction and provides immediate feedback. 6 sessions (once a week). **Control:** Sessions used remedial computer activities. No strategy training was provided.
Jao, H. P., & Lu, S. J. (1999)	2	14	4	**Intervention:** 2 times per week for 3 weeks. Problem-solving therapy. Treatment involves the use of graded activities interacting with the therapist and social situations. Practice on problem-solving exercises emphasized. **Control:** Treatment as usual. Individual therapy, industrial therapy, and group therapy were involved in treatment as usual.
Spaulding, W. D., Reed, D., Sullivan, M., Richardson, C., & Weiler, M. (1999)	5	12, 13, 14, 18	4	Participants were randomly assigned to 1 group with 6 months of intensive treatment followed by 1 year of continued psychiatric rehabilitation. Before, during, and after intensive treatment period, participants from both groups received standard psychiatric rehabilitation, including OT. **Intervention:** Integrated psychology therapy. **Control:** Supportive group therapy.
Wykes, T., Reeder, C., Corner, J., Williams, C., & Everitt, B. (1999)	5	14	4	**Group 1:** Daily sessions for 40 days. Intensive OT focused on activities: Relaxation, assertiveness training, life diary, comprehension of social information, and role playing. **Group 2:** Neuro-cognitive remediation program (did not specify type of therapist). Treatment consisted of numerous different tasks that were designed to address problem solving and complex planning.
Chen, S. H. A., Thomas, J. D., Glueckauf, R. L., & Bracy, O. L. (1997)	5	7	4	**Intervention:** Computer-assisted cognitive rehabilitation. **Control:** Receiving other treatments such as speech-language pathology and OT.
Cartwright, D. L., Madill, H. M., & Dennis, S. (1996)	1	8	4	General hospital inpatient OT and PT intervention.
Velligan, D., Mahurin, R., True, J., Lefton, R., & Flores, C. (1996)	5	14	4	Duration of treatment: 9 weeks. Standard psychosocial therapy group (included group psychotherapy, medication education, OT, socialization, and off-unit classes/work program). Cognitive adaptation training group (completed by trained nursing staff).
Bach, D., Bach, M., Bohmer, F., Fruhwald, T., & Grilc, B. (1995)	1	8	4	**Intervention:** 24-week duration. This group received functional rehabilitation plus reactivating OT. Reactivating OT (twice a week) within groups of 5 to 6, focusing on memory training, manual/creative activities for sensorimotor system, and self-management. **Control:** Received functional OT, PT, and speech-language pathology.
Brown, C., Harwood, K., Hays, C., Heckman, J., & Short, E. (1993)	5	14	5	**Intervention:** One-on-one OT cognitive rehabilitation program targeting basic deficits: Attention process training addresses different types of attention. 3 times per week over 12 weeks. **Control:** Traditional one-on-one OT cognitive skills training through task completion.

continued

Table 11-2 (continued)

Occupational Therapy Interventions Promoting Cognitive-Perceptual Outcomes

Author (Date)	Pop	DX	Setting	Intervention
Soderback, I. (1988)	5	7	4	14 weeks of treatment conducted by 4 different OTs for 4 different groups of participants were randomized to be: Intellectual function training program group plus regular rehabilitation. Intellectual housework training program plus regular rehabilitation. Intellectual function training plus intellectual housework training plus regular rehabilitation. Regular rehabilitation only.
Lincoln, N. B., Whiting, S. E., Cockburn, J., & Bhavnani, G. (1985)	5	3, 7	4	*Intervention:* Perceptual training group received practice in performing perceptual activities of the kind commonly seen in inpatient OT for 4 weeks. *Control:* Conventional OT. This group spent the same amount of time in activities that were not specifically designed to improve perceptual skills.
Carter, L., Howard, B., & O'Neil, W. (1983)	4	3	4	*Intervention:* 3- to 4-week duration, fluctuated based on time involved in stroke program. Standard practice plus cognitive skill remediation training. Tasks were drawn from the "Thinking Skills Workbook." *Control:* Standard practice (OT, speech-language pathology, social worker, rehabilitation nursing staff).

Population: 1=geriatric (65+); 2=adult (25 to 64); 3=young adult (18 to 24); 4=adult and geriatric; 5=young adult, adult, and geriatric.

Diagnosis: 3=stroke; 7=acquired brain injury; 8=dementia or Alzheimer's disease; 12=depression; 13=bipolar; 14=schizophrenia; 15=addiction/substance abuse; 18=other; 24=frail elderly.

Setting: 1=long-term care; 2=acute care; 3=home care; 4=rehabilitation; 5=primary care.

Table 11-3

EVIDENCE OF EFFECTIVENESS OF OCCUPATIONAL THERAPY ON COGNITIVE-PERCEPTUAL OUTCOMES

Author (Date)	Major Results	Study Design	Sample Size	Conclusions and Limitations
Positive Effects—Randomized Controlled Trial				
Wykes, T., Reeder, C., Williams, C., Corner, J., Rice, C., & Everitt, B. (2003)	Effects of cognitive remediation therapy (CRT) on cognition were still apparent at follow-up in memory domain higher than OT group but not statistically significant. Other areas noted improvements in both groups. CRT group had somewhat lower scores in regard to symptoms, but this was also not significant. No direct effect of therapy on social functioning, no effect of time of assessment, and no interaction.	RCT	28	*Conclusions:* Evidence supported the presence of CRT effects on memory at follow-up as well as improvements in social behavior and symptoms but did not display statistically significant differences from the improvements in OT group. *Limitations:* No report of evaluators or participants blinded to treatment, control group not described, small sample size, reason for dropouts not reported.
Hadas-Lidor, N., Katz, N., Tyano, S., & Weizman, A. (2001)	Significant differences between pre-test and post-test (p<0.001) were found for both memory and thought processes. All individual cognitive measures showed significant improvements, with the exception of the arithmetic exercises. Complex figure drawing test, proofreading, and arithmetic problems had p<0.05. Word memory and shape perception, p<0.01. Raven Work status changes were significant at follow-up, p<0.001.	RCT	58	*Conclusions:* The study addressed the impact of a specific program of cognitive rehabilitation on functional outcomes of individuals with schizophrenia and showed a positive influence on cognitive domains, living arrangements, and employment status. *Limitations:* No reports of evaluators or participants blinded to treatment, outcomes measures lack psychometric properties, no record of preventing contamination or co-intervention.
Dirette, D., & Hinojosa, J. (1999)	Control and experimental groups both improved significantly on weekly tests and pre-/post-evaluation p<0.001. There was no differential effect of treatment group on improvement in scores. 80% of all participants were found to have used compensatory strategies during tasks. Compensatory strategies had a significant positive impact on speed and had less erratic gain on accuracy measures.	RCT	30	*Conclusions:* The study examined literature on the efficacy of compensatory and remedial strategies for cognitive rehabilitation and found that the use of compensatory strategies does improve performance on cognitive tasks. *Limitations:* Possible volunteer bias from sample selection, some outcome measures lacked psychometric properties, dropouts not reported, no record of preventing contamination or co-intervention.

continued

Table 11-3 (continued)
EVIDENCE OF EFFECTIVENESS OF OCCUPATIONAL THERAPY ON COGNITIVE-PERCEPTUAL OUTCOMES

Author (Date)	Major Results	Study Design	Sample Size	Conclusions and Limitations
Positive Effects—Randomized Controlled Trial				
Spaulding, W. D., Reed, D., Sullivan, M., Richardson, C., & Weiler, M. (1999)	Integrated psychology therapy subjects showed greater gains compared to control group in terms of social competence, suggesting that procedures targeting cognitive impairments of schizophrenia can (in short term) enhance patients' response to standard psychiatric rehabilitation. There was also evidence for greater improvement in the integrated psychology therapy group on the BPRS (disorganization factor) and attentional processing. There was significant improvement in both conditions on measures of attention, memory, and executive functioning,	RCT	91	**Conclusions:** Therapy procedures that target impaired cognition may lead to improvement in social competence for severely disabled psychiatric patients. **Limitations:** Non-experimental design, the diagnostic heterogeneity of the subject sample requires careful interpretation of the general conclusions.
Wykes, T., Reeder, C., Corner, J., Williams, C., & Everitt, B. (1999)	Improvements in both treatment groups: In measures of cognitive flexibility and visual span task, memory, and planning tasks. There was some improvement in symptoms. In favor of Group 2 (neuro-cognitive remediation): Self-esteem showed significant improvements; overall, more people in neuro-cognitive remediation group reached "improved status" (cognitive flexibility and memory p<0.02). Functioning: Individuals who improved on measures of cognition also improved social functioning.	RCT	29	**Conclusions:** The study found that the neuro-cognitive remediation group showed more cognitive improvements compared to the intensive OT treatment group. **Limitations:** Reasons for dropouts not reported, no record of preventing contamination or co-intervention, possible volunteer bias, intervention not described, psychometric properties not documented for outcome measures.
Bach, D., Bach, M., Bohmer, F., Fruhwald, T., & Grilc, B. (1995)	At 12 weeks: Control and experimental within groups, statistically significant improvements in global and depressive symptoms. At 24 weeks: Control and experimental within groups, significant improvement in cognition related variables, visuomotor coordination, and symptoms of depression. At 12 weeks: Experimental group had significantly better symptom and cognition scores than control group. At 24 weeks: Experimental group had significantly better performance than control group on cognition, psychosocial functioning, well-being, and symptoms of depression.	RCT	44	**Conclusions:** Functional rehabilitation alone was found to be inferior to functional rehabilitation and reactivating OT on measures of cognition, psychosocial function, and contentedness. **Limitations:** Reasons for dropouts not reported, outcomes measures lack psychometric properties, small sample size, different therapists provided treatment.

continued

Table 11-3 (continued)

EVIDENCE OF EFFECTIVENESS OF OCCUPATIONAL THERAPY ON COGNITIVE-PERCEPTUAL OUTCOMES

Author (Date)	Major Results	Study Design	Sample Size	Conclusions and Limitations
Positive Effects—Randomized Controlled Trial				
Soderback, I. (1988)	Comparison between intellectual function training, intellectual housework training, and both groups with the regular rehabilitation group indicated areas of function (verbal [p<0.05], memory [p<0.05], and logical function [p<0.01]) where intellectual training was significantly more effective than regular rehabilitation of OT. The development of intellectual functions within each group was evident in most areas except for regular rehabilitation group.	RCT	67	***Conclusions:*** The study results demonstrated that the combination of any of the 4 training approaches are usable in OT rehabilitation for training in verbal, numerical, praxis, memory, and logical functions. ***Limitations:*** Small sample size, no record of preventing contamination or co-intervention, possible source bias for sample.
Carter, L., Howard, B., & O'Neil, W. (1983)	Experimental group showed significantly better performance on outcome measures than control group for all variables Scanning: p<0.005 Visual-spatial: p<0.005 Time judgment: p<0.05 Authors state the results support the incorporation of cognitive remediation training in acute phases of rehabilitation.	RCT	33	***Conclusions:*** The studies reviewed the prevalence of stroke and the importance of the targeted elements of cognition on functional tasks. The study found that cognitive remediation effectively increased cognitive ability compared to controls. ***Limitations:*** Potential for practice effects, outcomes do not measure change in functional ability, reasons for dropouts not reported, some outcome measures lacked psychometric properties.
Positive Effects—Non-Randomized Controlled Trial				
Campbell, L., Wilson, F. C., McCann, J., Kernahan, G., & Rogers, R. G. (2007)	At baseline, the notebook was not used. During intervention, mean daily notebook use was 8.1, and patient used notebook independently an average of 1.7 times per day. Post-intervention, the patient used the notebook unprompted an average of 8 times per day, and daily use increased over follow-up period to an average of 22 times per day. Increased usage was statistically significant. Prompts required to complete the tasks steadily decreased during intervention and follow-up. Levels of anxiety, caregiver strain, and memory impairment in both caregiver and patient were unchanged throughout the study.	Non-RCT	1	***Conclusions:*** Study shows the successful implementation of an errorless learning program delivered by a carer to manage everyday memory problems in a patient with severe memory post-brain injury. Maintenance of effects observed at 3-month follow-up beyond the cessation of the program. ***Limitations:*** Difficult to generalize results to practice because the technique required significant caregiver involvement.

continued

Table 11-3 (continued)

EVIDENCE OF EFFECTIVENESS OF OCCUPATIONAL THERAPY ON COGNITIVE-PERCEPTUAL OUTCOMES

Author (Date)	Major Results	Study Design	Sample Size	Conclusions and Limitations
Positive Effects—Non-Randomized Controlled Trial				
Ng, S., Lo, A., Lee, G., Lam, M., Yeong, E., Koo, M., et al. (2006)	Overall, participants improved in basic mental functions C-DRS (p=0.001), CMMSE (p=0.039), and mood GDS (p=0.007). Caregiver stress level was also shown to decrease, but was not statistically significant.	Non-RCT	45	***Conclusions:*** Results indicated that the community OT cognitive training programs were similar in nature and that participants showed improvements in cognitive abilities and mood that were sustained until 3-month follow-up. A positive effect was also seen on levels of caregiver stress. ***Limitations:*** Outcome measures lack psychometric properties, intervention not described, no reports of evaluators or participants blinded to treatment, reasons for dropouts not reported, small sample size, potential for practice effects.
Boman, I., Lindstedt, M., Hemmingsson, H., & Bartfai, A. (2004)	Impairment: Complex tasks showed significant improvements from pre-test to follow-up: Complex sustained attention p<0.05, selective attention p<0.05, and alternating attention p<0.01. No significant improvements were found on the more simple tasks. Memory: Participants showed no change in memory following training, but a significant effect was found at follow-up p<0.05. Activity: No significant improvements noted. Participation: No significant improvements were found on subtests.	Non-RCT	10	***Conclusions:*** Home intervention had a positive influence on some indices of impairment; these improvements did not extend to activity or participation levels. ***Limitations:*** Outcome measures may not have related to treatment goals, no reports of evaluators or participants blinded to treatment, small sample size, reasons for dropouts not reported.
Cicerone, K. D., Mott, T., Azulay, J., & Friel, J. C. (2004)	Both groups showed improvements on community integration scores, with intensive cognitive rehabilitation group exhibiting a significant treatment effect compared with standard neurorehabilitation group. Intensive cognitive rehabilitation participants also showed significant improvement in overall neuropsychologic functioning.	Non-RCT	56	***Conclusions:*** Individuals receiving intensive cognitive rehabilitation were more likely to be reintegrated into their communities than those receiving standard rehabilitation, demonstrating the effectiveness of this type of treatment. ***Limitations:*** Comparison groups were not equal and were not randomized, limited validity testing done for some outcome measures.

continued

Table 11-3 (continued)

EVIDENCE OF EFFECTIVENESS OF OCCUPATIONAL THERAPY ON COGNITIVE-PERCEPTUAL OUTCOMES

Author (Date)	Major Results	Study Design	Sample Size	Conclusions and Limitations
Positive Effects—Non-Randomized Controlled Trial				
Gutman, S., Diamond, H., Holness-Parchment, S., Brandofino, D., Pacheco, D., Jolly-Edouard, M., et al. (2004)	Overall performance: 21 of 26 (81%) of participants attained T-scores above 50 (goal area). Therefore, they achieved their most favorable outcomes. None of the participants received a score below 50. All participants achieved their goals at expected outcomes or greater. As a result, all women made gains toward personally directed goals.	Non-RCT	26	**Conclusions:** This study assesses the effectiveness of intervention for women who have experienced domestic violence and/or homelessness in regard to their attainment of their functional goals set in the program. All women who participated made gains toward personally desired goals and achieved or exceeded their expected outcomes. **Limitations:** Convenience sample, no random selection, small sample, no control group, short-term study without follow-up, limited disclosure of full client information.
Jao, H. P., & Lu, S. J. (1999)	Treatment group: Significant positive change in interpersonal problem-solving skills (p<0.05). Significant negative change in self-esteem (p<0.05). Comparison group: No significant changes on either measure between pre- and post-testing.	Non-RCT	18	**Conclusions:** The effectiveness of Siegel and Spivack's Problem-Solving Therapy for the Chronic Schizophrenic was analyzed in this study. The intervention was shown to be effective in increasing interpersonal problem solving, but it did not have a corresponding effect on self-esteem. **Limitations:** Psychometric properties of MEPS was valid for a language other than English, no record of preventing contamination or co-intervention, no reports of evaluators or participants blinded to treatment, small sample size.
Cartwright, D. L., Madill, H. M., & Dennis, S. (1996)	The sample was divided into severe and moderate impairment, based on admission MMSE. Overall, the total sample improved significantly in functional ability from admission to discharge (p<0.001). Results for each of the subscales of the motor and cognitive domains were significant (i.e., self-care p<0.001, social cognition p=0.015, communication p=0.013). There were no significant differences in the improvements between severity groups.	Non-RCT	65	**Conclusions:** Overall, patients demonstrated significant improvement in functional abilities across the intervention period, regardless of whether they were classified as moderately or severely cognitively impaired. **Limitations:** Lack of a control group.

continued

Table 11-3 (continued)

EVIDENCE OF EFFECTIVENESS OF OCCUPATIONAL THERAPY ON COGNITIVE-PERCEPTUAL OUTCOMES

Author (Date)	Major Results	Study Design	Sample Size	Conclusions and Limitations
Positive Effects—Non-Randomized Controlled Trial				
Velligan, D., Mahurin, R., True, J., Lefton, R., & Flores, C. (1996)	Adaptive function: Entire sample improved in adaptive function (p<0.001). Significant treatment by time interaction: p<0.01. Individuals in the cognitive adaptation group had a more substantial improvement compared to individuals in the standard treatment group. Positive and negative symptoms improved in both groups p<0.001. Individuals who were in the cognitive adaptation group increased their ability to initiate self-care tasks independently. Individuals whose performance on tasks pre-treatment showed impairment improved to non-impairment level post-treatment.	Non-RCT	40	**Conclusions:** The study found that, when compared to standard psychosocial treatment, the cognitive adaptation program had additional benefits on adaptive function that were both statistically and clinically meaningful. No differential benefits were found on positive or negative symptoms. **Limitations:** Some outcome measures lacked psychometric properties, potential for practice effects, evaluators were not blind to treatment, groups did not receive treatment concurrently.
No Effect				
Geusgens, C., van Heughten, C., Donkervoort, M., van den Ende, E., Jolles, J., & van den Heuvel, W. (2006)	No between-group differences found for amount of time in therapy or for ADL observation scores on trained and untrained tasks. Transfer of training: Both groups showed lower scores on non-trained tasks (post-training plus follow-up). Strategy group showed greater change scores post-training on non-trained tasks than the control group (p=0.040). Scores on trained tasks improved over time in both groups p=0.004 and for the strategy group at p=0.025. Change in ADL scores for control group did not change over time.	RCT	113	**Conclusions:** Evidence supported the presence of transfer of training; however, the effect was present in both groups, with the cognitive strategy training group achieving a higher level of transfer than the controls. **Limitations:** Some outcome measures lacked psychometric properties, possible source bias for sample, single-blinded study, intervention not described in order to be reproduced, no record of preventing contamination or co-intervention.
Edmans, J. A., & Webster, J. (2000)	No significant differences were found for any outcomes measured between the two treatment groups. Transfer of training group: p<0.05 on all but 5 perceptual tests. Functional group: p<0.05 on all but 7 perceptual tests. All participants showed significant improvements (p<0.001) on ADL function, on gross function, and perceptual abilities from pre- to post-testing. No improvements in 13 of transfer of training group and 15 functional group participants (non-significant).	RCT	79	**Conclusions:** No differences were found between the functional or transfer of training approach on perceptual abilities and function for post-stroke patients. **Limitations:** No record of preventing contamination or co-intervention, small sample size, outcome measures likely not sensitive enough.

continued

Table 11-3 (continued)

EVIDENCE OF EFFECTIVENESS OF OCCUPATIONAL THERAPY ON COGNITIVE-PERCEPTUAL OUTCOMES

Author (Date)	Major Results	Study Design	Sample Size	Conclusions and Limitations
No Effect				
Chen, S. H. A., Thomas, J. D., Glueckauf, R. L., & Bracy, O. L. (1997)	No significant differences found between groups. Experimental group made significant gains in 15 areas including memory, visual reproduction, verbal IQ, full-scale IQ, performance IQ, information, digit span, vocabulary, picture completion, object assembly, and digit symbol. The comparison group made gains in performance IQ, full-scale IQ, picture arrangement, block design, object assembly, and digit symbol.	Non-RCT	40	***Conclusions:*** The study described a comparison of computer-assisted cognitive rehabilitation to a group that received various other therapies including OT and speech/language/ pathology. No significant differences between groups. ***Limitations:*** Procedure not provided in terms of assessment delivery, no control group.
Brown, C., Harwood, K., Hays, C., Heckman, J., & Short, E. (1993)	No significant differences on test scores were found between the 2 treatment conditions. 10 of 11 parts of sorting task improved in both groups p<0.05; cognitively complex tasks showed no significant improvements. Self-confidence, motivation, and efficiency showed significant improvement in 4/5 tasks for attention process training. All measures of memory span improved following treatment in control/experimental group.	RCT	29	***Conclusions:*** Both the cognitive rehabilitation program interventions had equal effects on cognition and affective determinants of performance. ***Limitations:*** Potential for practice effects, no record of preventing contamination or co-intervention, reasons for dropouts not reported, small sample size.
Lincoln, N. B., Whiting, S. E., Cockburn, J., & Bhavnani, G. (1985)	There were no significant between-group differences on the RADL or RPAB tests, at baseline or post-intervention. Both groups improved from pre- to post-intervention assessment periods. On two of the tests (sequencing pictures and cancellation), the perceptual practice group demonstrated significant improvement across time (p<0.001), while the typical treatment group showed a non-significant decline. Both groups showed significant improvement in self-care tasks across time (p<0.001).	RCT	33	***Conclusions:*** Results indicated that there were no significant between-group differences on performance of perceptual tasks or ADL function before or after intervention between perceptual training vs. conventional OT treatment. ***Limitations:*** Small sample size, short intervention period.

BPRS=Brief Psychiatric Rating Scale, C-DRS=Chinese Dementia Rating Scale, CMMSE=Chinese Mini Mental Status Examination, GDS=Geriatric Depression Scale, MEPS=Means-Ends Problem-Solving Procedure, MMSE=Mini Mental Status Examination, RADL=Rivermead Activities of Daily Living Scale, RPAB=Rivermead Perceptual Assessment Battery.

Table 11-4

OUTCOME MEASURES USED TO CAPTURE COGNITIVE-PERCEPTUAL OUTCOMES

Author (Date)	Outcome(s) Investigated	Outcome Measure(s)	Method of Administration
Campbell, L., Wilson, F. C., McCann, J., Kernahan, G., & Rogers, R. G. (2007)	Level of notebook usage Level of prompting required Caregiver strain Depression and anxiety levels Perception of executive functioning Memory impairment	Daily checklist and review of notebook entries CSI HADS BADS RBMT	The patient's caregiver completed a daily checklist recording notebook use and prompting required and mailed it to the researchers. Notebook review was completed by the therapy team when meeting with patient and caregivers every 2 to 3 weeks. All assessments were completed at baseline, once the interventions were completed, and at 3-month follow-up.
Geusgens, C., van Heughten, C., Donkervoort, M., van den Ende, E., Jolles, J., & van den Heuvel, W. (2006)	ADL functioning Level of apraxia Motor functioning Understanding of Dutch language/verbal comprehension	ADL observations Apraxia test Functional motor test SAN	Measures were administered by an independent, blind assessor at baseline, post-intervention, and at 5-month follow-up.
Ng, S., Lo, A., Lee, G., Lam, M., Yeong, E., Koo, M., et al. (2006)	Basic mental functions Functional ability Mood Levels of caregiver stress	C-DRS CMMSE L-IADL BI GDS C-ZCSI	Measures were completed by an OT at pre-training, post-training, and 3-month follow-up.
Boman, I., Lindstedt, M., Hemmingsson, H., & Bartfai, A. (2004)	Impairment Activity Participation levels	WAIS-R CD RBMT AMPS Two IADL tasks EBIQ VAS	Outcome measures were administered (by therapist or self-report) pre-training, post-training, and at 3-month follow-up.
Cicerone, K. D., Mott, T., Azulay, J., & Friel, J. C. (2004)	Improvement in community integration Quality of life Neuropsychologic functioning	CIQ QCIQ Composite index derived from Trail Making Test A and B CVLT RCFT COWA Category Test	CIQ administered and scored before and after treatment; QCIQ administered by researchers at completion of treatment; neuropsychological battery administered by researchers at baseline and completion of treatment.
Gutman, S., Diamond, H., Holness-Parchment, S., Brandofino, D., Pacheco, D., Jolly-Edouard, M., et al. (2004)	Client-centered goal setting Knowledge base Life skills	GAS Pre- and post-tests were developed for each section Chart review	Pre- and post-treatment assessed by therapist and completed self-reported questionnaire.

continued

Table 11-4 (continued)

Outcome Measures Used to Capture Cognitive-Perceptual Outcomes

Author (Date)	Outcome(s) Investigated	Outcome Measure(s)	Method of Administration
Wykes, T., Reeder, C., Williams, C., Corner, J., Rice, C., & Everitt, B. (2003)	Cognition Symptoms Social functioning Self-esteem	WCST WAIS-R TLT HSCT HRB COWA SNST VST SST DST SET SBS PSE BPRS RSES	Assessed at baseline, post-treatment, and 6-month follow-up.
Hadas-Lidor, N., Katz, N., Tyano, S., & Weizman, A. (2001)	Memory and thought processes Self-concept Functional outcomes	LPAD RPM GATB FSCS IADL-Q WRSS	Tests were completed by the sameraters at all time points. Evaluations were completed pre-intervention and post-intervention. 6-month follow-up consisted of an interview that aimed to determine work and residence status.
Edmans, J. A., & Webster, J. (2000)	Perceptual ability Functional ability	RPAB BI EAI RMA	All outcome measures were administered pre/post (6 weeks). Ward PT completed RMA (pre and post); assessor blind to treatment group completed the post assessment for the RPAB, BI, and EAI; initial assessments were completed by the ward OT.
Dirette, D., & Hinojosa, J. (1999)	Visual processing	Pre-test/post-test Data entry tasks Computerized reading program Paced Auditory Serial Addition Task Matching Accuracy Test	Pre-test and post-test data collected by speech-language pathologist who was blind to group assignment. Pre-tests/post-tests measured at weeks 1 and 6. Weekly measurements completed at weeks 1 to 6.
Jao, H. P., & Lu, S. J. (1999)	Interpersonal problem solving skills Self-esteem	MEPS CFSEI-2	Tests were administered pre-intervention and post-intervention to both groups.

continued

Table 11-4 (continued)

OUTCOME MEASURES USED TO CAPTURE COGNITIVE-PERCEPTUAL OUTCOMES

Author (Date)	Outcome(s) Investigated	Outcome Measure(s)	Method of Administration
Spaulding, W. D., Reed, D., Sullivan, M., Richardson, C., & Weiler, M. (1999)	Assess social competence Cognitive competence Characterize participant sample	AIPSS, along with 4 additional role-playing skill assessments A battery of cognitive and neuro-psychological measures such as COGLAB cognitive assessment battery, trail-making test, tactile performance test, categories test, Rey auditory and visual learning tasks, Denman neuro-psychological memory test BPRS PNS Thought, Language, and Communication Scale	Measures were administered pre- and post-treatment. AIPSS and additional skill assessments were administered by trained clinical psychology graduate research assistants. The interview measures BPRS, PNS, and the Thought, Language, and Communication Scale were administered by 2 psychiatrists.
Wykes, T., Reeder, C., Corner, J., Williams, C., & Everitt, B. (1999)	Cognitive flexibility Planning Memory and working memory Symptoms and social functioning	HSCT HRB Response inhibition test COWFT SNST WCST SET TLT VST SST WAIS-R DST SBS PSE BPRS RSES	Outcomes measures were completed pre-treatment, post-treatment, and at 6-month follow-up; 6-month follow-up data are not reported in the study. Assessments of symptoms were completed by one person who was not aware of participant's allocation to groups.
Chen, S. H. A., Thomas, J. D., Glueckauf, R. L., & Bracy, O. L. (1997)	Cognitive function (such as, attention, visual spatial ability, memory, and problem solving)	WAIS-R WMS (in part) Other neurological subtests	N/A.
Cartwright, D. L., Madill, H. M., & Dennis, S. (1996)	Functional abilities Discharge location	FIM MMSE WoMS	Evaluations were performed by OT at admission and discharge. Baseline evaluations were conducted within 48 hours of admission and included the MMSE and FIM (FIM was re-administered the week prior to discharge).
Velligan, D., Mahurin, R., True, J., Lefton, R., & Flores, C. (1996)	Cognitive level Adaptive function Severity of positive symptoms Severity of negative symptoms	ACL FNA BPRS Negative symptom assessment	Measures were taken at baseline and post-treatment.
Bach, D., Bach, M., Bohmer, F., Fruhwald, T., & Grilc, B. (1995)	Cognitive performance Psychosocial functioning Degree of contentedness Subjective well-being Depression	SCAG HAMD DSI B-S BT GVG NAPI	All testing done at baseline, 12 weeks, and 24 weeks. Assessments either observer-rated clinical interview or self-reported.

continued

Table 11-4 (continued)

OUTCOME MEASURES USED TO CAPTURE COGNITIVE-PERCEPTUAL OUTCOMES

Author (Date)	Outcome(s) Investigated	Outcome Measure(s)	Method of Administration
Brown, C., Harwood, K., Hays, C., Heckman, J., & Short, E. (1993)	Attention (and memory) Functional performance	WAIS Halstead Reitan Neurological Test Battery: Trail Making Subtests A and B BaFPE	Outcomes were measured at baseline and at the end of treatment (12 weeks). Tests for attention were administered by psychology interns with supervision. Functional performance was measured by OTs blind to subject assignment.
Soderback, I. (1988)	Functional areas: Visuo-spatial Verbal Numerical Memory Logical attention Spatial and praxis functions	IFA IHA 15 other psychometric tests	Pre-test, post-test (14 weeks post-intervention), and follow-up (mean of 168 days after post-test measurement).
Lincoln, N. B., Whiting, S. E., Cockburn, J., & Bhavnani, G. (1985)	Visual perception ADL function	RPAB RADL	Prior to randomization, patients were assessed using the RPAB. Those with perceptual deficits were also assessed using the RADL. These assessments were conducted by an OT. Following the intervention, patients were reassessed by the same assessor, who was blinded to group belonging.
Carter, L., Howard, B., & O'Neil, W. (1983)	Scanning Visuo-spatial abilities Time Judgment	Letter cancellation task Visuo-spatial matching task Time judgment task Difference between subject's perception of 1 minute and actual time	Outcome measures were administered at baseline and at the end of treatment by the same tester. Outcome measures were only taken for individuals who scored <80% at baseline to avoid potential ceiling effect.

ACL=Allen Cognitive Level Test, AIPSS=Assessment of Interpersonal Problem-Solving Skills, AMPS=Assessment of Motor and Process Skills, BADS=Behavioural Assessment of Dysexecutive Syndrome (Dysexecutive Questionnaire), BaFPE=Bay Area Functional Performance Evaluation, BI=Barthel Index, BPRS=Brief Psychiatric Rating Scale, B-S=Scale of Well-Being, BT=Benton Test, CD=Claeson-Dahl Test, C-DRS=Chinese Dementia Rating Scale, CFSEI-2=Culture-Free Self-Esteem Inventories—Second Edition, CIQ=Community Integration Questionnaire, CMMSE=Chinese Mini Mental Status Examination, COGLAB=A cognitive assessment battery for various neurocognitive functions, COWA=Controlled Oral Word Association Test, COWFT=Controlled Oral Word Fluency Task, CSI=Caregiver Strain Index, CVLT=California Verbal Learning Test, C-ZCSI=Chinese Zarit Carer Stress Index, DSI=Depressive Scale Inventory, DST=Dual Span Test, EAI=Edmans ADL Index, EBIQ=European Brain Injury Questionnaire, FIM=Functional Independence Measure, FNA=Functional Needs Assessment, FSCS=Fitts Self-Concept Scale, GAS=Goal Attainment Scaling, GATB=General Aptitude Test Battery, GDS=Geriatric Depression Scale, GVG=Grunberger Verbal Memory Test, HADS=Hospital Anxiety and Depression Scale, HAMD=Hamilton Depression Rating Scale, HRB=Halstead Reitan Battery, HSCT=Hayling Sentence Completion Task, IADL-Q=Instrumental Activities of Daily Living Questionnaire, IFA=Intellectual Function Assessment, IHA=Intellectual Housework Assessment, L-IADL=Lawton Instrumental Activities of Daily Living Scale, LPAD=Learning Potential Assessment Device, MEPS=Means-Ends Problem-Solving Procedure, MMSE=Mini Mental Status Examination, NAPI=Nuremberg Aged Persons Inventory, PNS=Positive and Negative Syndrome Scale, PSE=Present State Examination, QCIQ=Quality of Community Integration Questionnaire, RADL=Rivermead Activities of Daily Living Scale, RBMT=Rivermead Behavioural Memory Test, RCFT=Rey Complex Figure Test, RMA=Rivermead Motor Assessment, RPAB=Rivermead Perceptual Assessment Battery, RPM=Raven Progressive Matrices, RSES=Rosenberg Self-Esteem Schedule, SAN=Standardized test assessing verbal comprehension used to monitor patient understanding of the Dutch language, SBS=Social Behaviour Schedule, SCAG=Clinical Assessment Geriatric Scale, SET=Six Elements Test, SNST=Stroop Neuropsychological Screening Test, SST=Sentence Span Test, TLT=Tower of London Test, VAS=Visual Analog Scale, VST=Visual Span Test, WAIS=Wechsler Adult Intelligence Scale, WAIS-R=Wechsler Adult Intelligence Scale-Revised, WCST=Wisconsin Card Sorting Test, WMS=Wechsler Memory Scale, WoMS=Workload Measurement System, WRSS=Work and Residence Status Scales.

and cognitive remediation. This study measured the impact of cognitive remediation while controlling for the therapist effect. The results indicated improvements in both groups and no short-term differences between interventions measuring outcomes of cognitive flexibility, planning, memory, symptoms, and social functioning. In a 6-month follow-up study, Wykes and colleagues (2003) compared the durability of the effects of cognitive remediation treatment to intensive occupational therapy activities. Once again, the researchers measured similar outcomes. Results showed that the cognitive remediation treatment group had increased memory and decreased symptoms in comparison to the control group, but the difference was not statistically significant (Wykes et al., 2003). A third study involving remediation as a treatment for people with schizophrenia was presented by Spaulding and colleagues (1999). This study evaluated the impact of a cognitive therapy group, integrated psychology therapy (IPT), in comparison to a control group providing supported group therapy. To determine if IPT enhanced cognitive abilities, both groups received standard intensive multidisciplinary psychiatric intervention, including occupational therapy (Spaulding et al., 1999). Short-term results showed both groups improving significantly on measures of attention, memory, and executive functioning, and IPT with greater gains in social competence, attentional processing, and decreased disorganization (Spaulding et al., 1999). These results show the benefits of cognitive remediation and standard intervention (including occupational therapy), which had a significant impact on cognitive outcomes.

In another standard multidisciplinary practice, occupational therapy was involved within both treatment arms of two studies evaluating cognitive skill remediation for a population of subjects post-stroke (Bach, Bach, Bohmer, Fruhwald, & Grilc, 1995; Carter, Howard, & O'Neil, 1983). The combination of standard practice with cognitive skill remediation therapy in comparison to standard practice only demonstrated statistically significant differences in scanning, visuospatial abilities, time, and judgment (Carter et al., 1983). In the study by Bach and colleagues (1995), although both treatment arms had significant within-group improvements in cognition-related outcomes post-intervention, the experimental group receiving both standard care and remediation had significantly better cognitive performance than the control group. Both studies support the incorporation of cognitive remediation training in acute phases of stroke rehabilitation.

Adaptive Approaches to Occupational Therapy Interventions

Systematic Reviews

Three reviews (two systematic reviews) examine specific adaptive approaches used by occupational therapy within intervention.

One review by Gagnon (1996) evaluated common treatment approaches for individuals with Alzheimer's disease, including adaptive approaches such as reality orientation therapy (RO). The conclusion from the review supports the uncertainty of the value of adaptive approaches, which included RO, and concluded that RO was unable to provide adequate observable changes for clients to support its implementation. A more recent Cochrane Review examining six randomized controlled trials evaluating RO in clients with dementia indicated significant cognitive and behavioral outcomes in favor of treatment (Spector, Orrell, Davies, & Woods, 2000).

In another Cochrane Review examining reminiscence therapy for people with dementia, occupational therapy was one of the multidisciplinary facilitators of this method (Woods, Spector, Jones, Orrell, & Davies, 2005). These results indicated that outcomes related to cognition, mood, and functional ability improved 4 to 6 weeks post-treatment, and caregivers participating reported lower strain. Each of these treatment approaches, RO and reminiscence therapy, which involve functional skill development, seem to have some benefits for cognitively impaired older adults.

Empirical Studies

In this review, several studies demonstrated evidence of occupational therapy involved in rehabilitation exclusively as adaptive strategies to address cognitive outcomes. Five empirical studies were relevant to occupational therapy practice involving adaptive approaches to improving cognitive-perceptual outcomes.

Two studies demonstrated occupational therapy involvement (independently and on a multidisciplinary team) in adaptive interventions that targeted functional skill development (Cartwright, Madill, & Dennis, 1996; Wallis, Baldwin, & Higginbotham, 1983). The studies differed in design but provided functional skills training for older adults with cognitive impairments. Cartwright and colleagues (1996) used a before-and-after design to evaluate a short-term occupational therapy/physical therapy/physiotherapy (OT/PT) functional skills training intervention for cognitively impaired older adults in a geriatric rehabilitation program. Results indicated that the total sample demonstrated statistically significant improvements in functional ability at discharge based on subscales of motor and cognitive domains (Cartwright et al., 1996). The other study was a randomized controlled trial by Wallis and colleagues (1983), which involved occupational therapy conducting RO for older adults with dementia. This intervention aims to address disorientation and confusion, symptoms of severe attention, and memory problems through specific skills training that aims to help a person feel connected to who he or she is (Toglia, 2003). In the study by Wallis and colleagues (1983), occupational therapists were trained to conduct RO in the treatment group with other occupational therapists facilitating the control group with a variety of activities. The results indicated that subjects benefited from both groups with RO faring better than the control group but differences were not statistically significant. These results are compromised by a small sample size (n=38) after a high number of dropouts (n=22).

Other adaptive methods of occupational therapy intervention involve both functional skills training with compensatory approaches to treatment. These seem to be common approaches in two studies that evaluate occupational therapy intervention for people with brain injuries (Dirette & Hinojosa, 1999; Gutman et al., 2004). In the randomized controlled trial by Dirette and Hinojosa (1999), the experimental group received compensatory strategy (verbalization, chunking, and pacing) instruction in addition to computer activities to address visual processing, which differed from the control group who received only computer activities. Both groups demonstrated significant improvements and no differential effects of treatment groups on post-intervention scores; however, further investigation of the results indicated that compensatory strategies were used by about 80% of both groups and contributed to improved scores (Dirette & Hinojosa, 1999). A less rigorous before-and-after design (n=26) evaluated occupational therapy intervention to address cognitive deficits for women who experienced domestic abuse (Gutman et al., 2004). Outcomes measuring goal attainment through treatment received in learning functional skills and using compensatory devices demonstrated results that all women achieved their goals and more than 80% exceeded their goal areas (Gutman et al., 2004).

A study by Velligan and colleagues (1996) pertained to an adaptive approach, focused on evaluating an intervention that used compensatory methods of treatment by adapting physical environment to overcome cognitive deficits and improve function. In this before-and-after design, occupational therapy was involved in a standard psychosocial therapy control group, which was compared to a cognitive compensatory training group, conducted by nursing. The results indicated that both groups showed improvements in schizophrenia symptoms and adaptive function (Velligan et al., 1996).

Comparing Remediation and Adaptive Approaches to Occupational Therapy Interventions

In the literature, the majority of studies providing intervention for cognitive or perceptual deficits compared remediation to adaptive approaches to rehabilitation. Nine empirical studies were selected.

Systematic Review

A systematic review of 32 studies evaluated the effectiveness of cognitive rehabilitation methods to improve outcomes of people with TBI (Carney, Chesnut, Maynard, Mann, Patterson, & Helfand, 1999). The outcomes of two of these studies demonstrated the involvement of occupational therapy intervention—one study compared remediation to adaptive approaches to treatment and the other combined remediation and adaptive approaches in comparison to a control group. Neither study demonstrated significance, possibly due to limitations from the study designs (Carney et al., 1999).

Empirical Studies

Nine empirical studies compared occupational therapy interventions that improved adaptive skills (functional skills training) to approaches to change body function (remediation of impaired components). Five of these studies demonstrated general cognitive-focused interventions involving occupational therapy only (Brown, Harwood, Hays, Heckman, & Short, 1993; Hadas-Lidor, Katz, Tyano, & Weizman, 2001; Jao & Lu, 1999) and occupational therapy on a multidisciplinary team (Chen, Thomas, Glueckauf, & Bracy, 1997; Cicerone, Mott, Azulay, & Friel, 2004). The common outcomes-measured interventions only involving occupational therapy included memory, self-esteem (or self-concept), and functional performance (Brown et al., 1993; Hadas-Lidor et al., 2001; Jao & Lu, 1999). The results of these studies varied, where both randomized controlled trials with a population of people with schizophrenia differed: Hadas-Lidor and colleagues (2001) showed a more significant impact of cognitive treatment than traditional-functional occupational therapy, and Brown and colleagues (1993) concluded that both interventions had equal effects of cognition.

Similar conflicting results were evident in the two multidisciplinary studies involving occupational therapy, which measured similar outcomes. Chen and colleagues (1997) concluded that there were no significant differences between groups, whereas Cicerone and colleagues (2004) showed improvements in both groups but statistically significant gains in intensive cognitive rehabilitation (remediation approach). Although the interventions compared in each of these studies were similar in approach, they differed in treatment content, which makes it difficult to compare in efficacy.

The remaining four studies comparing remediation and adaptive interventions focused on perceptual and cognitive components (Edmans & Webster, 2000; Geusgens, van Heughten, Donkervoort, van den Ende, Jolles, & van den Heuvel, 2006; Lincoln, Whiting, Cockburn, & Bhavnani, 1985; Soderback, 1988). In two studies where perceptual remediation was compared to functional, occupational therapy demonstrated significant improvements in each group post-intervention but no significant difference between groups (Edmans & Webster, 2000; Lincoln et al., 1985). Similarly, the studies by Soderback (1988) and Geusgens and colleagues (2006), which presented interventions addressing cognitive and perceptual outcomes, concluded that there were no significant differences between group outcomes.

Combination of Remediation and Adaptive Occupational Therapy Interventions

Combining remediation and adaptive approaches to occupational therapy intervention is an emerging approach within clinical practice (Lee et al., 2001). Two before-and-after design studies used combined treatment approaches to improve both functional ability and impairment deficits. Overall, both studies demonstrated significant improvements in basic mental functions (Ng et al., 2006) and impairment in complex tasks (Boman, Lindstedt, Hemmingsson, & Bartfai, 2004). Furthermore, gains were sustained for up to 3 months (Ng et al., 2006), and strategies were generalized and incorporated into daily activities (Boman et al., 2004). Impact of this type of treatment approach for the longer term benefit or transference could be further explored in future research.

Evidence for Neuro-Sensorimotor Outcomes

Empirical evidence that examines occupational therapy interventions impacting on neuro-sensorimotor outcomes included a total of 21 empirical studies. All of these studies detailed remediation strategies to address impairment-focused issues. This section is divided into outcomes focusing on improving neuro-motor abilities and sensory-based impairments. The full description of all neuro-sensorimotor empirical evidence is provided in greater detail in Tables 11-5 through 11-7.

Remediation of Neuro-Motor Abilities in Occupational Therapy Intervention

In the context of remedial and adaptive treatments for neuro-motor impairments, remedial approaches can help increase functional use of motor extremities through occupational demands that aim to increase reorganization of cortical motor areas, whereas adaptive treatments look to adapt and engage the clients' new abilities to their daily occupations (Cicinelli, Traversa & Rossini, 1997). Occupational therapy intervention can help enable a client through various adaptive and remedial intervention strategies. In our review, support was only evident for neuro-motor remediation interventions as demonstrated by one qualitative study, one meta-analysis, one systematic review, and 10 quantitative empirical studies.

Systematic Review

One example of neuro-motor treatments remediating function that is prominent in the literature is an intervention technique called constraint-induced movement therapy (CIMT) or constraint-induced therapy (CIT). This remediation strategy involves forcing the use of the affected or impaired limb by restricting the use of the unaffected limb (Kunkel et al., 1999). One qualitative study analyzed the perceptions of the experiences of two people with strokes who participated in CIMT within a neuro-based rehabilitation program (Gillot, Holder-Walls, Kurtz, & Varley, 2003). One theme generated from the interviews was "Perceived Changes in Function" post-intervention, and it was concluded that this occupational therapy treatment helped increase functional and quality of ability, satisfaction of performance, and decreased time to perform activities (Gillot et al., 2003). Further support for this treatment was evident in a meta-analysis of 11 studies looking at effectiveness of CIT (Bjorklund & Fecht, 2006). This review demonstrated CIT effectiveness for individuals with hemiplegia of an upper extremity post-stroke. Within this review, it was evident that occupational therapy did not exclusively conduct this intervention technique. One intervention study conducted only by occupational therapy showed significant client gains in functional ability (Dromerick, Edwards, & Hahn, 2000), and two treatment team studies (including OT/PT) demonstrated improvement of transferring motor ability to functional tasks (Page, Sisto, Johnston, & Levine, 2002; Page, Sisto, Levine, & McGrath, 2004).

Empirical Studies

This section highlights the diversity of interventions targeting neuro-motor outcomes within occupational therapy. Our search revealed 10 empirical

text continues on page 318

Table 11-5

OCCUPATIONAL THERAPY INTERVENTIONS PROMOTING NEURO-SENSORIMOTOR OUTCOMES

Author (Date)	Pop	DX	Setting	Intervention
Mullen, B., Champagne, T., Krishnamurty, S., Dickson, D., & Gao, R. X. (2008)	2, 3	21	N/A	**Intervention:** Participants underwent 5-minute intervals of treatment with and without a 30-lb weighted blanket. They received 5-minute breaks where they were taken out of the experiment room to complete surveys. During testing sessions, subjects were placed lying down in a simulated hospital room where their vitals were monitored.
Gilmore, P. E., & Spaulding, S. J. (2007)	4	3	4	**Intervention:** A 10-session treatment program combining videotaped feedback to augment a program of OT in order to teach participants how to don socks and shoes. **Control:** 10 sessions of only OT intervention to teach participants how to don socks and shoes.
Rice, M. S., & Hernandez, H. G. (2006)	2	1, 21	N/A	**Intervention:** Participants with developmental delay were randomized to either the 50% or 100% knowledge of results group and were age- and gender-matched with an average person as a control. During the skill acquisition phase, participants learned a motor skill and received feedback according to which group they were in. After a 10-minute break, they underwent the retention phase where they performed the motor skill and received no feedback on their performance.
Wolf, S. L., Winstein, C. J., Miller, J. P., Taub, E., Uswatte, G., Morris, D., et al. (2006)	5	3	4	**Intervention:** Group taught to apply a protective safety mitt and encouraged to wear it on their less impaired upper extremity for 90% of their awakened hours over a 2-week period. Also received adaptive task practice and standard task training of affected limb for up to 6 hours a day. **Control:** Usual and customary care ranging from no treatment to the application of mechanical interventions (e.g., orthotics) or various OT/PT approaches to intervention at home or in hospital.
Bonifer, N. M., Anderson, K. M., & Arciniegas, D. B. (2005)	5	3	4	21-day CIMT program using a soft mitt and sling for 90% of waking hours. Intervention included 6 hours of training, including shaping, massed practice, 1:1 therapist-client ratio, practice at home, daily practice diary. OT was one of the therapists involved in administering practice sessions, along with PT and rehab assistants.
Desrosiers, J., Bourbonnais, D., Corriveau, H., Gosselin, S., & Bravo, G. (2005)	1	3	4	**Intervention:** Usual arm therapy in addition to receiving an arm therapy OT and PT program (15 to 20 45-minute sessions) based on repetition of unilateral and bilateral symmetrical tasks. **Control:** Received usual arm therapy and additional usual arm therapy (of similar duration and frequency as experimental arm therapy program).
Flinn, N. A., Schamburg, S., Fetrow, J. M., & Flanigan, J. (2005)	4	3	4	CIMT: 28 hours treatment total at facility. Participants worked on a 30-minute work-rest ratio. Therapy was provided on one-on-one basis. For 30-minute therapy timeframes, patients chose between different activities that targeted specific movement difficulties. Patients were provided with mitts for the unaffected arm, independently donned and doffed.
Roberts, P. S., Vegher, J. A., Gilewski, M., Bender, A., & Riggs, R. V. (2005)	4	3	4	Education: 14-day intervention. Participants were taught how to don and doff the mitt and were required to wear the mitt for 90% of the time, except for tasks where there was a safety risk if participants were wearing the mitt. OT occurred in home and group settings. Group sessions 3 times a week and home-based sessions twice a week. Both types of sessions were based on shaping and practicing task activities.

continued

Table 11-5 (continued)
OCCUPATIONAL THERAPY INTERVENTIONS PROMOTING NEURO-SENSORIMOTOR OUTCOMES

Author (Date)	Pop	DX	Setting	Intervention
Unwin, R., & Ballinger, C. (2005)	2, 3	2, 5, 18	3	**Intervention:** Individual sensory integration training sessions were given for 10 to 40 minutes twice a week for 4 weeks. Training was given by 2 OTs and was centered on the patient's response, each session included training in tactile, vestibular, and proprioceptive sensory systems. Participants then completed a specific horticulture task after each training session.
Forbes, D. (2004)	1	8	4	2 groups received 8 sessions, one-on-one with same key worker (nurse, OT, or psychology assistant). **Intervention:** Individualized multisensory stimulation group. Multisensory stimulation matched patients' needs and interests and included light and sound effects and materials for touching and smelling. **Control:** Activity group. Playing cards, doing quizzes, and looking at photographs with no clear aim or focus to the task.
Kawahira, K., Shimodozono, M., Ogata, A., & Tanaka, N. (2004)	2	3, 7, 17, 18	4	All subjects received continuous conventional rehabilitation exercise (CRE) therapy for hemiplegia throughout the 8-week study period. In addition, the subjects participated in intensive repetition facilitation (IRF) sessions for the hemiplegic lower limb. 1 physician and 3 PTs participated in training sessions, compiled treatment specifications for CRE and IRF. OT (ADL, vocational, perceptual, and functional activity training), speech-language pathology, and recreational activity were also performed depending on the individual's needs.
McMenamy, C., Ralph, N., Auen, E., & Nelson, L. (2004)	2	16, 17, 20	4	Treatment duration varied from 15 to 22 days over 3 to 6 weeks. Multidisciplinary treatments on complex regional pain syndrome included PT; OT (sensory stimulation program and stress management); biofeedback; goal-oriented cognitively based individual, group, and family counseling; behavioral modification and pain management; nutritional education; and case management. Medications were also given and managed.
Cohen, H., & Kimball, K. (2003)	4	25	3	The 3 groups were given home programs with written instructions by OT investigator describing repetitive head movements to be performed 5 times per day over 4 weeks. For each program, the exercises were demonstrated, and subjects practiced them. **Group 1:** Slow head movements while seated. **Group 2:** Rapid head movements while seated and standing. **Group 3:** Rapid head movements plus attention.
Pfieffer, B., & Kinnealey, M. (2003)	2	25	4	Self-treatment program facilitated by OT. 3 major components of the intervention: Patient insight into sensory defensiveness, regular and daily sensory input, and engaging in physical activities of the patient's choice to provide sensory input. A sensory diet was prescribed to each individual client to be carried out independently over 4 weeks. Participants were contacted by OTs weekly.
Pierce, S. R., Gallagher, K. G., Schaumburg, S. W., Gershkoff, A. M., Gaughan, J. P., & Shutter, L. (2003)	4	3	4	Individualized programs consisting of 7 sessions composed of OT and PT. Therapy sessions were completed over a 2- to 3-week period and included instruction on use of a restraining mitt at home during functional activities (CIMT).

continued

Table 11-5 (continued)
Occupational Therapy Interventions Promoting Neuro-Sensorimotor Outcomes

Author (Date)	Pop	DX	Setting	Intervention
Page, S. J., Levine, P., Sisto, S., & Johnston, M. V. (2001)	4	3	4	All patients received 6 weeks of therapy administered by the same OTs and PTs. ***Intervention:*** In addition to regular therapy, they participated in 10-minute guided imagery sessions after each therapy session, as well as practicing imagery at home. ***Control:*** Patients participated in an intervention consisting of exposure to stroke information.
Oerlemans, H. M., Oostendorp, R. A., de Boo, T., van der Laan, L., Severens, J. L., & Goris, J. A. (2000)	5	20	4	Participants with complex regional pain syndrome were randomly allocated to 1 of 3 groups. ***PT Intervention:*** Control of pain, extinguishing the source of pain, improving skills. ***OT Intervention:*** Reducing symptoms of inflammation, normalizing sensibility, improving functional abilities of the arm/hand. ***Control:*** Social work.
Page, S. (2000)	4	3	4	***Intervention*** (OT and imagery treatment): 3 times per week for 4 weeks. OT treatment consisted of 40% neurodevelopmental theory techniques and 60% compensatory strategies requiring the use of the uninvolved limb. Imagery program included tape-recorded imagery intervention, focus on functional tasks targeted by OT. ***Control:*** Group that was not receiving imagery and only received OT treatment.
Volpe, B. T., Krebs, H. I., Hogan, N., Edelstein, L., Diels, C., & Aisen, M. (2000)	4	3	4	All patients experienced similar standard PT and OT post-stroke. Patients were randomly allocated to: ***Intervention:*** Patients also received training to participate in robot-aided sensorimotor stimulation. ***Control:*** Patients also received exposure to the robotic device without training.
Soper, G., & Thorley, C. R. (1996)	5	18	4	***Intervention:*** Weekly sessions for 1 year. Sensory integration-based treatment occurred in a sensory stimulation room, including various objects for the senses. Participants directed engagement with items in the sensory room, with therapist guidance. ***Control:*** Received sensory stimulation.
Paire, J., & Karney, R. (1984)	1	14, 24	4	***Intervention:*** 12-week duration. Treatment was provided by OT in 2 small groups: Sensory stimulation and staff attention. ***Control:*** Standard hospital treatment.

Population: 1=geriatric (65+); 2=adult (25 to 64); 3=young adult (18 to 24); 4=adult and geriatric; 5=young adult, adult, and geriatric.

Diagnosis: 1=developmental delay; 2=autism; 3=stroke; 5=multiple sclerosis; 7=acquired brain injury; 8=dementia or Alzheimer's disease; 14=schizophrenia; 16=upper extremity injury; 17=lower extremity; 18=other; 19=arthritis; 20=chronic pain; 21=no diagnosis; 24=frail elderly; 25=sensory impairment.

Setting: 1=long-term care; 2=acute care; 3=home care; 4=rehabilitation; 5=primary care; N/A=not applicable.

Table 11-6

EVIDENCE OF EFFECTIVENESS OF OCCUPATIONAL THERAPY ON NEURO-SENSORIMOTOR OUTCOMES

Author (Date)	Major Results	Study Design	Sample Size	Conclusion and Limitations
Positive Effects—Randomized Controlled Trial				
Rice, M. S., & Hernandez, H. G. (2006)	Results were considered significant at p=0.05 or p<0.05. In the population with developmental delay, analysis showed that the 100% feedback group performed better than the 50% group during the skill acquisition phase. During the retention phase, results were the opposite with subjects in the 50% feedback group performing better on the task. In both populations (average and developmentally delayed), results showed improvements in during the skill acquisition phase except for the developmentally delayed group with 100% feedback. During the retention phase, there were no significant differences in performance between populations or groups.	RCT	32	**Conclusions:** In subjects with developmental delay, high frequency of feedback improves performance during the learning process but has a negative impact on skill retention. This study shows that lower frequency of feedback has a significant improvement on retention of skills. **Limitations:** Small sample size and the task participants had to learn an "artificial occupation."
Wolf, S. L., Winstein, C. J., Miller, J. P., Taub, E., Uswatte, G., Morris, D., et al. (2006)	The CIMT group showed greater statistically significant improvements than the control group (from baseline to 12 months) in both UE performance time and in amount of arm use as well as quality of arm movement. The CIMT group also achieved a greater decrease in self-perceived hand function difficulty.	RCT	222	**Conclusions:** The CIMT group demonstrated statistically significant and clinically significant improvements in arm motor function that persisted for at least 12 months. **Limitations:** Less than half of the control group received other treatments through the year. Incomplete information provided regarding anatomical location of each stroke and use of medications.
Page, S. J., Levine, P., Sisto, S., & Johnston, M. V. (2001)	After intervention, FMA and ARA scores of patients in therapy-only group remained virtually the same; therapy plus imagery group scores improved by 13.4 and 16.8 points, respectively, on FMA and ARA (no p-values given).	RCT	13	**Conclusions:** Results indicate a greater increase in function in the intervention group than in control the group, suggesting that imagery is a feasible complement to standard stroke rehabilitation. **Limitations:** Statistical significance of difference in change scores unknown, small sample size.
Oerlemans, H. M., Oostendorp, R. A., de Boo, T., van der Laan, L., Severens, J. L., & Goris, J. A. (2000)	Both PT and, to a lesser extent, OT resulted in a significant and more rapid improvement in the ISS as compared with control group. On a disability level, a positive trend was found in favor of OT. Of PT, OT, and social work, PT was the most cost effective.	RCT	135	**Conclusions:** PT and, to a lesser extent, OT resulted in a significant and more rapid improvement in the ISS than the control group. PT was found to be more cost-effective, while OT was found more positive on a disability level. Both PT and OT contribute to recovery from complex regional pain syndrome/reflex sympathetic dystrophy. **Limitations:** No major limitations.

continued

Table 11-6 (continued)

EVIDENCE OF EFFECTIVENESS OF OCCUPATIONAL THERAPY ON NEURO-SENSORIMOTOR OUTCOMES

Author (Date)	Major Results	Study Design	Sample Size	Conclusions and Limitations
Positive Effects—Randomized Controlled Trial				
Volpe, B. T., Krebs, H. I., Hogan, N., Edelstein, L., Diels, C., & Aisen, M. (2000)	By end of treatment, experimental group demonstrated significant improvement in motor outcome for trained shoulder and elbow ($p<0.01$), but not the wrist and hand. Experimental group also demonstrated significantly improved functional outcome ($p<0.01$).	RCT	56	**Conclusions:** Robot-delivered sensorimotor training enhanced performance of exercised shoulder and elbow. Robot-treated group also demonstrated enhanced functional outcome. **Limitations:** Small sample size, heterogeneous groups compared because experimental group had less disability at the start of the trial.
Positive Effects—Non-Randomized Controlled Trial				
Bonifer, N. M., Anderson, K. M., & Arciniegas, D. B. (2005)	Statistically significant effect of treatment on UE motor impairment as assessed by FMA ($p<0.001$), GWFMT ($p<0.003$), and Motor Activity Log ($p<0.001$); improvements remained stable at 1-month follow-up.	Non-RCT	20	**Conclusions:** Participants took part in a 3-week CIMT program led by OTs and PTs. Results indicate significant improvement on outcome measures of upper limb function and impairment. **Limitations:** No control group, assessors were not blinded for 2/3 outcome measures, no long-term follow-up.
Flinn, N. A., Schamburg, S., Fetrow, J. M., & Flanigan, J. (2005)	Use of affected limb: Significant differences present pre- and post-treatment ($p=0.003$). UE coordination: No significant differences present pre- and post-treatment and at follow-up. Occupational performance: No significant differences present pre- and post-treatment and at follow-up for both average performance and satisfaction scores.	Non-RCT	11	**Conclusions:** Participants showed significant increases in the use of the affected UE in occupations following CIMT, although perception of their own performance did not improve significantly. **Limitations:** Small sample size, no record of preventing contamination or co-intervention.
Roberts, P. S., Vegher, J. A., Gilewski, M., Bender, A., & Riggs, R. V. (2005)	Significant improvements in weight lifted by affected arm from pre- to post-evaluation ($p=0.013$). Non-significant improvements for total time of activity and grip strength pre- to post-training. Non-significant improvements in total time of activity, weight lifted, and grip strength post-training to follow-up. Statistically significant improvement for perception of and satisfaction with performance from pre- to post-training. Decline in perception of performance and satisfaction from post-training to follow-up.	Non-RCT	5	**Conclusions:** For a specific sub-group of individuals with stroke, constraint-induced therapy resulted in positive post-treatment results on satisfaction and performance with life roles, which decreased significantly at follow-up assessment despite continued improvements in physical function. **Limitations:** Small sample size, many participants did not complete follow-up, no record of preventing contamination or co-intervention, some outcome measures lacked psychometric properties.

continued

Table 11-6 (continued)
EVIDENCE OF EFFECTIVENESS OF OCCUPATIONAL THERAPY ON NEURO-SENSORIMOTOR OUTCOMES

Author (Date)	Major Results	Study Design	Sample Size	Conclusions and Limitations
Positive Effects—Non-Randomized Controlled Trial				
Unwin, R., & Ballinger, C. (2005)	Visual and statistical data of the information for all participants shows that sensory integration therapy had a therapeutic effect and improved engagement, lowered maladaptive behavior, and increased functional ability. GAS scores for each participant showed significant improvement. Some improvements lasted throughout the intervention phase and persisted after withdrawing sensory integration therapy, indicating a possible carryover effect.	Non-RCT	5	***Conclusions:*** This study provides preliminary evidence that SIT can improve the functional behavior of adults with learning disabilities and tactile sensory modulation problems. Positive improvements during intervention indicated that SIT was effective. ***Limitations:*** The variability of the baseline data for each participant and the complex and highly individual nature of SIT make it difficult to describe.
Kawahira, K., Shimodozono, M., Ogata, A., & Tanaka, N. (2004)	Overall study results showed significant improvements in BRSH, FTT, and the strength of knee extension/flexion of the affected lower limb after the first conventional rehabilitation exercise (CRE) session and after the first and second intensive repetition facilitation (IRF) and CRE sessions. The improvements after IRF and CRE sessions were significantly greater than those after the preceding CRE sessions.	Non-RCT	24	***Conclusions:*** This multidisciplinary treatment involving intensive repetition of movement resulted in improved voluntary movement of a hemiplegic lower limb. ***Limitations:*** No control group (multiple-baseline design), small sample size, blind evaluations were not given.
McMenamy, C., Ralph, N., Auen, E., & Nelson, L. (2004)	Significant improvements on all 13 dependent variables were found between pre- and post-test scores. Vocational activity ($p<0.001$) and narcotic use ($p=0.006$) decreased significantly from pre-test to follow-up. Lower mean pain levels were reported at follow-up, but the difference was not significant.	Non-RCT	11	***Conclusions:*** Results indicate significant improvements on all dependent variables. ***Limitations:*** Small sample size, no control group.
Cohen, H., & Kimball, K. (2003)	Vertigo intensity and frequency decreased significantly ($p<0.001$). Independence in ADL improved significantly ($p<0.001$).	Non-RCT	53	***Conclusions:*** Evidence showed statistically significant support of a vestibular home program to decrease symptoms of vertigo and an improvement in independence of ADL. ***Limitations:*** None reported.

continued

Table 11-6 (continued)

EVIDENCE OF EFFECTIVENESS OF OCCUPATIONAL THERAPY ON NEURO-SENSORIMOTOR OUTCOMES

Author (Date)	Major Results	Study Design	Sample Size	Conclusions and Limitations
Positive Effects—Non-Randomized Controlled Trial				
Pfieffer, B., & Kinnealey, M. (2003)	Anxiety: Correlation was found between sensory defensiveness and anxiety (r=0.61, p=0.027). Effects of sensory integration self-treatment on sensory defensiveness and anxiety: Significant effects were found for both sensory defensiveness and anxiety post-treatment sensory defensiveness: p=0.048; anxiety: p=0.045.	Non-RCT	15	**Conclusions:** Preliminary evidence suggests that sensory integration has positive effects on anxiety and sensory defensiveness. More methodologically comprehensive research is required to support this initial evidence. **Limitations:** Small sample size, participants were largely self-referred to the study, while treatment was self-directed, it was provided in different settings and varying amounts of time for each participant, lack of masked and independent evaluation.
Pierce, S. R., Gallagher, K. G., Schaumburg, S. W., Gershkoff, A. M., Gaughan, J. P., & Shutter, L. (2003)	Patients demonstrated statistically significant improvements (p<0.05 corrected for multiple comparisons) in mean time for completion in 12 of 17 WMFT subtests when comparing baseline to post-treatment.	Non-RCT	17	**Conclusions:** Clients demonstrated significant improvements in UE function following treatment, suggesting that forced-use component of CIT may be effective when applied within a traditional outpatient rehabilitation program. **Limitations:** Unblinded outcome assessors, use of only one outcome measure, no control group.
Page, S. (2000)	Both groups improved in UE scores at post-evaluation: Control group: 21.15% improvement post-intervention. OT plus imagery group (experimental): 35.98% improvement. OT plus imagery groups had significantly greater improvements than OT-only group, p<0.05.	Non-RCT	16	**Conclusions:** Results from this study confirmed the hypothesis that adding imagery to OT has a more beneficial impact on physical impairment than OT alone for chronic stroke patients. **Limitations:** Outcome measures may not have related to all treatment goals, no record of preventing contamination or co-intervention, reasons for dropouts not reported.

continued

Table 11-6 (continued)

EVIDENCE OF EFFECTIVENESS OF OCCUPATIONAL THERAPY ON NEURO-SENSORIMOTOR OUTCOMES

Author (Date)	Major Results	Study Design	Sample Size	Conclusions and Limitations
Positive Effects—Non-Randomized Controlled Trial				
Soper, G., & Thorley, C. R. (1996)	Experimental (Exp) and control showed statistically significant improvements in clinical observations: Touch-Exp (p<0.001) and control (p<0.05); Movement-Exp (p<0.001); and Control (p<0.01); and total scores-Exp and Control (p<0.001). Significant improvements in behavioral responses for the Exp group in vestibular p<0.05, proprioception p<0.001, general responses p<0.01, and total scores p<0.025. Statistically significant difference between groups for proprioception (p<0.01) and total score (p<0.05) categories. Adaptive responses: Significant difference (p<0.025) found between experimental and control groups.	Non-RCT	28	**Conclusions:** The study investigated the impact of a sensory integration program on individuals with severe learning disabilities, when compared to controls. Results indicated that touch and movement scores yielded from the clinic environment improved in both groups with the experimental group performing significantly better for adaptive responses, proprioceptive, and total behavior scores. **Limitations:** Outcome measures lack psychometric properties, no reports of evaluators or participants blinded to treatment, intervention not described, small sample size.
Paire, J., & Karney, R. (1984)	All groups improved orientation and, the effects were maintained at follow-up (p<0.05). Self-care skills: No significant effects were noted with respect to grooming, toileting, and eating skills. Sensory stimulation group increased caring for personal hygiene at all time points. Staff attention group showed an increase at post-testing, followed by substantial drop at follow-up. Control group decreased from baseline at each evaluation point. Interpersonal skills: Helping on ward and individual response were unaffected by any group assignment.	Non-RCT	27	**Conclusions:** The results indicated that, when compared to an attention-only and control group, the sensory stimulation group showed a higher level of interest in hygiene and group activities. **Limitations:** No record of preventing contamination or co-intervention, no reports of evaluators or participants blinded to treatment, small sample size, outcome measures lack psychometric properties.
No Effect				
Mullen, B., Champagne, T., Krishnamurty, S., Dickson, D., & Gao, R. X. (2008)	No significant differences were found in participants' vital signs between sessions with blanket or without. Regardless of blanket order or test session, skin conductance values decreased significantly over time: 10/30 participants showed a larger drop in skin conductance while using the blanket, 4 had an increase in skin conductance, and 16 had no significant change. STAI-10 showed that the use of the weighted blanket was more effective in reducing self-perceived levels of anxiety though a small minority of subjects (3/30) experienced higher anxiety with the blanket.	Non-RCT	30	**Conclusions:** Using a 30-lb weighted blanket in a healthy adult population presented no danger to those who used it. 33% of subjects showed lower physical signs of anxiety, and 63% reported the blanket had a calming effect. **Limitations:** No consistent control to compare results. Absence of useful models to analyze skin conductance data to interpret this measure.

continued

Table 11-6 (continued)
EVIDENCE OF EFFECTIVENESS OF OCCUPATIONAL THERAPY ON NEURO-SENSORIMOTOR OUTCOMES

Author (Date)	Major Results	Study Design	Sample Size	Conclusions and Limitations
No Effect				
Gilmore, P. E., & Spaulding, S. J. (2007)	Donning socks: Both groups improved in their ability. No significant differences between groups for self-perception of performance and satisfaction over time. Donning shoes: Both groups improved in their ability. Significant differences between groups for self-perception of performance and satisfaction over time.	RCT	10	**Conclusions:** An intervention program including videotaped feedback with OT is not more effective in learning how to don socks and shoes post-stroke than OT only. **Limitations:** Small sample size and spontaneous post-stroke recovery not accounted for.
Desrosiers, J., Bourbonnais, D., Corriveau, H., Gosselin, S., & Bravo, G. (2005)	Both experimental and control groups improved similarly throughout the study. No significant difference between groups at end of study period for any dependent variables.	RCT	41	**Conclusions:** This RCT evaluated the effect of an arm training program emphasizing repeated symmetrical bilateral or unilateral movements in addition to standard arm therapy. Results do not support efficacy of repetitive program. **Limitations:** Small sample size.
Forbes, D. (2004)	Treatment groups did not differ in changes to behavior and mood post-treatment. At follow-up, cognition, behavior, or mood scores did not differ between groups.	RCT	136	**Conclusions:** Both groups received treatment twice a week for 4 weeks. No differences were found between groups on outcome measures of cognition, behavior, or mood. **Limitations:** Relatively short treatment duration, possible impact of co-intervention between groups because medication profiles of participants not reported.

ARA=Action Research Arm Test, BRSH=Brunnstrom Recovery Stage of Hemiplegia, FMA=Fugl-Meyer Assessment, FTT=Foot-Tap Test, GAS=Goal Attainment Scaling, ISS=Impairment Sum Score, STAI-10=State Trait Anxiety Inventory, WMFT=Wolf Motor Function Test.

Table 11-7

OUTCOME MEASURES USED TO CAPTURE NEURO-SENSORIMOTOR OUTCOMES

Author (Date)	Outcome(s) Investigated	Outcome Measure(s)	Method of Administration
Mullen, B., Champagne, T., Krishnamurty, S., Dickson, D., & Gao, R. X. (2008)	Pulse rate Pulse oximetry Blood pressure Electrodermal activity Anxiety levels	GE 4000 vital signs machine ProComp Skin Conductance sensor STAI-10	Vital signs and skin conductance were collected while patients underwent testing with or without the weighted blanket. Study subjects filled out the STAI-10 during 5-minute breaks between testing and as an exit survey once testing was completed.
Gilmore, P. E., & Spaulding, S. J. (2007)	Self-perception on ability to don socks and shoes Ability to don socks and shoes	COPM KB-ADL (socks and shoe subtests)	Measures were administered: Prior to intervention and following each of the 10 sessions.
Rice, M. S., & Hernandez, H. G. (2006)	Performance on motor skill task	CAE	Custom computer software monitored and recorded each participant's performance of the motor skill during testing.
Wolf, S. L., Winstein, C. J., Miller, J. P., Taub, E., Uswatte, G., Morris, D., et al. (2006)	Measure of UE motor function Interview of real-world arm use Hand function and physical function	WMFT MAL SIS	All testing was conducted on 5 occasions: Baseline; post-treatment; and 4, 8, 12 months follow-up. Trained assessors who were blinded to group assessment.
Bonifer, N. M., Anderson, K. M., & Arciniegas, D. B. (2005)	Motor performance (UE) Motor impairment (UE) Ability to perform daily tasks Cognitive state	FMA GWMFT MMSE	All assessments administered day before CIMT program began, at the end of treatment, and 1 month following treatment. FMA by OT; GWMFT via videotape by blinded OT and PT, not involved in study; motor assessment log by CIMT trainers as a semi-structured interview.
Desrosiers, J., Bourbonnais, D., Corriveau, H., Gosselin, S., & Bravo, G. (2005)	Arm impairments Arm disability in tasks related to daily activities Functional independence in ADL and IADL	FMA MV BBT PPT TEMPA F-FIM AMPS	Subjects evaluated before and after program by independent therapist blind to study condition. Evaluations completed in 1 or 2 sessions, depending on participants' tolerance.
Flinn, N. A., Schamburg, S., Fetrow, J. M., & Flanigan, J. (2005)	UE use in ADL UE coordination Occupational performance	MAL WMFT COPM	Measures were administered at baseline (1 to 3 weeks prior to intervention), last day of intervention, and follow-up (4 to 6 months post-intervention).
Roberts, P. S., Vegher, J. A., Gilewski, M., Bender, A., & Riggs, R. V. (2005)	Functional performance Subjective functional occupational performance	WMFT MAL COPM MODAPTS	Tests were administered by therapists at pre-training, post-training, and at follow-up (6 months).

continued

Table 11-7 (continued)

OUTCOME MEASURES USED TO CAPTURE NEURO-SENSORIMOTOR OUTCOMES

Author (Date)	Outcome(s) Investigated	Outcome Measure(s)	Method of Administration
Unwin, R., & Ballinger, C. (2005)	Engagement in task Engagement in maladaptive behaviors Functional ability while engaged in task	Time spent engaged in task Time spent engaged in maladaptive behaviors GAS	Participants were videotaped while performing the horticulture task, and tapes were later reviewed by research OTs.
Forbes, D. (2004)	Behavior and mood during and after sessions Cognition and behavior at home or on ward post-treatment Behavior on ward and at day hospital at 8 weeks Mood at home or on ward post-treatment and at 1-month follow-up	Interact rating form MMSE BRS BOIP REHS Baker Scale BMDS	Article does not state who administered assessments; interact rating form administered after each session; MMSE and BRS administered after 8 sessions; BOIP, REHS, and Baker Scale administered at 8 weeks; BMDS administered after 8 sessions and at 1-month follow-up.
Kawahira, K., Shimodozono, M., Ogata, A., & Tanaka, N. (2004)	Motor function of the affected lower limb Motor function of the foot Strength and flexion of knee Walking velocity	BRSH FTT Cybex 6000 machine Participants were timed with a stop watch (measures walking velocity)	During 8-week program, participants were evaluated at 2-week intervals (weeks 2, 4, 6, and 8) by the PT (Brunnstrom, walking velocity) and physician (foot tap, knee measurements). The PT and physician were blind to each other's measurements.
McMenamy, C., Ralph, N., Auen, E., & Nelson, L. (2004)	Assess depression and somatization levels Progress in affected area Pain-related functional levels Strength and endurance Satisfaction with program Work status Narcotic use	SCL-90R Thermometer PRC Strength and endurance Patient questionnaire	All measures were administered at baseline, discharge. At post-discharge follow-up (6 to 32 months), pain levels, vocational status, and narcotic use measures were re-administered. The SCL-90R, PRC, and patient questionnaires were self-reported. The strength and endurance and functional level tests were administered by the study personnel.
Cohen, H., & Kimball, K. (2003)	Vertigo intensity and frequency Independence in ADL	VSS VHQ VADL DHQ	Pre- and post-test evaluation.
Pfieffer, B., & Kinnealey, M. (2003)	Sensory defensiveness Anxiety	ASQ ASI BAI	Measures were administered pre-/post-intervention by the therapist.
Pierce, S. R., Gallagher, K. G., Schaumburg, S. W., Gershkoff, A. M., Gaughan, J. P., & Shutter, L. (2003)	UE impairment and function	WMFT	WMFT administered at by OT or PT at baseline, midway through treatment and post-treatment.

continued

Table 11-7 (continued)

OUTCOME MEASURES USED TO CAPTURE NEURO-SENSORIMOTOR OUTCOMES

Author (Date)	Outcome(s) Investigated	Outcome Measure(s)	Method of Administration
Page, S. J., Levine, P., Sisto, S., & Johnston, M. V. (2001)	UE impairment Grasp Grip Pinch Gross movement	FMA ARA	Both assessments administered as pre-tests, in separate sessions 1-week apart. Both assessments also administered after intervention complete.
Oerlemans, H. M., Oostendorp, R. A., de Boo, T., van der Laan, L., Severens, J. L., & Goris, J. A. (2000)	Impairment Disability Hand function Dexterity Daily activities and well-being	ISS RSQ RDT SIP	Not reported.
Page, S. (2000)	Physical impairment	FMA	Measure was administered both before and after intervention.
Volpe, B. T., Krebs, H. I., Hogan, N., Edelstein, L., Diels, C., & Aisen, M. (2000)	Motor impairment Functional independence	FMA MSS MPS FIM	At start and end of trial, same masked therapist administered motor impairment outcome measures. At start and end of trial, FIM-certified nurses or therapists masked to condition administered FIM.
Soper, G., & Thorley, C. R. (1996)	Sensory related profile Behavioral responses to sensory demands Level of adaptive responses	Clinical Observations Checklist Behavioral Checklist ASAR	Tests were administered both at baseline and post-intervention. Clinical observations checklist was completed by therapists. Behavioral checklist completed together by carer and therapist.
Paire, J., & Karney, R. (1984)	Orientation Interpersonal skills Self-care skills	GIES GRS	Outcome measures were administered pre-test, post-test, and at follow-up.

AMPS=Assessment of Motor and Process Skills, ARA=Action Research Arm Test, ASAR=Ayres Scale of Adaptive, ASI=Adult Sensory Interview, ASQ=Adult Sensory Questionnaire, BAI=Beck Anxiety Inventory, BBT=Box and Block Test, BMDS=Behaviour and Mood Disturbance Scale, BOIP=Behaviour Observation Scale for Intra-Mural Psychogeriatrics, BRS=Behavioural Rating Scale, BRSH=Brunnstrom Recovery Stage of Hemiplegia, CAE=Cumulative Absolute Error, COPM=Canadian Occupational Performance Measure, DHQ=Dizziness Handicap Questionnaire, F-FIM=Functional Independence Measure (French Version), FIM=Functional Independence Measure, FMA=Fugl-Meyer Assessment, FTT=Foot-Tap Test, GAS=Goal Attainment Scaling, GIES=Geriatric Interpersonal Evaluation Scale, GRS=Geriatric Rating Scale, GWMFT=Graded Wolf Motor Function Test, ISS=Impairment Sum Score, KB-ADL=Klein Bell Activities of Daily Living Scale, MAL=Motor Activity Log, MMSE=Mini Mental Status Examination, MODAPTS=Modular Arrangement of Predetermined Time Standards, MPS=Motor Power Score, MSS=Motor Status Score, MV=Martin Vigorimeter, PPT=Purdue Pegboard Test, PRC=PARC Rating Scale, RDT=Radboud Dexterity Test, REHS=Rehabilitation Evaluation Hall Scale, RSQ=Radboud Skills Questionnaire, SCL-90R=Symptom Checklist, SIP=Sickness Impact Profile, SIS=Stroke Impact Scale, STAI-10=State Trait Anxiety Inventory, TEMPA=Independence Measure-Upper Extremity (performance test for the elderly), VADL=Vestibular Disorders Activities of Daily Living, VHQ=Vertigo Handicap Questionnaire, VSS=Vertigo Symptom Scale, WMFT=Wolf Motor Function Test.

studies involving various neuro-motor interventions typically conducted by occupational therapy and two involving occupational therapy within a multidisciplinary team.

In our review, we found five empirical studies in the stroke literature that evaluated occupational therapy involved in improving neuro-motor outcomes through CIMT. Four of five studies were pre-post designs evaluating the effectiveness of CIMT without a control group (Bonifer, Anderson, & Arciniegas, 2005; Flinn, Schamburg, Fetrow, & Flanigan, 2005; Pierce, Gallagher, Schaumburg, Gershkoff, Gaughan, & Shutter, 2003; Roberts, Vegher, Gilewski, Bender, & Riggs, 2005). Studies by Flinn and colleagues (2005) and Roberts and colleagues (2005) evaluated occupational therapy intervention of CIMT and demonstrated significant improvements in occupational performance and upper extremity ability (coordination and strength) for the affected arm. Occupational therapy within a multidisciplinary team conducting CIMT also demonstrated significant improvements post-intervention in similar outcomes related to affected upper extremity function and motor performance (Bonifer et al., 2005; Pierce et al., 2003). The only randomized controlled trial evaluating CIMT compared a 2-week program of CIMT to a group receiving usual treatment, which ranged from no treatment to OT/PT treatment (Wolf et al., 2006). The results of the study indicated that "among patients who had a stroke within the previous 3 to 9 months, CIMT produced statistically significant and clinically relevant improvements in arm motor function that persisted for at least 1 year" (Wolf et al., 2006, p. 2095).

Therapy interventions other than CIMT have also been demonstrated in the literature and aimed to change body function for neuro-motor impairments of the upper extremity. A randomized controlled trial by Desrosiers and colleagues (2005) compared usual multidisciplinary (OT/PT) arm therapy to a specific arm therapy program based on repetition of arm exercises to improve motor impairment and functional independence. The results concluded that both groups improved similarly throughout the study but no significant differences were evident between groups (Desrosiers et al., 2005).

Another intervention approach involving occupational therapy to remediate neuro-motor impairments involves the use of motor learning theories, which promote learning of new motor skills by focusing on the process of skill acquisition (Miles Breslin, 1996). Four studies within the area of motor learning describe outcomes that evaluate motor skill development.

The first example of a motor theory-based approach is examined in a literature review, which described occupational therapy-based intervention to facilitate CNS plasticity by imaging and practicing movements mentally (Bell & Murray, 2004). Early evidence from the review indicated that physical function increased when treatment focused on physical practice was combined with mental imagery (Kelly & Shah, 2002). In our review, one cohort study was found by Page (2000) that compared treatment with only occupational therapy to occupational therapy combined with imagery for people with stroke. The results indicated improvements in both groups post-evaluation of physical upper extremity impairment, but additional imagery had a greater impact on physical impairment than occupational therapy intervention alone (Page, 2000). These results were supported by a randomized controlled case-series design that initially provided all subjects with 6 weeks of OT/PT treatment and then allocated subjects to either intervention (using guided imagery) or control group (exposure to stroke information) (Page, Levine, Sisto, & Johnston, 2001). Results indicated a greater increase in function (non-significant) within the therapy plus imagery group (Page et al., 2001).

In two other empirical studies (Gilmore & Spaulding, 2007; Rice & Hernandez, 2006), the focus of the intervention groups was on providing feedback in various ways, which emphasized one approach to the motor learning skill acquisition process. In the study by Rice and Hernandez (2006), a sample of people with developmental delay were allocated to two groups—an intervention group receiving 100% knowledge of results (KR) feedback versus 50% KR (control group) based on their performance on a motor skills task from their occupational therapist. The results indicated that the intervention group performed better in the skill acquisition phase only, whereas the control group improved more in the skill retention phase. In the study by Gilmore and Spaulding (2007), using a sample of people post-stroke, feedback was provided only within the intervention group in a videotaped format in conjunction with occupational therapy, whereas the control group received only occupational therapy. Overall, the results reported no significant differences in performance of specific motor tasks between groups; however, an improvement in self-perception of performance in the intervention group was statistically significant.

Multidisciplinary neuro-motor rehabilitation has also been used to address syndromes such as complex regional pain syndrome (CRPS), which are "characterized by pain out of proportion to injury, vasomotor and trophic changes, stiffness and decreased function" (Watson & Carlson, 1987, p. 779). Two studies examined OT/PT interventions aimed to increase skill and decrease pain symptoms. A before-and-after study (McMenamy, Ralph, Auen, & Nelson,

2004) and a randomized controlled trial (Oerlemans, Oostendorp, de Boo, van der Laan, Severens, & Goris, 2000) evaluated OT/PT interventions on clients with CRPS. Both studies demonstrated significant contributions of OT/PT treatment to improve impairment and disability (Oerlemans et al., 2000) and to improve strength, endurance, and other component areas to improve symptoms (McMenamy et al., 2004) to demonstrate effectiveness of treatment.

Remediation for Sensory-Based Occupational Therapy Intervention

Occupational therapy interventions aimed at changing body function with remedial treatments that are sensory-based are evident in nine empirical studies within our review. Sensory-focused interventions have been described in different formats such as specific occupational therapy led sensory stimulation or integration (Mullen, Champagne, Krishnamurty, Dickson, & Gao, 2008; Paire & Karney, 1984; Soper & Thorley, 1996; Unwin & Ballinger, 2005), home programs for vertigo or sensory diet (Cohen & Kimball, 2003; Pfeiffer & Kinnealey, 2003), or multidisciplinary sensory interventions (Forbes, 2004; Kawahira, Shimodozono, Ogata, & Tanaka, 2004; Volpe, Krebs, Hogan, Edelstein, Diels, & Aisen, 2000).

The four studies evaluating occupational therapy sensory intervention compared treatment to control groups using a cohort design (Paire & Karney, 1984; Soper & Thorley, 1996). Results from both studies demonstrated improvements in all groups for most outcomes measured. However, sensory intervention groups significantly improved and maintained their improvement across areas of personal hygiene and interest in group activities (Paire & Karney, 1984) and for proprioception, total behavioral scores, and adaptive responses (Soper & Thorley, 1996). A third study using a concurrent, nested, mixed methods design evaluated the safety and effectiveness of deep pressure stimulation from a weighted blanket (Mullen et al., 2008). The quantitative outcomes evaluated (e.g., skin conductance) were largely direct measures of sympathetic activity, which showed that 33% of the sample demonstrated a greater reduction in anxiety and preferred the weighted blanket as a calming modality. The implications of this study should be prefaced with the knowledge that the sample was a cohort of healthy participants. The fourth study relevant to sensory outcomes evaluated the outcomes of a sensory integration intervention (Unwin & Ballinger, 2005). Although the study indicated positive improvements in areas such as decreasing maladaptive behaviors and improving functional behaviors for a group of adults with learning disabilities and tactile sensory modulation prob-

lems, this study only provides preliminary evidence given the small sample (n=5) and the need for more rigorous methodology of the study design.

Occupational therapy-led home sensory programs (Cohen & Kimball, 2003; Pfeiffer & Kinnealey, 2003) demonstrated self-directed interventions that were facilitated or written by occupational therapists. Cohen and Kimball (2003) provided evidence that showed statistical significance of a vertigo home program to decrease symptoms and increase ADL independence. Pfeiffer and Kinnealey (2003) also concluded that a self-treatment program facilitated by an occupational therapy sensory diet had positive effects on anxiety and sensory defensiveness.

Multidisciplinary sensory-focused interventions involving occupational therapists were evident in addressing cognition and behavior (Forbes, 2004) and motor function or impairment (Kawahira et al., 2004; Volpe et al., 2000). In a large randomized controlled trial (n=136) by Forbes (2004), the evaluation of multisensory stimulation intervention for people with dementia demonstrated no differences in cognition, behavior, or mood scores from the control group. The impact of intervention could be the result of the shortened treatment duration (eight sessions). The remaining two multidisciplinary studies involved occupational therapy-targeted sensory areas for clients post-stroke (Kawahira et al., 2004; Volpe et al., 2000). In the randomized controlled trial by Volpe and colleagues (2000), sensorimotor stimulation that was robot-delivered in the experimental group improved significantly in comparison to control group's shoulder performance and functional outcome. The other study, a multiple baseline design, measured lower extremity performance (Kawahira et al., 2004). The results of this study reported that the facilitation technique, mainly proprioceptive neuromuscular facilitation pattern, stretch reflex, and skin-muscle reflex, resulted in improvements of the voluntary movement of a hemiplegic lower limb (Kawahira et al., 2004). In both studies, sensory-focused remediation intervention involving occupational therapy enabled participants to improve in outcomes related to the underlying impairments.

Measures Used to Capture Cognitive-Neurological Outcomes

Based on the evidence of the scoping reviews examining the outcomes sensitive to cognitive-neurological occupational therapy intervention, there are some distinctions between cognitive-perceptual and

Table 11-8

OUTCOME MEASURES TO ASSESS COGNITIVE-PERCEPTUAL INTERVENTIONS

Measure	Population	Content Domains	Reliability and Validity
Brief Psychiatric Rating Scale (BPRS)	Adult and geriatric	Measures symptoms related to mental health issues (specifically schizophrenia).	Well-established reliability and validity data in literature for both measures.
Functional Independence Measure (FIM)	Geriatric	Functional ability in terms of disability and cognition.	Studies reported strong internal consistency and inter-rater reliability, as well as good content, convergent, predictive, and construct validity (Law, Baum, & Dunn, 2005).
Mini Mental Status Examination (MMSE)	Adult and geriatric	Cognitive state and basic mental functions.	Studies demonstrate test-retest and intra-rater and inter-rater reliability. Furthermore, validity has been measured in terms of concurrent, construct, predictive, and content (Molloy, Alemayehu, & Roberts, 1991).
Wechsler Adult Intelligence Scale (WAIS/WAIS-Revised)	Young adult, adult, older adult, and geriatric	Various cognitive abilities and function (level of impairment), such as attention, memory, problem solving, and visual abilities.	Well-established reliability and validity data in literature for both measures.

neuro-sensorimotor treatment evaluation approaches. For cognitive-perceptual interventions, outcomes measuring changing body functions (remediation) and/or modifying the skills or task were prominent (adaptive). In terms of occupational therapy focusing on neuro-sensorimotor interventions, outcomes were largely related to changing body functions (remediation).

Cognitive-Perceptual Outcome Measurement

For cognitive or perceptual occupational therapy intervention, the following outcomes were evaluated.

Impairment level focus to change body functions:
▲ Cognitive abilities (e.g., attention, memory, problem solving)
▲ Perceptual abilities (e.g., visual-spatial abilities, scanning)
    Functional focus to modify skill/task:
▲ Abilities related to ADL or independence

Neuro-Sensorimotor Outcome Measurement

For occupational therapy interventions focused on sensory or neuro-motor approaches, the strategy of remediation at the impairment level was emphasized;

however, outcomes were on occasion measured at both the impairment and functional level.

Impairment level focus to change body functions:
▲ Neuro-motor abilities (e.g., motor performance, pain)
▲ Sensory abilities (e.g., sensory defensiveness, vestibular)
    Functional focus to modify skill/task:
▲ Abilities related to activities of daily living or independence

Outcome Measures to Assess Cognitive-Neurological Interventions

From the scoping reviews of cognitive-perceptual interventions, the areas of outcomes measurement that were best evaluated by a combination of measures included the Mini Mental Status Examination (MMSE), Wechsler Adult Intelligence Scale (WAIS/WAIS-Revised), and Brief Psychiatric Rating Scale (BPRS) for impairment-focused assessments, as well as the Functional Independence Measure (FIM) to evaluate intervention impacting at the level of function. See Table 11-8 for a full description of the measures.

The scoping reviews also demonstrated that most outcome measures focusing on changes at the impairment level included the Mini Mental Status Examination (MMSE), Fugl-Meyer Assessment (FMA), Wolf Motor Function Test (WMFT), and the

Table 11-9
OUTCOME MEASURES TO ASSESS NEURO-SENSORIMOTOR INTERVENTIONS

Measure	Population	Content Domains	Reliability and Validity
Functional Independence Measure (FIM)	Geriatric	Functional ADL independence in terms of personal care.	Studies reported strong internal consistency and inter-rater reliability, as well as good content, convergent, predictive, and construct validity (Law, Baum, & Dunn, 2005).
Fugl-Meyer Assessment (FMA)	Adult and geriatric	Physical impairment (e.g., upper extremity motor components or arm deficits).	Studies provided inter-rater reliability of assessment (Sanford, Moreland, Swanson, Stratford, & Gowland, 1993).
Motor Activity Log (MAL)	Adult and geriatric	Structured participant interview of real-world arm use. Can be provided to caregiver if necessary.	Studies did not indicate psychometric properties of this outcome measure.
Mini Mental Status Examination (MMSE)	Adult and geriatric	Cognitive state and basic mental functions, which is also a concern when considering neuro-sensorimotor deficits.	Studies demonstrate test-retest and intra-rater and inter-rater reliability. Furthermore, validity has been measured in terms of concurrent, construct, predictive, and content (Molloy et al., 1991).
Wolf Motor Function Test (WMFT)	Adult and geriatric	15 functional tasks that are timed and rated by using a 6-point functional ability scale.	Studies have reported high inter-rater reliability, internal consistency, and test-retest reliability (Morris, Uswatte, Crago, Cook, & Taub, 2001), as well as construct and criterion validity (Wolf, Catlin, Ellis, Link Archer, Morgan, & Piacentino, 2001).

Motor Activity Log (MAL). On occasion, occupational therapy research used function-based assessments to evaluate neuro-sensorimotor interventions, such as the Functional Independence Measure (FIM). See Table 11-9 for a full description of the measures.

Conclusions and Recommendations for Future Research

Research pertaining to cognitive-neurological occupational therapy interventions is mainly focused on either remediating body function deficits or adapting the client's skills/task to enable improved function. Very few studies measure the combination of remediation and adaptive strategies used in cognitive-neurological interventions. In addition, outcome measures that were used focused mainly on evaluating at the impairment level, and only on occasion were they coupled with functional assessments.

In light of the increasing frequency of more occupational therapy interventions that combine remediation with adaptive approaches, future outcome measures could focus on function or occupation-based evaluation, for instance, the Assessment for Motor and Processing Scales (AMPS), which is an occupation-based assessment that has been moderately (positively) correlated with a measure of body function (impairment level), namely the Allen Cognitive Level (ACL) Test (Marom, Jarus, & Josman, 2006). More research on evaluating the components remediating client abilities and adaptive approaches to function individually and collectively can help determine the weighting of each approach in occupational therapy intervention.

References

Bach, D., Bach, M., Bohmer, F., Fruhwald, T., & Grilc, B. (1995). Reactivating occupational therapy: A method to improve cognitive performance in geriatric patients. *Age and Ageing, 24*, 222-226.

Baum, C. M., & Christiansen, C. H. (2005). Person-environment-occupation-performance: An occupation-based framework for practice. In C. H. Christiansen, C. M. Baum, & J. Bass-Haugen (Eds.), *Occupational therapy: Performance, participation, and well-being* (3rd ed.). Thorofare, NJ: SLACK Incorporated.

Bell, A., & Murray, B. (2004). Improvement in upper limb motor performance following stroke: The use of mental practice. *British Journal of Occupational Therapy, 67*, 501-507.

Bjorklund, A., & Fecht, A. (2006). The effectiveness of constraint induced therapy as a stroke intervention: A meta-analysis. *Occupational Therapy in Health Care, 20*, 31-49.

Boman, I., Lindstedt, M., Hemmingsson, H., & Bartfai, A. (2004). Cognitive training in home environment. *Brain Injury, 18*(10), 985-995.

Bonifer, N. M., Anderson, K. M., & Arciniegas, D. B. (2005). Constraint-induced movement therapy after stroke: Efficacy for patients with minimal upper-extremity motor ability. *Archives of Physical Medicine and Rehabilitation, 86*(9), 1867-1873.

Bowen, A., Lincoln, N. B., & Dewey, M. (2002). Cognitive rehabilitation for spatial neglect following stroke. *Cochrane Database of Systematic Reviews*. Issue 2. Art No.: CD003586. DOI: 10.1002/14651858.CD003586.

Brown, C., Harwood, K., Hays, C., Heckman, J., & Short, E. (1993). Effectiveness of cognitive rehabilitation for improving attention in patients with schizophrenia. *Occupational Therapy Journal of Research, 13*(2), 71-86.

Campbell, L., Wilson, F. C., McCann, J., Kernahan, G., & Rogers, R. G. (2007). Single case experimental design study of carer facilitated errorless learning in a patient with severe memory impairment following TBI. *Neurorehabilitation, 22*(4), 325-333.

Carney, N., Chesnut, R., Maynard, H., Mann, N., Patterson, P., & Helfand, M. (1999). Effect of cognitive rehabilitation on outcomes for persons with traumatic brain injury: A systematic review. *Journal of Head Trauma Rehabilitation, 14*, 277-307.

Carter, L., Howard, B., & O'Neil, W. (1983). Effectiveness of cognitive skill remediation in acute stroke patients. *American Journal of Occupational Therapy, 37*(5), 320-326.

Cartwright, D. L., Madill, H. M., & Dennis, S. (1996). Cognitive impairment and functional performance of patients admitted to a geriatric assessment and rehabilitation centre. *Physical and Occupational Therapy in Geriatrics, 14*, 1-21.

Chen, S. H. A., Thomas, J. D., Glueckauf, R. L., & Bracy, O. L. (1997). The effectiveness of computer-assisted cognitive rehabilitation for persons with traumatic brain injury. *Brain Injury, 11*(3), 197-209.

Cicerone, K. D., Mott, T., Azulay, J., & Friel, J. C. (2004). Community integration and satisfaction with functioning after intensive cognitive rehabilitation for traumatic brain injury. *Archives of Physical Medicine and Rehabilitation, 85*(6), 943-950.

Cicinelli, P., Traversa, R., & Rossini, P. M. (1997). Post-stroke reorganization of brain motor output to the hand: A 2-4 month follow-up with focal magnetic transcranial stimulation. *Electroencephalography and Clinical Neurophysiology, 105*, 438-450.

Cohen, H., & Kimball, K. (2003). Increased independence and decreased vertigo after vestibular rehabilitation. *Otolaryngology—Head and Neck Surgery, 128*, 60-70.

Desrosiers, J., Bourbonnais, D., Corriveau, H., Gosselin, S., & Bravo, G. (2005). Effectiveness of unilateral and symmetrical bilateral task training for arm during the subacute phase after stroke: A randomized controlled trial. *Clinical Rehabilitation, 19*(6), 581-593.

Dirette, D., & Hinojosa, J. (1999). The effects of a compensatory intervention on processing deficits of adults with acquired brain injuries. *Occupational Therapy Journal of Research, 19*(4), 223-238.

Dolhi, C., Leibold, M. L., & Schreiber, J. (2003). Sensorimotor techniques. In E. Crepeau, E. Cohn, & B. Boyt Schell (Eds.), *Willard & Spackman's occupational therapy* (10th ed., pp. 595-606). Philadelphia, PA: Lippincott Williams & Wilkins.

Doornhein, K., & deHaan, E. H. F. (1998). Cognitive training for memory deficits in stroke patients. *Neuropsychological Rehabilitation, 8*(4), 393-400.

Dromerick, A. W., Edwards, D. F., & Hahn, M. (2000). Does the application of constraint induced movement therapy during acute rehabilitation reduce arm impairment after ischemic stroke? *Stroke, 31*, 2984-2988.

Edmans, J. A., & Webster, J. (2000). A comparison of two approaches in the treatment of perceptual problems after stroke. *Clinical Rehabilitation, 14*, 230-243.

Flinn, N. A., Schamburg, S., Fetrow, J. M., & Flanigan, J. (2005). The effect of constraint-induced movement treatment on occupational performance and satisfaction in stroke survivors. *OTJR: Occupation, Participation, and Health, 25*(3), 119-127.

Forbes, D. (2004). Multisensory stimulation was not better than usual activities for changing cognition, behaviour, and mood in dementia. *Evidence-Based Nursing, 7*(2), 55.

Gagnon, D. L. (1996). A review of reality orientation (RO), validation therapy (VT), and reminiscence therapy (RT) with the Alzheimer's client. *Physical and Occupational Therapy in Geriatrics, 14*(2), 661-675.

Geusgens, C., van Heughten, C., Donkervoort, M., van den Ende, E., Jolles, J., & van den Heuvel, W. (2006). Transfer of training effects in stroke patients with apraxia: An exploratory study. *Neuropsychological Rehabilitation, 16*(2), 213-229.

Gillot, A., Holder-Walls, A., Kurtz, J., & Varley, N. (2003). Perceptions and experiences of two survivors of stroke who participated in constraint-induced movement therapy home programs. *American Journal of Occupational Therapy, 57*, 168-176.

Gilmore, P. E., & Spaulding, S. J. (2007). Motor learning and the use of videotape feedback after stroke. *Topics in Stroke Rehabilitation, 14*, 28-36.

Giuffrida, C. G. (2003). Motor control theories and models guiding occupational performance interventions principles and assumptions. In E. Crepeau, E. Cohn, B. Boyt Schell (Eds.). *Willard & Spackman's occupational therapy* (10th ed., pp. 587-594). Philadelphia, PA: Lippincott Williams & Wilkins.

Greenhalgh, T. (2006). *How to read a paper: The basics of evidence-based medicine* (3rd ed.). London, England: Blackwell Publishing Ltd.

Gutman, S., Diamond, H., Holness-Parchment, S., Brandofino, D., Pacheco, D., Jolly-Edouard, M., et al. (2004). Enhancing independence in women experiencing domestic violence and possible brain injury: An assessment of an occupational therapy intervention. *Occupational Therapy in Mental Health, 20*(1), 49-79.

Hadas-Lidor, N., Katz, N., Tyano, S., & Weizman, A. (2001). Effectiveness of dynamic cognitive intervention in rehabilitation of clients with schizophrenia. *Clinical Rehabilitation, 15*(4), 349-359.

Hayes, R. L., & McGrath, J. J. (2000). Cognitive rehabilitation for people with schizophrenia and related conditions. *Cochrane Database of Systematic Reviews, 3*, 1-29.

Jao, H. P., & Lu, S. J. (1999). The acquisition of problem-solving skills through the instruction in Siegel and Spivack's problem-solving therapy for the chronic schizophrenic. *Occupational Therapy in Mental Health, 14*(4), 47-63.

Kawahira, K., Shimodozono, M., Ogata, A., & Tanaka, N. (2004). Addition of intensive repetition of facilitation exercise to multidisciplinary rehabilitation promotes motor functional recovery of the hemiplegic lower limb. *Journal of Rehabilitation Medicine, 36*(4), 159-164.

Kelly, M., & Shah, S. (2002). Axonal sprouting and neuronal connectivity following central nervous system insult: Implications for occupational therapy. *British Journal of Occupational Therapy, 65*(10), 469-475.

Kunkel, A., Kopp, B., Muller, G., Villringer, K., Villringer, A., Taub, E., & Flor, H. (1999). Constraint-induced movement therapy for motor recovery in chronic stroke patients. *Archives of Physical Medicine and Rehabilitation, 80*, 624-628.

Lamport, N. K., Coffey, M. S., & Hersch, G. I. (2001). *Activity analysis and application* (4th ed.). Thorofare, NJ: SLACK Incorporated.

Law, M., Baum, C., & Dunn, W. (2005). *Measuring occupational performance: Supporting best practice in occupational therapy* (2nd ed.). Thorofare, NJ: SLACK Incorporated.

Lee, S. S., Powell, N. J., & Esdaile, S. (2001). A functional model of cognitive rehabilitation in occupational therapy. *Canadian Journal of Occupational Therapy, 68*, 41-50.

Lincoln, N. B., Whiting, S. E., Cockburn, J., & Bhavnani, G. (1985). An evaluation of perceptual retraining. *International Rehabilitation Medicine, 7*, 99-110.

Ma, H. I., & Trombly, C. A. (2002). A synthesis of the effects of occupational therapy for persons with stroke, part II: Remediation of impairments. *American Journal of Occupational Therapy, 56*(3), 260-274.

Majid, M. J., Lincoln, N. B., & Weyman, N. (2000). Cognitive rehabilitation for memory deficits following stroke. *Cochrane Database of Systematic Reviews*. Issue 3. Art. No.: CD002293. DOI: 10.1002/14651858.CD002293.

Marom, B., Jarus, T., & Josman, N. (2006). The relationship between the assessment of motor and process skills (AMPS) and the Large Allen Cognitive Level (LACL) Test in clients with stroke. *Physical and Occupational Therapy in Geriatrics, 24*, 33-50.

McColl, M. A. (2002). Introduction: A basis for theory in occupational therapy. In M. A. McColl, M. Law, D. Stewart, L. Doubt, N. Pollock,

& T. Krupa (Eds.). *Theoretical basis of occupational therapy* (2nd ed., pp. 1-6). Thorofare, NJ: SLACK Incorporated.

McMenamy, C., Ralph, N., Auen, E., & Nelson, L. (2004). Treatment of complex regional pain syndrome in a multidisciplinary chronic pain program. *American Journal of Pain Management, 14*(2), 56-62.

Miles Breslin, D. M. (1996). Motor-learning theory and the neuro-developmental treatment approach: A comparative analysis. *Occupational Therapy in Health Care, 10,* 25-40.

Molloy, D., Alemayehu, M. B., & Roberts, R. (1991). Reliability of a standardized mini-mental state examination compared with the traditional mini-mental state examination. *American Journal of Psychiatry, 148,* 102-105.

Morris, D. M., Uswatte, G., Crago, J. E., Cook, E. W., & Taub, E. (2001). The reliability of the Wolf Motor Function Test for assessing upper extremity function in stroke. *Archives of Physical Medicine and Rehabilitation, 82,* 750-755.

Mullen, B., Champagne, T., Krishnamurty, S., Dickson, D., & Gao, R. X. (2008). Exploring the safety and therapeutic effects of deep pressure stimulation, using a weighted blanket. *Occupational Therapy in Mental Health, 24*(1), 65.

Ng, S., Lo, A., Lee, G., Lam, M., Yeong, E., Koo, M., et al. (2006). Report of the outcomes of occupational therapy programmes for elderly persons with mild cognitive impairment (MCI) in community elder centres. *Hong Kong Journal of Occupational Therapy, 16,* 16-22.

Oerlemans, H. M., Oostendorp, R. A., de Boo, T., van der Laan, L., Severens, J. L., & Goris, J. A. (2000). Adjuvant physical therapy versus occupational therapy in patients with reflex sympathetic dystrophy/complex regional pain syndrome type I. *Archives of Physical Medicine and Rehabilitation, 81*(1), 49-56.

Page, S. (2000). Imagery improves upper extremity motor function in chronic stroke patients: A pilot study. *Occupational Therapy Journal of Research, 20*(3), 200-215.

Page, S. J., Levine, P., Sisto, S., & Johnston, M. V. (2001). A randomized efficacy and feasibility study of imagery in acute stroke. *Clinical Rehabilitation, 15*(3), 233-240.

Page, S. J., Sisto, S., Johnston, M. V., & Levine, P. (2002). Modified constraint-induced therapy after subacute stroke: A preliminary study. *Neurorehabilitation and Neural Repair, 16,* 290-295.

Page, S. J., Sisto, S., Levine, P., & McGrath, R. E. (2004). Efficacy of modified constraint-induced movement therapy in chronic stroke: A single-blinded randomized controlled trial. *Archives of Physical Medicine and Rehabilitation, 85,* 14-18.

Paire, J., & Karney, R. (1984). The effectiveness of sensory stimulation for geropsychiatric inpatients. *American Journal of Occupational Therapy, 38*(8), 505-509.

Pfeiffer, B., & Kinnealey, M. (2003). Treatment of sensory defensiveness in adults. *Occupational Therapy International, 10*(3), 175-184.

Pierce, S. R., Gallagher, K. G., Schaumburg, S. W., Gershkoff, A. M., Gaughan, J. P., & Shutter, L. (2003). Home forced use in an outpatient rehabilitation program for adults with hemiplegia: A pilot study. *Neurorehabilitation and Neural Repair, 17*(4), 214-219.

Rice, M. S., & Hernandez, H. G. (2006). Frequency of knowledge of results and motor learning in persons with developmental delay. *Occupational Therapy International, 13*(1), 35-48.

Roberts, P. S., Vegher, J. A., Gilewski, M., Bender, A., & Riggs, R. V. (2005). Client-centered occupational therapy using constraint-induced therapy. *Journal of Stroke and Cerebrovascular Diseases, 14*(3), 115-121.

Sanford, J., Moreland, J., Swanson, L. R., Stratford, P. W., & Gowland, C. (1993). Reliability of the Fugl-Meyer assessment for testing motor performance in patients following stroke. *Physical Therapy, 73,* 447-454.

Soderback, I. (1988). The effectiveness of training intellectual functions in adults with acquired brain injury. *Scandinavian Journal of Rehabilitation Medicine, 20,* 47-56.

Soper, G., & Thorley, C. R. (1996). Effectiveness of an occupational therapy programme based on sensory integration theory for adults with severe learning disabilities. *British Journal of Occupational Therapy, 59*(10), 475-482.

Spaulding, W. D., Reed, D., Sullivan, M., Richardson, C., & Weiler, M. (1999). Effects of cognitive treatment in psychiatric rehabilitation. *Schizophrenia Bulletin, 25*(4), 657-676.

Spector, A. E., Orrell, M., Davies, S. P., & Woods, B. (2000). Reality orientation for dementia. *Cochrane Database of Systematic Reviews.* Issue 3. Art. No.: CD001119. DOI: 10.1002/14651858.CD001119.pub2.

Sterr, A., Szameitat, A., Shen, S., & Freivogel, S. (2006). Application of the CIT concept in the clinical environment: Hurdles, practicalities and clinical nenefits. *Cognitive and Behvioral Neurology, 19*(1), 48-54.

Toglia, J. (2003). Cognitive-perceptual retraining and rehabilitation. In E. Crepeau, E. Cohn, & B. Boyt Schell (Eds.), *Willard & Spackman's occupational therapy* (10th ed., pp. 607-629). Philadelphia, PA: Lippincott Williams & Wilkins.

Unwin, R., & Ballinger, C. (2005). The effectiveness of sensory integration therapy to improve functional behaviour in adults with learning disabilities: Five single-case experimental designs. *British Journal of Occupational Therapy, 68*(2), 56-66.

Uomoto, J. M. (1992). Neuropsychological assessment and cognitive rehabilitation after brain injury. *Physical Medicine and Rehabilitation Clinics of North America, 3,* 291-318.

Velligan, D., Mahurin, R., True, J., Lefton, R., & Flores, C. (1996). Preliminary evaluation of adaptation to training to compensate for cognitive deficits in schizophrenia. *Psychiatric Services, 47*(4), 415-417.

Volpe, B. T., Krebs, H. I., Hogan, N., Edelstein, L., Diels, C., & Aisen, M. (2000). A novel approach to stroke rehabilitation: Robot-aided sensorimotor stimulation. *Neurology, 54*(10), 1938-1944.

Wallis, G. G., Baldwin, M., & Higginbotham, P. (1983). Reality orientation therapy: A controlled trial. *British Journal of Medical Psychology, 56,* 271-277.

Watson, H. K., & Carlson, L. (1987). Treatment of reflex sympathetic dystrophy of the hand with an active "stress loading" program. *Journal of Hand Surgery, 12A,* 779-785.

Wolf, S. L., Catlin, P. A., Ellis, M., Link Archer, A., Morgan, B., & Piacentino, A. (2001). Assessing Wolf Motor Function Test as outcome measure for research in patients after stroke. *Stroke, 32,* 1635-1639.

Wolf, S. L., Winstein, C. J., Miller, J. P., Taub, E., Uswatte, G., Morris, D., et al. (2006). Effect of constraint-induced movement therapy on upper extremity function 3 to 9 months after stroke. *Journal of the American Medical Association, 296,* 2095-2104.

Woods, B., Spector, A., Jones, C., Orrell, M., & Davies, S. (2005). Reminiscence therapy for dementia. *Cochrane Database of Systematic Reviews.* Issue 2. Art. No.: CD001120. DOI:10.1002/14651858.CD001120. pub2.

World Health Organization. (2001). *International classification of functioning, disability and health.* Geneva, Switzerland: Author.

Wykes, T., Reeder, C., Corner, J., Williams, C., & Everitt, B. (1999). The effects of neurocognitive remediation on executive processing in patients with schizophrenia. *Schizophrenia Bulletin, 25*(2), 291-307.

Wykes, T., Reeder, C., Williams, C., Corner, J., Rice, C., & Everitt, B. (2003). Are the effects of cognitive remediation therapy (CRT) durable? Results from an exploratory trial in schizophrenia. *Schizophrenia Research, 61,* 163-174.

12

CONCLUSION AND RECOMMENDATIONS

Mary Law, PhD, FCAOT and Mary Ann McColl, PhD, MTS

The purpose of this book was to assemble and discuss evidence about the effectiveness of occupational therapy for adults. The scoping review methodology (Arksey & O'Malley, 2005) was used to identify the most rigorous research published internationally related to occupational therapy outcomes. The specific objectives for the scoping review were

▲ To identify a finite set of **interventions** with which occupational therapists are most often associated and to provide details of those intervention approaches

▲ To identify where the research evidence shows that occupational therapists can achieve specific **effects** as a result of those interventions

▲ To identify the **outcome** measures most commonly and reliably used by researchers to demonstrate the effects of occupational therapy interventions

The scoping review identified 467 studies that described and evaluated occupational therapy interventions. The results of the scoping review were summarized in nine chapters, corresponding to the nine areas where occupational therapy can be shown to make a difference. Each chapter focuses on

▲ **Interventions:** The ways occupational therapists purposefully interact with their clients to improve

occupation. These interventions can be provided by occupational therapists alone or by occupational therapists working within an inter-professional team.

▲ **Effects:** The evidence that occupational therapy can be successful in achieving positive changes as a result of intervention.

▲ **Outcomes:** The measures that occupational therapists use to show where occupational therapy has made a difference.

Interventions and Effects

A considerable body of knowledge has accrued during the past 28 years about the effects of occupational therapy interventions. For this book, we have classified occupational therapy interventions using a taxonomy of eight categories. These intervention categories are intended to help occupational therapists think about their practice as a composite of a finite set of these interventions. In this way, it may be possible to validate sets of interventions or intervention approaches, rather than having to validate every

M. Law & M. A. McColl (Eds.)
Interventions, Effects, and Outcomes in Occupational Therapy:
Adults and Older Adults (pp. 325-330)
© 2010 SLACK Incorporated

distinct intervention in every possible setting. Rather, we hope to show the relative effectiveness of particular occupational therapy interventions for particular aspects of practice.

The book is organized to cover three areas of occupation (self-care, productivity, and leisure), overall participation (a synthesis of the three areas of occupation), and five determinants of occupation (physical, cognitive-neurological, psychological-emotional, socio-cultural, and environmental). A summary of the findings of the scoping review is described below.

Self-Care, Productivity, and Leisure

The scoping review found 29 systematic reviews, 57 studies, and four qualitative studies relating to **self-care** outcomes. The results indicate that occupational therapy intervention can have positive effects on personal care, functional mobility, and community management across several diagnostic categories (e.g., stroke, arthritis, multiple sclerosis, hip fracture/replacement) and for both institutional and community settings. Occupational therapy as part of early supported discharge leads to improved activities of daily living, decreased incidence of depression, and decreased cost. The interventions reported most frequently in the literature are training, skill development, education, task and environmental modification, and provision of support through equipment.

For **productivity and work**, we reviewed 16 systematic reviews and 22 quantitative research studies. Occupational therapy interventions led to significant improvements in knowledge and use of appropriate body mechanics and postures. There is rigorous evidence that a mental health team approach including occupational therapy leads to improved work skills and work participation. These studies include research with assertive community treatment (ACT) teams, supported employment, transitional employment programs, paid work placement, case management, and social skills training. Four randomized controlled trials found that multidisciplinary programs (including occupational therapy) improved work participation. Participants in these studies had chronic pain (two studies), soft tissue injury, or arthritis.

In the area of **leisure**, the scoping review found only three systematic reviews, nine quantitative studies, and one qualitative study. Two clinical trials demonstrated that occupational therapy intervention of home and community programs increased leisure participation and life satisfaction among older adults. Occupational therapy interventions used to promote leisure participation or satisfaction tended to be relatively brief and non-intensive and consist of a mixture of skills teaching, task adaptation, and tool provision.

Participation

For the chapter on **participation in daily occupations**, we reviewed 13 systematic reviews, 27 quantitative studies, and one qualitative study. The interventions used in this research include education and occupational development as part of self-management programs for older adults with chronic disease, task adaptation, and skill development. Evidence from systematic reviews indicates that occupational therapy intervention is effective in improving participation in daily occupations for adults across a range of diagnostic groups and in a variety of intervention settings. Furthermore, systematic reviews indicate that intervention that uses activity and occupation enhances client motivation and leads to improved functional outcomes. Areas of participation where the evidence of effectiveness is strongest include the areas of self-care, domestic life, major life areas, and community, social, and civic life. The amount of research focused on participation in a range of occupations is growing as outcomes increasingly focus on measurement at the level of participation. There have been two recent clinical trials demonstrating significant positive outcomes for occupational therapy prevention programs for older adults.

Determinants of Occupation

Chapters 8 through 11 focused on interventions to change the person-related determinants of occupation—cognitive-neurological, physical, psycho-emotional, and socio-cultural. Chapter 7 focused on environmental determinants.

Interventions for **cognitive-neurological** determinants of occupation tend to either remediate body function deficits or adapt the client's skills/task to enable improved function. The scoping review found 13 systematic reviews, 42 quantitative studies, and one qualitative study. Very few studies measure the combination of remediation and adaptive strategies. Research regarding cognitive remediation after stroke is inconclusive. A recent Cochrane Review evaluating reality orientation in clients with dementia indicated significant cognitive and behavioral outcomes. There is high level evidence that constraint-induced therapy leads to significant changes in movement and functional abilities for people after stroke.

In the area of **psycho-emotional** determinants, the scoping review found nine systematic reviews, 22 quantitative studies, and one qualitative study. Occupational therapy intervention, either individually or as a part of a multidisciplinary team, tends to focus on improving pain, motivation, mood, anxiety, and interpersonal interactions. The interventions studied fall into three categories—comprehensive occupation-based programs, cognitive behavioral programs with a focus on self-management and pacing, and occupational therapy as part of a mental health team. Evidence from two systematic reviews and several clinical trials indicate that occupational therapy has a positive impact on psychosocial well-being (including depressive symptoms) and interaction skills. Multidisciplinary cognitive-behavioral interventions (including occupational therapy) for people with chronic pain have been shown to be effective. A meta-analysis and several clinical trials have found significant improvements that ACT results in a greater reduction in homelessness and greater improvement in psychiatric symptoms such as anxiety, depression, and thought disturbances compared with standard case management treatment.

In the area of the **physical** determinants of occupation, the review identified 33 systematic reviews, 97 quantitative studies, and two qualitative studies. Occupational therapy interventions have focused primarily on training, education, skill development, occupational development, and environmental adaptations, such as wheelchairs, seating, and splints. The most effective areas of occupational therapy intervention for physical impairment appear to be:

▲ Occupationally embedded activity used for training of range of movement, strength, and dexterity

▲ Energy conservation and joint protection using educational-behavioral approaches to improve function, enhance energy, and manage pain

There was no consensus about the effectiveness of splinting, but there was a suggestion that custom splinting may not produce results commensurate with its resource intensity.

With regard to the **socio-cultural** determinants of occupation, this review found only 15 quantitative studies. These studies show that training in social and communication skills can be successful in promoting the development of social interactions, but there is no assurance that these skills will generalize to other social situations. The combination of skills training with purposeful activity appears to promote confidence and lead to a belief in improved ability to participate in social situations. The one study dealing with role development suggests that role functioning can be improved using an educational approach and, furthermore, that this learning is durable over time.

Occupational therapy intervention focuses on removing **environmental** barriers and increasing supports in order to maximize an individual's occupational performance or participation. This review found 14 systematic reviews, 34 quantitative studies, and two qualitative studies on this area. There

is evidence to support the impact of occupational therapy on the following environmental outcomes: safety and prevention, use of adaptive equipment, environmental modification, and equipment/devices. The most significant effects of environmental interventions occurred when programs combined home modifications and education for the client and/or caregiver. Findings indicate that environmental interventions for older adults living at home led to reduced institutional and health care costs.

Another focus of occupational therapy that has been shown to be successful is intervention directed to caregivers (e.g., adapting the home environment to support client functioning, promoting self-efficacy among caregivers, moderating stress and mood, decreasing burden with extra assistance in the home). Several studies demonstrated the effectiveness of caregiver education and training. These interventions focused on training caregivers to improve their skills in using the physical and social environment to maintain client functioning and to address troublesome behavior for family members with dementia.

Outcomes

The incorporation of a valid outcome measure is an essential part of evidence-based occupational therapy. In each chapter of this review, we have recorded the outcome measures used most frequently to measure the effects of intervention. Table 12-1 provides a summary list of the outcome measures that demonstrated positive impacts of occupational therapy intervention. The outcome measures have been divided into those that assess at the level of occupation, environment, or determinants of occupation.

The most notable finding with regard to outcomes is the vast number of measures used across the studies. Many studies used unpublished and unstandardized measures, thereby making their results less readily comparable or understandable to the wide array of readers. Furthermore, there is a lack of consistency in the choice of instruments for measuring the same outcomes. In response to this problem, the National Institutes of Health (2009) have recently begun developing a suite of outcome measures for use in clinical trials.

Recommendations

The foregoing discussion has highlighted the findings of the scoping review and has demonstrated that there are many positive outcomes that can be shown to result from occupational therapy intervention. In Chapter 1, we included a brief review of goal setting

Table 12-1

MOST FREQUENTLY REPORTED OUTCOME MEASURES

Intervention Effects	*Outcome Measures*
Occupation	Assessment of Motor and Process Skills (AMPS)
	Barthel Index (BI)
	Canadian Occupational Performance Measure (COPM)
	Community Integration Measure
	Community Integration Questionnaire (CIQ)
	Craig Handicap Assessment (CHART)
	European Quality of Life (EuroQol)
	Functional Independence Measure (FIM)
	Functional Status Questionnaire
	Health Assessment Questionnaire (HAQ)
	Independent Living Skills Scale (ILSS)
	Life Habits Assessment (LIFE-H)
	Life Satisfaction Scale (LSS)
	Life Satisfaction Index (LSI)
	Number of leisure occupations
	Number of work days
	OARS Multidimensional Functional Assessment Questionnaire
	Return to Normal Living Index (RNLI)
	Short Form Health Survey (SF-36)
	Sickness Impact Profile (SIP)
	Worker Role Interview (WRI)
Environmental determinant	Craig Hospital Inventory of Environmental Factors (CHIEF)
	Environmental Functional Independence Measure (EnviroFIM)
	Home Falls and Accidents Screening Tool (HOME FAST)
	Modified Falls Efficacy Scale (MFES)
	Safety Assessment of Function and the Environment for Rehabilitation (SAFER)
	Work Environment Impact Scale
	Zarit Caregiver Burden Scale (ZCBS)
Determinants of occupation	Brief Psychiatric Rating Scale (BPRS)
	Fugl-Meyer Assessment (FMA)
	Interpersonal Communication Inventory
	Mini Mental Status Examination (MMSE)
	Motor Activity Log (MAL)
	Pain assessments
	Social communication questionnaire
	Social Functioning Scale
	Strength/endurance/range of motion
	Wolf Motor Function Test (WMFT)

because, throughout the book, we assume that occupational therapy uses a goal-oriented client-centered approach. Starting intervention through a structured process of goal setting improves motivation and facilitates a structured therapy intervention focused on the most important occupational performance issues. Research in both occupational therapy and other disciplines indicates that goal setting can have a positive impact on client motivation and outcomes. Thus, the inclusion of a validated approach to goal setting within occupational therapy practice is suggested.

Using the taxonomy developed for this book, and expounded in Chapter 1, interventions have been classified into eight categories that demonstrate both the breadth and the focus of occupational therapy. While this taxonomy cannot be considered completely comprehensive or mutually exclusive, it is a useful starting place for discussion on where occupational therapists have their greatest impact. We urge readers to consider interventions with which they are involved and assess whether they can be classified according to this taxonomy. As has been shown in the preceding review, one seldom finds an intervention that is a pure example of one type. Rather, we tend to see hybrids and combinations of several of these basic intervention approaches used together in practice.

Wherever possible in this review, we have attempted to show where the research validates the theoretical basis of occupational therapy. However, our review noted that many studies did not include an explicit discussion of the theory underpinning the interventions studied, the effects sought, or the outcome measured. It is important to note that it is impossible to validate the practice of occupational therapy—that would require us to literally evaluate every maneuver an occupational therapist might make. Instead, we must seek to validate the theory linking specific occupational therapy interventions to outcomes, or actions to consequences. This is exactly what theory gives us—a way of understanding why we would expect a certain therapeutic maneuver to be associated with a particular desired outcome. Therefore, we recommend that researchers include a discussion of the theory that drove them to design an intervention the way they did, with the expectation of effecting specific outcomes. Further, we encourage researchers to be explicit about the theoretical implications of their conclusions, as well as the practical or clinical implications.

With regard to specific outcomes, leisure warrants some further mention in these conclusions. As one of the core elements of occupation, it is disappointing to find so little research promoting the effectiveness of occupational therapy in this area. As discussed, this may be a function of its usual placement late in the course of rehabilitation; however, given all we know about the need for a balanced lifestyle, it seems essential that occupational therapists focus attention on leisure. Particularly for children and older adults, the impact of leisure occupations becomes increasingly important for health and well-being.

There are also several areas where it would be gratifying to see more creative programming that makes use of the many aspects of occupation and the multi-dimensional nature of occupational therapy. The socio-cultural area is an example where there is considerable opportunity to demonstrate the many unique and varied approaches occupational therapists have at their disposal. Concepts like role performance, time use, cultural sensitivity, and spirituality are highly promising areas for occupational therapy intervention that have a rich history and hopefully a bright future.

Most of the research reviewed for this book centers on remediation and adaptation/compensation as the primary purpose of the occupational therapy intervention. According to Christiansen, Baum, and Bass-Haugen (2005), these are only two of the three main intervention approaches used in occupational therapy. The third approach they call "making the best fit," referring to interventions focused on the broader environment within which individuals exist. Studies focused on advocacy or prevention have been emerging over the past decade, but there has to date been little evidence in the literature for their effectiveness in promoting changes in occupational performance. We look forward to seeing the results of research on some of these less traditional approaches.

The scoping review has provided some information about the intensity of occupational therapy intervention needed to positively impact outcomes. Studies that focused on specific modifications to a few areas of the home, such as a bathroom, demonstrated significant differences after two to three visits. Environmental interventions that were more extensive need to combine education and modifications and have four to eight visits to be effective (see Chapter 7). Community home care interventions of up to 10 times over 6 weeks were effective in improving functional performance for people after stroke (see Chapter 4). In Chapter 4, we cite several studies that indicate that a greater intensity of occupational therapy alone or as part of a multidisciplinary intervention leads to significantly improved functional outcomes. In many studies, the occupational therapy intervention ranged from two to three visits or one to two visits per month. These levels of intensity of intervention are not always enough to effect significant changes in outcome.

It was also noted in several instances that relatively brief and superficial interventions were expected to produce profound and far-reaching outcomes. For example, in the area of leisure, it was noted that interventions of only a few hours in some cases were assessed for their ability to produce far-reaching effects, such as resolving depression or promoting life satisfaction. While it is arguable that these general outcomes may well be associated with a satisfying leisure profile, it is misleading to evaluate leisure interventions on the basis of outcomes so remote from the intervention itself.

The findings also indicate that combinations of more than one intervention strategy are more likely to be effective. For example, studies reviewed in Chapter 7 on the environment indicate that home modification plus education work best. In Chapter 4, we found that self-care intervention is effective when combining training, skill development, and task adaptation.

Research designs have become more rigorous, and substantial evidence exists to support specific areas of occupational therapy intervention. There remains a need for more research with adequate sample sizes in some areas of intervention. Furthermore, research in occupational therapy would benefit greatly from the delineation of a finite set of outcome measures that are sensitive to occupational therapy outcomes and that meet international standards for psychometric rigor. Our recommendation is that the occupational therapist work toward identifying a finite set of outcome measures to use in occupational therapy intervention research. The data from this scoping review indicate that the outcome measures shown in Table 12-1 are used most often in occupational therapy intervention research, measure important constructs for occupational therapy outcomes, and have adequate evidence of reliability and validity. Over the past two decades, the development of outcome measures for use in occupational therapy research has been excellent. It is our hope that we can now move toward consensus about which measures to use and continue the development of measures for the areas in need of further research.

Another problem noted across a number of the studies in the scoping review is the tendency to evaluate relatively distal outcomes of the interventions studied. In addition to measuring the more proximal or direct outcomes sought in response to a particular intervention, occupational therapy research also often assesses more distal measures, such as mood, well-being, or life satisfaction.

For example, in the area of leisure, studies tended to invoke the assumption that greater involvement in leisure activities would lead to improved mood and general well-being. On the basis of that assumption,

investigators would use these distal measures as the outcomes of interest in evaluating the intervention. While it is useful to monitor these broad, general outcomes, it is more pertinent to discover if the intervention produced the direct effects it intended—effects such as increasing the number, frequency, or satisfaction with particular leisure activities. It is also fairer to the intervention in question to evaluate it on outcomes toward which it actually dedicated resources. It is considerably more likely to be productive in terms of research results.

A Final Word—Knowledge Exchange and Transfer

Evidence-based occupational therapy can enhance health and is valued by consumers and policy makers. Many barriers limit effective translation of knowledge into practice. For students and practitioners, the inability to quickly find and evaluate quality research is the most common barrier. The volume of information and research is too much for a student or practitioner to manage.

The evidence summarized in this scoping review addresses some of the limitations in knowledge exchange and transfer. This book includes evidence about occupational therapy intervention research for adults and older adults that has been systematically searched, reviewed, and summarized. The data are accessible and credible. However, making evidence-based knowledge available does not guarantee that it will be used to inform decision making. Our challenge to each reader is to actively use the findings from this review for your study and use in practice. Work together with your colleagues to discern the interventions for which there is evidence. Use outcome measures in your practice to assess the changes after therapy intervention. Everyone can contribute to the growing body of evidence about the effect of occupational therapy intervention.

References

Arksey, H., & O'Malley, L. (2005). Scoping studies: Towards a methodological framework. *International Journal of Social Research Methodology, 8*(1), 19-32.

Christiansen, C., Baum, C., & Bass-Haugen, J. (2005). *Occupational therapy: Performance, participation, and well-being* (3rd ed.). Thorofare, NJ: SLACK Incorporated.

National Institutes of Health. (2009). Patient reported outcomes measurement information system. Retrieved from www.nihpromis.org/default.aspx on March 2, 2009.

ANNOTATED BIBLIOGRAPHY

Akalin, E., El O., Peker, O., Senocak, O., Tamci, S., Gulbahar, S., et al. (2002). Treatment of carpal tunnel syndrome with nerve and tendon gliding exercises. *American Journal of Physical Medicine and Rehabilitation, 81*, 108-113.

    Keywords: carpal tunnel syndrome, gliding exercises, tinels sign, phalens sign

    The aim of this study was to assess the effect of nerve and tendon gliding exercises in carpal tunnel syndrome. This study discusses other studies that have examined conservative treatments of carpal tunnel syndrome. There were no significant differences between a splint and exercises compared with just a splint. There were statistically significant improvements in both groups measured by many assessments. Further investigations are necessary to discover the role of nerve and tendon gliding exercises in the treatment of carpal tunnel syndrome.

Aldehag, A. S., Jonsson, H., & Ansved, T. (2005). Effects of a hand training programme in five patients with myotonic dystrophy type 1. *Occupational Therapy International, 12*(1), 14-27.

    Keywords: myotonic dystrophy, hand training, occupational performance

    The aim of this study was to assess hand function and self-rated occupational performance in patients with myotonic dystrophy type I before and after completing a hand training program. The training program focused on resistance training, and participants completed exercises with a therapeutic silicone-based putty three times a week for 3 months. Hand function increased significantly after completion of the training program, and a positive change in self-rated occupational performance was observed.

Alexander, H., Bugge, C., & Hagen, S. (2001). What is the association between the different components of stroke rehabilitation and health outcomes? *Clinical Rehabilitation, 15*, 207-215.

    Keywords: rehabilitation, health outcomes

    This study examined the association between the different components of stroke. Study aims were to investigate the relationship between different types of rehabilitation following stroke in order to examine impact on health status and level of disability at 1, 3, and 6 months post-stroke. Results indicate that those with the poorest health status received the greatest amount of rehabilitation. Additionally, some types of rehab (occupational therapy, community nursing) are correlated with specific health outcomes.

Alexander, J. A., Lichtenstein, R., Jinnet, K., Wells, R., Zazzeli, J., & Liu, D. (2005). Cross-functional team processes and patient functional improvement. *Health Services Research, 40*, 1335-1355.

    Keywords: cross-functional team, activities of daily living, team functioning, participation

    The purpose of this study was to examine correlations between processes of a multidisciplinary (cross-functional) team and clients' functional status as measured by ADL performance. A multi-level, longitudinal analysis was used, as opposed to a randomized controlled trial, in an attempt to better address specific team processes. Key results indicate that level of team participation is positively correlated with ADL progress/performance over time. Possibilities for future research include examination of other team processes, such as conflict resolution. As well, an attempt to further understand the impact of team functioning may be possible by examining differences between team function and performance.

Alvund, K., Jepsen, E., Vass, M., & Lundemark, H. (2002). Effects of comprehensive follow-up home visits after hospitalization on functional ability and readmissions in older people. A randomized controlled study. *Scandinavian Journal of Occupational Therapy, 9*, 17-22.

    Keywords: comprehensive geriatric assessment, readmissions, elderly, home visits, geriatric team

    The purpose of this study was to investigate whether home visits from interdisciplinary teams after discharge from hospital impacted older people's functional abilities and readmission status. Results were largely non-significant in terms of demonstrating any impact of the intervention on readmission and functional ability, when examining controls versus intervention groups. However, those discharged from medical units did show an effect of intervention compared to controls from medical units. Researchers concluded that those significant results might be related to the fact that standard discharge procedures in acute, short-stay units are not adequate. They suggest a need to examine discharge planning procedures for older adults from other types of wards and with different diagnoses.

Arnetz, B. (1985). Gerontic occupational therapy—psychological and social predictors of participation and therapeutic benefits. *American Journal of Occupational Therapy, 39*(7), 460-465.

    Keywords: activity programs, aged, geriatrics, institutionalization, services, occupational therapy

    The article begins by highlighting the impact of social under-stimulation among older adults who are institutionalized as a physiological stressor that can impact their health and well-being. A study reports the impact of a gerontic occupational therapy (social activation) program aimed at improving mood and loneliness to increase activity level. One of the major findings of the study was that subjects who initially had a low social activity level increased their participation the most after the initiation of the program. The author concluded that gerontic occupational therapy plays an important role in preventing unnecessary social isolation in institutional living.

Austin, J., Williams, R., Ross, L., Moseley, L., & Hutchison, S. (2005). Randomised controlled trial of cardiac rehabilitation in elderly patients with heart failure. *European Journal of Heart Failure, 7*(3 special issue), 411-417.

    Keywords: heart failure, elderly, cardiac rehabilitation, health-related quality of life, multidisciplinary intervention

    The aim of this study was to determine whether a cardiac rehabilitation program led to improved outcomes for stroke patients over the age of 60 compared to a standard care program. Participants in the experimental group received standard care plus the cardiac rehabilitation program, which consisted of education, exercise, and counseling from a multidisciplinary team that included occupational therapy, dietetics, and psychology/social work. Significant improvements for the cardiac rehabilitation group were seen for health-related quality of life, functional status, and functional performance. In addition, the number of hospital admissions and length of stay once admitted decreased for this group. The study concluded that a multidisciplinary cardiac rehabilitation program offers an effective model of care for older patients with heart failure as it can improve symptoms, functional performance, and health-related quality of life and decrease hospital admissions due to heart disease.

Bach, D., Bach, M., Bohmer, F., Fruhwald, T., & Grilc, B. (1995). Reactivating occupational therapy: A method to improve cognitive performance in geriatric patients. *Age and Ageing, 24*, 222-226.

> *Keywords*: reactivating occupational therapy
>
> The article opens by highlighting the processes required for the engagement in activities and the purpose of conventional versus reactivating occupational therapy for a geriatric population. The study aimed to determine whether the addition of reactivating occupational therapy to functional rehabilitation would result in increased cognitive and psychosocial function and levels of contentedness. Functional rehabilitation alone was found to be inferior to functional rehabilitation and reactivating occupational therapy on measures of cognition, psychosocial function, and contentedness.

Bailey, A., Starr, L., Alderson, M., & Moreland, J. (1999). A comparative evaluation of a (No Suggestions) rehabilitation program. *Arthritis Care and Research, 12*(5), 336-340.

> *Keywords*: fibromyalgia, interdisciplinary
>
> This article looks at the Fibro-Fit program run by an occupational therapist, physiotherapist, and a social worker for people with fibromyalgia. The program is based on education and exercise within small groups, which focuses on three previous study findings by other researchers. The results showed significant changes in almost all outcomes investigated and stated that improvement in overall disability was clinically significant.

Barry, M. A., Purser, J., Hazleman, R., McLean, A., & Hazleman, B. L. (1994). Effect of energy conservation and joint protection education in rheumatoid arthritis. *British Journal of Rheumatology, 33*(12), 1171-1174.

> *Keywords*: occupational therapy, rheumatoid arthritis
>
> This article describes a study conducted to determine the effect of occupational therapy intervention on clients with rheumatoid arthritis. The intervention involved instruction on joint protection and energy conservation maneuvers. The study concludes that occupational therapy intervention is effective in improving client knowledge and performance, and this is sustained for at least 6 months.

Baskett, J. J., Broad, J. B., Reekie, G., Hocking, C., & Green, G. (1999). Shared responsibility for ongoing rehabilitation: A new approach to home-based therapy after stroke. *Clinical Rehabilitation, 13*(1), 23-33.

> This study reports on the results of a randomized controlled trial with stroke survivors participating in rehabilitation exercises. Subjects were grouped into an experimental group consisting of weekly home visits by an occupational therapist or physiotherapist to plan exercises and activities, or rehabilitation in an outpatient clinic. The authors conclude that there are no statistically significant differences in the effects of either intervention.

Bendix, T., Bendix, A., Labriola, M., Haestrup, C., & Ebbenhoj, N. (2000). Functional restoration versus outpatient physical training in chronic low back pain. *Spine, 25*(19), 2429-2500.

> *Keywords*: chronic lower back pain, functional restoration, outpatient physical training
>
> The study compares functional restoration with outpatient physical training for adults with lower back pain living in Denmark. The functional restoration is a multidisciplinary approach with an occupational therapist and physiotherapist involved in the team. Many variables such as work capability and back pain were measured using self-report tools. The study shows that the two rehabilitation approaches are only statistically significant in their overall assessment with functional restoration being more favorable and that both are beneficial for this population.

Bendstrup, K. E., Ingemann Jensen, J., Holm, S., & Bengtsson, B. (1997). Out-patient rehabilitation improves activities of daily living, quality of life and exercise tolerance in chronic obstructive pulmonary disease. *European Respiratory Journal, 10*(12), 2801-2806.

> *Keywords*: activities of daily living, chronic obstructive pulmonary disease, controlled, randomized design, quality of life, rehabilitation, six minute walking test
>
> This study examines the effects of a 12-week outpatient rehabilitation intervention program for people with chronic obstructive pulmonary disease (COPD) on activities of daily living (ADL), quality of life, exercise tolerance, and spirometry. The intervention group took part in a 12-week program containing exercise therapy, occupational therapy, education about COPD, and help with smoking cessation (if wanted by participants who were smokers). Results indicated that the outpatient rehabilitation program improved ADL, quality of life, and exercise tolerance for people with COPD. The study concluded that a comprehensive outpatient rehabilitation program can produce long-term improvement in ADL, quality of life, and exercise tolerance in patients with moderate-to-severe COPD.

Bishop, S. A., Bulla, N., DiLellio, E., Dy, M., Koski, J. H., Linnemeyer, C. B., et al. (1999). The effects of low-cost wheelchair cushions and body-type on dynamic sitting pressure in nursing home residents. *Physical and Occupational Therapy in Geriatrics, 17*(1), 29-41.

> *Keywords*: physical disabilities, rehabilitation, wheelchair cushions, gerontology, pressure sores, ulcers
>
> The article begins with a discussion of pressure sores in the elderly population due to extended periods of time spent sitting. It then examines four different low-cost wheelchair pads to see if there is a difference in the amount of pressure recorded for each while sitting in a variety of positions and to see if different pads are better for certain body types. Although no significant differences for seated pressure were found between the four wheelchairs, some descriptive trends may have shown that certain wheelchair pads are more favorable for certain body types. The authors conclude that more research in this area needs to be completed.

Bode, R. K., Heinemann, A. W., Semik, P., & Mallinson, T. (2004). Relative importance of rehabilitation therapy characteristics on functional outcomes for persons with stroke. *Stroke, 35*, 2537-2542.

> *Keywords*: rehabilitation, stroke, stroke outcome
>
> The major aim of this study was to investigate the impact of a number of clinical variables such as therapy focus and intensity and length of hospital stay on "greater than expected" functional gains, in patients who experienced their first stroke. Researchers suggested that using "raw gains" to assess functional outcomes often made the contribution of therapy (to outcomes) unclear because admission status is such a strong predictor of functional ability at discharge. Thus, research used residual change scores to examine the impact of variables on responses to therapy because of the idea that it allows for a clearer picture of the impact of therapy on functional outcomes. Results indicated that when controlling for severity of stroke, longer hospital stays and more intense function-focused therapy was associated with greater-than-expected gains in mobility and self-care. The researchers conclude that residual change scores provide stronger evidence of the dose-response relationship (i.e., therapy intensity to functional gains) than has been previously found using raw gains.

Bohannon, R. W., Ahlquist, M., Lee, N., & Maljanian, R. (2003). Functional gains during acute hospitalization for stroke. *Neurorehabilitation and Neural Repair, 17*, 192-195.

> *Keywords*: stroke, hospital, measurement, outcomes
>
> The purpose of the study was to examine the impact of variables, such as therapy (or therapy units), on discharge function and change in functional independence between admission and discharge. This was deemed important, as the length of acute hospitalization has decreased and rehabilitation has increasingly been moved to post-hospital settings. Results suggest that the strongest predictor of discharge function is function at admission. However, discharge function and functional change over the course of hospitalization were weakly, but significantly predicted by therapy units. Thus, researchers suggest that the study offers limited support for the utility of rehabilitation service in acute care settings.

Bolin, I., Bodin, P., & Kreuter, M. (2000). Sitting position—posture and performance in C5-C6 tetraplegia. *Spinal Cord, 38*(7), 425-434.

> *Keywords*: tetraplegia, wheelchair, posture, balance, sitting position

This article begins by discussing some of the common ergonomic challenges when fitting a wheelchair for a client with a spinal cord injury. It then describes a small cohort study of interventions to reduce kyphotic posture and pelvic obliquity. The authors conclude that the interventions improved the sitting posture and performance of the subjects, although client self-report contradicted some of the results from the outcome measures.

Boman, I., Lindstedt, M., Hemmingsson, H., & Bartfai, A. (2004). Cognitive training in home environment. *Brain Injury, 18*(10), 985-995.
> The study aimed to determine the effectiveness of providing cognitive training in the home or work environment. The study found that home intervention had a positive influence on some indices of impairment; these improvements did not extend to activity or participation levels.

Bonifer, N. M., Anderson, K. M., & Arciniegas, D. B. (2005). Constraint-induced movement therapy after stroke: Efficacy for patients with minimal upper-extremity motor ability. *Archives of Physical Medicine and Rehabilitation, 86*(9), 1867-1873.
> *Keywords*: hemiparesis, rehabilitation, stroke
> This article explores the effects of constraint-induced movement therapy (CIMT) on motor function in the affected limb after stroke. Participants took part in a 3-week CIMT program led by occupational and physical therapists. Results indicate significant improvement on outcome measures of upper limb function and impairment.

Boswell, S. (1989). A social support group for depressed people. *Australian Occupational Therapy Journal, 36*(1), 34-41.
> *Keywords*: depression, mutual support networks, communication skills, evaluation
> The purpose of this study was to set up a support group for depressed patients to help them develop social support networks and to work on communication skills and improving self-perceptions. Statistical improvements were seen for depression and anxiety scores over the course of the program. Participants also began to form supportive relationships (some with each other, some joined community organizations, etc.). The author concluded that the program was beneficial but offered suggestions on how to make improvements in the future.

Braverman, S. E., Spector, J., Warden, D. L., Wilson, B. C., Ellis, T. E., Bamdad, M. J., et al. (1999). A multidisciplinary TBI inpatient rehabilitation programme for active duty service members as part of a randomized clinical trial. *Brain Injury, 13*(6), 405-415.
> *Keywords*: TBI, return to work, military
> The article looks at interdisciplinary intervention for military personnel with moderate traumatic brain injuries based on an inpatient milieu-oriented neuropsychological focus. The intervention, which ran for 10 hours a day for 8 weeks, involved many professionals including an occupational therapist. Although no results were reported statistically, at 12 months follow-up, 96% of the population returned to work in military, and 66% returned to active duty.

Brosseau, L., Philippe, P., Potvin, L., & Boulanger, Y. L. (1996). Post-stroke inpatient rehabilitation. I. predicting length of stay. *American Journal of Physical Medicine and Rehabilitation, 75*, 422-430.
> *Keywords*: length of stay, stroke, rehabilitation, path analysis
> The purpose of this study was to examine factors that may impact length of stay in an inpatient rehabilitation unit for patients with stroke. Results indicated that age positively predicted length of stay, in that older patients had longer lengths of stay. Better functional status 1 week after admission to rehabilitation and balance status were associated with shorter lengths of stay. Additionally, perceptual status was a significant contributor to length of stay. Those with perceptual problems had longer stays than those with higher perceptual abilities.

Brown, C., Harwood, K., Hays, C., Heckman, J., & Short, E. (1993). Effectiveness of cognitive rehabilitation for improving attention in patients with schizophrenia. *Occupational Therapy Journal of Research, 13*(2), 71-86.
> *Keywords*: cognitive retraining, attention, psychiatric occupational therapy, schizophrenia

The study aimed to determine the effects of two different cognitive rehabilitation programs on attention processes and affective determinants of performance. A literature review supported the importance of attention to cognitive training for individuals with schizophrenia. Both interventions had equal effects on cognition and affective determinants of performance. A comprehensive approach was recommended for addressing cognition.

Buchain, P. C., Vizzotto, A. D., Henna Neto, J., & Elkis, H. (2003). Randomized controlled trial of occupational therapy in patients with treatment-resistant schizophrenia. *Revista Brasileira de Psiquiatria, 25*(1), 26-30.
> *Keywords*: schizophrenia, treatment-resistant schizophrenia (TRS)
> This study investigates the effectiveness of occupational therapy added to psychopharmalogical treatment in treating patients with treatment-resistant schizophrenia. The combination of occupational therapy and Clozapine was shown to be more effective than Clozapine on its own.

Buri, H. (1997). A group programme to prevent falls in elderly hospital patients. *British Journal of Therapy and Rehabilitation, 4*, 550-556.
> This article initially discusses the complexity of the etiology of falls for older adults. A pre-test/post-test study was presented that delivered two falls prevention group interventions with some receiving a group education program and an information booklet while others received the information booklet only. Results indicated that subjects receiving the booklet and education program were most likely to show a very high knowledge score in terms of falls prevention strategies but little changed between groups in regard to their attitudes/behavior toward risk-taking 1 month after discharge.

Callinan, N. J., & Mathiowetz, V. (1996). Soft versus hard resting hand splints in rheumatoid arthritis: Pain relief, preference, and compliance. *American Journal of Occupational Therapy, 50*(5), 347-353.
> *Keywords*: hand functions, orthotic devices, rehabilitation, hand
> This article discussed the benefits of hand splints for people with rheumatoid arthritis but also the problems with patient compliance in wearing their splints due to a variety of factors. The study compared two different types of splints (hard and soft) against each other as well as against a no-splint condition to see the effects on pain, hand function, and splint preference. Findings indicate that "resting hand splints are effective for pain relief and that persons with rheumatoid arthritis are more likely to prefer and comply with soft splint use for this purpose."

Campbell, A. J., Robertson, M. C., La Grow, S. J., Kerse, N. M., Sanderson, G. F., Jacobs, R. J., et al. (2005). Randomised controlled trial of prevention of falls in people aged 75 with severe visual impairment: The VIP trial. *British Medical Journal, 331*, 817-823.
> *Keywords*: visual impairment, elderly
> This article aimed to assess the efficacy and cost effectiveness of a home safety program and a home exercise program to reduce falls and injuries in older people with visual impairment. The study shows that the home safety program reduces falls and injuries, but the exercise program does not, possibly due to low levels of adherence.

Campbell, L., Wilson, F. C., McCann, J., Kernahan, G., & Rogers, R. G. (2007). Single case experimental design study of carer facilitated errorless learning in a patient with severe memory impairment following TBI. *Neurorehabilitation, 22*(4), 325-333.
> *Keywords*: memory rehabilitation, errorless learning, family and carers, brain injury
> The objective of this study was to determine if errorless learning given by a carer could reduce the frequency of everyday memory problems. A patient with severe memory deficits as a result of traumatic brain injury was recruited from an outpatient clinic. The patient's carer was trained in the treatment by an occupational therapist. Frequency of memory lapses was significantly reduced, and treatment effect was maintained at 3-month follow-up.

Caplan, G. A., Williams, A. J., Daly, B., & Abraham, K. (2004). A randomized, controlled trial of comprehensive geriatric assessment and multidisciplinary intervention after discharge of elderly from the emergency department—the DEED II study. *Journal of the American Geriatrics Society, 52*, 1417-1423.

Keywords: emergency service, hospital, geriatric assessment, activities of daily living, cognition, patient re-admission

The purpose of this study was to assess health and functional outcomes of geriatric patients who were discharged from the emergency department and received either usual care upon discharge or comprehensive geriatric assessment from a multidisciplinary team. Results indicated that those receiving the intervention had an overall decrease in admissions to hospital, compared to controls, as well as slower decline in both physical and cognitive functions.

Carlton, R. S. (1987). The effects of body mechanics instruction on work performance. *American Journal of Occupational Therapy, 41*(1), 16-20.

Keywords: body mechanics, patient education, work functions

This article examined whether an occupational teaching session on proper body mechanics while lifting and lowering at work, for a group of food service workers, would be effective in teaching body mechanics principles and whether any techniques learned would be implemented in the workplace. Results indicated that participants who received body mechanics testing performed better than those who received no training during lab testing of lifting and lowering but not better in their work environment. The authors conclude that further research is needed on the use of body mechanics instruction in the work environment.

Carter, L., Howard, B., & O'Neil, W. (1983). Effectiveness of cognitive skill remediation in acute stroke patients. *American Journal of Occupational Therapy, 37*(5), 320-326.

The study aimed to examine the ability of a cognitive training program to increase cognition for acute stroke patients. The study reviewed the prevalence of stroke and the importance of the targeted elements of cognition on functional tasks. The study found that cognitive remediation effectively increased cognitive ability compared to controls.

Cartwright, D. L., Madill, H. M., & Dennis, S. (1996). Cognitive impairment and functional performance of patients admitted to a geriatric assessment and rehabilitation centre. *Physical and Occupational Therapy in Geriatrics, 14*, 1-21.

Keywords: rehabilitation, cognitive impairment functional performance

The purpose of this study was to investigate the effectiveness of interventions for cognitively impaired elderly people who were admitted to a geriatric assessment and rehabilitation program. The main outcome measure was functional status. Overall, patients demonstrated significant improvement in functional abilities across the intervention period, regardless of whether they were classified as moderately or severely cognitively impaired. Thus, cognitively impaired people can benefit from intervention in a geriatric rehabilitation setting.

Case-Smith, J. (2003). Outcomes in hand rehabilitation using occupational therapy services. *American Journal of Occupational Therapy, 57*, 499-506.

Keywords: upper-extremity, occupational therapy, outpatient, functional outcome

The aim of this study was to measure functional outcomes after outpatient occupational therapy for clients who had upper extremity injury or surgery or both with the COPM, DASH, SF-36, and CIQ. The study reviews each of these outcome measurements as well as their psychometric properties. The final result was that clients with upper extremity injury or surgery made strong, positive gains in functional measures following client-centered occupational therapy services. The COPM was the most sensitive to change, then the DASH, and then the SF-36.

Chamberlain, M. A., Thornley, G., Stow, J., & Wright, V. (1981). Evaluation of aids and equipment for the bath: II. A possible solution to the problem. *Rheumatology and Rehabilitation, 20*, 38-43.

One hundred patients needing bath aids leaving the hospital were randomly allocated into control and treated groups. Prompt, correct prescription of aids and supervision of their use in bathing shortly after discharge by a hospital-based occupational therapist resulted in safe bathing by all treated subjects, compared to only 82% of control subjects.

Chen, S. H. A., Thomas, J. D., Glueckauf, R. L., & Bracy, O. L. (1997). The effectiveness of computer-assisted cognitive rehabilitation for persons with traumatic brain injury. *Brain Injury, 11*(3), 197-209.

The article described the two major categories of cognitive rehabilitation techniques—traditional and computer assisted. The study described a comparison of computer-assisted cognitive rehabilitation to a group that received various other therapies including occupational therapy and speech-language pathology. Results indicated that there were no significant differences between groups. Both groups demonstrated gains in cognitive function: The computer-assisted group showed significant gains in 15 measures and the traditional group presented significant improvements in seven measures.

Chiu, C. W. Y., & Man, D. W. K. (2004). The effect of training older adults with stroke to use home-based assistive devices. *OTJR: Occupation, Participation, and Health, 24*, 113-120.

Keywords: bathing devices, usage rate, functional independence

This study assessed whether additional home visits and training would improve usage rates and satisfaction with assistive bathing devices after discharge from hospital for people who had a stroke. A prospective pre-test/post-test design was used. Results indicated that functional independence and satisfaction with and use of bathing devices improved for patients who received home visits.

Christensen, O. M., Kunov, A., Hansen, F. F., Christiansen, T. C., & Krasheninnikoff, M. (2001). Occupational therapy and Colles' fractures. *International Orthopaedics, 25*, 43-45.

Keywords: Colles' fracture, upper extremity, occupational therapy, exercise

The aim of this study was to see the effectiveness of instructions in exercises compared to instructions as well as occupational therapy at 5 weeks and 3 and 9 months. The results are that there are no significant differences between the two groups at the specified time periods. In conclusion, for non-surgically treated patients with a distal radius fracture, only instructions are necessary.

Cicerone, K. D., Mott, T., Azulay, J., & Friel, J. C. (2004). Community integration and satisfaction with functioning after intensive cognitive rehabilitation for traumatic brain injury. *Archives of Physical Medicine and Rehabilitation, 85*(6), 943-950.

Keywords: brain injuries, outcome and process assessment (healthcare), quality of life, rehabilitation

This article describes a study in which individuals with brain injury were given either standard neurorehabilitation or intensive cognitive rehabilitation. Results indicate that individuals receiving intensive cognitive rehabilitation were more likely to be reintegrated into their communities than those receiving standard rehabilitation, demonstrating the effectiveness of this type of treatment.

Clemson, L., Cumming, R. G., Kendig, H., Swann, M., Heard, R., & Taylor, K. (2004). The effectiveness of a community-based program for reducing the incidence of falls in the elderly: A randomized trial. *Journal of the American Geriatrics Society, 52*(9), 1487-1494.

Keywords: accidental falls, elderly, prevention, cognitive-behavioral, small-group intervention

The study discussed a falls prevention program, Stepping On, to be tested in a randomized controlled trial. Results indicated that subjects involved in a cognitive-behavioral program called Stepping On experienced at 31% reduction in falls. These results demonstrate the success of the Stepping On group to the idea that learning in a small-group environment can reduce falls.

Clark, F., Azen, S. P., Carlson, M., Mandel, D., LaBree, L., Hay, J., et al. (2001). Embedding health-promoting changes into the daily lives of independent-living older adults: Long-term follow-up of occupational therapy intervention. *Journals of Gerontology. Series B: Psychological Sciences and Social Sciences, 56B*(1), P60-P63.

Keywords: preventative OT, long term, health, overall health, psychological health, health relevant behaviors, transportation, personal safety, social relationships, cultural awareness, finances, independent living

The article begins by noting the increase in the elderly population and identifies the need to find effective interventions that prevent age-related decline. Included is a study that reports on the long-term effectiveness of an occupational therapy intervention aimed at reducing health-related declines of independently urban-living elderly adults. The study identified long-term health benefits related to preventative occupational therapy.

Clark, F., Azen, S. P., Zemke, R., Jackson, J., Carlson, M., Mandel, D., et al. (1997). Occupational therapy for independent-living older adults. A randomized controlled trial. *Journal of the American Medical Association, 278*(16), 1321-1326.

Keywords: well elderly, community, preventative, aging

The article begins by describing the aging population and the need to provide quality of life for longer life spans. A case is made for preventative health approaches as a means of maintaining quality of life in aging populations. Next, a study is presented that investigates the efficacy of a preventative occupational therapy program (well elderly study) for older adults. The study demonstrates preventative occupational therapy as a means to improving quality of life for an aging population.

Close, J., Ellis, M., Hooper, R., Glucksman, E., Jackson, S., & Swift, C. (1999). Prevention of falls in the elderly trial (PROFET): A randomised controlled trial. *Lancet, 353*, 93-97.

Keywords: falls prevention, elderly, multidisciplinary

The aims of this study were to assess the benefits of a structured interdisciplinary assessment of a geriatric population with a history of falls in terms of further falls. This study shows positive results for a multidisciplinary assessment in this population in terms of the number of falls, recurrent falls, hospital admission, and function. The study concluded that the reduction in falls from this intervention was promising and that proven falls and injury prevention strategies should be implemented into clinical service due to this study's evidence.

Cohen, H., & Kimball, K. (2003). Increased independence and decreased vertigo after vestibular rehabilitation. *Otolaryngology—Head and Neck Surgery, 128*, 60-70.

The authors sought to determine the effectiveness in decreasing vertigo symptoms and increasing functional performance post-vestibular rehabilitation. Evidence showed statistically significant support of a vestibular home program to decrease symptoms of vertigo and an improvement in independence of activities of daily living (ADL). Therefore, a simple vestibular habituation home program can reduce symptoms and increase independence in ADL.

Cole, M. B., & Greene, L. R. (1988). A preference for activity: A comparative study of psychotherapy groups vs. occupational therapy groups for psychotic and borderline inpatients. *Occupational Therapy in Mental Health, 8*(3), 53-67.

The article discusses the importance of group treatment in people with mental health issues and details psychotherapy and occupational therapy-focused group treatment. The study compares participant preference between unstructured psychotherapy with structured occupational therapy groups. Results demonstrated preference for occupational therapy groups over psychotherapeutic groups by all subjects involved. Conclusions call for possible integration of conceptualizations between psychoanalytic psychology and occupational therapy theories.

Comella, C. L., Stebbins, G. T., Brown-Toms, N., & Goetz, C. G. (1994). Physical therapy and Parkinson's disease: A controlled clinical trial. *Neurology, 44*(3 Pt 1), 376-378.

The purpose of this single-blind cross-over study was to evaluate the impact of a physical therapy program on clinical functional outcomes of Parkinson's disease patients. Results indicated that immediately after the intervention, patients showed improvement in various outcomes such as motor and activities of daily living function. No improve-

ments were seen in depression, and, at a 6-month evaluation, functional abilities had returned to baseline.

Conine, T. A., Hershler, C., Daechsel, D., Peel, C., & Pearson, A. (1994). Pressure ulcer prophylaxis in elderly patients using polyurethane foam of Jay wheelchair cushions. *International Journal of Rehabilitation Research, 17*, 123-137.

The article provides an overview of pressure ulcers and the cushions used to help relieve/prevent them. Foam cushions are inexpensive and do not require training to use, while the Jay cushion is more expensive and has been marketed as a better option, without evidence. This study compares two types of cushions (foam versus Jay) on elderly patients and hypothesizes that no differences will be found for factors like incidence, location, severity, and healing over a 3-month period. The Jay group did, however, experience less pressure ulcer formation during the observation period compared to the foam group, but no differences were found on the location, severity, or healing duration of the ulcers. The Jay cushion was considered more uncomfortable than the foam cushion, leading some participants to reject this cushion.

Corcoran, M. A., & Gitlin, L. N. (2001). Family caregiver acceptance and use of environmental strategies provided in an occupational therapy intervention. *Physical and Occupational Therapy in Geriatrics, 19*, 1-20.

Keywords: Alzheimer's disease, family care, environmental intervention

The article discusses the environmental interventions occupational therapists use to support caregivers who care for family with dementia. The study provides results that caregivers utilize about 81% of recommended strategies involving modification of the task, social, and physical environment. It is concluded that caregivers are receptive to and utilize environmental strategies offered by occupational therapists.

Corey, D. T., Koepfler, L., Etlin, D., & Day, H. (1996). A limited functional restoration program for injured workers: A randomized trial. *Journal of Occupational Rehabilitation, 6*(4), 239-249.

Keywords: functional restoration, pain management, treatment outcome, soft tissues injury, multidisciplinary approach

This randomized controlled trial compared a multidisciplinary functional restoration treatment with usual care for clients with soft tissue injuries associated with the Worker's Compensation Board. The functional restoration may involve occupational therapy but it is not stated explicitly within the article. The article finds the functional restoration program favorable to improve sleep and increase probability of return to work. Patients reported less pain than usual care.

Cron, L., & Sprigle, S. (1993). Clinical evaluation of the hemi wheelchair cushion. *American Journal of Occupational Therapy, 47*(2), 141-144.

Keywords: posture, seats, adjusted, wheelchairs, and accessories

This article begins by describing the importance of proper seating for people using wheelchairs. It continues with a description of a study undertaken to assess the effectiveness of the hemi wheelchair cushion for people who propel with one leg. Although the results are not statistically significant, the authors conclude that the hemi cushion is just as effective as other cushions and could be a viable low-cost alternative for this population.

Cumming, R. G., Thomas, M., Szonyi, G., Salkeld, G., O'Neill, E., Westbury, C., et al. (1999). Home visits by an occupational therapist for assessment and modification of environmental hazards: A randomized trial of falls prevention. *Journal of the American Geriatrics Society, 47*(12), 1397-1402.

Keywords: accidental falls, environment design, randomized controlled trial, occupational therapy, safety management

The article discusses the importance of reducing environmental hazards to prevent falls for older adults, but effectiveness for home modification is unproven. A study was introduced that compared occupational therapy home assessment and modifications with usual care. Results indicated that participants from the intervention group were less likely to have a fall in the year following occupational therapy treatment versus those who only received usual treatment. This randomized trial showed that a home visit by an occupational therapist can prevent falls among older people who have fallen in the previous year.

Dahlin Ivanoff, S., Sonn, U., & Svensson, E. (2002). A health education program for elderly persons with visual impairments and perceived security in the performance of daily occupations: A randomized study. *American Journal of Occupational Therapy, 56*(3), 322-330.

> **Keywords**: macular degeneration, self-efficacy, perceived security, ADL performance
>
> The article begins with a brief discussion of macular degeneration and its effect on activities of daily living (ADL) performance and perceived security in ADL performance. Next, a study is presented that evaluates occupational therapist-led health education groups aimed at improving ADL performance for seniors with macular degeneration. Results indicate that occupational therapist-led groups are effective at improving perceived security in ADL performance for adults with macular degeneration.

Dam, M., Tonin, P., Ermani, M., Pizzolato, G., Iaia, V., & Battistin, L. (1993). The effects of long-term rehabilitation therapy on post-stroke hemiplegic patients. *Stroke, 24*, 1186-1191.

> **Keywords**: hemiplegia, rehabilitation, stroke outcome
>
> The purpose of this study was to investigate the impacts of long-term rehabilitation on participants with stroke. Results indicated significant functional and neurological improvements in a "consistent" number of patients receiving rehabilitation during the first year after stroke for those receiving rehabilitation. Some improvements were seen during the second year following stroke for some individuals (results were not significant).

Daniel, A., & Manigandan, C. (2005). Efficacy of leisure intervention groups and their impact on quality of life among people with spinal cord injury. *International Journal of Rehabilitation Research, 28*(1), 43-48.

> **Keywords**: rehabilitation, spinal cord injury, leisure intervention, group therapy, quality of life
>
> The purpose of this study was to determine the impact of leisure activities on quality of life in spinal cord injury patients and the effectiveness of group therapy to increase leisure participation. The study included 25 people in an inpatient rehabilitation program who were paraplegic and able to communicate and had no serious co-morbid conditions. The study found that group therapy was an effective method of changing patients' understanding of leisure and thus improving their participation in and satisfaction with their leisure activities. This, in turn, led to an increase in quality of life scores.

Darragh, A., Harrison, H., & Kenny, S. (2008). Effect of an ergonomics intervention on workstations of microscope workers. *American Journal of Occupational Therapy, 62*(1), 61-69.

> **Keywords**: ergonomics, microscope, occupational therapy, work
>
> The aim of this study was to examine the effect of a preventative occupational therapy ergonomics intervention on workstation design and body positioning in microscope workers. Subjects were selected from a fiberoptics company and randomized to receive one of three interventions according to their workstation. Results showed that providing subjects with informational material and conducting information sessions was the most effective way to influence work habits.

Davison, J., Bond, J., Dawson, P., Steen, I. N., & Kenny, R. A. (2005). Patients with recurrent falls attending accident and emergency benefit from multifactorial intervention—a randomised controlled trial. *Age and Ageing, 34*(2), 162-168.

> **Keywords**: recurrent falls, older person, accident & emergency, fall-related injury, randomized controlled trial, elderly, treatment
>
> This study recruited elderly patients from emergency departments who had suffered more than one fall in the preceding 12 months and had no medical explanation for their fall. The aim of the study was to investigate whether a multidisci-

plinary falls prevention program including comprehensive medical assessment, physical therapy, and occupational therapy would be successful in reducing the number of falls experienced by the subjects. The study concluded that the intervention reduced the cumulative number of falls in the intervention group but did not reduce the proportion of patients who fell. A significant reduction in fear of falling was also observed.

de Buck, P., Le Cessie, S., van den Hout, W. B., Peeters, A., Ronday, H. K., Westedt, M., et al. (2005). Randomized comparison of a multidisciplinary job-retention vocational rehabilitation program with usual outpatient care in patients with chronic arthritis at risk for job loss. *Arthritis and Rheumatism: Arthritis Care and Research, 53*(5), 682-690.

> **Keywords**: arthritis, work disability, vocational rehabilitation
>
> This study investigated the use of a multidisciplinary team approach to a job retention vocational rehabilitation program for clients with rheumatoid diseases. The primary outcome investigated was the occurrence of job loss, which indicated after 24 months of follow-up no significant difference between the rehabilitation program and the usual care. The study discussion compares the findings to another study, which found positive results using a similar vocational rehabilitation program.

DeCarlo, J., & Mann, W. (1985). The effectiveness of verbal versus activity groups in improving self-perceptions of interpersonal communication skills. *American Journal of Occupational Therapy, 39*(1), 20-26.

> **Keywords**: communication, group processes, occupational therapy, social interaction
>
> The article begins with a discussion regarding the need for interpersonal communication skills for people with mental health issues and how psychiatric day treatment (group) programs conducted by occupational therapists often address these needs. A randomized controlled study is then presented that compares the efficacy of a verbal group with that of an activity group in an occupational therapy clinic during the treatment of interpersonal communication skills. Findings indicate that a significantly higher level of interpersonal communication skills was attained by the activity group; however, comparisons between both groups and the control group showed no significant differences. As a result, these findings suggest, rather than provide, conclusive evidence that activity groups are more effective in improving self-perceptions of interpersonal communication skills than are verbal groups during occupational therapy in a psychiatric day program.

De Craen, A., Gussekloo, J., Blauw, G. J., Willems, C. G., & Westendorp, R. (2006). Randomised controlled trial of unsolicited occupational therapy in community-dwelling elderly people: The LOTIS trial. *PLoS Clinical Trials, 1*(1), e2.

> The objective of this trial was to determine if unsolicited occupational therapy for elderly people living in the community (compared to no therapy) could slow down the increase in disability experienced by this population. Participants in the intervention group were visited in their homes by an occupational therapist and received training on existing assistive devices as well as recommendations for new equipment and/or home modifications. Both intervention and control groups experienced an increase in disability throughout the course of the study; however, no significant difference was found between the two groups. There were also no significant differences in any other secondary outcome measures.

Desrosiers, J., Bourbonnais, D., Corriveau, H., Gosselin, S., & Bravo, G. (2005). Effectiveness of unilateral and symmetrical bilateral task training for arm during the subacute phase after stroke: A randomized controlled trial. *Clinical Rehabilitation, 19*(6), 581-593.

> The purpose of this study was to evaluate the effect of an arm training program emphasizing repeated symmetrical bilateral or unilateral movements in addition to standard arm therapy. A randomized controlled trial in which half the clients received this therapy and the other half received

standard care with matching additional hours of therapy time is presented. Results do not support efficacy of repetitive program.

Desrosiers, J., Malouin, F., Richards, C., Bourbonnais, D., Rochette, A., & Bravo, G. (2003). Comparison of changes in upper and lower extremity impairments and disabilities after stroke. *International Journal of Rehabilitation Research, 26*(2), 109-116.

> **Keywords**: recovery after stroke, cerebrovascular accident
> This study investigates the differences in rates of recovery of impairment and disability in the upper and lower extremity following post-stroke active rehabilitation. Using a prospective cohort study design, the authors investigated the differences in recovery based on changes in motor function and coordination and differences in performance on a functional assessment. The authors concluded that the level of motor improvement of the upper and lower extremities is similar during active rehabilitation, but the upper extremity has a higher rate of motor recovery after discharge.

Desrosiers, J., Noreau, L., Rochette, A., Carbonneau, H., Fontaine, L., Viscogliosi, C., et al. (2007). Effect of a home leisure education program after stroke: A randomized controlled trial. *Archives of Physical Medicine and Rehabilitation, 88*, 1095-1100.

> **Keywords**: depressive symptoms, leisure activities, quality of life, rehabilitation, stroke
> The study initially discusses the importance of leisure on quality of life and how stroke impacts on this occupation. Because the effect of leisure-based education programs has not been well studied, the study aims to evaluate the effect of a home leisure education program with an emphasis on empowerment for people with a stroke. The study concludes that an empowerment-focused home leisure education program had positive effects on mainly leisure satisfaction and participation.

DeWilliams, C. A. C., Nicholas, M. K., Richardson, P. H., Pither, C. E., Justins, D. M., Chamberlain, J. H., et al. (1993). Evaluation of a cognitive behavioural programme for rehabilitating patients with chronic pain. *British Journal of General Practice, 43*(377), 513-518.

> **Keywords**: chronic pain, rehabilitation, cognitive therapy, behavior therapy, management of disease
> This study describes an inpatient cognitive-behavioral program for patients with chronic pain. Improvements in patients' physical functioning and self-reported emotional functioning between pre-treatment and follow-up interviews indicate that the program was effective in reducing impact of pain on functioning. Patients also reduced their use of analgesic medications over this time period, and results stayed steady to the 6-month follow-up.

DiFabio, R. P., Choi, T., Soderberg, J., & Hansen, C. R. (1997). Health-related quality of life for patients with progressive multiple sclerosis: Influence of rehabilitation. *Physical Therapy, 77*(12), 1704-1716.

> **Keywords**: multiple sclerosis, outpatient treatment, quality of life, rehabilitation
> This article examines the effects of a 1-year outpatient rehabilitation program on the health-related quality of life and functional abilities for people with progressive multiple sclerosis. The before-and-after scores of the participants in the program were compared with the scores of multiple sclerosis patients who were on the waiting list to enter the same program. The program was beneficial to participants with multiple sclerosis, especially in the areas of physical health, bodily pain, energy/fatigue, social support, cognitive ability, and overall positive change in general health.

DiFabio, R. P., Soderberg, J., Choi, T., Hansen, C. R., & Schapiro, R. T. (1998). Extended outpatient rehabilitation: Its influence on symptom frequency, fatigue and functional status for persons with progressive multiple sclerosis. *Archives of Physical Medicine and Rehabilitation, 79*, 141-146.

> **Keywords**: multiple sclerosis, extended outpatient rehabilitation
> The purpose of the study was to understand the impact of extended outpatient rehabilitation services in a group of patients with multiple sclerosis. The design was a non-equivalent, pre-test/post-test control group design. The control group was composed of individuals on a waiting list who had not received extended outpatient rehabilitation. Results indicate that participants who participated in the rehabilitation program had fewer reported symptoms, lower rates of physical decline, and less fatigue than controls at the 1-year evaluation. Results are discussed both in terms of the treatment effects on functional ability, as well as concept of "environmental mastery," specifically as it relates to fatigue.

Dirette, D., & Hinojosa, J. (1999). The effects of a compensatory intervention on processing deficits of adults with acquired brain injuries. *Occupational Therapy Journal of Research, 19*(4), 223-238.

> **Keywords**: cognitive rehabilitation, strategies, computers, attention, visual processing
> The study examined literature on the efficacy of compensatory and remedial strategies for cognitive rehabilitation. The current study found that the use of compensatory strategies does improve performance on cognitive tasks. However, the use of compensatory strategies is not limited to individuals who receive formal instruction on their use. The study supports that individuals may improve many months post-injury, despite severity of injury.

Dohnke, B., Knauper, B., & Muller-Fahrnow, W. (2005). Perceived self-efficacy gained from, and health effects of, a rehabilitation program after hip joint replacement. *Arthritis and Rheumatism, 53*(4), 585-592.

> **Keywords**: self-efficacy, routine multidisciplinary rehabilitation, hip joint replacement, disability, pain, depressive symptoms
> The objective of this study was to assess whether an inpatient multidisciplinary rehabilitation program can increase self-efficacy and to determine the effect of self-efficacy on health status in patients who have undergone hip joint replacement. Patients were admitted to the rehabilitation program after surgery and were evaluated on disability, pain, depressive symptoms, and coping self-efficacy at admission, discharge, and 6-month follow-up. Significant improvements in all outcomes were observed, and higher self-efficacy at admission and larger increases in self-efficacy were found to predict larger positive improvements in health status.

Donnelly, C. J., & Wilton, J. (2002). The effect of massage to scars on active range of motion and skin mobility. *British Journal of Hand Therapy, 7*(1), 5-11.

> **Keywords**: scar management, hand therapy
> This article begins by discussing how scars can be managed by therapists. The purpose is to determine if scar massage in combination with standard therapies are effective to improve active range of motion and skin mobility. The study showed that massage in conjunction with hand therapy does improve active range of motion and not skin mobility, but these results should be observed with caution due to the limitations of the study.

Dooley, N. R., & Hinojosa, J. (2004). Improving quality of life for persons with Alzheimer's disease and their family caregivers: Brief occupational therapy intervention. *American Journal of Occupational Therapy, 58*(5), 561-569.

> **Keywords**: dementia, Alzheimer's, home, recommendations
> The article begins with a thorough discussion of Alzheimer-related quality of life and caregiver burden. A study is then presented that examines the effect of occupational therapy interventions (assessment and care recommendations) aimed at improving care recipient quality of life and function. Findings indicate that occupational therapy intervention can significantly increase aspects of care recipients' quality of life and function, while decreasing caregiver burden.

Dortch, H. L., & Trombly, C. A. (1990). The effects of education on hand use with industrial workers in repetitive jobs. *American Journal of Occupational Therapy, 44*(9), 777-782.

> **Keywords**: hand functions, patient education
> This study looked at the effects of two educational interventions on the number of risky hand movements performed by workers who were at risk for developing cumulative trauma disorder. In one of the intervention groups, participants received handouts of less risky hand movements while the

other intervention group received the handout and practiced the preferred movements. No differences were found between the educational intervention groups but the number of risky hand motions and right-hand usage decreased significantly in the groups that received education versus the control group. The authors concluded that, "the number of at-risk repetitive motions performed by employees during work tasks decreases immediately following preventative educational programs."

Drummond, A. E. R., Miller, N., Colquohoun, M., & Logan, P. C. (1996). The effects of a stroke unit on activities of daily living. *Clinical Rehabilitation, 10*, 12-22.

The purpose of this randomized controlled trial was to evaluate whether performance of activities of daily living (ADL) were improved, to a greater extent, after treatment on a specialized stroke unit compared to conventional ward in patients with stroke. Results suggested that those in the stroke unit were more independent in many areas of personal and instrumental ADL, specifically feeding, dressing, making a snack, and using money. However, some significant effects seemed to decrease over time, and thus researchers recommended further research on how to maintain results over time.

Drummond, A., & Walker, M. (1995). A randomized controlled trial of leisure rehabilitation after stroke. *Clinical Rehabilitation, 9*, 283-290.

This article discusses the common decrease in leisure participation that occurs post-stroke. Therefore, it examines the effects of a leisure performance occupational therapy intervention on the mood and functional performance of people who have suffered a stroke. Results showed improved leisure scores in the intervention group only.

Edmans, J. A., & Webster, J. (2000). A comparison of two approaches in the treatment of perceptual problems after stroke. *Clinical Rehabilitation, 14*, 230-243.

Keywords: perceptual abilities, stroke, transfer of training approach, functional approach, ADLs

The study analyzed the differential impact between two different treatments for perceptual abilities in individuals post-stroke. The study did not find any difference between the functional or transfer of training approach on perceptual abilities and function.

Egan, M., Kessler, D., Laporte, L., Metcalfe, V., & Carter, M. (2007). A pilot randomized controlled trial of community-based occupational therapy in late stroke rehabilitation. *Topics in Stroke Rehabilitation, 14*(5), 37-45.

Keywords: chronic disease, occupational therapy, outcomes, participation, stroke

The aim of this study was to investigate whether a brief period of client-centered occupational therapy would improve participation in valued activities for patients in the later stages of stroke recovery. Study participants identified up to five activities they wished to improve prior to the intervention and rated both their performance and satisfaction with the activities pre- and post-intervention. Results show that both groups rated their performance of the activities equally but the intervention group showed higher satisfaction with their participation.

Eklund, M. (1999). Outcome of occupational therapy in a psychiatric day care unit for long-term mentally ill patients. *Occupational Therapy in Mental Health, 14*(4), 21-45.

Keywords: schizophrenia, group therapy, activity, occupational performance, MOHO

This study investigates the effects of an occupational therapy program in psychiatric day care. This occupational therapy program was shown to be beneficial for improvement for some psychiatric patients on a variety of outcome variables covering occupational performance, global mental health, and psychiatric symptoms.

Elinge, E., Lofgren, B., Gagerman, E., & Nyberg, L. (2003). A group learning programme for old people with hip fracture: A randomized study. *Scandinavian Journal of Occupational Therapy, 10*(1), 27-33.

Keywords: activity performance, occupational therapy, participation, rehabilitation

The study aimed at examining whether a multidisciplinary group learning program (including occupational therapy) would influence subjects' perceived activity performance and ability to participate in social life post-hip fracture. Results indicated that there were no significant differences within the control and intervention groups post-group and 12 months post-group. However, between groups, the intervention program demonstrated statistically significant improvements in participating in activities with families and friends and in regaining their perceived ability to take part in social life (not evident in control group). The study concludes that the group learning program had a positive effect on the participant's activity performance and participation.

Fange, A., & Iwarsson, S. (2005). Changes in accessibility and usability in housing: An exploration of the housing adaptation process. *Occupational Therapy International, 12*(1), 44-59.

Keywords: housing accessibility, environmental barriers, housing adaptations

The purpose of this study was to explore changes in accessibility and usability for clients who had received home modifications. The study assessed home accessibility before modifications and at 2 and 8 months after modifications. Significant decreases in the number of environmental barriers and increases in clients' perceptions of usability were observed after modification.

Finlayson, M. (2005). Pilot study of an energy conservation education program delivered by telephone conference call to people with multiple sclerosis. *Neurorehabilitation, 20*(4), 267-277.

Keywords: multiple sclerosis, fatigue management, occupational therapy

This article describes the modification of an energy conservation program for people with multiple sclerosis. Using the guiding question "Is delivery of energy conservation education by telephone teleconference efficacious for persons with MS?" the researchers assessed outcomes related to fatigue impact and severity before and after the intervention. Results were not statistically significant, but the researchers concluded that the results support the need for more rigorous studies on this topic.

Finlayson, M., & Havixbeck, K. (1992). A post-discharge study on the use of assistive devices. *Canadian Journal of Occupational Therapy, 59*, 201-207.

Keywords: consumer satisfaction, quality assurance, occupational therapy, self-help devices

The article begins by reviewing the importance of educating clients on how to use assistive devices. A study is reported that reports the satisfaction and use of prescribed assistive devices. The study concluded that, although 97% of the subjects were satisfied with the education they provided for using assistive devices and demonstrated a high rate of equipment utilization (75% overall), further research is needed.

Finnerty, J. P., Keeping, I., Bullough, R. G. N., & Jones, J. (2001). The effectiveness of outpatient pulmonary rehabilitation in chronic lung disease: A randomized control trial. *Chest, 119*, 1705-1710.

Keywords: lung diseases, pulmonary rehabilitation, quality of life

The purpose of the study was to assess the impacts of an outpatient pulmonary rehabilitation program on quality of life for patients with chronic obstructive pulmonary disease, as most previous research has focused on inpatient rehabilitation for this population. Researchers concluded that the 6-week outpatient pulmonary rehabilitation program significantly improved quality of life. These changes remained apparent after 24 weeks, as measured.

Fischer, T., Nagy, L., & Buechler, U. (2003). Restoration of pinch grip in ulnar nerve paralysis: Extensor carpi radialis longus to adductor pollicis and abductor pollicis longus to first dorsal interosseus tendon transfers. *Journal of Hand Surgery (British and European Volume), 28B*, 28-32.

Keywords: tendon transfer, ulnar nerve paralysis

The aim of this study was to measure the change in strength and functional performance after tendon transfers for ulnar paralysis. The results show that there are improvements in overall function, return to work, and wrist extension strength. No statistical significance was provided.

Fisher, K., & Hardie, R. J. (2002). Goal attainment scaling in evaluating a multidisciplinary pain management programme. *Clinical Rehabilitation, 16*(8), 871-877.

>This article examines the validity of Goal Attainment Scaling (GAS) as an outcome measure for chronic back pain. A study in which results for GAS are compared with results of established pain impairment measures is presented. Results indicate a correlation between goal attainment and physical mobility.

Fleming, S. A., Blake, H., Gladman, J. R. F., Hart, E., Lymbery, M., Dewey, M. E., et al. (2004). A randomised controlled trial of care home rehabilitation service to reduce long-term institutionalisation for elderly people. *Age and Ageing, 33*, 384-390.

>**Keywords**: health services for the aged, rehabilitation, care homes, elderly, randomised controlled trial
>
>The study investigated the impact of care home rehabilitation services on institutionalization, health outcomes, and service use in elderly people. Based on results, the researchers concluded that care home rehabilitation services did not reduce institutionalization. There was a reduction in the number of patients receiving hospital care, but there was an increase in those receiving social services. This shift in hospital to social services did not appear to have significant impacts on well-being and activity levels.

Fletchall, S., & Hickerson, W. L. (1991). Early upper-extremity prosthetic fit in patients with burns. *Journal of Burn Care and Rehabilitation, 12*(3), 234-236.

>This study described the benefits of early prosthetic fit for patients requiring amputation. This study followed patients requiring an upper extremity amputation from the pre-surgery assessment by a multidisciplinary team through the rehabilitation process where patients were being fitted with a prosthesis and learning how to use it. The authors concluded that early prosthetic fit is beneficial "as evidenced by decrease in edema, good stump shape, transference of phantom sensation to the prosthesis, no skin breakdown, and an independent return to pre-amputation activities."

Flinn, N. A., Schamburg, S., Fetrow, J. M., & Flanigan, J. (2005). The effect of constraint-induced movement treatment on occupational performance and satisfaction in stroke survivors. *OTJR: Occupation, Participation, and Health, 25*(3), 119-127.

>**Keywords**: stroke rehabilitation, occupational performance, constraint-induced movement treatment
>
>The study analyzed the benefits of completing a constraint-induced movement treatment for individuals affected by stroke who had some active movement in the affected upper extremity. The study found that participants had significant increases in the use of the affected upper extremity in occupations following treatment, although participants' perception of their performance did not improve significantly.

Forbes, D. (2004). Multisensory stimulation was not better than usual activities for changing cognition, behaviour, and mood in dementia. *Evidence-Based Nursing, 7*(2), 55.

>**Keywords**: psychogeriatrics, dementia
>
>This article reported on a study comparing multisensory stimulation to activities for older adults with dementia. Both groups received treatment twice a week for 4 weeks. No differences were found between groups on outcome measures of cognition, behavior, or mood.

Freeman, J. A., Langdon, D. W., Hobart, J. C., & Thompson, A. J. (1999). Inpatient rehabilitation in multiple sclerosis: Do the benefits carry over into the community? *Neurology, 52*, 50-56.

>**Keywords**: multiple sclerosis, disability, handicap
>
>The purpose of this study was to determine the carry-over and benefits of short-term inpatient rehabilitation for people with multiple sclerosis; this was deemed to be important because few studies have examined outcomes after discharge from rehab in order to see if results are sustained in clients' environments. Results indicated that improvements in disability, handicap, health-related quality of life, and emotional well-being were made during rehabilitation. Although these improvements declined after discharge, they were maintained to some degree, compared to

baseline, despite decreasing neurological function. Results point to the need for continuity of care services between inpatient rehabilitation and community, in order to ensure that benefits are sustained. Researchers also suggest that the high degree of individual variation seen in the results indicate that services need be flexible to help meet needs of individuals.

Furst, G. P., Gerber, L. H., Smith, C. C., & Fisher, S. (1987). A program for improving energy conservation behaviors in adults with rheumatoid arthritis. *American Journal of Occupational Therapy, 41*(2), 102-111.

>**Keywords**: arthritis, rheumatoid, patient education, research
>
>This article reports the results of a randomized controlled trial comparing two energy conservation programs—a standard program and a program based on a model of educational diagnosis (educational-behavior). The results were not statistically significant, though the authors did note improvements in the experimental group. The authors conclude that more formal research evaluation of energy conservations programs is needed.

Furth, H. J., Holm, M. B., & James, A. (1994). Reinjury prevention follow-through for clients with cumulative trauma disorders. *American Journal of Occupational Therapy, 48*(10), 890-898.

>**Keywords**: patient education
>
>The article begins with a discussion of the occupational therapist's role in training and educating patients with cumulative trauma disorder to help them return to work and also prevent re-injury. It examined whether occupational therapist recommendations made to participants during an occupational therapy session would be followed and would help to lower the chance of re-injury. Results showed a lower level of recommendation follow-through than expected, leading authors to conclude that further research into re-injury prevention is needed.

Gentry, T. (2008). PDAs as cognitive aids for people with multiple sclerosis. *American Journal of Occupational Therapy, 62*(1), 18-27.

>**Keywords**: assistive technology, cognition, multiple sclerosis, occupational therapy, personal digital assistant (PDA)
>
>This study evaluated an occupational therapy-based patient education program that trained patients with cognitive impairment related to multiple sclerosis to use personal digital assistants (PDAs) as assistive devices. Training was delivered in patients' homes by an experienced occupational therapist, and the main outcome measure was functional performance and frequency of use of the PDA. Results showed that all participants were able to learn to use the PDA and experienced a significant increase in functional performance. These effects also lasted until the end of the 8-week follow-up period.

Gerber, L., Furst, G., Shulman, B., Smith, C., Thornton, B., Liang, M., et al. (1987). Patient education program to teach energy conservation behaviors to patients with rheumatoid arthritis: A pilot study. *Archives of Physical Medicine and Rehabilitation, 68*, 442-445.

>**Keywords**: education, occupational therapy, patient, rheumatoid arthritis
>
>The purpose of this randomized controlled trial was to determine if the use of a workbook intervention for people with rheumatoid arthritis would facilitate behavioral change, in terms of impacting outcomes such as decreasing pain and fatigue, as well as increasing participation in physical activity and use of rest periods during activities. Researchers conclude that the significant differences between groups, in terms of activity level and rest periods, may suggest that a "systematic" approach to education is successful in changing behavior.

Geusgens, C., van Heughten, C., Donkervoort, M., van den Ende, E., Jolles, J., & van den Heuvel, W. (2006). Transfer of training effects in stroke patients with apraxia: An exploratory study. *Neuropsychological Rehabilitation, 16*(2), 213-229.

>The authors aimed to determine whether a cognitive strategy-based approach was effective in producing transfer of training effects between trained and non-trained tasks. Evidence supported the presence of transfer of training;

however, the effect was present in both groups, with the strategy training group achieving a higher level of transfer.

Gilbertson, L., & Langhorne, P. (2000). Home-based occupational therapy: Stroke patients' satisfaction with occupational performance and service provision. *British Journal of Occupational Therapy, 63*(10), 464-468.

Keywords: adult, stroke, home, RCT, COPM
The article begins by describing some challenges of adults living in the community post-stroke. A case is made for offering home-based services aimed at easing the transition to independent living following hospital discharge. Next, a study is presented that investigates the efficacy of a home-based support program for post-stoke adults. The study shows increases in perceived occupational performance and performance satisfaction, as well as emotional condition, and service level satisfaction in the treatment group.

Gillen, G., Berger, S. M., Lotia, S., Morreale, J., Siber, M. I., & Trudo, W. J. (2007). Improving community skills after lower extremity joint replacement. *Physical and Occupational Therapy in Geriatrics, 25*(4), 41-54.

Keywords: orthopedic rehabilitation, total hip replacement, total knee replacement, community
The purpose of this study was to determine the effect of a community reintegration intervention on community skills in people who had a lower extremity joint replacement. Subjects were evaluated on performance of community skills, satisfaction with performance, confidence, and self-rated performance of five community skills immediately before and after the intervention. Scores on all three measures and self-rated performance of individual community skills were significantly higher after the intervention.

Gilmore, P. E., & Spaulding, S. J. (2007). Motor learning and the use of videotape feedback after stroke. *Topics in Stroke Rehabilitation, 14*, 28-36.

Keywords: cerebral vascular event, feedback, motor learning, occupational therapy, stroke
The study examined the benefits of using videotaping to help facilitate feedback within occupational therapy intervention for the motor learning of donning socks and shoes for adults post-stroke. The study randomly allocated participants into either a group receiving occupational therapy only or occupational therapy with videotaped feedback. The results indicated that there were no differences in outcomes between groups in sock donning. However, the perception and satisfaction of donning shoes was significantly higher in the group that received videotaped feedback. This lends support to the conclusion that videotaped feedback may lead to improved satisfaction with performance.

Gitlin, L. N., Corcoran, M., Winter, L., Boyce, A., & Hauck, W. W. (2001). A randomized, controlled trial of a home environmental intervention: Effect on efficacy and upset in caregivers and on daily function of persons with dementia. *Gerontologist, 41*(1), 4-14.

Keywords: clinical trial, home modification, home care
This article begins by reviewing literature on interventions for people with dementia and their caregivers and points to a need for research on interventions targeting the home environment. The authors then outline a randomized controlled trial investigating the effects of a home environmental intervention on people with dementia and their caregivers. Although the results are not statistically significant, the authors conclude that the environmental program appears to have a modest effect on dementia patients' instrumental activities of daily living dependence; among certain subgroups of caregivers, the program improves self-efficacy and reduces upset in specific areas of caregiving.

Gitlin, L. N., Hauck, W. W., Dennis, M. P., & Winter, L. (2005). Maintenance of effects of the home environmental skill-building program for family caregivers and individuals with Alzheimer's disease and related disorders. *Journals of Gerontology. Series A: Biological Sciences and Medical Sciences, 60*(3), 368-374.

This article reports on the 12-month results of an environmental skill-building program for caregivers of people with dementia. The only statistically significant improvement for the experimental group was in the area of caregiver affect.

The authors conclude that more frequent professional contact and on-going skills training may be necessary to maintain positive intervention effects in the long-term.

Gitlin, L., Hauck, W., Winter, L., Dennis, M., & Schulz, R. (2006). Effect of an in-home occupational and physical therapy intervention on reducing mortality in functionally vulnerable older people: Preliminary findings. *Journal of the American Geriatrics Society, 54*(6), 950-955.

Keywords: older adults, home modification, frailty, home care
This article looks at occupational therapy and physiotherapy in-home interventions to reduce mortality of the vulnerable older adult population. Although the article does not state how many participants received or did not receive the in-home interventions, the article states that those who did receive the intervention were given home modifications as well as strategies for cognition, behavior, and physical strategies. The main study finding was that there was significantly less mortality in the group that received the in-home intervention.

Gitlin, L. N., Miller, K. S., & Boyce, A. (1999). Bathroom modifications for frail elderly renters: Outcomes of a community-based program. *Technology and Disability, 10*(3), 141-149.

Keywords: self-care, home modifications, chronic conditions
This article begins by describing the relation of home modifications to functional independence for frail elders and discusses some of the issues facing non-homeowners. The authors then describe a community-based study of the impact of occupational therapy assessment and equipment provision on activities of daily living (ADL) and instrumental ADL performance for female elders who live in rental units. The resulting improvement in ADL performance, and in particular bathing, points to the efficacy of occupational therapy assessment and follow-up in home modifications.

Gitlin, L. N., Winter, L., Corcoran, M., Dennis, M. P., Schinfeld, S., & Hauck, W. W. (2003). Effects of the home environmental skill-building program on the caregiver-care recipient dyad: 6-month outcomes from the Philadelphia REACH initiative. *Gerontologist, 43*(4), 532-546.

Keywords: clinical trial, home modification, home care
This article describes the 6-month post-intervention results of an environmental skill-building program for caregivers of people with dementia. Compared to the control group, the intervention group had statistically significant improvements in the following areas: Memory-related behaviors, less need for assistance from others, and better affect. The authors conclude that the intervention is beneficial in certain domains, and that it affects certain subgroups more than others.

Gitlin, L. N., Winter, L., Dennis, M. P., Corcoran, M., Schinfeld, S., & Hauck, W. W. (2006). A randomized trial of a multi-component home intervention to reduce functional difficulties in older adults. *Journal of the American Geriatrics Society, 54*, 809-816.

Keywords: home care, home modification, rehabilitation, disability, frailty
The study aimed to test the efficacy of a multi-component intervention to reduce functional difficulties, fear of falling, and home hazards and enhance self-efficacy and adaptive coping in older adults with chronic conditions. The study noted that the current intervention could provide an alternative approach for those unable or unwilling to attend group sessions in the community. The study concluded that functional difficulties imposed by chronic health problems are a primary threat to quality of life and that modifying environmental and behavioral factors can ameliorate functional difficulties and concerns, such as fear of falling, poor self-efficacy, and home hazards.

Gladman, J. R., Lincoln, N. B., & Barer, D. H. (1993). A randomized controlled trial of domiciliary and hospital-based rehabilitation for stroke patients after discharge from hospital. *Journal of Neurology, Neurosurgery and Psychiatry, 56*, 960-966.

Keywords: stroke, functional recovery, domiciliary rehabilitation

This randomized controlled study examined functional recovery and perceived health in stroke patients who received service from a "domiciliary rehabilitation service" compared to those who received conventional hospital-based services after discharge from the hospital. Overall, there were no significant differences between groups who received home-based rehabilitation versus hospital-based services in terms of functional recovery or perceived health status; one exception to this was the sub-group of patients discharged from the stroke unit to home care. There were also no significant differences between groups on any of the caregiving measures.

Gosman-Hedstrom, G., Claesson, L., & Blomstrand, C. (2002). Assistive devices in elderly people after stroke: A longitudinal, randomized study—the Goteborg 70+ Stroke Study. *Scandinavian Journal of Occupational Therapy, 9*, 109-118.

Keywords: assistive devices, cost, daily activities, elderly, intervention, occupational therapy, outcomes, randomization, stroke unit

This study focused on assistive devices in the different stages of the rehabilitation process, and the main outcome of interest was the impact of assistive devices in daily activities for older adults who had a stroke. Results indicated that, although there was no significant difference between the groups regarding the impact of assistive devices, the prescription of assistive devices in both groups increased the ability for subjects to perform daily activities.

Graff, M., Adang, E., Vernooij-Dassen, M., Dekker, J., Jonsson, L., Thijssen, M., et al. (2008). Community occupational therapy for older patients with dementia and their care givers: Cost effectiveness study. *British Medical Journal, 336*(7636), 134-138.

The purpose of this study was to assess the effectiveness and cost-effectiveness of community-based occupational therapy in dementia patients and their caregivers as compared with usual care. Subjects in the treatment group received 10 sessions of occupational therapy over 5 weeks, while those in the control group were free to receive any care except occupational therapy. Results showed that the occupational therapy program was successful in improving patients' functional ability and reducing caregiver burden and was also more cost-effective (lower costs) than usual care.

Graff, M. J., Vernooij-Dassen, M. J., Thijssen, M., Dekker, J., Hoefnagels, W. H., & Rikkert, M. G. (2006). Community based occupational therapy for patients with dementia and their caregivers: Randomised controlled trial. *British Medical Journal, 333*(7580), 1196.

Keywords: dementia, home, care giver, care recipient, ADL, competence

The article begins with a brief discussion on activities of daily living (ADL) performance challenges related to dementia, caregiver burden, and treatment options. Next, a study is presented that evaluates in-home occupational therapy as an intervention aimed at improving care-recipient ADL performance and care-provider confidence. Results indicate that in-home occupational therapy is effective at both improving care-recipient ADL performance and care-provider confidence.

Greenberg, S., & Fowler, R. S., Jr. (1980). Kinesthetic biofeedback: A treatment modality for elbow range of motion in hemiplegia. *American Journal of Occupational Therapy, 34*(11), 738-743.

Keywords: kinesthesia

This article begins by differentiating biofeedback for muscle re-education from kinesthetic biofeedback. The authors then describe a randomized controlled trial comparing kinesthetic biofeedback to conventional occupational therapy as a treatment for increasing elbow flexion in clients with hemiplegia. The results are not statistically significant, but the authors state that kinesthetic biofeedback should be considered for use in conjunction with other modalities in stroke rehabilitation.

Griffiths, T., Burr, M., Campbell, I., Lewis-Jenkins, V., Mullins, J., Shiels, K., et al. (2000). Results at 1 year of outpatient multidisciplinary pulmonary rehabilitation: A randomized controlled trial. *Lancet, 355*(9201), 362-368.

Keywords: multidisciplinary, chronic obstructive pulmonary disease, outpatient

This article looks at a multidisciplinary approach, with an occupational therapist, physiotherapist, and dietitian, to rehabilitation for people with chronic obstructive pulmonary disease. The rehabilitation program included an education component, an exercise component, and a psychological component. Overall, there was some evidence for the program to be used, but this was limited.

Gruwsved, A., Soderback, I., & Fernholm, C. (1996). Evaluation of a vocational training programme in primary health care rehabilitation: A case study. *Work, 7*, 47-61.

Keywords: job analyses, musculoskeletal pain, occupation, self-estimated pain assessment, rehabilitation, temporal adaptation, video-feedback, vocational training, work

This article studies a group of people with musculoskeletal pain within an occupational therapy program focused on work capacity and pattern of engagement in daily occupations. The study evaluates the outcomes of 4 of 38 participants within the program, which indicates that 2 of 4 subjects decreased their resting time and 3 of 4 subjects performed activities previously avoided due to pain and achieved their occupational goals.

Gutman, S., Diamond, H., Holness-Parchment, S., Brandofino, D., Pacheco, D., Jolly-Edouard, M., et al. (2004). Enhancing independence in women experiencing domestic violence and possible brain injury: An assessment of an occupational therapy intervention. *Occupational Therapy in Mental Health, 20*(1), 49-79.

Keywords: abuse, cognitive impairment, head injury, homelessness

The article initially discusses the link between domestic abuse and brain injury. This can result in impairment of specific cognitive skills due to brain injury, which can prevent these women from planning to leave abusive situations. This study assesses the effectiveness of intervention for women who have experienced domestic violence and/or homelessness in regard to attainment of their functional goals set in the program. Results indicated that all women who participated made gains toward personally desired goals and achieved their expected outcomes or exceeded them. Self-reported results indicate that 81% of participants achieved their most favorable outcome and 19% their expected outcome. The participants expressed a high degree of satisfaction with the intervention and cited that it was client-centered and helped them learn new skills gradually.

Hadas-Lidor, N., Katz, N., Tyano, S., & Weizman, A. (2001). Effectiveness of dynamic cognitive intervention in rehabilitation of clients with schizophrenia. *Clinical Rehabilitation, 15*(4), 349-359.

Keywords: cognitive rehabilitation, schizophrenia, long-term treatment, functional outcomes

The study addressed the impact of a specific program of cognitive rehabilitation on functional outcomes of individuals with schizophrenia. The researchers found a positive influence on cognitive domains, living arrangements, and employment status.

Haines, T., Bennell, K., Osborne, R., & Hill, K. (2004). Effectiveness of targeted falls prevention in sub-acute hospital setting: Randomised controlled trial. *British Medical Journal, 328*, 676-679.

Keywords: falls prevention, sub-acute hospital setting, multiple intervention programme

The article begins with providing an overview of the incidence of falling among the elderly in sub-acute hospitals. An intervention plan is then studied for its efficacy against patient falls. The study finds that the intervention plan decreases the number and/or severity of falls among intervention participants.

Hammond, A. (1994). Joint protection behavior in patients with rheumatoid arthritis following an education program: A pilot study. *Arthritis Care and Research, 7*, 5-9.

Keywords: joint protection, behavioral assessment, rheumatoid arthritis

The purpose of this study was to assess whether hand movement patterns changed in patients with rheumatoid arthritis after an education program on joint protection. Based on the results, researchers concluded that the joint protection education did not lead to significant change in behavior in terms of the activities that were assessed.

Hammond, A., & Freeman, K. (2001). One-year outcomes of a randomized controlled trial of an educational-behavioural joint protection programme for people with rheumatoid arthritis. *Rheumatology (Oxford, England), 40*(9), 1044-1051.

> **Keywords**: rheumatoid arthritis, joint protection, patient education, occupational therapy
>
> This article begins by describing previous research on joint protection and the effectiveness of educational programs. The researchers describe the method and intervention used in the current study. They conclude that the study provides support for the use of joint protection programs that follow an educational-behavioral approach.

Hammond, A., & Freeman, K. (2004). The long-term outcomes from a randomized controlled trial of an educational behavioural joint protection programme for people with rheumatoid arthritis. *Clinical Rehabilitation, 18*(5), 520-528.

> **Keywords**: rheumatoid arthritis, joint protection, patient education, occupational therapy
>
> This article describes the 4-year follow-up of a randomized controlled trial on joint protection programs. The researchers compared a standard program and a program based on an educational-behavioral approach. Similar to the 1-year follow-up, the 4-year follow-up provides support for the use of joint protection programs that follow an educational-behavioral approach.

Hammond, A., Jefferson, P., Jones, N., Gallagher, J., & Jones, T. (2002). Clinical applicability of an educational-behavioural joint protection programme for people with rheumatoid arthritis. *British Journal of Occupational Therapy, 65*(9), 405-412.

> **Keywords**: rheumatoid arthritis, joint protection, patient education, occupational therapy
>
> This article describes the results from a study assessing the effectiveness of occupational therapy-delivered educational-behavioral joint protection program for people with rheumatoid arthritis. Results from the study show that this approach is effective in increasing adherence to joint protection techniques, yet results were less strong that in a previous randomized controlled trial by the same authors.

Hammond, A., Young, A., & Kidao, R. (2004). A randomised controlled trial of occupational therapy for people with early rheumatoid arthritis. *Annals of the Rheumatic Diseases, 63*(1), 23-30.

> The purpose of this study was to assess the effects of a pragmatic, comprehensive occupational therapy program on self-management and health status of early rheumatoid arthritis patients. A randomized controlled trial was carried out with outcomes measured at study entry and 6, 12, and 24 months by a blinded assessor. Self-management increased significantly in the intervention group, but there were no significant differences in any other outcome measures either over time or between groups.

Hartman, D., Borrie, M. J., Davison, E., & Stolee, P. (1997). Use of goal attainment scaling in a dementia special care unit. *American Journal of Alzheimer's Disease, 12*(3), 111-116.

> **Keywords**: dementia, Alzheimer's disease, goal attainment scaling, GAS, client-centered practice
>
> This study used Goal Attainment Scaling (GAS) to set individualized functional and recreation goals for 10 residents with Alzheimer's disease in a chronic care hospital. GAS was found to be an effective means of measuring client goals, was very client-centered, and can be a valuable tool in maximizing quality of life for people with dementia.

Hartman-Maeir, A., Eliad, Y., Kizoni, R., Nahaloni, I., Kelberman, H., & Katz, N. (2007). Evaluation of a long-term community based rehabilitation program for adult stroke survivors. *Neurorehabilitation, 22*(4), 295-301.

> **Keywords**: stroke rehabilitation outcome, participation, life satisfaction
>
> The objective of this study was to evaluate functional ability, leisure activity, and life satisfaction in adult stroke survivors attending a community rehabilitation program compared to those receiving no rehabilitation. Subjects in the study were

stroke survivors who had received inpatient rehabilitation and were living at home at least 1 year post-onset. Results showed that the patients attending the program had severe disability due to stroke and low functional ability; however, the intervention significantly increased leisure participation and life satisfaction.

Haskett, S. Backman, C., Porter, B., Goyert, J., & Palejko, G. (2004). A crossover trial of custom-made and commercially available wrist splints in adults with inflammatory arthritis. *Arthritis and Rheumatism, 51*, 792-799.

> **Keywords**: arthritis, splint, wrist pain, hand function, occupational therapy
>
> The aim of this study was to compare the effect of three different wrist splints on perceived wrist pain, hand function, and perceived upper extremity function in adults with inflammatory arthritis. The result was that pain was significantly reduced, and aspects of hand function were as well. In conclusion, after 4 weeks' use, wrist splints reduce pain, improve strength, and do not compromise dexterity. The leather and Rolyan splint had similar improvements and were superior to the Anatech splint.

Hastings, J., Gowans, S., & Watson, D. E. (2004). Effectiveness of occupational therapy following organ transplantation. *Canadian Journal of Occupational Therapy, 71*(4), 238-242.

> **Keywords**: organ transplantation, evidence-based occupational therapy, outcomes research
>
> The article briefly describes typical functional results post-organ transplant surgeries. Functional status of patients was examined in an inpatient setting where occupational therapy interventions were given. Functional Independence Measure (FIM) scores improved significantly with positive correlation with occupational therapy attendance and time spent with the occupational therapist. Individuals with lower function received more occupational therapy.

Hayes, R., Halford, W., & Varghese, F. (1991). Generalization of the effects of activity therapy and social skills training on the social behavior of low functioning schizophrenic patients. *Occupational Therapy in Mental Health, 11*(4), 3-20.

> The article begins by describing two forms of therapy that occupational therapists use to improve social deficits for people with schizophrenia, activity groups, and social skills training. A study is presented that investigates the comparison of activity group therapy with social skills training, with the emphasis on the extent of generalizing those skills. The study shows that social skills improved significantly in the social skills training group but not during the activity group. However, there was no evidence that either phase impacted on the level of social engagement of subjects in a naturalistic social setting.

Heinemann, A. W., Hamilton, B., Linacre, J. M., Wright, B. D., & Granger, C. (1995). Status and therapeutic intensity during inpatient rehabilitation. *American Journal of Physical Medicine and Rehabilitation, 74*, 315-326.

> **Keywords**: traumatic brain injury, spinal cord injury, therapy intensity, functional status, medical rehabilitation
>
> The purpose of this study was to examine (a) the interaction between therapy intensity and functional change, (b) how efficiently potential gains in function were mathematically calculated, and (c) efficiency in functional gains. The population consisted of patients with spinal cord injury (SCI) and traumatic brain injury (TBI) who were receiving inpatient medical rehabilitation. Results showed that occupational, physical, and speech therapy did not significantly predict any outcomes in those with SCI or TBI. Psychology was significantly associated with better cognitive outcomes in the group with TBI.

Helewa, A., Goldsmith, C. H., Lee, P., Bombardier, C., Hanes, B., Smythe, H. A., et al. (1991). Effects of occupational therapy home service on patients with rheumatoid arthritis. *Lancet, 337*(8755), 1453-1456.

> **Keywords**: rheumatoid arthritis, home, splint, education, ADL, IADL, assistive device
>
> The article begins by briefly outlining some of the functional challenges associated with rheumatoid arthritis. Next, a study is presented that evaluates the effectiveness of a

comprehensive in-home occupational therapy program for adults with rheumatoid arthritis. Results indicate that the program is effective at increasing the functional status of adults affected with rheumatoid arthritis.

Helfrich, C., Aviles, A., Badiani, C., Walens, D., & Sabol, P. (2006). Life skill interventions with homeless youth, domestic violence victims, and adults with mental illness. *Occupational Therapy in Health Care, 20*, 189-207.

> **Keywords**: homelessness, mental illness, domestic violence, youth, life skills
>
> This paper presents three exploratory studies of life skills interventions (employment, money management, or food/nutrition) with 73 homeless individuals from four shelters and supportive housing programs located in the urban Midwest for youth, victims of domestic violence, and adults with mental illness. The Ansell Casey Life Skills Assessment was administered prior to the eight group and individual sessions. Quizzes and post-tests indicated clinical change in all groups, with statistical significance in the domestic violence group. The intervention implementation, challenges encountered, and strategies developed for implementing shelter-based interventions are discussed. Recommendations for successfully providing collaborative university-shelter clinical interventions are provided.

Hendriks, M. R. C., van Haastregt, J. C. M., Diederiks, J. P. M., Evers, S. M. A. A., Crebolder, H. F. J. M., & van Eijk, J. T. M. (2005). Effectiveness and cost-effectiveness of a multidisciplinary intervention programme to prevent new falls and functional decline among elderly persons at risk: Design of a replicated randomised controlled trial. *BMC Public Health, 5*, 6.

> The aim of this study is to describe the design of a replication study evaluating a multidisciplinary intervention program on recurrent falls and functional decline among elderly people at risk. This study, which is an alteration of a previous randomized controlled trial, will provide new information about the effectiveness in a Dutch situation. Economic evaluation will provide details into the intervention's cost effectiveness and the effects on quality of life.

Hildebrandt, J., Pfingsten, M., Saur, P., & Jansen, J. (1997). Prediction of success from a multidisciplinary treatment program for chronic low back pain. *Spine, 22*(9), 990-1001.

> **Keywords**: low back pain, rehabilitation program, outpatient
>
> The article looked at a program for people with chronic lower back pain to return to work. The program included exercise and education components. There is evidence that this program is effective for the low back pain population.

Holm, M. B., Santangelo, M. A., Fromuth, D. J., Brown, S. O., & Walter, H. (2000). Effectiveness of everyday occupations for changing client behaviours in a community living arrangement. *American Journal of Occupational Therapy, 54*, 361-371.

> **Keywords**: child developmental disorders, planning techniques (programs), psychiatry
>
> The study discusses the movement toward community-based programs, namely the Community Living Arrangement (CLA) program for people with psychiatric diagnoses. A multiple-baseline study design was reported that compared three conditions, including occupation-based intervention in conjunction with the CLA program aimed at reducing dysfunctional behaviors in two women with dual developmental psychiatric conditions. Results showed significant improvements in functional and decreases in dysfunctional behaviors when using everyday occupations as interventions in conjunction with positive reinforcement.

Hooten, W. M., Townsend, C., Sletten, C., Bruce, B., & Rome, J. D. (2007). Treatment outcomes after multidisciplinary pain rehabilitation with analgesic medication withdrawal for patients with fibromyalgia. *Pain Med, 8*(1), 8-16.

> **Keywords**: fibromyalgia, multidisciplinary pain rehabilitation, analgesic medication
>
> The objective of this study was to assess whether a program of multidisciplinary pain rehabilitation with concurrent withdrawal of analgesic pain medication would improve post-treatment measures of psychosocial functioning, health attributes, negative pain-related emotions, and depressive symptoms in patients with fibromyalgia. The study took place at a tertiary referral medical center and examined 159 consecutive patients admitted to the 3-week outpatient program. Results showed a significantly favorable response to treatment and a significant reduction in the use of pain medications in patients who went through the program.

Hoppes, S. (1997). Can play increase standing tolerance? A pilot-study. *Physical and Occupational Therapy in Geriatrics, 15*(1), 65-73.

> The article discusses the positive effects of play for geriatric patients as play allows freedom, creativity, and decision making. A study is then discussed that looks at whether patients who are unable to maintain a functional standing position are able to stand up for longer periods of time after playing a game versus taking part in a non-playful activity such as reading. Game-playing was shown to increase standing tolerance for participants in the study.

Horowitz, B. P., & Chang, P. F. (2004). Promoting well-being and engagement in life through occupational therapy lifestyle redesign: A pilot study within adult day programs. *Topics in Geriatric Rehabilitation, 20*(1), 46-58.

> **Keywords**: health, lifestyle redesign, medical model adult day program, preventive occupational therapy, well-being
>
> The article begins with an in-depth discussion of preventive occupational therapy and notes its recorded success with elderly populations. Next, a study is presented that evaluates occupational therapist-led lifestyle redesign programs aimed at limiting seniors' functional, physical, and mental decline. A limited sample size was attributed to the inability to note statistically significant differences between participant groups.

Hsieh, C. L., Nelson, D. L., Smith, D. A., & Peterson, C. Q. (1996). A comparison of performance in added-purpose occupations and rote exercise for dynamic standing balance in persons with hemiplegia. *American Journal of Occupational Therapy, 50*(1), 10-16.

> **Keywords**: human activities and occupations, motivation
>
> "This study examined whether 21 subjects with hemiplegia performed more exercise repetitions in two added-purpose occupations than in a rote exercise. The results showed that the subjects did significantly more exercise repetitions in the added-purpose occupations than in the rote exercise, suggesting that purpose may be effectively added to an exercise through the use of actual material or through the use of imagery. These results help to substantiate one of occupational therapy's basic tenets, that added-purpose occupation is a motivating factor in performance."

Huebner, R. A., Johnson, K., Bennett, C. M., & Schneck, C. (2003). Community participation and quality of life outcomes after adult traumatic brain injury. *American Journal of Occupational Therapy, 57*(2), 177-185.

> **Keywords**: activity limitation, community integration, occupational performance
>
> This study examined outcomes after traumatic brain injury in adults salient to occupational therapy. Demographic and functional ability data were collected retrospectively through a medical chart review, and a follow-up was completed an average of 21 months later that measured disability, community participation, quality of life, and satisfaction with occupational therapy. Results support the premise that participation is associated with a high quality of life, yet people with brain injury have significant needs for long-term occupational therapy.

Hui, E., Lum, C. M., Woo, J., Or, K. H., & Kay, R. L. (1995). Outcomes of elderly stroke patients: Day hospital versus conventional medical management. *Stroke, 26*, 1616-1619.

> **Keywords**: elderly, stroke outcome, hospitalization, rehabilitation
>
> The goals of this study were to evaluate stroke outcomes (function, emotional well-being) and cost-effectiveness when using a geriatric team at a day hospital versus conventional inpatient treatment in elderly patients with stroke. Conclusions from the study suggest that although both approaches to treatment improve functional outcomes in stroke patients, treatment with a geriatric team at a day

hospital may speed recovery with fewer outpatient visits. There were no significant differences in cost between the two types of treatment.

Indredavik, B., Bakke, F., Solberg, R., Rokseth, R., Lund Haaheim, L., & Holme, I. (1991). Benefit of a stroke unit: A randomized control trial. *Stroke, 22,* 1026-1031.

> *Keywords*: stroke unit, general medical wards
>
> The aim of this study was to help determine the value of stroke units by conducting a randomized controlled trial that compared clinical outcomes from 6 weeks of treatment in a stroke unit versus treatment in general medical wards. All outcomes (functional status, mortality, neurological scores, and home/institutional stays) were significant at 6 weeks, with more positive outcomes seen in those treated in stroke units. At 52 weeks, all aforementioned outcomes remained significant, in favor of the stroke unit group, with the exception of morality rates. At 1 year, there were no differences between groups in terms of mortality rate.

Ip, W. M., Woo, J., Yue, S. Y., Kwan, M., Sum, S. M., Kwok, T., et al. (2006). Evaluation of the effect of energy conservation techniques in the performance of activity of daily living tasks. *Clinical Rehabilitation, 20*(3), 254-261.

> This study evaluated the effectiveness of energy conservation techniques in lowering the energy expenditure during completion of common activities of daily living and documented participants' subjective comments regarding perceived level of effort. Members were recruited from the community and staff of the rehabilitation hospital where the study took place. Participants completed three tasks with and without the use of energy conservation techniques. Energy expenditure was measured throughout by a portable calorimetry system, and patients were interviewed afterwards on levels of dyspnea, fatigue, and perceived exertion. Reduction in energy expenditure by using the energy conservation techniques was observed for a few of the tasks in younger subjects only, although older subjects reported less perceived effort.

Jao, H. P., & Lu, S. J. (1999). The acquisition of problem-solving skills through the instruction in Siegel and Spivack's Problem-Solving Therapy for the chronic schizophrenic. *Occupational Therapy in Mental Health, 14*(4), 47-63.

> The effectiveness of Siegel and Spivack's Problem-Solving Therapy for the chronic schizophrenic was analyzed in this study. The intervention was shown to be effective in increasing interpersonal problem solving, but it did not have a corresponding effect on self-esteem.

Jarus, T., Shavit, S., & Ratzon, N. (2000). From hand twister to mind twister: Computer-aided treatment in traumatic wrist fracture. *American Journal of Occupational Therapy, 54,* 176-182.

> *Keywords*: hand functions, physical disabilities, occupational therapy, technology
>
> The aim of the study was to examine the use of computers as a treatment modality in the occupational therapy hand clinic by comparing it to a low technology treatment alternative. The study also justified the application of such devices. Significant improvements in range of motion, grip strength, and edema across 5 weeks were seen for all participants. No significant differences were found between the two groups in range of motion, grip strength, and edema. The computer-aided group showed significantly more interest in treatment than did the brush machine group. In conclusion, the potential for more interesting motor treatment and rehabilitation of the wrist through the use of computer games is there.

Johansson, A., & Bjorklund, A. (2005). Occupational adaptation or well-tried, professional experience in rehabilitation of the disabled elderly at home. *Activities, Adaptation and Aging, 30*(1), 1-21.

> *Keywords*: OAM, home rehabilitation, seniors, experienced health, FIM, home-rehabilitation, IAM, independence, SF-36, semi-structured interviews
>
> The article begins by reviewing a model of practice. Next, a study is presented that evaluates treatment effectiveness under that model of practice against a control group that is treated under a combination of other models. Outcomes indicate that the investigated model of practice generates superior outcomes on the measures employed.

Johansson, K., Lindgren, I., Widner, H., & Wiklund, I. (1993). Can sensory stimulation improve the functional outcome in stroke patients? *Neurology, 43,* 2189-2192.

> *Keywords*: acupuncture, stroke
>
> The purpose of this study was to address three questions: a) Can acupuncture improve or speed up the motor recovery in patients post-stroke; b) Do patients receiving acupuncture achieve greater independence in activities of daily living (ADL) function compared to controls; and c) Can acupuncture improve quality of life of patients who have experienced stroke? The results revealed that those in the acupuncture group had faster and greater improvements in balance, mobility, ADL function, and quality of life compared to controls. Researchers suggest that the degree to which acupuncture is responsible for these differences requires more research.

Jones, G. R., Miller, T. A., & Petrella, R. J. (2002). Evaluation of rehabilitation outcomes for older patients with hip fractures. *American Journal of Physical Medicine and Rehabilitation, 81,* 489-497.

> *Keywords*: rehabilitation, aging, outcome measures, hip fracture
>
> The aim of this study was to evaluate functional outcomes as well as rehabilitation efficacy for older patients with hip fractures who participated in an inpatient rehabilitation program. Results indicated that inpatient rehabilitation was associated with improvements in functional abilities, particularly in the areas of self-care. Improvements in functional ability were seen to be maintained in a sub-sample who participated in follow-up 6 weeks after discharge from the hospital.

Jongbloed, L. (1993). Evaluating the efficacy of OT intervention related to leisure activities. *Canadian Journal of Rehabilitation, 7*(1), 19-20.

> The purpose of this study was to evaluate the effect of five leisure facilitation sessions by an occupational therapist for patients who had experienced a stroke. Forty participants were randomly allocated to receive leisure facilitation or general discussion about leisure (control group). Results indicated that there were no significant differences between the two groups for the outcomes of activity involvement and satisfaction.

Jongbloed, L., & Morgan, D. (1991). An investigation of involvement in leisure activities after a stroke. *American Journal of Occupational Therapy, 45*(5), 420-427.

> *Keywords*: adaptation, psychological, cerebrovascular disorders, leisure activities, occupational therapy services, social adjustment
>
> This article examined an occupational therapy intervention for stroke survivors to see if the intervention would impact leisure activity involvement or satisfaction with the leisure activities. Participants received either a 5-week therapy intervention (intervention group) or a 5-week talk/question session (control group) with an occupational therapist. Overall, improvement was shown for both groups in activity involvement and satisfaction with this involvement but no statistically significant differences were found between the groups.

Jongbloed, L., Stacey, S., & Brighton, C. (1989). Stroke rehabilitation: Sensorimotor integrative treatment versus functional treatment. *American Journal of Occupational Therapy, 43*(6), 391-397.

> *Keywords*: cerebrovascular disorder, modalities, occupational therapy, rehabilitation, sensorimotor therapy
>
> This article discussed two different occupational therapy approaches—the sensorimotor integrative approach and the more traditional functional approach. It then examined the effectiveness of the two types of therapy on the self-care, mobility, and functional performance for people with cerebrovascular accident. No performance differences were found between the groups leading the researchers to conclude that "any differences between the effectiveness of the two approaches are small."

Jousset, N., Fanello, S., Bontoux, L., Dubus, V., Billabert, C., Vielle, B., et al. (2004). Effects of functional restoration versus 3 hours physical therapy: A randomized control trial. *Spine, 29,* 487-494.

Keywords: functional restoration, low back pain, physical therapy, psychotherapy, occupational therapy, rehabilitation, randomized control trial

The purpose of this randomized controlled trial was to compare treatment in a functional restoration program (FRP) to that of active individual therapy (AIT), in terms of impacting number of sick days (and other functional outcomes) in patients with chronic low back pain. Conclusion were drawn that support the effectiveness of FRP, compared to AIT, in reducing number of sick days, when adjusting for a variable related to workplace ergonomics. FRP participants also improved on a number of physical capacity variables, when compared both between and within groups.

Kaapa, E. H., Frantsi, K., Sarna, S., & Malmivaara, A. (2006). Multidisciplinary group rehabilitation versus individual physiotherapy for chronic nonspecific low back pain: A randomized trial. *Spine, 31*(4), 371-376.

Keywords: chronic low back pain, female, multidisciplinary rehabilitation

This article begins by looking at systematic review evidence that intense multidisciplinary rehabilitation is effective for chronic lower back pain. The study compares a multidisciplinary approach to rehabilitation versus regular physiotherapy care. Overall, the study found that there is no benefit for semi-light multidisciplinary rehabilitation for women with chronic low back pain in an outpatient setting compared to physiotherapy.

Kalra, L. (1994). The influence of stroke unit rehabilitation on functional recovery from stroke. *Stroke, 25*, 821-825.

Keywords: hospitalization, rehabilitation

The purpose of this study was to compare rates of functional change and therapy "inputs" for stroke patients receiving care in a stroke unit compared to general wards. The rate of change compared to length of stay was also examined. In this study, significantly more and faster rates of change were seen in patients receiving care in the stroke unit compared to general wards. Length of stay was also significantly shorter for those in the stroke unit versus the general ward.

Kawahira, K., Shimodozono, M., Ogata, A., & Tanaka, N. (2004). Addition of intensive repetition of facilitation exercise to multidisciplinary rehabilitation promotes motor functional recovery of the hemiplegic lower limb. *Journal of Rehabilitation Medicine, 36*(4), 159-164.

This article discusses different approaches used for stroke rehabilitation before evaluating the effect of an 8-week multidisciplinary program that utilized intensive repetition of movements on voluntary movements of a hemiplegic lower limb. Not all participants in this study received occupational therapy. The authors conclude that "intensive repetition of movement elicited by the facilitation technique (chiefly proprioceptive neuromuscular facilitation pattern, stretch reflex, and skin-muscle reflex) improved voluntary movement of a hemiplegic lower limb in patients with brain damage."

Keren, O., Motin, M., Heinemann, A. W., O'Reilly, C. M., Bode, R. K., Semik, P., et al. (2004). Relationship between rehabilitation therapies and outcome of stroke patients in Israel: A preliminary study. *Israel Medical Association Journal, 6*, 736-741.

Keywords: stroke, intensity of therapies, improvement of impairment, rehabilitation

The purpose of this study was to evaluate the effectiveness of inpatient rehabilitation for post-stroke patients, specifically in terms of the relationship between intensity of therapies and functional outcomes at the time of discharge. Researchers concluded that, based on results, there was a significant reduction of impairment between admission and discharge. Functional abilities, as measured by the Functional Independence Measure (FIM), were also improved. Specifically relevant to occupational therapy was the fact that intensity of this therapy was positively correlated with motor and cognitive functions.

Kielhofner, G., Braveman, B., Finlyason, M., Paul-Ward, A., Goldbaum, L., & Goldstein, K. (2004). Outcomes of a vocational program for persons with AIDS. *American Journal of Occupational Therapy, 58*, 64-72.

In this study, a vocational rehabilitation program was developed and given to unemployed people with AIDS to assess the outcomes of the program in terms of which aspects of the program were most helpful and whether certain participant characteristics were related to better outcomes. The outcomes for people who completed the program were good—67% of completers achieved success. People's narratives (their interpretation of their life and events as positive or negative) were found to be associated with program completion and with successful outcomes.

Kielhofner, G., Braveman, B., Fogg, L., & Levin, M. (2008). A controlled study of services to enhance productive participation among people with HIV/AIDS. *American Journal of Occupational Therapy, 62*(1), 36-45.

Keywords: HIV/AIDS, Model of Human Occupation, occupational therapy, work rehabilitation

The objective of this study was to assess the effectiveness of an intervention designed to increase productive participation in HIV/AIDS patients living in supportive living facilities. Participants were non-randomly assigned to receive either standard care or the intervention and were followed for 9 months. Results showed that participants in the intervention group had significantly more involvement in productive participation and were twice as likely to be engaged in productive activity than controls throughout follow-up.

King, T. I. (1993). Hand strengthening with a computer for purposeful activity. *American Journal of Occupational Therapy, 47*(7), 635-637.

Keywords: computer-assisted therapy, hand occupational therapy, motivation

This study examined the effects of purposeful versus non-purposeful activity on the number of times a patient requiring hand therapy could grip or pinch a strengthening device. The number of times the participant gripped or pinched while he or she played a videogame (purposeful) versus when he or she was asked to see how many times he or she could complete the exercise (non-purposeful) were compared. Participants did much better when completing a purposeful activity. The authors suggest that the use of computer games may be valuable for treatment-related activities like dexterity and range of motion.

Kohlmeyer, K. M., Hill, J. P., Yarkony, G. M., & Jaeger, R. J. (1996). Electrical stimulation and biofeedback effect on recovery of tenodesis grasp: A controlled study. *Archives of Physical Medicine and Rehabilitation, 77*, 702-706.

Keywords: spinal cord injury, inpatient, occupational therapy, tenodesis grasp

The aim of this study was to evaluate the effectiveness of electrical stimulation and biofeedback on the recovery of tenodesis grasp in tetraplegic individuals during the initial phase of acute rehabilitation. The results were that electrical stimulation and biofeedback were no more effective than conventional treatment. However, it is possible that there are individual patients who would benefit substantially and preferentially from electrical stimulation and/or biofeedback.

Kool, J., Bachmann, S., Oesch, P., Knuesel, O., Ambergen, T., de Bie, R., et al. (2007). Function-centred rehabilitation increases workdays in patients with nonacute nonspecific low back pain: 1 year results from a randomized trial. *Archives of Physical Medicine and Rehabilitation, 88*(9), 1089-1094.

Keywords: exercise therapy, low back pain, occupational diseases, outcome assessment (health care), randomized controlled trial, rehabilitation, sick leave, vocational rehabilitation

This article begins by emphasizing the importance of multidisciplinary rehabilitation to treated people with chronic back pain. The study compares two different multidisciplinary interventions for people with low back pain—function centred rehabilitation (FCR) and pain-centered treatment (PCT)—to assist with return to work. The results showed that FCT is more effective than PCT for increasing workdays.

Koppenhaver, D., Erickson, K., Harris, B., McLellan, J., Skotko, G., & Newton, R. (2001). Storybook-based communication intervention for girls with Rett syndrome and their mothers. *Disability and Rehabilitation, 23*, 149-159.

> The article begins by reporting how storybook reading provides a natural support to early symbolic communication for children. The study describes the impact of hand splints, light augmentative communication systems, and basic parenting training on the symbolic communication and labeling behaviors of six girls with Rett syndrome. Results indicated that the girls became more active and successful participants during storybook reading, which demonstrated how the intervention could enhance early participation and communication.

Lamb, A., Finlayson, M., Mathiowetz, V., & Chen, H. Y. (2005). The outcomes of using self-study modules in energy conservation education for people with multiple sclerosis. *Clinical Rehabilitation, 19*(5), 475-481.

> To evaluate the effectiveness of an energy conservation program facilitated by an occupational therapist compared to self-study program completed in the patient's home. This was completed as a secondary analysis of a larger trial with the intervention and control groups being formed from those who completed the entire program and patients who had missed one or more sessions. Participants who missed sessions of the course and completed self-study modules and participants who completed the entire course all experienced the same benefits from the energy conservation program.

Lambert, R. A., Harvey, I., & Poland, F. (2007). A pragmatic, unblinded randomised controlled trial comparing an occupational therapy-led lifestyle approach and routine GP care for panic disorder treatment in primary care. *Journal of Affective Disorders, 99*(1-3), 63-71.

> ***Keywords***: clinical trial, panic disorder, lifestyle, primary care, occupational therapy, pragmatic
>
> The aim of this study was to assess if an occupational therapy-led lifestyle approach to the treatment of panic disorders was as clinically effective as routine general practitioner-led care. Patients enrolled in the intervention received an occupational therapy-led treatment that consisted of a review of current lifestyle, negotiation of positive changes between the therapist and patient, and monitoring and review of the impact of those changes. The primary outcome measure was the Beck Anxiety Inventory (BAI). Results showed significantly lower BAI scores in the lifestyle treatment group at 20 weeks, but the difference in BAI scores was non-significant at 10-month follow-up. More than 60% of patients who received the intervention were panic free at 20 weeks and 10-month follow-up.

Landi, F., Cesari, M., Onder, G., Tafani, A., Zamboni, V., & Cocchi, A. (2006). Effects of an occupational therapy program on functional outcomes in older stroke patients. *Gerontology, 52*(2), 85-91.

> ***Keywords***: function, stroke, older adults
>
> The study examined the efficacy of occupational therapy programs on patients with recent stroke because of the increasing importance of occupational therapy as a component of rehabilitation. A brief discussion of function and rehabilitation teams was included. Older adults who have had strokes fared better in their level of independence in activities of daily living after receiving occupational therapy intervention than those who did not.

Lannin, N., Clemson, L., McCluskey, A., Lin, C., Cameron, I., & Barras, S. (2007). Feasibility and results of a randomised pilot-study of pre-discharge occupational therapy home visits. *BMC Health Services Research, 7*(1), 42.

> The aim of this pilot study was to determine how feasible a controlled trial comparing pre-discharge home visits to standard in-hospital visits would be and the effect on functional ability. Ten participants were recruited to the study over 3 months and were randomized to receive the intervention (home visit) or be in the control group. The study showed that a larger trial would be feasible; however, any observed increase in functional ability was not significant as the sample size was too small.

Lannin, N., Cusick, A., McCluskey, A., & Herbert, R. (2007). Effects of splinting on wrist contracture after stroke: A randomized controlled trial. *Stroke, 38*(1), 111-116.

> ***Keywords***: function, pain, occupational therapy, upper limb disability, spasticity
>
> The aim of this study was to evaluate the use of splints that kept the wrist in an extended or neutral position in preventing wrist contracture in the hemiplegic arm after stroke. Adults that had experienced a stroke within the previous 8 weeks were selected to participate in the study and were randomized to a control group that received only routine therapy or an intervention group that received routine therapy and wore a splint in the neutral or extended position nightly. Splint use did not have any clinically or statistically significant effect on extension of the wrist or long finger flexor muscles.

Lannin, N. A., Horsley, S. A., Herbert, R., McCluskey, A., & Cusick, A. (2003). Splinting the hand in the functional position after brain impairment: A randomized, controlled trial. *Archives of Physical Medicine and Rehabilitation, 84*, 297-302.

> ***Keywords***: contracture, hemiplegia, occupational therapy, rehabilitation, spasticity
>
> The aim of this study was to evaluate the effects of 4 weeks of hand splinting on the length of finger and wrist flexor muscles, hand function, and pain in the people with acquired brain impairment. The main result was that effects of splinting were statistically non-significant and clinically unimportant. At follow-up, estimates of treatment effects slightly favored the control group. In conclusion, use of overnight splints with the affected hand in the functional position does not produce clinically beneficial effects in adults with acquired brain impairment.

Lee, H., Tan, H., Ma, H., Tsai, C., & Liu, Y. (2006). Effectiveness of a work-related stress management program in patients with chronic schizophrenia. *American Journal of Occupational Therapy, 60*(4), 435-441.

> This study evaluated the effectiveness of a work-related stress management program in patients with chronic schizophrenia. Inpatients who were engaged in low-wage work within the psychiatric hospital were recruited to participate in the study and were randomly assigned to receive 12 weeks of intervention followed by 12 weeks of no treatment or vice versa. Results showed that the intervention had very significant short-term positive effects on subjects' work-related stress but once the treatment was withdrawn nearly all subjects experience significant deterioration.

Li, E., Li-Tsang, C., Lam, C., Hui, K., & Chan, C. (2006). The effect of a "training on work readiness" program for workers with musculoskeletal injuries: A randomized control trial (RCT) study. *Journal of Occupational Rehabilitation, 16*(4), 529-541.

> ***Keywords***: return to work, musculoskeletal injuries, work readiness, long term sick leave
>
> The objective of this study was to evaluate the effectiveness of a multidisciplinary 3-week training program for workers with musculoskeletal injuries. The program consisted of group therapy and individualized training sessions, and its main purpose was to change participant's attitudes toward injury and return to work. Results showed the program was effective in reducing subjects' anxiety toward returning to work and improving their motivation and readiness to seek re-employment.

Li, L., Davis, A., Lineker, S., Coyte, P., & Bombardier, C. (2005). Outcomes of home-based rehabilitation provided by primary therapists for patients with rheumatoid arthritis: Pilot study. *Physiotherapy Canada, 57*(4), 255-264.

> ***Keywords***: home-based rehabilitation, primary therapist model, rheumatoid arthritis
>
> This pilot study discusses how a primary therapist can be beneficial with the trends in health care today. The primary therapist acts as a case manager and generalist rather than specializing in his or her profession. The study shows that there is a trend toward improvement through use of a primary therapist model for adults with rheumatoid arthritis.

Li, L. C., Davis, A. M., Lineker, S. C., Coyte, P. C., & Bombardier, C. (2006). Effectiveness of the primary therapist model for rheumatoid arthritis rehabilitation: A randomized controlled trial. *Arthritis and Rheumatism, 55*(1), 42-52.

Keywords: rheumatoid arthritis, primary therapist model
This article is a randomized controlled trial comparing a primary therapist model to a traditional treatment model for people with rheumatoid arthritis. The primary service model is used by the Arthritis Society, whereas the traditional treatment model was used in other outpatient rehabilitation settings. There is some evidence to show that the primary therapist model is beneficial for people with rheumatoid arthritis, although the study had a high attrition rate.

Li, S., Liu, L., Miyazaki, M., & Warren, S. (1999). Effectiveness of splinting for work-related carpal tunnel syndrome: A three-month follow-up study. *Technology and Disability, 11*, 51-64.

Keywords: splinting, work-related CTS, symptom severity, functional status
The article begins by discussing the prevalence of carpal tunnel syndrome (CTS) in the workplace and the evidence of splinting to reduce symptoms in the short-term. The study intended to explore the long-term (3-month) impact of splinting on clients with work-related CTS. The researchers concluded that splinting for 3 months was effective in relieving CTS symptoms and improved functional status for subjects in the study.

Liberman, R. P., Wallace, C. J., Blackwell, G., Kopelowicz, A., Vaccaro, J. V., & Mintz, J. (1998). Skills training versus psychosocial occupational therapy for persons with persistent schizophrenia. *American Journal of Psychiatry, 155*(8), 1087-1091.

Keywords: schizophrenia, skills training, psychosocial occupational therapy, outpatient
The article begins with a brief discussion of the effectiveness of life skills training for mental health clientele. In the opening discussion, the authors note that the effectiveness of skills training has not been examined against other "active approaches." Next, a study is presented that examines the effect of skills training for clients with persistent schizophrenia versus psychosocial occupational therapy interventions. Results indicate that the group who received skills training scored significantly better on all scales that indicated improvement in both groups and on some scales where the psychosocial group did not improve.

Liddle, J., March, L., Carfrae, B., Finnegan, T., Druce, J., Schwarz, J., et al. (1996). Can occupational therapy intervention play a part in maintaining independence and quality of life in older people? A randomized controlled trial. *Australian and New Zealand Journal of Public Health, 20*, 574-578.

The study aims to see if older people could maintain their quality of life and independence after their homes had been modified and they used community services as recommended by occupational therapy. The article describes how quality of life and functional outcomes were assessed for both the control group and the group who received intervention, which did not demonstrate differences between groups but showed improvements within groups. From the results of this study after 6 months of follow-up, it does not seem that in the short term acting on occupational therapy recommendations appears to improve outcomes in this population.

Lin, J. H., Chang, C. M., Liu, C. K., Huang, M. H., & Lin, Y. T. (2000). Efficiency and effectiveness of stroke rehabilitation after first stroke. *Journal of the Formosan Medical Association, 99*, 483-490.

Keywords: stroke, rehabilitation, functional recovery
The purpose of this study was to look at variables associated with the efficiency and effectiveness of inpatient multidisciplinary rehabilitation in patients with stroke. Results indicated that shorter inpatient stay and higher arm motor recovery stage predicted better rehabilitation efficiency, although a large amount of variance remained unaccounted for. Younger age and higher arm motor recovery stage was associated with better rehabilitation effectiveness.

Lincoln, N. B., Walker, M. F., Dixon, A., & Knights, P. (2004). Evaluation of a multiprofessional community stroke team: A randomized controlled trial. *Clinical Rehabilitation, 18*, 40-47.

Keywords: community stroke team, randomization, caregiver

The aim of this study was to compare conventional outpatient post-stroke rehabilitation to care provided by a specialized multi-professional team, in regard to outcomes such as mood, functional abilities, quality of life, and satisfaction with services. Through the use of a randomized control trial, researchers found that functional outcomes and mood did not significantly differ based on whether patients received rehabilitation from the community stroke team or a more routine form of care. However, those receiving services from the community stroke team reported feeling significantly more supported emotionally than those in the conventional care group. Caregivers of those in the community stroke group reported feeling significantly less strain.

Lincoln, N. B., Whiting, S. E., Cockburn, J., & Bhavnani, G. (1985). An evaluation of perceptual retraining. *International Rehabilitation Medicine, 7*, 99-110.

Keywords: cognitive rehabilitation, perception, occupational therapy
A randomized controlled trial involving stroke patients and those with head injury was conducted to evaluate the effectiveness of perceptual training versus conventional occupational therapy treatment. Outcome measures included visual perception and independence in activities of daily living (ADL). Results indicated that there were no significant between-group differences on performance of perceptual tasks or ADL function before or after intervention. Both groups improved on most perceptual tasks across time. Both groups also improved significantly in self-care from baseline to post-intervention assessments. Therefore, perceptual training failed to be shown as more or less effective than conventional occupational therapy in terms of impacting the outcome measures.

Lindh, M., Lurie, M., & Sanne, H. (1997). A randomized prospective study of vocational outcome in rehabilitation of patients with non-specific musculoskeletal pain: A multidisciplinary approach to patients identified after 90 days of sick-leave. *Scandinavian Journal of Rehabilitative Medicine, 29*(2), 103-112.

Keywords: musculoskeletal pain, return to work, re-sick listing
This article outlines a multidisciplinary approach for people with generalized chronic musculoskeletal pain to return to work and remain at work. The study followed up both a control group with no therapy and a group with therapy for 5 years to determine if they were working. The results were not strongly stated, although there was some indication that there is improvement for Swedish workers who did receive early rehabilitation to be working more consistently.

Lippert-Gruner, M., Wedekind, C., & Klug, N. (2002). Functional and psychosocial outcome one year after severe traumatic brain injury and early-onset rehabilitation therapy. *Journal of Rehabilitation Medicine, 34*(5), 211-214.

Keywords: traumatic brain injury, outcome, rehabilitation, occupational reintegration
This prospective study begins by outlining increased interest in functional outcomes for clients with traumatic brain injuries. Study methods are reviewed, selected outcome measures are outlined, and the results are presented. The majority of clients reached high levels of independence in their activities of daily living, but many continued to have behavioral and speech deficits that impacted reintegration into school and work life. The authors attempt to compare their results with similar types of studies, but note limitations due to methodological variability.

Liu, K. P., Chan, C. C., Lee, T. M., & Hui-Chan, C. W. (2004). Mental imagery for promoting relearning for people after stroke. *Archives of Physical Medicine and Rehabilitation, 85*, 1403-1408.

Keywords: imagery (psychotherapy), mental disorders, rehabilitation, stroke, randomized controlled trial
The purpose of this randomized controlled trial was to evaluate the efficacy of mental imagery for relearning of tasks in patients with stroke. The results indicate a significant impact of mental imagery in improving task performance on "trained" as well as new tasks compared to patients in a control group.

Logan, P. A., Ahern, J., Gladman, J. R., & Lincoln, N. B. (1997). A randomized controlled trial of enhanced social service occupational therapy for stroke patients. *Clinical Rehabilitation, 11*(2), 107-113.

> **Keywords**: stroke, discharge, home, outpatient
> The article begins by briefly outlining a poverty of services available for patients being discharged after acute stroke. Next, a study is presented that evaluates the effectiveness of occupational therapy-based services for patients being discharged after acute stroke. Results indicate that the program is effective at increasing function and reducing health declines for care providers.

Logan, P. A., Gladman, J. R., Avery, A., Walker, M. F., Dyas, J., & Groom, L. (2004). Randomised controlled trial of an occupational therapy intervention to increase outdoor mobility after stroke. *British Medical Journal, 329*(7479), 1372-1375.

> The objective of this paper was to evaluate an occupational therapy intervention designed to improve outdoor mobility after stroke. A randomized controlled trial was implemented, and 168 community-dwelling people with clinical diagnosis of stroke in the previous 36 months were recruited to participate. Results suggest that a targeted occupational therapy intervention delivered in the client's home increases outdoor mobility in people after stroke.

Lushbough, R. S., Priddy, J. M., Sewell, H. H., Lovett, S. B., & Jones, T. C. (1988). The effectiveness of an occupational therapy program in an inpatient geropsychiatric setting. *Physical and Occupational Therapy in Geriatrics, 6*(2), 63-73.

> **Keywords**: OT, psychosocial groups
> The study reviewed the literature about occupational therapy and psychosocial interventions for people with psychiatric disorders. The methods, results, and study limitations were reviewed. The authors concluded that the occupational therapy and psychosocial groups resulted in clinical improvements evident in improved Comprehensive Occupational Therapy Evaluation (COTE) scores, voluntary group attendance, peer interaction, and engagement in tasks. No significant changes were observed in the Nurses Observation Scale for Inpatient Evaluation (NOSIE) and Brief Psychiatric Rating Scale (BPRS).

Luukinen, H., Lehtola, S., Jokelainen, J., Vaananen-Sainio, R., Lotvonen, S., & Koistinen, P. (2007). Pragmatic exercise-oriented prevention of falls among the elderly: A population-based, randomized, controlled trial. *Preventive Medicine, 44*(3), 265-271.

> The purpose of this study was to assess the effectiveness of a fall prevention program implemented by regional geriatric care teams. The study was conducted among home-dwelling people aged 85 years or older who were randomized to receive either routine care or a program consisting of home exercise and self-care training. The total number of falls and time to first four falls did not differ significantly between the two groups; however, the program was effective in slowing down the reduction of balance performance.

Lynch, D., Ferraro, M., Krol, J., Trudell, C. M., Christos, P., & Volpe, B. T. (2005). Continuous passive motion improves shoulder joint integrity following stroke. *Clinical Rehabilitation, 19*(6), 594-599.

> This article describes a study comparing device-delivered continuous passive range of motion exercises with self-administered, therapist-observed exercises. All participants had recently had their first stroke. Though the statistical significance of the results is weak, the authors conclude that they provide support for the use of continuous passive motion devices, noting their low cost in rehabilitation units.

MacPhee, A. H., Kirby, R. L., Coolen, A. L., Smith, C., MacLeod, D. A., & Dupuis, D. J. (2004). Wheelchair skills training program: A randomized clinical trial of wheelchair users undergoing initial rehabilitation. *Archives of Physical Medicine and Rehabilitation, 85*(1), 41-50.

> **Keywords**: assistive technology, motor skills, rehabilitation, wheelchairs
> This study examined the safety and effectiveness of a wheelchair skills training program. It concluded that "the WSTP is safe and practical and has a clinically significant effect on the independent wheeled mobility of new wheelchair users.

These findings have implications for the standards of care in rehabilitation programs."

Maeshima, S., Ueyoshi, A., Osawa, A., Ishida, K., Kunimoto, K., Shimamoto, Y., et al. (2003). Mobility and muscle strength contralateral to hemiplegia from stroke: Benefit from self-training with family support. *American Journal of Physical Medicine and Rehabilitation, 82*(6), 456-462.

> **Keywords**: stroke, hemiparesis, family, muscle strength
> This article focuses on self-training with family support for clients with hemiplegia from a stroke. The study compared regular occupational therapy and physiotherapy to regular therapy with the addition of family-supported therapy. The study found that there were no significant results at first evaluation, but with further statistical testing, patients' strength and mobility improved with family participation.

Mairs, H., & Bradshaw, T. (2004). Life skills training in schizophrenia. *British Journal of Occupational Therapy, 67*(5), 217-224.

> The article begins with a brief discussion on the deficits of social functioning that accompany a diagnosis of schizophrenia and the life skill approaches that aim to promote the acquisition of life skills through occupational therapy. A pilot study is presented that aims to assess the impact of a life skills training program for individuals with schizophrenia. Results indicate that individuals participating in the intervention had a reduction in negative symptoms and overall levels of general psychopathology, although this was not reflected in social functioning.

Malcus-Johnson, P., Carlqvist, C., Sturesson, A., & Eberhardt, K. (2005). Occupational therapy during the first 10 years of rheumatoid arthritis. *Scandinavian Journal of Occupational Therapy, 12*(3), 128-135.

> **Keywords**: assistive devices, comprehensive care, hand function, occupational therapy, patient education, rheumatoid arthritis
> This study evaluated the effects of consistent occupational therapy during the first 10 years of rheumatoid arthritis and assessed patients' experiences with occupational therapy and conventional care. Patients in the very early stages of rheumatoid arthritis were selected and followed up for 10 years with regular therapist visits and assessments. The majority of the visits to the therapist resulted in interventions, and impairments in hand function were generally mild to moderate and remained that way with activity limitations only showing a slight increase.

Mann, W. C., Ottenbacher, K. J., Fraas, L., Tomita, M., & Granger, C. V. (1999). Effectiveness of assistive technology and environmental interventions in maintaining independence and reducing home care costs for the frail elderly. A randomized controlled trial. *Archives of Family Medicine, 8*(3), 210-217.

> **Keywords:** function, assistive technology
> The purpose of this randomized trial was to evaluate the effectiveness of an occupational therapy program that included comprehensive functional assessment, evaluation of the home environment, and provision of environmental interventions and assistive technology to maintain function. The control group received usual care. Findings indicated that function in the intervention group declined but significantly less than the control group. Mann and colleagues demonstrated that provision of environmental interventions and assistive technology for older adults living at home led to physical environmental changes and associated reduced institutional and nurse/case manager costs.

Masiero, S., Boniolo, A., Wassermann, L., Machiedo, H., Volante, D., & Punzi, L. (2007). Effects of an educational–behavioural joint protection program on people with moderate to severe rheumatoid arthritis: A randomized controlled trial. *Clinical Rheumatology, 26*(12), 2043-2050.

> **Keywords**: activities of daily living, disability evaluation, exercise, joint, rehabilitation, rheumatoid arthritis
> The purpose of this study was to assess the effects of a joint protection training program on pain, disability, and health status in a group of moderate to severe rheumatoid arthritis patients. The patients were in treatment with anti-TNF-α drugs and were randomized to receive routine care or the

joint education program. After attending the program, patients showed significantly less pain and disability and increased social and health status.

Mathiowetz, V., Bolding, D. J., & Trombly, C. A. (1983). Immediate effects of positioning devices on the normal and spastic hand measured by electromyography. *American Journal of Occupational Therapy, 37*(4), 247-254.

Keywords: volar splint, cone, finger spreader, CVA, hypertonus

This article discussed the clinical controversy surrounding the best type of positioning devices to use to decrease spasticity. The study compared a volar resting splint, a finger spreader, a firm cone, and no device in a sample of normal and hemiplegic patients. There were no significant positive effects found between the use of any of the positioning devices versus using no device for the hemiplegic patients, and, in fact, use of the volar resting splint appeared to increase spasticity for hemiplegic patients in this study.

Mathiowetz, V. G., Finlayson, M. L., Matuska, K. M., Chen, H. Y., & Luo, P. (2005). Randomized controlled trial of an energy conservation course for persons with multiple sclerosis. *Multiple Sclerosis, 11*(5), 592-601.

Keywords: energy effectiveness, fatigue, occupational therapy, outcomes, quality of life, rehabilitation, self-efficacy, work simplification

This article reports the results of a randomized controlled trial assessing the effectiveness of an energy conservation program for people with multiple sclerosis. The researchers used a crossover design and found significant improvements in fatigue impact, some areas of quality of life, and self-efficacy. The researchers conclude that the results support the use of energy conservation courses as non-pharmacological approaches to managing fatigue in people with multiple sclerosis.

Mathiowetz, V., & Matuska, K. M. (1998). Effectiveness of inpatient rehabilitation on self-care abilities of individuals with multiple sclerosis. *Neurorehabilitation, 11*(2), 141-151.

Keywords: activities of daily living, functional outcomes, adapted equipment, multiple sclerosis

This study evaluated the effectiveness of inpatient rehabilitation on self-care ability of people who have multiple sclerosis. Those who received the rehabilitation program improved significantly between discharge and 6 weeks post-discharge for most self-care activities. All (100%) participants were satisfied with occupational therapy services and felt the equipment was effective.

Mathiowetz, V., Matuska, K. M., & Murphy, M. E. (2001). Efficacy of an energy conservation course for persons with multiple sclerosis. *Archives of Physical Medicine and Rehabilitation, 82*(4), 449-456.

Keywords: conservation of energy resources, fatigue, multiple sclerosis, rehabilitation

This article investigates the efficacy of an energy conservation program for people with multiple sclerosis. Using a repeated measures design, the researchers looked for changes in fatigue impact, self-efficacy, and quality of life. The researchers conclude that the results provide strong evidence for the efficacy the program.

Matuska, K., Giles-Heinz, A., Flinn, N., Neighbor, M., & Bass-Haugen, J. (2003). Outcomes of a pilot occupational therapy wellness program for older adults. *American Journal of Occupational Therapy, 57*(2), 220-224.

Keywords: community participation, prevention, quality of life, older adults

This article evaluates a pilot occupational therapy wellness program designed to teach older adults the importance of participation to their quality of life. The study measured health-related quality of life and frequencies of social and community participation. The results concluded that, following participation, subject scores on the vitality, social functioning, and mental health subscales of the quality of life measure significantly improved. Furthermore, increases in the frequency of socialization and community participation improved post-program.

Matuska, K., Mathiowetz, V., & Finlayson, M. (2007). Use and perceived effectiveness of energy conservation strategies for managing multiple sclerosis fatigue. *American Journal of Occupational Therapy, 61*(1), 62-69.

Keywords: energy conservation, fatigue, multiple sclerosis

This study describes the use and perceived effectiveness of energy conservation strategies by people with multiple sclerosis after participating in an energy conservation course. Participants were surveyed about their use of energy conservation strategies and their perception of the program after completing the training program. Approximately half the participants used the strategies and rated them effective, the most common reason for not using a strategy was that the patient was already using the technique.

Mayo, N. E., Wood-Dauphinee, S., Cote, R., Gayton, D., Carlton, J., Buttery, J., et al. (2000). There's no place like home: An evaluation of early supported discharge for stroke. *Stroke, 31*, 1016-1023.

Keywords: outcome assessment, randomized control trials, rehabilitation, quality of life

The goal of this study was to evaluate the effectiveness of prompt discharge to home for stroke patients, in terms of an impact on reintegration, functional abilities, and health-related quality of life measures. The underlying logic that was presented suggested that the earlier a patient was discharged to home, the more quickly the processes of reintegration could be initiated. Results of this randomized controlled trial indicated that the home group had better performance on physical health and reintegration measures, as well as instrumental activities of daily living functions (before adjustments for multiple comparisons). Thus, "prompt" discharge and home rehabilitation may lead to better physical health and more satisfaction with community reintegration after stroke.

McCabe, P., Nason, F., Turco, P. D., Friedman, D., & Seddon, J. M. (2000). Evaluating the effectiveness of a vision rehabilitation intervention using an objective and subjective measure of functional performance. *Ophthalmic Epidemiology, 7*, 259-270.

Keywords: activities of daily living, vision rehabilitation, visual function, vision impairment, low vision outcome measure

The purpose of this study was to assess vision rehabilitation involving optometrists, occupational therapists, and social workers. Outcomes examined objective measures of patients' functional abilities within a rehabilitation setting, as well as self-report measures of daily functional activities. Additionally, this study sought to determine whether family involvement in the rehabilitation process affected functional outcomes of patients. Results suggested that patients benefited from the rehabilitation, as measured through observation and self-report of functional abilities. There were no significant differences, in terms of functional outcomes, between the group with and the group without involvement of family members.

McClain, L., & Todd, C. (1990). Food store accessibility. *American Journal of Occupational Therapy, 44*, 487-491.

Keywords: architectural accessibility, environmental design

The article begins by discussing the accessibility issues faced by many people who use wheelchairs. A study is described where occupational therapists assessed the accessibility of 20 grocery and convenience stores and provided constructive feedback to the managers as to how they could make their stores more accessible. Results indicate that five of 20 stores made changes based on occupational therapist recommendations. In conclusion, occupational therapists can be effective advocates for accessibility and thus provide a vital link to productive living for people in wheelchairs.

McDermott, C., Richards, S. C. M., Ankers, S., Harmer, J., & Moran, C. J. (2004). An evaluation of a chronic fatigue lifestyle management programme focusing on the outcome of return to work or training. *British Journal of Occupational Therapy, 67*(6), 269-273.

The study examined an occupational therapy lifestyle management program for people with chronic fatigue syndrome to see if the program had an impact on ability to return to paid or volunteer work. It also aimed to look at whether demographic variables such as age and severity of condition were related to the ability to return to employment. The authors concluded that lifestyle management programs may be beneficial but that a randomized controlled trial is needed to be sure.

McGruder, J., Cors, D., Tiernan, A. M., & Tomlin, G. (2003). Weighted wrist cuffs for tremor reduction during eating in adults with static brain lesions. *American Journal of Occupational Therapy, 57*(5), 507-516.

Keywords: intention tremor, rehabilitation, traumatic brain injury

The article discusses a study that aims to provide a test of the therapeutic principle of weighting the distal upper extremity to decrease tremor or its effects on skilled movement. The results partially support this principle because three of five participants improved their feeding performance on one or more variables studied. These observations suggest that weights used to reduce tremors are effective both because of the increased proprioceptive input and for purely biomechanical reasons.

McMenamy, C., Ralph, N., Auen, E., & Nelson, L. (2004). Treatment of complex regional pain syndrome in a multidisciplinary chronic pain program. *American Journal of Pain Management, 14*(2), 56-62.

Keywords: CRPS, multidisciplinary treatment, outcome assessment, pain, pain treatment, RSD

This article begins with a thorough discussion of the treatments used with complex regional pain syndrome (CRPS). It then examines the effects of a complex multidisciplinary treatment program for patients with CRPS. Results indicate significant improvements on all dependent variables indicating that "multidisciplinary treatment of CPRS is effective in the improvement of symptomatology."

McNaughton, H., DeJong, G., Smout, R. J., Melvin, J. L., & Brandstater, M. (2005). A comparison of stroke rehabilitation practice and outcomes between New Zealand and United States facilities. *Archives of Physical Medicine and Rehabilitation, 86*(12 Suppl), S115-S120.

Keywords: outcome assessment (health care), cerebrovascular accident, health care systems, rehabilitation

The purpose of this prospective cohort study was to determine if there were differences between rehabilitation practices in the United States and New Zealand and if any potential differences impacted outcomes following stroke, in terms of functional ability and discharge placement. Results indicated that US patients had shorter lengths of stay and more intense rehabilitation compared to NZ patients. US participants also demonstrated greater change in functional and stroke severity measures during admission. At discharge, however, the two groups' Functional Independence Measure (FIM) scores were not significantly different.

Melin, A. L., & Bygren, L. O. (1992). Efficacy of the rehabilitation of elderly primary health care after short-stay hospital treatment. *Medical Care, 30*, 1004-1015.

Keywords: early intervention, rehabilitation, elderly, activities of daily living, primary care, home care

The purpose of this study was to evaluate the impact of primary home care services on medical and functional outcomes in elderly patients with chronic illness. Results indicated the home care program did appear to be significantly related to better medical and functional outcomes compared to typical care experienced by controls. Specifically, those in the treatment group had better instrumental activities of daily living function and fewer medical diagnoses than controls at 6 months.

Mendelsohn, M. E., Overend, T. J., & Petrella, R. J. (2004). Effect of rehabilitation on hip and knee proprioception in older adults after hip fracture: A pilot study. *American Journal of Physical Medicine and Rehabilitation, 83*(8), 624-632.

Keywords: hip fracture, proprioception, aging

The purpose of this pilot study is to determine if proprioception of the hip and knee are improved by rehabilitation for older adults with a hip fracture. The article describes in very little detail the intervention carried out by an occupational therapist and physiotherapist. The findings of the study show that there is a statistically significant increase in hip and knee proprioception in the injured limb as a result of rehabilitation.

Montgomery Orr, P., & Bratton, G. N. (1992). The effect of an inpatient arthritis rehabilitation program on self-assessed functional ability. *Rehabilitation Nursing, 17*, 306-310.

Keywords: self-assessment, arthritis

The goal of this study was to help determine if a short-term inpatient, multidisciplinary rehabilitation program would help patients with arthritis to improve functionally and have decreased pain. Based on patients' self-assessments, there were significant increases in functional ability following the rehabilitation program. Patients also reported significant decreases in pain and need for assistance in daily activities, as assessed at the time of discharge.

Mullen, B., Champagne, T., Krishnamurty, S., Dickson, D., & Gao, R. X. (2008). Exploring the safety and therapeutic effects of deep pressure stimulation, using a weighted blanket. *Occupational Therapy in Mental Health, 24*(1), 65.

Keywords: sensory modulation, weighted blanket, deep pressure touch stimulation, skin conductance, electrodermal activity

This paper presents the results of an exploratory study on the safety and effectiveness of the use of a 30-pound weighted blanket in a convenience sample of 32 adults. Safety was assessed using patients' vital signs, while effectiveness was measured using electrodermal activity (EDA) and self-reported anxiety. Results show that use of the 30-pound blanket while lying down was safe. One third (33%) of subjects showed lower EDA, and 68% reported lower anxiety levels.

Naglie, G., Tansey, C., Kirkland, J. L., Ogilvie-Harris, D. J., Detsky, A. S., Etchells, E., et al. (2002). Interdisciplinary inpatient care for elderly people with hip fracture: A randomized controlled trial. *Canadian Medical Association Journal, 167*, 25-32.

Keywords: interdisciplinary inpatient care, hip fracture

The purpose of this study was to compare effectiveness of inpatient interdisciplinary care to usual care received by elderly patients with hip fractures. This randomized controlled trial failed to find significant differences between interdisciplinary and typical care, in terms of mortality rates, residential change, mobility, transfers, and activities of daily living function at 3 and 6 months postoperatively. Lack of significant finding was attributed, in part, to a possible lack of statistical power.

Neistadt, M. E. (1994). The effects of different treatment activities on functional fine motor coordination in adults with brain injury. *American Journal of Occupational Therapy, 48*(10), 877-882.

Keywords: brain injuries, tests, by title, Jebsen-Taylor Test of Hand Function

This study discusses the idea that therapy involving repeating a motor task again and again via a tabletop activity might not translate into more functional activities as the movement patterns used may differ. It examined the effects of therapy using a tabletop puzzle versus therapy teaching kitchen skills on the fine motor coordination of participants with dexterity deficits due to a brain injury. The findings showed that "functional activities may be better than tabletop activities for fine motor coordination with this population."

Nelson, D. L., Konosky, K., Fleharty, K., Webb, R., Newer, K., Hazboun, V. P., et al. (1996). The effects of an occupationally embedded exercise on bilaterally assisted supination in persons with hemiplegia. *American Journal of Occupational Therapy, 50*(8), 639-646.

Keywords: cerebrovascular disorders, neurodevelopmental theory, therapeutic exercise

This article begins by reviewing literature on the importance of using occupations to enhance rehabilitation. The authors describe the results of a randomized controlled trial comparing an occupationally embedded exercise to a rote exercise in increasing supination in clients with hemiplegia. The results are statistically significant, and the authors conclude that occupationally embedded exercise is more effective in increasing supination and occupational therapists should incorporate occupationally embedded exercises in rehabilitation.

Ng, S., Chu, M., Wu, A., & Cheung, P. (2005). Effectiveness of home-based occupational therapy for early discharged patients with stroke. *Hong Kong Journal of Occupational Therapy, 15*, 27-36.

Keywords: stroke, discharge, home, outpatient

The article begins by briefly outlining a poverty of services available for patients being discharged after acute stroke. Next, the article discusses theoretical frameworks that support providing occupational therapy-based services for patients being discharged after acute stroke. Next, a study is presented that evaluates the effectiveness occupational therapy-based services for patients being discharged after acute stroke. Results indicate that the program is effective at increasing function and reducing environmental risk.

Ng, S., Lo, A., Lee, G., Lam, M., Yeong, E., Koo, M., et al. (2006). Report of the outcomes of occupational therapy programmes for elderly persons with mild cognitive impairment (MCI) in community elder centres. *Hong Kong Journal of Occupational Therapy, 16*, 16-22.

Keywords: mild cognitive impairment, community elderly center, occupational therapy program

The study aimed to compare, evaluate, and determine the effectiveness of cognitive training programs offered by occupational therapists in community centers. Results indicated that the programs were similar in nature and that participants showed improvements in cognitive abilities and mood that were sustained until the 3-month follow-up. A positive effect was also seen on levels of caregiver stress.

Nieuwenhuijsen, E. R. (2004). Health behavior change among office workers: An exploratory study to prevent repetitive strain injuries. *Work, 23*(3), 215-224.

Keywords: prevention, repetitive strain injury

This article looks at a multifaceted intervention in the workplace to prevent repetitive strain injuries, such as carpal tunnel syndrome. By assessing the approach on a group of 40 airline workers, the authors devised a theoretical path model of factors that affect health-related change. These include self-efficacy, intention, health status, and health behavior.

Nikolaus, T., Specht-Leible, N., Bach, M., Oster, P., & Schlierf, G. (1999). A randomized trial of comprehensive geriatric assessment and home intervention in the care of hospitalized patients. *Age and Ageing, 28*, 543-550.

Keywords: comprehensive geriatric assessment, functional status, home intervention, nursing home placement, re-hospitalization

The purpose of this study was to evaluate the effectiveness of geriatric evaluation for elderly people in hospitals, as well as the impact of home intervention by an interdisciplinary team. Results of this randomized controlled trial were gathered from measures that examined functional status, direct cost of care over 1 year, and re-hospitalization. Conclusions drawn include the fact that geriatric assessment in combination with an interdisciplinary home health team does not increase survival rates but does improve functional outcomes and lead to decreased lengths of stay in the hospital. This intervention also demonstrated an ability to reduce direct cost of care for hospitalized patients.

Niva, B., & Skar, L. (2006). A pilot study of the activity patterns of five elderly persons after a housing adaptation. *Occupational Therapy International, 13*(1), 21-34.

Keywords: housing adaptations, accessibility, activity patterns of elderly people

The aim of this study was to describe the activity patterns of five elderly people before and after they received home modifications. The results showed that, after housing modifications, the subjects performed more and new activities, increased activity, and took fewer rest periods during the day.

Nobili, A., Riva, E., Tettamanti, M., Lucca, U., Liscio, M., Petrucci, B., et al. (2004). The effect of a structured intervention on caregivers of patients with dementia and problem behaviors: A randomized controlled pilot study. *Alzheimer's Disease and Associated Disorders, 18*(2), 75-82.

Keywords: dementia, caregiver stress, problem behaviors, randomized controlled trial

This article begins by describing the effect of caregiver stress on institutionalization of individuals with dementia. A study measuring the effect of a structured intervention on caregiver stress follows. Results indicate that this intervention lowered problem behaviors in clients, but did not reduce caregiver stress directly.

Nordmark, B., Blomqvist, P., Andersson, B., Hagerstrom, M., Nordh-Grate, K., Ronnqvist, R., et al. (2006). A two-year follow-up of work capacity in early rheumatoid arthritis: A study of multidisciplinary team care with emphasis on vocational support. *Scandinavian Journal of Rheumatology, 35*(1), 7-14.

Keywords: rheumatoid arthritis, return to work, vocational rehabilitation, multidisciplinary

This article follows a group of people in Sweden with rheumatoid arthritis getting a combination intervention of pharmacological treatment for their rheumatoid arthritis as well as vocational rehabilitation from a nurse, occupational therapist, physiotherapist, social worker, and a consultative rheumatologist. The results of the study show a trend toward improvement for people with rheumatoid arthritis to continue to work or improve working status with vocational group in addition to pharmacological treatment. The article divides participants into groups depending on where they are in terms of work at 24 months.

Oerlemans, H. M., Oostendorp, R. A., de Boo, T., van der Laan, L., Severens, J. L., & Goris, J. A. (2000). Adjuvant physical therapy versus occupational therapy in patients with reflex sympathetic dystrophy/complex regional pain syndrome type I. *Archives of Physical Medicine and Rehabilitation, 81*(1), 49-56.

Keywords: reflex sympathetic dystrophy, RSD, complex regional pain syndrome type I, CRPS

This randomized controlled trial investigates the effectiveness and cost of physical therapy and occupational therapy in patients with complex regional pain syndrome (CRPS)/reflex sympathetic dystrophy (RSD). Results indicate that physical therapy and, to a lesser extent, occupational therapy resulted in a significant and more rapid improvement in the ISS compared with the control group. Physical therapy was found to be more cost effective, while occupational therapy was found to be more positive on a disability level. Both physical therapy and occupational therapy contribute to recovery from CRPS/RSD.

Ostrow, P., Parente, R., Ottenbacher, K. J., & Bonder, B. (1989). Functional outcomes and rehabilitation: An acute care field. *Journal of Rehabilitation Research and Development, 26*(3), 17-26.

Keywords: measurement, occupational therapy, treatment efficacy

The study looked at the effectiveness of rehabilitation services and occupational therapy in particular by comparing acute care patients who received occupational therapy services as part of their hospital rehabilitation program to those who did not on functional outcomes and discharge status. While no differences in function were found between the groups, participants who received occupational therapy as part of their rehabilitation program were more often discharged to their homes. The authors indicate that "future outcome research should be designed to investigate the nature and type of support services that are required to maintain home placement."

Ozdemir, F., Birtane, M., Tabatabaei, R., Kokino, S., & Ekuklu, G. (2001). Comparing stroke rehabilitation outcomes between acute inpatient and nonintense home settings. *Archives of Physical Medicine and Rehabilitation, 82*(10), 1375-1379.

Keywords: inpatient rehabilitation, stroke, home care

This article begins by discussing the cost and bed use in hospitals by stroke patients. The article compares rehabilitation time for people with strokes either in the hospital or at home. The results of the study indicate that it is more favorable for clients with strokes to have inpatient rehabilitation services.

Paes Lourencao, M. I., Battistella, L. R., Moran de Brito, C. M., Tsukimoto, G. R., & Miyazaki, M. H. (2008). Effect of biofeedback accompanying occupational therapy and functional electrical stimulation in hemiplegic patients. *International Journal of Rehabilitation Research, 31*(1), 33-41.

> **Keywords**: electric stimulation, electromyography, hemiplegia, occupational therapy, rehabilitation
>
> The objective of this study was to determine the effect of electromyographic biofeedback (EMG-BFB) in conjunction with occupational therapy and functional electric stimulation (FES) on range of motion, spasticity, and upper extremity function in hemiplegic stroke patients. A total of 59 patients were recruited from a rehabilitation center and randomized to receive either occupational therapy and FES twice a week or occupational therapy and FES in conjunction with weekly EMG-BFB. Results show that patients receiving EMG-BFB as well as occupational therapy and FES had a greater improvement in range of motion and greater recovery of upper extremity function.

Page, S. (2000). Imagery improves upper extremity motor function in chronic stroke patients: A pilot study. *Occupational Therapy Journal of Research, 20*(3), 200-215.

> **Keywords**: imagery, functional motor recovery, stroke, Fugl-Meyer
>
> This study opened by reviewing literature about treatment approaches for individuals who have stroke. Results from their study confirmed the hypothesis that adding imagery to occupational therapy has a more beneficial impact on physical impairment than occupational therapy alone for chronic stroke patients.

Page, S. J., Levine, P., Sisto, S., & Johnston, M. V. (2001). A randomized efficacy and feasibility study of imagery in acute stroke. *Clinical Rehabilitation, 15*(3), 233-240.

> This article describes a feasibility study of the use of imagery in addition to standard upper-extremity therapy following stroke. Results indicate a greater increase in function in the intervention group than in the control group, suggesting that imagery is a feasible complement to standard stroke rehabilitation.

Pagnotta, A., Baron, M., & Korner-Bitensky, N. (1998). The effect of a static wrist orthosis on hand function in individuals with rheumatoid arthritis. *Journal of Rheumatology, 25*(5), 879-885.

> **Keywords**: rheumatoid arthritis, hand, hand strength, orthotic devices, static splint
>
> The article begins by briefly reviewing literature that discusses the benefits and limitations of wrist orthoses for people with rheumatoid arthritis. Next, a study is presented that evaluates the effect of wrist orthoses on hand output. The study concluded that while splints decrease pain, they also decrease hand output.

Pagnotta, A., Korner-Bitensky, N., Mazer, B., Baron, M., & Wood-Dauphinee, S. (2005). Static wrist splint use in the performance of daily activities by individuals with rheumatoid arthritis. *Journal of Rheumatology, 32*(11), 2136-2143.

> **Keywords**: rheumatoid arthritis, hand, hand strength, orthotic devices, static splint
>
> The article begins by briefly reviewing literature that discusses the benefits and limitations of wrist orthoses for people with rheumatoid arthritis. Next, a study is presented that evaluates the use of commercially available working wrist splints on pain, work performance, endurance, and perceived task difficulty for 10 standardized tasks. Results suggest that commercially available working wrist splints subjectively decrease task difficulty and generally reduce pain without negatively affecting work performance.

Paire, J., & Karney, R. (1984). The effectiveness of sensory stimulation for geropsychiatric inpatients. *American Journal of Occupational Therapy, 38*(8), 505-509.

> **Keywords**: geriatrics, nursing homes, occupational therapy
> The effectiveness of sensory stimulation on interpersonal functioning, orientation, and self-care skills was examined in this study. The results indicated that, when compared to an attention-only and control group, the sensory stimulation group showed a higher level of interest in hygiene and group activities.

Pang, M., Harris, J., & Eng, J. (2006). A community-based upper-extrem-ity group exercise program improves motor function and performance of functional activities in chronic stroke: A randomized controlled trial. *Archives of Physical Medicine and Rehabilitation, 87*(1), 1-9.

> **Keywords**: arm, cerebrovascular accident, exercise, rehabilitation
>
> The purpose of this study was to evaluate the effectiveness of a community-based exercise program on recovery of motor function and functional ability in the upper extremities of stroke patients. A sample of adults with chronic stroke 1-year post-onset was randomized to receive a lower extremity or upper extremity exercise program based in the community. Results showed that the arm exercise group had significant improvements in functional ability and motor function compared to the control.

Pankow, L., Luchins, D., Studebaker, J., & Chettleburgh, D. (2004). Evaluation of a vision rehabilitation program for older adults with visual impairment. *Topics in Geriatric Rehabilitation, 20*, 223-232.

> **Keywords**: goal attainment, vision rehabilitation, older adults
>
> The purpose of this study was to assess a vision rehabilitation program to determine its impact on functional independence. Rehabilitative impacts on psychological variables were also examined. Results indicated significant improvement in functional and psychological variables for the treatment group, compared to the control group. Thus, researchers support the need for vision rehabilitation in increasing independence, as well as a need for insurance coverage for these services.

Parker, C. J., Gladman, C. R. F., & Drummond, A. E. R. (2001). A multicentre randomized controlled trial of leisure therapy and conventional occupational therapy after stroke. *Clinical Rehabilitation, 15*, 42-52.

> The aim of this study was to determine the effects of two different occupational therapy interventions (leisure therapy or conventional occupational therapy) versus no occupational therapy intervention on mood, activities of daily living (ADL) performance, and leisure participation of stroke patients who had been discharged from the hospital. Patients were randomized to one of three groups—leisure intervention, ADL intervention, and no intervention. Results did not show any significant differences between the three groups, and the authors conclude that "the use of either leisure or ADL-based occupational therapy for stroke patients in the community after discharge from hospital" was not supported.

Parruti, G., Manzoli, L., Giansante, A., Deramo, C., Re, V., Graziani, R. V., et al. (2007). Occupational therapy for advanced HIV patients at a home care facility: A pilot study. *AIDS Care, 19*(4), 467-470.

> This paper presents the findings of a 5-year study of a comprehensive intervention for people with advanced HIV and multiple disabilities. The program consisted of drug therapy, psychiatric support, and occupational therapy all aimed at reducing social stress and increasing social and occupational functioning. Results showed the program was highly effective in both reducing social stress and increasing social functioning, and some participants were able to find and maintain employment positions outside of the facility they were living in as a result of the intervention.

Parush, S., & Hahn-Markowitz, J. (1997). The efficacy of an early prevention program facilitated by occupational therapists: A follow-up study. *American Journal of Occupational Therapy, 51*(4), 247-251.

> **Keywords**: infant, mother-child relations, preventative health services (community)
>
> The article begins with review of the need to educate new mothers about child development and how an occupational therapy program in Israel helps to educate mothers in helping their children reach their developmental milestones. This study examines the long-term follow-up (1 to 2 years) post-intervention. The study concludes that the effect of a primary prevention program during the first year of a child's life can be sustained for 1 to 2 years.

Patti, F., Reggio, A., Nicoletti, F., Sellaroli, T., Deinite, G., & Nicoletti, F. (1996). Effects of rehabilitation therapy on Parkinson's disability and functional independence. *Journal of Neurologic Rehabilitation, 10*, 223-231.

> **Keywords**: physiotherapy, rehabilitation, Parkinson's disease, independence, disability
>
> The purpose of these two parallel studies was to assess the impact of a short course of inpatient rehabilitation on individuals with Parkinson's disease. Outcome measures focused on level of disability and impairment as well as functional abilities related to activities of daily living performance. Overall, results indicated that the rehabilitation program had beneficial impacts on decreasing levels of disability and increasing functional ability, both relative to baseline as well as controls. However, results also suggested that stopping the rehabilitation program led to deterioration over time.

Pellow, T. R. (1999). A comparison of interface pressure readings to wheelchair cushions and positioning: A pilot study. *Canadian Journal of Occupational Therapy, 66*(3), 140-149.

> **Keywords**: cushions—wheelchairs, posture and positioning evaluation, pressure
>
> This study begins by describing the causes and effects of pressure sores for people using wheelchairs. It continues by describing the need for occupational therapists to have evidence supporting their seating interventions. It then describes a pilot study comparing cushions and positioning, in which the ROHO cushion and tilt position are shown to provide the best pressure relief.

Persson, E., Rivano Fischer, M., & Eklund, M. (2004). Evaluation of changes in occupational performance among patients in a pain management program. *Journal of Rehabilitation Medicine, 36*(2), 85-91.

> **Keywords**: pain management, occupational therapy, occupational performance, outcomes
>
> This article begins with a discussion of the importance of involving clients in setting their own goals in a rehabilitation setting. A study in which clients with chronic pain use the Canadian Occupational Performance Measure (COPM) to set their own goals is then presented. Results demonstrate that clients overall, but especially those receiving sickness compensation and those with a profile of interpersonal distress, significantly increase their self-perceived occupational performance following a multidisciplinary pain treatment program.

Petersson, I., Lilja, M., Hammel, J., & Kottorp, A. (2008). Impact of home modification services on ability in everyday life for people ageing with disabilities. *Journal of Rehabilitation Medicine, 40*(4), 253-260.

> **Keywords**: community living, occupational therapy, environmental intervention, ADL, differential item function, Rasch analysis
>
> The purpose of this study was to examine the impact of home modifications on self-rated ability in various aspects of everyday life. The study compared outcomes between a group of subjects who had received their home modifications and a group still on the waiting list. Home modifications were found to have a positive impact on self-rated ability in a number of areas both in and out of the home and also increased perceptions of safety.

Pfeiffer, A., Thompson, J. M., Nelson, A., Tucker, S., Luedtke, C., Finnie, S., et al. (2003). Effects of a 1.5-day multidisciplinary outpatient treatment program for fibromyalgia: A pilot study. *American Journal of Physical Medicine and Rehabilitation, 82*(3), 186-191.

> **Keywords**: fibromyalgia, treatment outcomes, multidisciplinary treatment, patient education
>
> The article outlines the rationale for developing a 1.5-day multi-modality treatment program. It describes the program for newly diagnosed clients, the methods involved in the pilot study, and the rationale for selected outcome measures. Statistically significant improvements were identified in the FIQ. The authors further analyzed the scores of subjects who entered the program depressed and discovered that they were able to benefit from the program, similar to subjects who did not have depression.

Pfeiffer, B., & Kinnealey, M. (2003). Treatment of sensory defensiveness in adults. *Occupational Therapy International, 10*(3), 175-184.

> **Keywords**: sensory defensiveness, anxiety, Adult Sensory Interview
>
> A pilot study was conducted with two purposes: To provide further support for the idea that sensory defensiveness is correlated to anxiety and to determine the effectiveness of a sensory integration treatment on anxiety and sensory defensiveness. Preliminary evidence suggests that sensory integration has positive effects on anxiety and sensory defensiveness. More methodologically comprehensive research is required to support this initial evidence.

Pierce, S. R., Gallagher, K. G., Schaumburg, S. W., Gershkoff, A. M., Gaughan, J. P., & Shutter, L. (2003). Home forced use in an outpatient rehabilitation program for adults with hemiplegia: A pilot study. *Neurorehabilitation and Neural Repair, 17*(4), 214-219.

> **Keywords**: rehabilitation, arm, cerebrovascular accident, motor skills
>
> This study examines the efficacy of the home restraint portion of constraint-induced movement therapy on upper extremity motor function in patients who have had a stroke. Clients demonstrated significant improvements in upper extremity function following treatment, suggesting that forced-use component of constraint-induced therapy may be effective when applied within a traditional outpatient rehabilitation program.

Pizzi, A., Carlucci, G., Falsini, C., Verdesca, S., & Grippo, A. (2005). Application of a volar static splint in post stroke spasticity of the upper limb. *Archives of Physical Medicine and Rehabilitation, 86*(9), 1855-1859.

> **Keywords**: arm, hemiplegia, H-reflex, muscle spasticity, rehabilitation, splints
>
> The article begins by briefly reviewing literature that discusses the potential benefits and limitations of static resting splints for patients with hemiplegia secondary to cerebrovascular accident (CVA). Next, a study is presented that evaluates the effectiveness of a custom-made volar resting splint for patients with hemiplegia secondary to CVA. Results indicate that a static resting splint produces statistically significant benefits for patients with hemiplegia secondary to CVA.

Poole, J. L., Whitney, S. L., Hangeland, N., & Baker, C. (1990). The effectiveness of inflatable pressure splints on motor function in stroke patients. *Occupational Therapy Journal of Research, 10*(6), 360-366.

> **Keywords**: CVA, upper extremity, splint
>
> The article begins with a brief description on the use of inflatable pressure splints with cerebrovascular accident (CVA) patients. Next, a study is presented that evaluates the effect of inflatable pressure splints on upper extremity motor function in subjects with hemiparesis secondary to CVA. No statistically significant differences between control and experimental groups were found.

Popovic, M. R., Thrasher, T. A., Adams, M. E., Takes, V., Zivanovic, V., & Tonack, M. I. (2006). Functional electrical therapy: Retraining grasping in spinal cord injury. *Spinal Cord, 44*(3), 143-151.

> **Keywords**: neuroprosthesis, functional electrical stimulation, functional electrical therapy, spinal cord injury, quadriplegia, grasping, and hand functions
>
> This article begins by reviewing the use of functional electrical therapy (FET) and points to the lack of studies on the use of FET in spinal cord injury rehabilitation. The article then describes a randomized controlled trial comparing the effectiveness of FET and conventional occupational therapy. Though the results are not statistically significant, the authors conclude that FET is a practical and efficient occupational therapy modality and that further studies with larger sample sizes are needed to demonstrate its effectiveness.

Pratt, J., McFadyen, A., Hall, G., Campbell, M., & McLay, D. (1997). A review of the initial outcomes of a return-to-work programme for police officers following injury or illness. *British Journal of Occupational Therapy, 60*(6), 253-258.

> This article presents preliminary results of a study intended to describe outcomes of a return-to-work program for ill or injured police officers. It finds that the program was positively associated with return to work, lifting capacity, and

grip strength. No correlations were found between length of time since diagnosis, age, or number of sessions attended.

Przybylski, B. R., Dumont, E. D., Watkins, M. E., Warren, S. A., Beaulne, A. P., & Lier, D. A. (1996). Outcomes of enhanced physical and occupational therapy service in a nursing home setting. *Archives of Physical Medicine and Rehabilitation, 77*, 554-561.

> **Keywords**: Functional Assessment Measure (FAM), nursing home, functional status
>
> The aim of this study was to evaluate whether differences in occupational therapy/physical therapy staff to patient ratio (1.0 full-time equivalent [FTE] physical therapist and 1 FTE occupational therapist per 50 beds compared to 1 FTE physical therapist and 1 FTE occupational therapist for 200 beds) impacted functional status of nursing home residents. Results indicated that the treatment group, which received more occupational therapy/physical therapy services, had better functional status, both overall as well as on many functional components, compared to the control group. Additionally, cost analysis revealed a cost savings in the enhanced care group compared to routine care.

Raweh, D. V., & Katz, N. (1999). Treatment effectiveness of Allen's cognitive disabilities model with adult schizophrenic outpatients: A pilot study. *Occupational Therapy in Mental Health, 14*(4), 65-77.

> **Keywords**: schizophrenia, Allen's Cognitive Disabilities Model
>
> The purpose of this study was to determine the effectiveness of the Allen's Cognitive Disabilities Model on patients with schizophrenia. Results showed that the study group had improved significantly in cognitive functional ability (ACL-90 level) in comparison to the control. The study group also showed greater improvement in ability to perform routine tasks (RTI-2 level).

Reeder, C., Newton, E., Frangou, S., & Wykes, T. (2004). Which executive skills should we target to affect social functioning and symptom change? A study of a cognitive remediation therapy program. *Schizophrenia Bulletin, 30*, 87-100.

> **Keywords**: cognitive remediation therapy, executive functioning, social functioning, symptoms, schizophrenia
>
> The aim of this study was to determine the effect of individualized cognitive remediation therapy (CRT) on cognitive factors, psychological symptoms, and social functioning for adults with schizophrenia. This study describes a randomized controlled design that allocated participants to either CRT as the intervention group (n=18), a control group using occupational therapy activities (n=14), or a "treatment as usual" group (n=19). The results indicate that CRT was associated with significant improvement in verbal working memory, but no effect in regard to social behavior. In addition, there was no effect in the occupational therapy activity group on social behavioral outcomes.

Rice, M. S., & Hernandez, H. G. (2006). Frequency of knowledge of results and motor learning in persons with developmental delay. *Occupational Therapy International, 13*(1), 35-48.

> **Keywords**: knowledge of results, motor learning, mental retardation
>
> The purpose of this study was to compare the effects of high or low frequency knowledge of results on learning a motor skill in a group of developmentally delayed adults. Sixteen participants with developmental delay were age- and gender-matched with average individuals and randomized to receive 50% or 100% feedback while learning a motor skill. Results show that both populations that received 50% feedback during skill acquisition retained the information more effectively and performed the skill better when asked to demonstrate it.

Richards, S. H., Coast, J., Gunnell, D. J., Peters, T. J., Pounsford, J., & Darlow, M. A. (1998). Randomized controlled trial comparing effectiveness and acceptability of an early discharge, hospital at home scheme with acute hospital care. *British Medical Journal, 316*(7147), 1796-1801.

> **Keywords**: home care, inpatient, older adult
>
> This article looks at a hospital at-home care compared to usual inpatient care after acute care. The article includes occupational therapy in home care, but does not describe

the intervention in detail. The results of the study indicate that in hospital care reduces the amount of treatment time.

Ring, H., & Rosenthal, N. (2005). Controlled study of neuroprosthetic functional electrical stimulation in sub-acute post-stroke rehabilitation. *Journal of Rehabilitation Medicine, 37*(1), 32-36.

> **Keywords**: hemiplegia, neuroplasticity, electric stimulation therapy, orthotic devices
>
> This study looked at clients who had hemiplegia at 3 to 6 months post-stroke. The study compares usual rehabilitation care to rehabilitation care in addition to neuroprosthesis intervention. Results conclude some positive results indicating that daily home neuroprosthetic activation may be beneficial for stroke clients with hemiplegia.

Roberts, A. H., Sternbach, R. A., & Polich, J. (1993). Behavioral management of chronic pain and excess disability: Long-term follow-up of an outpatient program. *Clinical Journal of Pain, 9*, 41-48.

> **Keywords**: chronic pain, excess disability, rehabilitation, behavioral medicine, behavioral therapy
>
> The purpose of this study was to assess the effectiveness of an outpatient behavioral rehabilitation program for individuals with chronic pain and "excess disability." Results indicated that patients experienced decreased pain in a number of domains, such as sitting, standing, walking, and playing, over the treatment period. There was also a decrease in terms of pain interference on work- and home-related activities. Results of decreased pain lasted over the course of the 2-year follow-up, with non-significant trends back to baseline results, in some areas, at 24 months.

Roberts, P. S., Vegher, J. A., Gilewski, M., Bender, A., & Riggs, R. V. (2005). Client-centered occupational therapy using constraint-induced therapy. *Journal of Stroke and Cerebrovascular Diseases, 14*(3), 115-121.

> **Keywords**: stroke, rehabilitation, upper extremity, therapy, motor control, behavior
>
> The study aimed to determine the effects of constraint-induced therapy for a specific subgroup of individuals with stroke on their satisfaction and performance with life roles. The study found positive post-treatment results on satisfaction and performance with life roles, which decreased significantly at follow-up assessment despite continued improvements in physical function.

Rodgers, H., Mackintosh, J., Price, C., Wood, R., McNamee, P., Fearon, T., et al. (2003). Does an early increased-intensity interdisciplinary upper limb therapy programme following acute stroke improve outcome? *Clinical Rehabilitation, 17*(6), 579-589.

> **Keywords**: stroke, upper limb impairment
>
> This article compares inpatient rehabilitation for clients with a stroke with a specialized increased intensity upper limb therapy program. The intervention involved both an occupational therapist and a physiotherapist. The results show that the increased intensity program is not effective.

Rosenberg, N. K., & Hougaard, E. (2005). Cognitive-behavioural group treatment of panic disorder and agoraphobia in a psychiatric setting: A naturalistic study of effectiveness. *Nordic Journal of Psychiatry, 59*(3), 198-204.

> **Keywords:** agoraphobia, cognitive-behavioral therapy, group therapy, panic disorder
>
> The purpose of this study was to investigate the effectiveness of cognitive-behavioral group therapy of panic disorder and agoraphobia. A naturalistic comparison between a group receiving this intervention and a waiting list control group found that significantly more members of the intervention group were panic-free after the study than members of the waiting list control group.

Rosenstein, L., Ridgel, A. L., Thota, A., Samame, B., & Alberts, J. (2008). Effects of combined robotic therapy and repetitive-task practice on upper-extremity function in a patient with chronic stroke. *American Journal of Occupational Therapy, 62*(1), 28-35.

> **Keywords**: assistive technology, occupational therapy, robotics, stroke, upper extremity, wrist movement
>
> This article describes the effect of a robotic device combined with repetitive task practice on upper extremity function in a 32-year-old woman 11 months after stroke. The patient received approximately 48 hours of rehabilitation

split evenly between a robotic device (the Hand Mentor) and repetitive task training. Improvements were seen in upper extremity function and functional performance of activities of daily living as well as active range of motion.

Ryan, T., Enderby, P., & Rigby, A. S. (2006). A randomized controlled trial to evaluate intensity of community-based rehabilitation provision following stroke or hip fracture in old age. *Clinical Rehabilitation, 20*, 123-131.

> The purpose of this randomized controlled trial was to assess the impacts of intensive versus non-intensive in-home rehabilitation on outcomes such as function, impairment, and quality of life in a group a geriatric patients who had experienced either stroke or hip fracture. Results indicated significant benefits of intensive therapy, in terms of social participation and quality of life, for those with stroke. Those with hip fracture did not show similar significant benefits of more intense intervention. However, after making adjustments for missing data, both stroke and hip fracture participants in the intensive group showed significantly better outcomes on the depression measure, compared to the less intensive group.

Saltvedt, I., Opdahl Mo, E. S., Fayers, P., Kaasa, S., & Sletvold, O. (2002). Reduced mortality in treating acutely sick, frail older patients in a geriatric evaluation and management unit. A prospective randomized trial. *Journal of the American Geriatrics Society, 50*, 792-798.

> ***Keywords***: geriatrics, acute care, frail, mortality, hospital
> The aim of this study was to assess whether treatment of frail, acutely ill elderly in a geriatric evaluation and management unit (GEMU) would reduce mortality compared to traditional intervention in the Department of Internal Medicine. Results revealed that treatment in the GEMU significantly reduced mortality during the first year of follow-up.

Sandin-Aldehag, A., & Jonsson, H. (2003). Evaluation of a hand-training programme for patients with welander distal myopathy. *Scandinavian Journal of Occupational Therapy, 10*(4), 188-192.

> ***Keywords***: activities of daily living, hand training, occupational therapy, Welander distal myopathy, life satisfaction
> The article begins by briefly identifying that people who have neuromuscular diseases often have hand limitations as a result of muscular weakness. Next, a study is presented that evaluates the effectiveness of a hand-therapy program for people affected with a neuromuscular disease. The study concludes that specific interventions may be beneficial in restoring hand function for people affected with neuromuscular diseases.

Sandqvist, G., Akesson, A., & Eklund, M. (2004). Evaluation of paraffin bath treatment in patients with systemic sclerosis. *Disability and Rehabilitation, 26*(16), 981-987.

> The study investigates the effects of treatment with paraffin bath in patients with systemic sclerosis (scleroderma). Results of the study indicate that improvements in function were significantly greater in the hand that was treated with paraffin bath and exercise than in the hand treated with exercise only, concerning extension deficit, perceived stiffness, and skin elasticity.

Sanford, J. A., Griffiths, P. C., Richardson, P., Hargraves, K., Butterfield, T., & Hoenig, H. (2006). The effects of in-home rehabilitation on task self-efficacy in mobility-impaired adults: A randomized clinical trial. *Journal of the American Geriatrics Society, 54*(11), 1641-1648.

> ***Keywords***: assistive technology, home modification, in-home services, OT, PT, telerehabilitation, self-efficacy, activities of daily living
> The study examined whether mobility self-efficacy in a group of mobility impaired adults could be changed through in-home occupational/physical therapy interventions that consisted of using teletechnology therapists or traditional in-home visits by therapists. The study methods are detailed, and the results presented. The study indicates that occupational/physical therapy interventions increased overall self-efficacy for the treatment group.

Sang, L. S., & Ying Eria, L. P. (2005). Outcome evaluation of work hardening program for manual workers with work-related back injury. *Work, 25*(4), 297-305.

> ***Keywords***: outcome measurement, work hardening, return to work
> This article discusses vocational rehabilitation for people with work-related back injuries and examines the effectiveness of a 12-week work hardening program, designed for back-injured workers and based on the overloading principle, in terms of improved strength and return to work. The study showed comparable rates of return to work as reported in previous studies. However, improvements in physical demand characteristic levels (strength) were shown, leading authors to conclude that using the overloading principle in work hardening programs may be beneficial.

Sarajuuri, J., Kaipio, M., Koskinen, S., Niemela, M., Servo, A., & Vilkki, J. (2005). Outcome of a comprehensive neurorehabilitation program for patients with traumatic brain injury. *Archives of Physical Medicine and Rehabilitation, 86*(12), 2296-2302.

> ***Keywords***: brain injuries, neuropsychology, outcome assessment (health care), rehabilitation
> The aim of this study was to evaluate the effectiveness of a comprehensive, multidisciplinary neurorehabilitation program in patients with traumatic brain injury. Nineteen adults who underwent the program were compared with 20 matched controls who received conventional care. Subjects were evaluated on the outcome of productivity (defined as working, volunteering, or studying), and they were evaluated through questionnaires completed by them and their caregivers. Results from the study showed that a significantly larger percentage of patients in the intervention (89% compared to 55% in control) were engaged in productive activity at 2-year follow-up.

Schene, A., Koeter, M., Kikkert, M., Swinkels, J., & McCrone, P. (2007). Adjuvant occupational therapy for work-related major depression works: Randomized trial including economic evaluation. *Psychological Medicine, 37*(3), 351-362.

> This study evaluated the effectiveness of usual care for work-related major depression coupled with occupational therapy compared with usual care alone. Patients with a diagnosis of major depression and significant absenteeism were recruited for the study and were randomized to intervention and control groups. The main outcome measures were depression, work resumption, and work-related stress, and subjects were evaluated at baseline and 3, 6, 12, and 42 months. Results of the study show that occupational therapy in conjunction with usual care for depression had no impact on depressive symptoms or work stress but enabled a faster return to work and resulted in fewer lost days of productivity.

Schweitzer, J. A., Mann, W. C., Nochajski, S., & Tomita, M. (1999). Patterns of engagement in leisure activity by older adults using assistive devices. *Technology and Disability, 11*, 103-117.

> ***Keywords***: aging, assistive devices, leisure, occupational therapy
> The purpose of the study was to look at whether participation in leisure activities at home could be increased through the use of assistive devices in older adults with physical and/or sensory disabilities. Participants reported increases in active involvement in at least one leisure activity. Participants were quite satisfied with commercially and publicly available assistive devices leading the authors to conclude that it may not be necessary to provide custom-adapted devices for most people—perhaps just those people for which a device can't be found otherwise.

Sellwood, W., Thomas, C. S., Tarrier, N., Jones, S., Clewes, J., James, A., et al. (1999). A randomised controlled trial of home-based rehabilitation versus outpatient-based rehabilitation for patients suffering from chronic schizophrenia. *Social Psychiatry and Psychiatric Epidemiology, 34*(5), 250-253.

> The study aimed to determine the differential impact of home and outpatient rehabilitation on outcomes for individuals with chronic schizophrenia. Significant differences between the two groups at the 9-month follow-up were not found. The home group spent fewer (non-significant) days in the hospital, and the savings that resulted nearly accounted for the wages of the study staff.

Shechtman, O., Hanson, C. S., Garrett, D., & Dunn, P. (2001). Comparing wheelchair cushions for effectiveness of pressure relief: A pilot study. *Occupational Therapy Journal of Research, 21*(1), 29-48.

> **Keywords**: wheelchair cushions, pressure mapping system, cushion comfort
>
> This article begins by reviewing literature on pressure-relieving cushions and the role of occupational therapy in pressure relief. It describes a study comparing the pressure relieving effectiveness of six different wheelchair cushions with participants with a variety of diagnoses. The authors conclude that the ROHO high and low cushions were the most effective in reducing pressure and received the highest comfort ratings.

Sietsema, J. M., Nelson, D. L., Mulder, R. M., Mervau-Scheidel, D., & White, B. E. (1993). The use of a game to promote arm reach in persons with traumatic brain injury. *American Journal of Occupational Therapy, 47*(1), 19-24.

> **Keywords**: developmental tasks, motor control, movement analysis, neurodevelopmental therapy
>
> This article begins by reviewing the literature supporting the use of occupationally embedded exercise in occupational therapy interventions. It describes a study comparing the use of a computer-controlled game with rote exercise in increasing range of motion for people with traumatic brain injuries. The authors conclude that occupationally embedded exercise can increase range of motion in the upper limb and call for more research into the effects of this approach.

Soderback, I. (1988). The effectiveness of training intellectual functions in adults with acquired brain injury. *Scandinavian Journal of Rehabilitation Medicine, 20*, 47-56.

> **Keywords**: brain injury, intellectual functions, occupational therapy, rehabilitation, stroke, training
>
> The authors wanted to evaluate the effectiveness and maintenance of occupational therapy training of intellectual functions. The study subjects underwent training in one of four groups, including a control group (regular occupational therapy rehabilitation), which resulted in more effective intellectual training in the three training groups in comparison to the regular occupational therapy rehabilitation group. The study concluded that the combination of any of the training approaches are usable in occupational therapy rehabilitation for training in verbal, numerical, praxis, memory, and logical functions.

Sood, J. R., Cisek, E., Zimmerman, J., Zaleski, E. H., & Fillmore, H. H. (2003). Treatment of depressive symptoms during short-term rehabilitation: An attempted replication of the DOUR project. *Rehabilitation Psychology, 48*(1), 44-49.

> **Keywords**: older adults, depression, CBT, quality of life
>
> This study investigated the effectiveness of the geriatric wellness program (GWP) to reduce depression among clients in short-term rehabilitation through cognitive-behavioral therapy and pleasant events. While differences between the control group receiving standard occupational therapy and the treatment group receiving the GWP are not statistically significant, there was a difference in depressive symptoms between both groups, which is encouraging. The authors are eager to investigate the GWP with a larger sample size.

Soper, G., & Thorley, C. R. (1996). Effectiveness of an occupational therapy programme based on sensory integration theory for adults with severe learning disabilities. *British Journal of Occupational Therapy, 59*(10), 475-482.

> The authors of the study aimed to determine the beneficial impact of a sensory integration program on individuals with severe learning disabilities, when compared to controls. Results indicated that touch and movement scores yielded from the clinic environment improved in both groups, and the experimental group had performed significantly better for adaptive responses and proprioceptive and total behavior scores.

Spadaro, A., De Luca, T., Massimiani, M., Ceccarelli, F., Riccieri, V., & Valesini, G. (2008). Occupational therapy in ankylosing spondylitis: Short-term prospective study in patients treated with anti-TNF-alpha drugs. *Joint Bone Spine, 75*(1), 29-33.

> **Keywords**: occupational therapy, ankylosing spondylitis, anti-TNF-alpha drugs
>
> The purpose of this study was to assess the effectiveness of occupational therapy in ankylosing spondylitis patients treated with anti-TNF-alpha drugs. Patients were randomized to receive occupational therapy and drug treatment or drug treatment alone. Results show that combined treatment with occupational therapy and anti-TNF-alpha drugs was beneficial and reduced pain and disability while improving function.

Spalding, N. J. (1995). A comparative study of the effectiveness of a preoperative education programme for total hip replacement patients. *British Journal of Occupational Therapy, 58*(12), 526-531.

> In this study, it was hypothesized that patients who attended an education session before total hip replacement surgery (compared with those who did not receive the education) would be less anxious after surgery and, thus, experience less pain, would be able to exercise sooner after surgery and, thus, reach independence more quickly, and would be more knowledgeable about what to expect postoperatively and, thus, be able to plan ahead to meet their needs when they return home. The length of hospitalization was reduced for people who took part in the education session leading authors to suggest that preoperative educational programs may have cost-saving benefits.

Spaulding, W. D., Reed, D., Sullivan, M., Richardson, C., & Weiler, M. (1999). Effects of cognitive treatment in psychiatric rehabilitation. *Schizophrenia Bulletin, 25*(4), 657-676.

> **Keywords**: schizophrenia, neuropsychology, neurocognition, treatment, psychiatric rehabilitation, cognitive remediation
>
> This study compared the cognitive component of integrated psychological therapy, a group-therapy modality intended to re-establish basic neurocognitive functions, with supportive therapy in terms of their effect on social competence and cognitive functioning. The results of the study "support the hypothesis that therapy procedures that target impaired cognition enhance improvement in social competence during comprehensive psychiatric rehabilitation of severely disabled psychiatric patients."

Stark, S. (2004). Removing environmental barriers in the homes of older adults with disabilities improves occupational performance. *OTJR: Occupation, Participation, and Health, 24*(1), 32-39.

> **Keywords**: environment, home modifications, occupational performance
>
> This study examines the effectiveness of an occupational therapy home modification intervention program for older adults with various impairments. Results indicated that the overall mean scores for all participants had a positive change from before to after intervention based on self-perception of performance and satisfaction of occupational performance issues. The removal of environmental barriers from the homes of older adults with functional limitations can significantly improve their occupational performance.

Stenvall, M., Olofsson, B., Lundstrom, M., Englund, U., Borssen, B., Svensson, O., et al. (2007). A multidisciplinary, multifactorial intervention program reduces postoperative falls and injuries after femoral neck fracture. *Osteoporosis International, 18*(2), 167-175.

> **Keywords**: accidental falls, elderly, hip fracture, in-hospital, intervention
>
> This study evaluates whether a postoperative multidisciplinary rehabilitation program could reduce inpatient falls and fall-related injuries after a femoral neck fracture. The program featured systematic assessment and treatment of fall risk factors and active prevention, detection, and treatment of postoperative complications. The program implemented by a team successfully prevented inpatient falls and fall-related injuries even in patients with dementia.

Stern, E. B., Ytterberg, S. R., Krug, H. E., & Mahowald, M. L. (1996). Finger dexterity and hand function: Effect of three commercial wrist extensor orthoses on patients with rheumatoid arthritis. *Arthritis Care and Research, 9*(3), 197-205.

> **Keywords**: rheumatoid arthritis, hand, hand strength, orthotic devices, working splint

The article begins by briefly reviewing literature that discusses the benefits and limitations of wrist orthoses for people with rheumatoid arthritis. Next, a study is presented that evaluates the effect of three different wrist orthoses on dexterity and hand function. The study concludes that none of the orthoses are more effective than any of the others at improving hand function or dexterity. The study also concludes that wrist orthoses negatively affect hand function and dexterity.

Stern, E. B., Ytterberg, S. R., Krug, H. E., Mullin, G. T., & Mahowald, M. L. (1996). Immediate and short-term effects of three commercial wrist extensor orthoses on grip strength and function in patients with rheumatoid arthritis. *Arthritis Care and Research, 9*(1), 42-50.

> **Keywords**: rheumatoid arthritis, hand, hand strength, orthotic splint, working splint
>
> The article begins by briefly reviewing literature that discusses the benefits and limitations of wrist orthoses for people with rheumatoid arthritis. Next, a study is presented that evaluates the effect of three different wrist orthoses on seven daily activities and grip strength. The study concludes that one orthoses may be slightly more effective than the two others.

Sterner, Y., Lofgren, M., Nyberg, V., Karlsson, A. K., Bergstrom, M., & Gerdle, B. (2001). Early interdisciplinary rehabilitation programme for whiplash associated disorders. *Disability and Rehabilitation, 23*(10), 422-429.

> **Keywords**: whiplash-associated disorders, multidisciplinary rehabilitation
>
> The purpose of this pilot study was to assess the clinical outcomes of a multidisciplinary rehabilitation program for early intervention of chronic whiplash-associated disorders. The study included both retrospective and prospective data of programs that were run in 1997 and 1998. The study concluded that some positive effects for the program were seen retrospectively, although these results do not differ greatly from the prospective data of the same programs.

Storr, L. K., Sorensen, P. S., & Ravnborg, M. (2006). The efficacy of multidisciplinary rehabilitation in stable multiple sclerosis patients. *Multiple Sclerosis, 12*(2), 235-242.

> **Keywords**: EDSS, disability, FAMS, impairment, inpatient, LASQ, MSIS, multiple sclerosis, quality of life, rehabilitation
>
> The purpose of this study was to evaluate the short-term efficacy of multidisciplinary, inpatient rehabilitation in stable patients with multiple sclerosis. It aimed to examine the impact of inpatient rehab on those with multiple sclerosis, primarily in terms of quality of life and activity level. A double-blind, randomized, parallel group design was used, and the intervention offered comprehensive multidisciplinary rehabilitation while the control group received no treatment related to the study. No statistically significant differences between the two groups were found on any outcome measures. This randomized controlled trial was unable to find significant effect of treatment on the outcome measures selected.

Strong, J., Cramond, T., & Maas, F. (1989). The effectiveness of relaxation techniques with patients who have chronic low back pain. *Occupational Therapy Journal of Research, 9*(3), 184-192.

> **Keywords**: relaxation, pain, biofeedback
>
> This study investigates the use of relaxation and biofeedback to benefit female patients with chronic low back pain. Results show that the addition of EMG biofeedback to applied relaxation training has a long-term benefit.

Studenski, S., Duncan, P., Perera, S., Reker, D., Lai, S. M., & Richards, L. (2005). Daily functioning and quality of life in a randomized controlled trial of therapeutic exercise for subacute stroke survivors. *Stroke, 36*(8), 1764-1770.

> **Keywords**: disability, exercise, quality of life, rehabilitation, stroke
>
> This paper evaluates the ability of therapeutic exercise after stroke to improve daily functioning and quality of life in subacute stroke survivors. Secondary analysis of a single-blind randomized controlled trial of a 12-week program versus usual care was carried out. The rehabilitation exercise program led to more rapid improvement in aspects of physical, social, and role function than usual care.

Sulch, D., Perez, I., Melbourne, A., & Kalra, L. (2000). Randomized control trial of integrated (managed) care pathway for stroke rehabilitation. *Stroke, 31*, 1929-1934.

> **Keywords**: integrated care pathways, effectiveness, rehabilitation, stroke
>
> A randomized controlled trial was established to evaluate the effectiveness of integrated care pathways (ICP) versus conventional care. The main outcome measure was length of stay. Conclusions suggest no benefit of ICP compared to conventional care, with a multidisciplinary approach in those receiving stroke rehabilitation. Those patients in the conventional group experienced a faster functional improvement between 4- and 12-week assessments, as well as significantly higher quality of life scores by the final assessment.

Thomas, J. J. (1996). Comparison of patient education methods: Effects on knowledge of cardiac rehabilitation principles. *Occupational Therapy Journal of Research, 16*(3), 166-178.

> **Keywords**: pretesting effect, adult learning, inpatient education
>
> This article begins by discussing the role of occupational therapists in educating clients. The author continues by describing a study comparing a traditional client education program to a collaborative, client-centered education program. The results show no difference between the two approaches; however, the author concludes that more research should be conducted on this subject and on the effects of pretesting in patient education.

Thomas, L. J., & Thomas, B. J. (1995). Early mobilization method for surgically repaired zone III extensor tendons. *Journal of Hand Therapy, 8*, 195-198.

> This article outlines a 6-week occupational therapy splinting technique used for the mobilization of extensor tendons after surgery. "The central theme of this article is early controlled motion beginning within 4 days of surgical repair. A critical element to the successful outcome is the resting position." The technique helped to reduce pain and re-establish early hand use.

Thorsen, A., Widen Holmqvist, L., de Pedro-Cuesta, J., & von Koch, L. (2005). A randomized controlled trial of early supported discharge and continued rehabilitation at home after stroke: Five-year follow-up of patient outcome. *Stroke, 36*, 297-302.

> **Keywords**: cerebrovascular accident, home care services, randomized controlled trials, rehabilitation, outcome assessment
>
> This randomized controlled trial assessed survival and various functional outcomes of stroke patients who received home rehabilitation, through an early supported discharge framework, compared to those who received conventional rehab. The study followed participants for 5 years post-stroke, and results indicated a significantly better outcome for extended activities of daily living performance for those within the home rehabilitation group compared to conventional group. At 5 years, survival rates were not significantly different, but these results were significantly different (in favor of the home rehab group) at 46 months.

Tijhuis, G. J., Vliet Vlieland, T. P., Zwinderman, A. H., & Hazes, J. M. (1998). A comparison of the futuro wrist orthosis with a synthetic thermo-Lyn orthosis: Utility and clinical effectiveness. *Arthritis Care and Research, 11*(3), 217-222.

> **Keywords**: rheumatoid arthritis, hand, hand strength, orthotic devices, static splint, wrist splint
>
> The article begins by briefly reviewing literature that discusses the benefits and limitations of wrist orthoses for people with rheumatoid arthritis. Next, a study is presented that evaluates the difference in effectiveness of two static wrist splints (pre-fabricated and custom made). No statistically significant differences were observed between the two splints. The authors conclude the increased cost of a custom-made orthoses is not justified by the results of the study.

Tippet, C. (2001). Broken neck of femur: Does rehabilitation improve function? *British Journal of Therapy and Rehabilitation, 8*(11), 410-417.

This article discusses the permanent problems that elderly patients can experience after hip fracture such as dependency, permanent disability, isolation, and depression. It then examines the benefits of a multidisciplinary hospital rehabilitation program involving occupational therapy, physical therapy, and nursing on the patient's functional ability. All participants improved in terms of function, a high number were able to return to their own home, and length of hospital stay (as compared with other studies) was shorter.

Tolley, L., & Atwal, A. (2003). Determining the effectiveness of a falls prevention programme to enhance quality of life: An occupational therapy perspective. *British Journal of Occupational Therapy, 66*(6), 269-276.

This study aimed to determine whether occupational therapy as part of a multifaceted falls prevention program could enhance quality of life by educating people of the risks of falling. Results indicated that participants reported noticeable improvements in their abilities to do specific activities of daily living (ADL) safely and reduce their anxiety after their fall. Participants also demonstrated their increased ability to implement advice provided by occupational therapy post-program. These results suggest that occupational therapy in a falls prevention program can reduce the impact of falls by enhancing ability and confidence in doing ADL, which can in turn increase their quality of life.

Trend, P., Kaye, J., Gage, H., Owen, C., & Wade, D. (2002). Short-term effectiveness of intensive multidisciplinary rehabilitation for people with Parkinson's disease and their carers. *Clinical Rehabilitation, 16,* 717-725.

Keywords: Parkinson's disease, multidisciplinary rehabilitation, day hospital

This before-and-after study examined the impacts of a multidisciplinary treatment program for patients with Parkinson's disease and their caregivers. Outcomes evaluated included mobility, speech, psychological well-being, and health-related quality of life, etc. Results indicated that, after treatment, patients demonstrated improvement in a number of measures including mobility, gait, speech, depression, and health-related quality of life. Caregivers did not demonstrate a significant effect of treatment, in terms of outcomes such as depression and anxiety.

Trombly, C. A., Thayer-Nason, L., Bliss, G., Girard, C. A., Lyrist, L. A., & Brexa-Hooson, A. (1986). The effectiveness of therapy in improving finger extension in stroke patients. *American Journal of Occupational Therapy, 40*(9), 612-617.

Keywords: CVA, stoke, hemiparesis, hand, flexion

The article begins by briefly describing literature that suggests exercise may reduce flexion synergy in the hand following cerebrovascular accident. Next, a study is presented that evaluates three hand exercises on hand function versus no exercises. No statistical differences were observed between treatment and control.

Tsuji, T., Liu, M., Hase, K., Masakado, Y., Takahashi, H., Hara, Y., et al. (2004). Physical fitness in persons with hemiparetic stroke: Its structure and longitudinal changes during an inpatient rehabilitation programme. *Clinical Rehabilitation, 18*(4), 450-460.

Keywords: stroke, multidisciplinary, inpatient

This study is a before-and-after study with participants who had recent-onset, first-time hemispheric strokes. The study found that fitness in this population can be categorized into activities of daily living/paresis, muscular function, metabolic function, and cardiopulmonary function. Overall, the clinical message is that emphasis should be placed on fitness promotion.

Turk, D. C., Okifuji, A., Sinclair, J. D., & Starz, T. W. (1998). Interdisciplinary treatment for fibromyalgia syndrome: Clinical and statistical significance. *Arthritis Care and Research, 11*(3), 186-195.

Keywords: fibromyalgia syndrome (FMS), interdisciplinary treatment, outpatient program, physical therapy, occupational therapy, psychologic therapy, medical treatment

The study evaluated the efficacy of a 4-week outpatient interdisciplinary treatment program for people with fibromyalgia syndrome. Pre-treatment and post-treatment measures revealed significant improvements in pain severity, life interference, sense of control, affective distress, depression, perceived physical impairment, fatigue, and anxiety. A 6-month follow-up indicated continued treatment gains in pain, life interference, sense of control, affective distress, and depression. The authors conclude the outpatient interdisciplinary treatment program was effective in reducing many fibromyalgia syndrome symptoms.

Unsworth, C. A., & Duncombe, D. (2005). A comparison of client outcomes from two acute care neurological services using self-care data from the Australian therapy outcome measures for occupational therapy (AusTOMs-OT). *British Journal of Occupational Therapy, 68*(10), 477-482.

Keywords: neurological services, Australian Therapy Outcome Measures for Occupational Therapy (AusTOMs-OT)

The article begins by describing the AusTOMs-OT scales. It was found that more client contact resulted in better self-care scores. AusTOMs-OT can be used to establish clinical benchmarks when comparing client outcomes.

Unwin, R., & Ballinger, C. (2005). The effectiveness of sensory integration therapy to improve functional behaviour in adults with learning disabilities: Five single-case experimental designs. *British Journal of Occupational Therapy, 68*(2), 56-66.

The aim of this paper was to explore the effect of sensory integration therapy on level of engagement, maladaptive behavior, and function in learning-disabled adults with sensory modulation disorders. Participants received individually tailored sensory integration therapy delivered by two occupational therapists over a 4-week period. Results show that sensory integration therapy significantly decreased maladaptive behavior in all participants, and, upon withdrawal of treatment, significant losses in level of engagement and goal attainment were observed in four of the five participants.

van der Giesen, F. J., Nelissen, R., Rozing, P., Arendzen, J., de Jong, Z., Wolterbeek, R., et al. (2007). A multidisciplinary hand clinic for patients with rheumatic diseases: A pilot study. *Journal of Hand Therapy, 20*(3), 251-261.

The aim of this study was to describe the characteristics, management strategies, and outcomes of patients with rheumatic diseases referred to a multidisciplinary hand clinic. The most common impairments related to grip, pain, and grip strength, and the most common intervention was conservative therapy followed by surgery. On average, all of the patients showed improvements in grip strength and hand function.

van Houten, P., Achterberg, W., & Ribbe, M. (2007). Urinary incontinence in disabled elderly women: A randomized clinical trial on the effect of training mobility and toileting skills to achieve independent toileting. *Gerontology, 53*(4), 205-210.

Keywords: incontinence, mobility disorders, toileting skills, nursing homes, randomized clinical trial, urinary incontinence

The objective of this study was to determine the feasibility and effect of training mobility and toileting skills on the severity of urinary incontinence in elderly dependent women. In a randomized, single-blinded trial, women were randomized to receive no treatment or an individualized 8-week training program. The intervention resulted in a 37.7% reduction in the daily amount of urine loss and increased independent toileting in a number of women in the intervention group.

VanLeit, B., & Crowe, T. (2002). Outcomes of an occupational therapy program for mothers of children with disabilities: Impact on satisfaction with time use and occupational performance. *American Journal of Occupational Therapy, 56,* 402-410.

Keywords: health promotion, psychosocial practice, quality of life

The study evaluates the impact of an 8-week psychosocial occupational therapy intervention program for mothers of children with disabilities. The intervention was designed to facilitate increased perceptions of satisfaction with time use and occupational performance. Significant differences between the control and intervention groups were demonstrated on the Canadian Occupational Performance Measure (COPM) Satisfaction subscale. The study suggests that attending to the time and occupational concerns of mothers of children with disabilities can have a positive impact on their satisfaction with occupational performance.

Velligan, D., Mahurin, R., True, J., Lefton, R., & Flores, C. (1996). Preliminary evaluation of adaptation to training to compensate for cognitive deficits in schizophrenia. *Psychiatric Services, 47*(4), 415-417.

> **Keywords**: depression, health behaviors, immune function, multimodal pain programs, pain

The study evaluated the effects of a program aimed to compensate for the cognitive deficits experienced by individuals with schizophrenia. The study found that, when compared to standard psychosocial treatment, the cognitive adaptation program had additional benefits on adaptive function that were both statistically and clinically meaningful. No differential benefits were found on positive or negative symptoms.

Vines, S. W., Ng, A. K., Breggia, A., & Mahoney, R. (2000). Multimodal chronic pain rehabilitation program: Its effect on immune function, depression, and health behaviors. *Rehabilitation Nursing, 25*(5), 185-191.

> **Keywords**: depression, health behaviors, immune function, multimodal pain programs, pain

This article begins with a discussion of the hypothesized relationship between chronic pain and immunosuppression. A study of 23 patients is then described in which immune function, depression, and health behaviors are measured before and after a multimodal pain program. Blood test results fail to support a relationship between multimodal pain rehabilitation and improved immune response, although a decrease in depression scores was noted.

Volpe, B. T., Krebs, H. I., Hogan, N., Edelstein, L., Diels, C., & Aisen, M. (2000). A novel approach to stroke rehabilitation: Robot-aided sensorimotor stimulation. *Neurology, 54*(10), 1938-1944.

> **Keywords**: robotics, robot, aids, stroke, motor recovery

In patients with stroke, authors tested whether additional sensorimotor training of paralyzed or paretic upper limb provided by a robotic device enhanced motor outcome. Robot-delivered sensorimotor training enhanced performance of exercised shoulder and elbow. Robot-treated group also demonstrated enhanced functional outcome.

Von Koch, L., de Pedro-Cuesta, J., Kostulas, V., Almazan, J., & Holmqvist, L. W. (2001). Randomized controlled trial of rehabilitation at home after stroke: One-year follow-up of patient outcome, resource use and cost. *Cerebrovascular Diseases, 12*, 131-138.

> **Keywords**: randomized controlled trial, stroke management, stroke outcome

The purpose of this randomized controlled trial was to assess patient and resource outcomes, at least 6 months after the end of the stroke rehabilitation period, in groups receiving either routine care or home care, through early supported discharge. Results revealed no significant differences between groups in terms of patient outcomes related to activities of daily living function, mobility, etc. There were significant between-group differences in length of hospital stay and where services were accessed. Cost of care after 1 year was less for the home rehabilitation group when examined on a per-patient basis.

von Renteln-Kruse, W., & Krause, T. (2007). Incidence of in-hospital falls in geriatric patients before and after the introduction of an interdisciplinary team-based fall-prevention intervention. *Journal of the American Geriatrics Society, 55*(12), 2068-2074.

> **Keywords**: in-hospital falls, geriatric patients, fall prevention

This article describes a fall prevention program and its effects on the incidence of falls in geriatric hospital wards. The intervention included a fall-risk assessment on admission and reassessment after a fall, risk alert, additional supervision, and assistance with patient transfers and use of the toilet. After the intervention was implemented, there was a significant reduction in falls but no reduction in injuries related to fall.

Wade, D. T., Gage, H., Owen, C., Trend, P., Grossmith, C., & Kaye, J. (2003). Multidisciplinary rehabilitation for people with Parkinson's disease: A randomised controlled study. *Journal of Neurology, Neurosurgery and Psychiatry, 74*, 158-162.

> **Keywords**: crossover trial, Parkinson's disease

The purpose of this randomized cross-over study was to evaluate the impact of interdisciplinary outpatient rehabilitation on various patient and caregiver outcomes, 4 months after intervention had ceased. Results suggest that the strongest predictor of discharge function is function at admission. However, discharge function and functional change over the course of hospitalization were weakly, but significantly predicted by therapy units. Thus, researchers suggest that the study offers limited support for the utility of rehabilitation service in acute care settings.

Wahi Michener, S. K., Olson, A. L., Humphrey, B. A., Reed, J. E., Stepp, D. R., Sutton, A. M., et al. (2001). Relationship among grip strength, functional outcomes, and work performance following hand trauma. *Work, 16*(3), 209-217.

> **Keywords**: grip strength, functional outcomes, work performance, hand trauma, Michigan Hand Outcomes Questionnaire

The article begins by briefly discussing the importance of measuring outcomes in hand therapy. Next, the article discusses theoretical underpinnings of the relationship between hand function and grip strength post-therapy. Next, a study is presented that examines the link between gains in grip strength and hand function. A mild but statistically insignificant correlation is observed between gains in grip strength and hand function post-occupational therapy intervention.

WaiShan Louie, S. (2004). The effects of guided imagery relaxation in people with COPD. *Occupational Therapy International, 11*(3), 145-159.

> **Keywords**: guided imagery, COPD, anxiety-coping strategies

This study investigated the effectiveness of guided imagery relaxation at reducing anxiety-induced physiological symptoms in people with chronic obstructive pulmonary disease. Results indicated that, in terms of partial percentage of oxygen saturation, a significant improvement occurred for the treatment group after the relaxation intervention. The author concludes that exploring psychological effects of guided imagery would be helpful. Also, she suggests that personal traits and individualized coping styles should be considered when planning to use imagery relaxation as an intervention.

Walsh, D. A., Kelly, S. J., Johnson, P. S., Rajkumar, S., & Bennetts, K. (2004). Performance problems of patients with chronic low-back pain and the measurement of patient-centered outcome. *Spine, 29*(1), 87-93.

> **Keywords**: chronic low back pain, multidisciplinary

This before-and-after study looks at the effects of a rehabilitation program on people with chronic low back pain. The study found that all outcomes measured were statistically improved, and self-reported improvements in performance and satisfaction were associated with observed improvement in performance and increased self-efficacy.

Ward, C. D., Turpin, G., Dewey, M. E., Fleming, S., Hurwitz, B., Ratib, S., et al. (2004). Education for people with progressive neurological conditions can have negative effects: Evidence from a randomized controlled trial. *Clinical Rehabilitation, 18*(7), 717-725.

This article begins by reviewing some of the evidence supporting education as an intervention for people with progressive neurological conditions. It proceeds to describe a randomized controlled trial comparing a comprehensive educational intervention and a control intervention of providing printed educational material. The experimental group had more negative effects (falls, skin sores) than the control group, prompting the authors to caution against the assumption that all educational interventions are beneficial for these populations.

Weatherall, M. (2004). A targeted falls prevention programme plus usual care significantly reduces falls in elderly people during hospital stays. *Evidence-Based Healthcare and Public Health, 8*(5), 273-275.

Keywords: falls, fall prevention, elderly, accident prevention, risk factors, hospitals, systematic review
The study looked to see if a targeted falls prevention program could reduce falls and falls-related injuries when compared with a usual care program. Results indicated that targeted falls prevention program plus usual care significantly reduced the rate of falls by 30% compared to usual care alone (0.004). A combination of the programs during the hospital stay can reduce falls in older adults.

Weiss, Z., Snir, D., Klein, B., Avraham, I., Shani, R., Zetler, H., et al. (2004). Effectiveness of home rehabilitation after stroke in Israel. *International Journal of Rehabilitation Research, 27,* 119-125.

Keywords: home rehabilitation, institutional rehabilitation
The purpose of this study was to examine the effectiveness of home rehabilitation, using a multidisciplinary approach, in terms of an impact on mobility, range of motion, and activities of daily living function after stroke. Impact on activity involvement and cost-effectiveness were also examined. Results indicated that the home rehabilitation group improved in many aspects of these aforementioned outcomes, relative to pre-intervention status. Compared to a group receiving inpatient rehabilitation, the home rehabilitation group also had marginally higher scores on the Frenchay Activities Index (FAI). Overall, the authors conclude that home rehabilitation can provide functional benefits and is cost effective for the population studied.

Wennemer, H. K., Borg-Stein, J., Gomba, L., Delaney, B., Rothmund, A., Barlow, D., et al. (2006). Functionally oriented rehabilitation program for patients with fibromyalgia: Preliminary results. *American Journal of Physical Medicine and Rehabilitation, 85*(8), 659-666.

Keywords: fibromyalgia, exercise, pain, rehabilitation, treatment
The aim of this study was to evaluate function and disability in patients with fibromyalgia before and after participation in a functionally oriented multidisciplinary 8-week exercise treatment program. A total of 23 patients who met American College of Rheumatology criteria for the diagnosis of fibromyalgia were enrolled in the study. All subjects completed the program without injury, and there was a significant improvement in physical function with a non-significant trend toward improvement in general health status.

Werner, R. A., & Kessler, S. (1996). Effectiveness of an intensive outpatient rehabilitation program for post acute stroke patients. *American Journal of Physical Medicine and Rehabilitation, 75,* 114-120.

Keywords: occupational therapy, physical therapy, outcomes rehabilitation, cerebral vascular disease, outcomes
The purpose of this study was to investigate the impact of outpatient rehabilitation for those who have experienced stroke at least 1 year earlier. Neuromuscular facilitation as well as functional tasks, composed therapeutic activities, and outcomes evaluated functional abilities as well as psychological variables such as self-esteem and depression. Results of this randomized controlled trial suggest that outpatient intervention does lead to significant improvement in functional abilities, especially in some aspects of self-care. Improvements were also seen in self-esteem for the treatment group and non-significantly in depression. Researchers suggested that benefits may be seen for up to 6 months after intervention.

Wheeler, S. D., Lane, S. J., & McMahon, B. T. (2007). Community participation and life satisfaction following intensive, community-based rehabilitation using a life skills training approach. *OTJR: Occupation, Participation, and Health, 27*(1), 13-22.

Keywords: traumatic brain injury, life skills training, community integration
This pilot study investigated the effect of an intensive life skills training program on community integration and life satisfaction in adults with traumatic brain injury. The program was delivered by a trained specialist as a supplement to usual rehabilitative care that included occupational, physical, and speech therapy among other things. Results show that subjects receiving the life skills training had significantly higher scores on the Community Integration Questionnaire

(CIQ), but no significant improvement in life satisfaction was found in either the intervention or control group.

Widen Holmqvist, L. W., von Koch, L., Kostulas, V., Holm, M., Widsell, G., Tegler, H., et al. (1998). A randomized controlled trial of rehabilitation at home after stroke in southwest Stockholm. *Stroke, 29,* 591-597.

Keywords: clinical trials, stroke management, stroke outcomes, stroke rehabilitation
The purpose of this randomized controlled trial was to examine the effects of home rehabilitation, with early supported discharge, on functional outcomes of stroke patients, as well use of rehabilitation and hospital resources. The home rehabilitation group was compared to a group receiving routine rehabilitation, and the results indicated that there were non-significant differences in terms of functional patient outcomes such as walking and activities of daily living performance. Those in the home rehabilitation group had fewer days in hospital and significantly poorer subjective impairment scores, especially in the areas of communication and emotional behavior.

Wolf, S. L., Winstein, C. J., Miller, J. P., Taub, E., Uswatte, G., Morris, D., et al. (2006). Effect of constraint-induced movement therapy on upper extremity function 3 to 9 months after stroke. *Journal of the American Medical Association, 296,* 2095-2104.

The purpose of this study was to compare the effects of a 2-week multi-site program of constraint-induced movement therapy (CIMT) versus usual and customary care in improving upper extremity function for participants. A randomized controlled trial was presented for allocating participants who had a first stroke within the previous 3 to 9 months to either group and were followed for 12 months. Results indicated that CIMT produced statistically significant and clinically relevant improvements in arm motor function that persisted for at least 12 months.

Wressle, E., Filipsson, V., Andersson, L., Jacobsson, B., Martinsson, K., & Engel, K. (2006). Evaluation of occupational therapy interventions for elderly patients in Swedish acute care: A pilot study. *Scandinavian Journal of Occupational Therapy, 13*(4), 203-210.

Keywords: acute care, intervention, discharge home
The article begins with a brief discussion of the noted benefits of providing elderly patients with occupational therapy services in acute care settings. A study is presented that aims to measure the degree to which occupational therapy services offered to elderly patients in acute care can improve perceived ability to manage at home. Results returned no significant differences between the control and experimental group. The authors note indications that suggest further study is warranted under a larger sample size.

Wu, C-Y. (2001). Facilitating intrinsic motivation in individuals with psychiatric illness: A study on the effectiveness of an occupational therapy intervention. *Occupational Therapy Journal of Research, 21,* 142-167.

Keywords: psychiatric rehabilitation, outcome study, applied scientific inquiry
The purpose of this mixed-effects, nested design study was to assess whether occupational therapy intervention, using a motivational frame of reference, would improve intrinsic motivation and related behaviors in patients with psychiatric illnesses. Results suggested that occupational therapy intervention was effective in facilitating intrinsic motivation in individuals with various motivational styles, such as those with autonomy-oriented, control-oriented, and impersonal types. There was also a significant positive correlation between intrinsic motivation and changed social behaviors.

Wykes, T., Reeder, C., Corner, J., Williams, C., & Everitt, B. (1999). The effects of neurocognitive remediation on executive processing in patients with schizophrenia. *Schizophrenia Bulletin, 25*(2), 291-307.

Keywords: cognition, remediation
The study aimed to evaluate the differential benefits of intensive occupational therapy and neurocognitive remediation on cognition, symptom presentation, and social functioning. The study found that the neurocognitive remediation group showed more cognitive improvements compared to

the intensive occupational therapy treatment group. The authors suggested that changes in social functioning are related to a threshold change in cognitive functioning.

Wykes, T., Reeder, C., Williams, C., Corner, J., Rice, C., & Everitt, B. (2003). Are the effects of cognitive remediation therapy (CRT) durable? Results from an exploratory trial in schizophrenia. *Schizophrenia Research, 61*, 163-174.

> **Keywords**: cognitive remediation therapy, patient, schizophrenia
>
> The authors investigated the durability effects of cognitive remediation therapy (CRT) in comparison to intensive occupational therapy activities. Evidence supported the presence of CRT effects on memory at follow-up as well as improvements in social behavior and symptoms but did not display statistically significant differences from the improvements in the occupational therapy group.

Yagura, H., Miyai, I., Suzuki, T., & Yanagihara, T. (2005). Patients with severe stroke benefit most by interdisciplinary rehabilitation team approach. *Cerebrovascular Diseases, 20*, 258-263.

> **Keywords**: interdisciplinary rehabilitation, multidisciplinary rehabilitation, stroke rehabilitation unit, general rehabilitation ward
>
> The purpose of this study was to assess functional outcomes of stroke patients who were treated by an interdisciplinary team in either a stroke rehabilitation unit or general rehabilitation unit. The difference between these units was the existence of weekly interdisciplinary team conferences, which occurred on the stroke rehabilitation unit, but not on the general rehabilitation unit. In the general unit, these team conferences occurred only as needed. Results indicated that, overall, there were no between-group differences in terms of functional outcomes at discharge. However, those with severe disabilities in the stroke unit were more likely to be discharged home compared to those with severe disabilities in the general rehabilitation ward. Researchers suggest that this difference in "discharge disposition" may be related to comprehensive discharge planning on the stroke unit, associated with the weekly team meetings.

Yang, J. J., Mann, W. C., Nochajski, S., & Tomita, M. R. (1997). Use of assistive devices among elders with cognitive impairment: A follow-up study. *Topics in Geriatric Rehabilitation, 13*, 13-31.

> **Keywords**: aging, caregivers, dementia, frail older persons, occupational therapy
>
> This article presents the follow-up results after 1 to 2 years of receiving occupational therapy interventions involving assistive devices. Overall, participants experienced functional, physical, and cognitive decline since intervention, as well as a decline in assistive device use and ownership. It was concluded that although participants had degenerative changes in health and abilities, occupational therapy interventions appeared to be helpful for small study sample.

Yuen, H. K., Huang, P., Burik, J. K., & Smith, T. G. (2008). Impact of participating in volunteer activities for residents living in long-term-care facilities. *American Journal of Occupational Therapy, 62*(1), 71.

> **Keywords:** aged, health surveys, long-term care, mentorship, voluntary workers
>
> This study investigated the effect of volunteer activity on self-reported levels of well-being in elderly long-term care residents. Residents from five different care facilities were randomized to a mentoring group where they tutored English-as-a-second-language students twice a week or a usual care control group. Assessment after the intervention showed that residents who participated in the mentoring reported significantly higher levels of well-being than controls, and these effects were maintained at 3 months of follow-up.

Yuen, H. K., Nelson, D. L., Peterson, C. Q., & Dickinson, A. (1994). Prosthesis training as a context for studying occupational forms and motoric adaptation. *American Journal of Occupational Therapy, 48*(1), 55-61.

> **Keywords**: motor skills, prosthesis, training, object-oriented
>
> The article begins by briefly reviewing literature from other professions that recognize the benefits of object-oriented motor control/movement training. Next, the article evaluates the use of object-oriented motor control training in prosthesis training. The study concludes that object-oriented motor training is more effective than non-object-oriented motor training.

Zijlstra, T. R., Heijnsdijk-Rouwenhorst, L., & Rasker, J. J. (2004). Silver ring splints improve dexterity in patients with rheumatoid arthritis. *Arthritis and Rheumatism, 51*(6), 947-951.

> **Keywords**: silver ring splint, rheumatoid arthritis, dexterity, hand function, SODA
>
> The article begins by briefly reviewing literature that discusses the potential benefits of silver ring splints (SRS) for people with rheumatoid arthritis. Next, a study is introduced that examines the effectiveness of SRS on functional outcomes for patients with rheumatoid arthritis. The article concludes that SRS can be an effective treatment method for certain individuals after following a careful screening process.

INDEX

ABI. See acquired brain injury

acculturation, as benefit of leisure, 146

ACL. See Allen Cognitive Level Test

acquired brain injury, 10–11, 113–114, 157, 287

ACS. See Activity Card Sort

activities of daily living, 2, 47–49, 109–112, 158, 179, 240, 242, 257

Activity Card Sort, 153

acute inpatient geriatric admission, 20

addiction, 20

ADL. See activities of daily living

AIDS, 137, 248

Allen Cognitive Level Test, 321

Alzheimer's disease, 20, 31, 42, 59, 162, 164, 178–179, 265, 291, 303

American Occupational Therapy Association, 1–2, 242

AMPS. See Assessment of Motor and Process Skills

amputations, 20

anxiety, 20

AOTA. See American Occupational Therapy Association

arthritis, 20

    impact measurement scale, 241

    self-efficacy scale, 241

arthroplasty of hip/knee, 20

assertive community treatment, 138, 262, 277, 279–280

Assessment of Motor and Process Skills, 321, 328

at-risk older adults, 20

autism, 20

back pain, 20

Barthel Index, 48, 110–111, 114, 241, 328

BBS. See Berg Balance Scale

Bells Test, 114

belonging, as benefit of leisure, 146

Berg Balance Scale, 241

BI. See Barthel Index

bipolar disorder, 20

BPRS. See Brief Psychiatric Rating Scale

Brief Psychiatric Rating Scale, 320, 328

burns, 20

Canadian Association of Occupational Therapists, 1, 23, 119–120, 261

Canadian Model of Occupational Performance, 5–6, 16

Canadian Occupational Performance Measure, 43, 114, 180, 257, 328

Canadian Occupational Performance Measure: An Annotated Bibliography and Research Resource, 16

CAOT. See Canadian Association of Occupational Therapists

cardiac conditions, 20

categories of leisure, 145

CBT. See cognitive-behavioral therapy

central nervous system, 285–323

characteristics of leisure, 146

Charron Test, 114

CHIEF. See Craig Hospital Inventory of Environmental Factors

chronic obstructive pulmonary disease, 20

chronic pain, 20

CIMT. See constraint-induced movement therapy

CIQ. See Community Integration Questionnaire

client perception, of occupational therapy services, 10

clinical SOAP notes, 112

CMOP. See Canadian Model of Occupational Performance

CNS. See central nervous system

Cochrane Collaboration Publications, 288

cognitive-behavioral therapy, 262, 277, 279

cognitive-neurological outcomes, 8, 285–323, 326

    adaptive approaches to occupational therapy interventions, 303–304

    cognitive-perceptual outcomes, 286–287

    comparing remediation, adaptive approaches, 304–305

    effects of occupational therapy in promoting, 288–319

    evidence for cognitive outcomes, 288

    interventions to improve, 286–287

    measures to capture, 319–321

    neuro-sensorimotor outcome, 320

neuro-sensorimotor outcomes, 287, 305
    interventions to improve, 286
  remediation, adaptive, combined, 305
  remediation-based therapy interventions, 288–303
  remediation for sensory-based occupational therapy, 319
  remediation of neuro-motor abilities, 305–319
cognitive outcomes, interventions to improve, 286
cognitive stimulation, leisure as opportunity for, 146
collating findings of selected studies, 18
communication, 24
community, social, and civic life, 24
community engagement, as benefit of leisure, 146
Community Integration Measure, 328
Community Integration Questionnaire, 328
community management, 48
Complex Reaction Time, 114
complex regional pain syndrome, 318–319
constraint-induced movement therapy, 305
COPM. See Canadian Occupational Performance Measure
Craig Handicap Assessment, 44, 328
Craig Hospital Inventory of Environmental Factors, 180, 328
CRPS. See complex regional pain syndrome

daily occupational participation, 23–45
  empirical studies, 26–43
  participation outcomes
    effects of occupational therapy in promoting, 26–43
    interventions to improve, 25–26
    measures to capture, 43
  systematic reviews, 26
dementia, 20, 31, 42, 59, 162, 164, 178–179, 265, 291, 303
depression, 20
detailed analysis, selecting studies for, 16–18
determinants of occupation, 8, 326–327
developmental delay, 20
direction sense, 114
discretionary characteristic of leisure, 146
diversionary leisure, 146
domestic life, 24

EADL. See extended activities of daily living
early supported discharge, 49, 110–111
elderly, 20
endurance, 328
Enviro-FIM. See Environmental Functional Independence Measure

environmental change, 155–182
  effects of occupational therapy in promoting, 158–179
  interventions to improve, 156–158
  measures to capture, 179–180
  physical environment, 158–179
    interventions to improve, 156–157
  social environment, 179
    interventions to improve, 157–158
Environmental Functional Independence Measure, 180, 328
ESD. See early supported discharge
European Quality of Life, 328
EuroQol. See European Quality of Life
experimentation, leisure as opportunity for, 146
extended activities of daily living, 48, 109, 113

FAI. See Frenchay Activities Index
Falls Efficacy Scale, 241
Fatigue Impact Scale, 241
FES. See Falls Efficacy Scale
FIM. See Functional Independence Measure
FIS. See Fatigue Impact Scale
FMA. See Fugl-Meyer Assessment
fracture of hip/knee, 20
freely chosen characteristic of leisure, 146
Frenchay Activities Index, 110
Fugl-Meyer Assessment, 241, 320, 328
Functional Independence Measure, 111–112, 114, 241, 320–321, 328
functional mobility, 48
Functional Status Questionnaire, 328

General Health Questionnaire, Short Form 36, 110
general tasks and demands, 24
gustatory impairment, 20

HAQ. See Health Assessment Questionnaire
Health Assessment Questionnaire, 241, 328
hearing impairment, 20
hip arthroplasty, 20
HIV, 137, 248
home care, 4
Home Falls and Accidents Screening Tool, 180, 328
HOME FAST. See Home Falls and Accidents Screening Tool
How to Read a Paper: The Basics of Evidence-Based Medicine, 17

ICF. See International Classification of Functioning, Disability, and Health

ILSS. See Independent Living Skills Scale

imagination, leisure as opportunity for, 146

Independent Living Skills Scale, 328

initial study selection criteria, 16–17

instrumental activities of daily living, 2, 47–48, 110, 115, 119, 179, 240, 257

integrated psychology therapy, 303

interest checklist, 153

International Classification of Functioning, Disability, and Health, 7, 16, 23–24, 139, 155, 287

Interpersonal Communication Inventory, 328

interpersonal interactions, 24

interventions, 2–4, 325–327
    areas of practice, 4
    client-centered practice, 3
    enabling process, 2–3
    goal setting, 3–4
    types of occupational therapy interventions, 4

intrinsically rewarding characteristic of leisure, 146

IPT. See integrated psychology therapy

Jebsen Hand Function Test, 241

JHFT. See Jebsen Hand Function Test

joint injury, 20

key concepts, charting data according to, 18

knee arthroplasty, 20

knowledge exchange, 330

LCM. See Leisure Competence Measure

LDB. See Leisure Diagnostic Battery

Leisure Competence Measure, 153

Leisure Diagnostic Battery, 153

leisure occupations, 328

leisure outcomes, 145–154
    effects of occupational therapy in promoting, 148
    interventions to improve, 147–148
    measures to capture, 148–153

Leisure Satisfaction Scale, 153

LIFE-H. See Life Habits Assessment

Life Habits Assessment, 44, 328

Life Satisfaction Index, 180, 328

Life Satisfaction Scale, 328

literature search, 15–21

long-term care, 4

lower extremity injury, 20

LSI. See Life Satisfaction Index

LSS. See Leisure Satisfaction Scale

macular degeneration, 26, 33, 113

major life areas, 24

MAL. See Motor Activity Log

MAS. See Motor Assessment Scale

mastery, leisure as opportunity for, 146

McGill Pain Questionnaire, 241

Meyer, Adolph, 248

MFES. See Modified Falls Efficacy Scale

Mini Mental Status Examination, 320, 328

Ministry of Health and Long Term Care, Ontario, 280

MMSE. See Mini Mental Status Examination

model of human occupation, 248

Modified Falls Efficacy Scale, 328

Money Road Map Test of Direction Sense, 114

Motor Activity Log, 320–321, 328

Motor Assessment Scale, 241, 243

Motor-Free Visual Perception Test, 114

MPI. See Multidimensional Pain Inventory

MPQ. See McGill Pain Questionnaire

Multidimensional Pain Inventory, 241

multiple sclerosis, 20

MVPT. See Motor-Free Visual Perception Test

neuro-sensorimotor outcomes, interventions to improve, 286

non-obligatory characteristic of leisure, 146

Nottingham Scale, 114

OARS Multidimensional Functional Assessment Questionnaire, 328

Occupational Performance Process Model, 3

Occupational Therapy Practice Framework, 2

older adult acute hospital intake, 20

OPPM. See Occupational Performance Process Model

pain assessments, 328

Parkinson's disease, 20

PEO Model. See Person-Environment-Occupation Model

Person-Environment-Occupation Model, 5–6, 120

personal care, 47

personal fulfillment, as benefit of leisure, 146

personal meaning, from leisure, 146

physical determinants of occupation, 8, 183–246, 327
    educational approach, 240, 249
    effects of occupational therapy, 240–241
    interventions to improve, 184–240
    measures to capture, 241–242
    skill development, 240
    training, 184–185

physical environment, interventions to improve, 156–157

primary health care, 4
productivity, 119–143
    summarizing findings of selected studies
        comprehensive programs, 121–139
        education, 121, 137
        effects of occupational therapy in pro-
            moting, 137–139
        interventions to improve, 121–137
        measures to capture, 139–140
        work task modification, 121, 137
psycho-emotional outcomes, 8, 261–283, 326–327
    cognitive-behavioral training interventions,
        277, 279
    effects of occupational therapy in promoting,
        277–280
    interventions to improve, 262–277
    measures to capture, 280
    occupation-based programs, 277–279
    outcome measures, 280

QLI. See quality of life index
quality of life index, 111

range of motion, 328
reality orientation therapy, 303
recommendations, 325–330
relevant studies, identifying, 15–16
removing environmental barriers, 327
research question, identifying, 15
Return to Normal Living Index, 110, 241, 328
RNLI. See Return to Normal Living Index
RO therapy. See reality orientation therapy

SAFER. See Safety Assessment of Function and
    Environment for Rehabilitation
Safety Assessment of Function and Environment for
    Rehabilitation, 180, 328
SAS. See Social Activities Scale
SBS. See Social Behavior Schedule
schizophrenia, 20, 26, 31, 33, 113, 125, 139, 248, 258, 262,
    277–278, 288, 303–304
SDRS. See Social Dysfunction Rating Scale
secondary study selection criteria, 17–18
self-care, 24, 47–118
    community management outcomes
        effects of occupational therapy in pro-
            moting, 113–114
        interventions to improve, 113
    comprehensive occupational therapy, 48, 109–
        110
    development of occupations, 109, 111–112

early supported discharge, 49, 110–111
    effects of occupational therapy in promoting,
        109–112
    environmental modification, 112–113, 185–240
    functional mobility outcomes
        effects of occupational therapy in pro-
            moting, 112–113
        interventions to improve, 112
    interventions to improve, 48–109
    productivity, and leisure, 7, 326
    self-care outcomes, measures to capture, 114–
        115
    skill development, 49–109, 111, 113–114
    training for driving, 113–114
self-concept, as benefit of leisure, 146
self-expression, leisure as opportunity for, 146
sensory impairment, 20
sensual enjoyment, leisure as opportunity for, 146
SF-36. See General Health Questionnaire, Short Form
    36
SFS. See Social Functioning Scale
Short Form Health Survey, 243, 328
Sickness Impact Profile, 180, 241, 328
Single and Double Letter Cancellation Test, 114
SIP. See Sickness Impact Profile
Social Activities Scale, 257
Social Behaviour Schedule, 257
Social Communication Questionnaire, 328
Social Dysfunction Rating Scale, 257
social environment, 8
    interventions to improve, 157–158
Social Functioning Scale, 257, 328
social meaning, from leisure, 146
social relationships, as benefit of leisure, 146
socio-cultural determinants of occupation, 8, 247–259,
    327
    effects of occupational therapy, 249–257
    interventions to improve, 248–249
    measures to capture, 257–258
    skills development, 248–249
    support provision, enhancement, 249
spinal cord injury, 20
spiritual meaning, from leisure, 146
stroke, 20, 26–27, 48–49, 109–114, 148, 288
substance abuse, 20

tactile impairment, 20
task adaptation, 5
TENS. See transcutaneous electrical stimulation
Test of Everyday Attention results, 114
Theoretical Basis of Occupational Therapy, 16

Time Perception Inventory, 180
Time Use Analyzer, 180
Timed Up and Go Test, 110, 241
TMT. See Trail Making Test
TPI. See Time Perception Inventory
Trail Making Test, 114
transcutaneous electrical stimulation, 242
transfer of knowledge, 330
traumatic brain injury, 26, 139, 281, 287–288
TUA. See Time Use Analyzer
TUG. See Timed Up and Go Test
types of leisure activity, 146

upper extremity injury, 20

VAS. See Visual Analog Scale
vestibular impairment, 20
vicarious competition, leisure as opportunity for, 146
Visual Analog Scale, 241, 243
visual impairment, 20
voluntary characteristic of leisure, 146

WAIS/WAIS-Revised. See Wechsler Adult Intelligence Scale
Wechsler Adult Intelligence Scale, 320
WHO. See World Health Organization
WMFT. See Wolf Motor Function Test
Wolf Motor Function Test, 320, 328
Work Environment Impact Scale, 328
work tasks and activities, modification of, 121, 137
Worker Role Interview, 328
World Health Organization, 156, 287
    Disability Schedule II, 44
        International Classification of Functioning, Disability, and Health, 7–8, 16, 23–24, 139, 155, 287
WRI. See Worker Role Interview

Zarit Caregiver Burden Scale, 180, 328
ZCBS. See Zarit Caregiver Burden Scale

Wait...There's More!

SLACK Incorporated's Health Care Books and Journals offers a wide selection of books in the field of Athletic Training. We are dedicated to providing important works that educate, inform and improve the knowledge of our customers. Don't miss out on our other informative titles that will enhance your collection.

Measuring Occupational Performance: Supporting Best Practice in Occupational Therapy, Second Edition

Mary Law PhD, OT Reg. (Ont.), FCAOT; Carolyn M. Baum PhD, OTR/C, FAOTA; Winnie Dunn PhD, OTR, FAOTA

440 pp., Hard Cover, 2005, ISBN 13 978-1-55642-683-4, Order #36836, $57.95

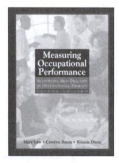

As the profession of occupational therapy continues to mature and expand its practice, the measurement of occupational performance is one of the key avenues that all practicing clinicians will need to explore and master. A complex subject for the new and practicing occupational therapist, each step in the evaluation process from assessment to interpretation to intervention is critical. Having one solid, evidence-based textbook to teach and guide in the measurement process is welcome.

Interventions, Effects, and Outcomes in Occupational Therapy: Adults and Older Adults

Mary Law PhD, OT Reg.(Ont.); Mary Ann McColl PhD, MTS

400 pp., Hard Cover, 2010, ISBN 13 978-1-55642-880-7, Order #38807, $52.95

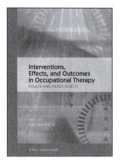

Drs. Mary Law and Mary Ann McColl have comprehensively reviewed all of the intervention effectiveness literature for occupational therapy provided for adults. The material reviewed crosses all diagnostic categories and areas of practice for adults and older adults. Analysis of over 500 research studies and systematic reviews form the basis for this book.

Evidence-Based Rehabilitation: A Guide to Practice, Second Edition

Mary Law PhD, OT Reg. (Ont.); Joy MacDermid PT, PhD

448 pp., Hard Cover, 2008, ISBN 13 978-1-55642-768-8, Order #37689, $49.95

This is a comprehensive and well-organized text that provides the most up-to-date information on evidence-based

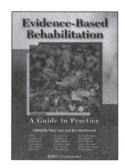

practice, the concepts underlying evidence-based practice, and implementing evidence into the rehabilitation practice. This text is organized by the steps of the process of evidence-based practice—introduction to evidence-based practice, finding the evidence, assessing the evidence, and using the evidence.

Quick Reference Dictionary for Occupational Therapy, Fifth Edition

Karen Jacobs EdD, OTR/L, CPE, FAOTA; Laela Jacobs OTR

632 pp., Soft Cover, 2009, ISBN 13 978-1-55642-865-4, Order #38654, $39.95

Occupational Therapy: Performance, Participation, and Well-Being, Third Edition

Charles H. Christiansen EdD, OTR, OT(C), FAOTA; Carolyn M. Baum PhD, OTR/L, FAOTA; Julie Bass Haugen PhD, OTR/L, FAOTA

680 pp., Hard Cover, 2005, ISBN 13 978-1-55642-530-1, Order #35309, $77.95

Please visit **www.slackbooks.com** to order any of the above titles!

24 Hours a Day...7 Days a Week!

Attention Industry Partners!

Whether you are interested in buying multiple copies of a book, chapter reprints, or looking for something new and different — we are able to accommodate your needs.

MULTIPLE COPIES

At attractive discounts starting for purchases as low as 25 copies for a single title, SLACK Incorporated will be able to meet all your of your needs.

CHAPTER REPRINTS

SLACK Incorporated is able to offer the chapters you want in a format that will lead to success. Bound with an attractive cover, use the chapters that are a fit specifically for your company Available for quantities of 100 or more.

CUSTOMIZE

SLACK Incorporated is able to create a specialized custom version of any of our products specifically for your company.

Please contact the Marketing Communications Director for further details on multiple copy purchases, chapter reprints or custom printing at 1-800-257-8290 or 1-856-848-1000.

*Please note all conditions are subject to change.

SLACK® INCORPORATED

Health Care Books and Journals • 6900 Grove Road • Thorofare, NJ 08086

1-800-257-8290
Fax: 1-856-848-6091
E-mail: orders@slackinc.com

www.slackbooks.com

3 5282 00685 8172